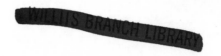

Veterinary Notes
for Horse Owners

VETERINARY NOTES
FOR
HORSE OWNERS

M. HORACE HAYES, FRCVS

Eighteenth Edition
Revised and Enlarged

Edited by Roy Knightbridge
Co-Trustee of the Hayes Literary Estate

Technical Consultant Peter Rossdale
OBE, MA, PhD, DmedVet (Berne), FACVSc, DESM, FRCVS

Illustrations by Fiona Silver

SIMON &
SCHUSTER

Simon & Schuster
Rockefeller Center
1230 Avenue of the Americas
New York, New York 10020

First edition 1877
Second edition 1880
Third edition 1884
Fourth edition 1889
Fifth edition 1897
Sixth edition 1903
Seventh edition 1906
Eighth editin 1915
Ninth edition 1921
Tenth edition 1924
Eleventh edition 1929
Twelfth edition 1934
Thirteenth edition 1938
Fourteenth enlarged edition 1950
Fifteenth edition 1964
Sixteenth edition 1968
Seventeenth revised edition 1987

Originally published in Great Britain by Stanley Paul Ltd.
Previous edition published n the U.S.A by Arco Publishing, Inc.

SIMON & SCHUSTER and colophons are registered trademarks
of Simon & Schuster Inc.

A former Prentice Hall Press Book

Library of Congress Catalog Card Number: 87-062114

ISBN 0 09 186277 9

Printed in Great Britain

10 9 8 7 6 5 4 3 2 1

CONTENTS

The Musculoskeletal System

The Reproductive System

Infectious Diseases

Medical and Surgical Matters

Management and Husbandry

Miscellaneous

Appendices

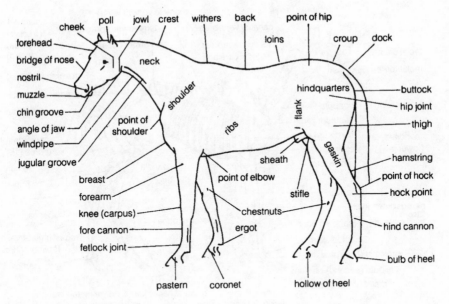

Figure 1 The points of a horse

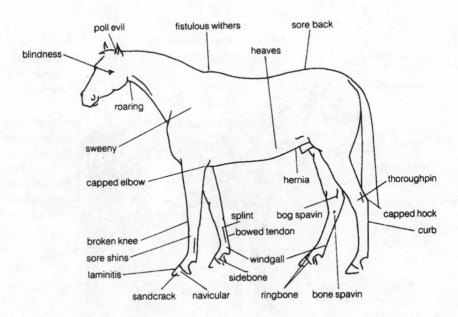

Figure 2 Location of unsoundness and blemishes

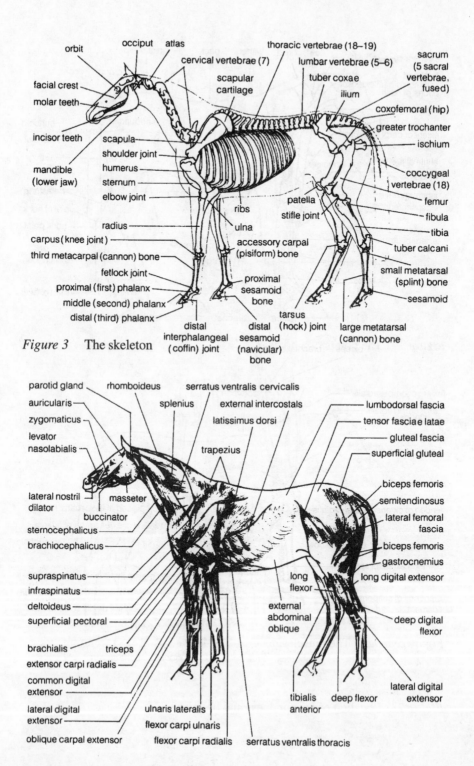

Figure 3   The skeleton

orbit
occiput   atlas
facial crest
molar teeth
incisor teeth
mandible (lower jaw)
scapula
shoulder joint
humerus
sternum
elbow joint
radius
carpus (knee joint)
third metacarpal (cannon) bone
fetlock joint
proximal (first) phalanx
middle (second) phalanx
distal (third) phalanx
cervical vertebrae (7)
scapular cartilage
thoracic vertebrae (18–19)
lumbar vertebrae (5–6)
tuber coxae
ilium
sacrum (5 sacral vertebrae, fused)
coxofemoral (hip)
greater trochanter
ischium
coccygeal vertebrae (18)
femur
fibula
tibia
tuber calcani
small metatarsal (splint) bone
sesamoid
ribs
ulna
accessory carpal (pisiform) bone
proximal sesamoid bone
patella
stifle joint
distal interphalangeal (coffin) joint
distal sesamoid (navicular) bone
tarsus (hock) joint
large metatarsal (cannon) bone

Figure 4   The muscle system

parotid gland
auricularis
zygomaticus
levator nasolabialis
lateral nostril dilator
masseter
buccinator
sternocephalicus
brachiocephalicus
supraspinatus
infraspinatus
deltoideus
superficial pectoral
brachialis   triceps
extensor carpi radialis
common digital extensor
lateral digital extensor
oblique carpal extensor
ulnaris lateralis
flexor carpi ulnaris
flexor carpi radialis
rhomboideus
splenius
serratus ventralis cervicalis
external intercostals
latissimus dorsi
trapezius
lumbodorsal fascia
tensor fasciae latae
gluteal fascia
superficial gluteal
biceps femoris
semitendinosus
lateral femoral fascia
biceps femoris
gastrocnemius
long digital extensor
deep digital flexor
lateral digital extensor
long flexor
external abdominal oblique
tibialis anterior
deep flexor
serratus ventralis thoracis

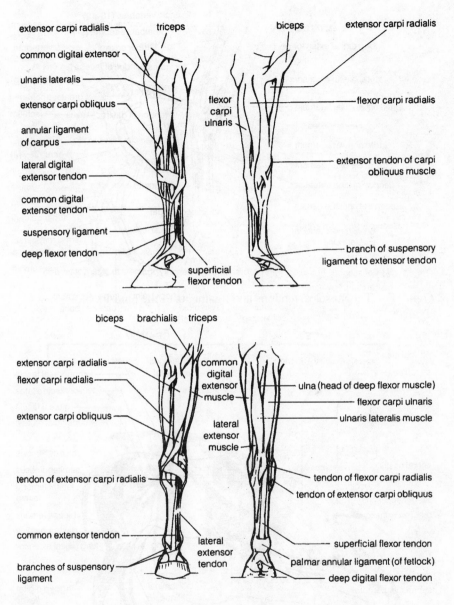

extensor carpi radialis
triceps
biceps
extensor carpi radialis
common digital extensor
ulnaris lateralis
flexor carpi radialis
extensor carpi obliquus
flexor
carpi
ulnaris
annular ligament
of carpus
extensor tendon of carpi
obliquus muscle
lateral digital
extensor tendon
common digital
extensor tendon
suspensory ligament
deep flexor tendon
branch of suspensory
ligament to extensor tendon
superficial
flexor tendon

biceps   brachialis   triceps
extensor carpi radialis
common
digital
extensor
muscle
flexor carpi radialis
ulna (head of deep flexor muscle)
flexor carpi ulnaris
extensor carpi obliquus
ulnaris lateralis muscle
lateral
extensor
muscle
tendon of extensor carpi radialis
tendon of flexor carpi radialis
tendon of extensor carpi obliquus
common extensor tendon
lateral
extensor
tendon
superficial flexor tendon
branches of suspensory
ligament
palmar annular ligament (of fetlock)
deep digital flexor tendon

Figure 5 and 6   The muscles, tendons and ligaments of the forelimb

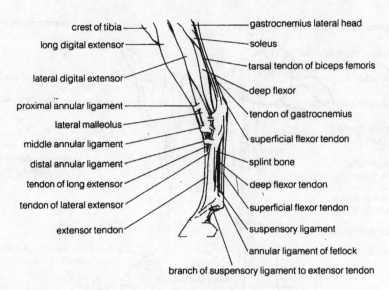

crest of tibia
long digital extensor
lateral digital extensor
proximal annular ligament
lateral malleolus
middle annular ligament
distal annular ligament
tendon of long extensor
tendon of lateral extensor
extensor tendon

gastrocnemius lateral head
soleus
tarsal tendon of biceps femoris
deep flexor
tendon of gastrocnemius
superficial flexor tendon
splint bone
deep flexor tendon
superficial flexor tendon
suspensory ligament
annular ligament of fetlock
branch of suspensory ligament to extensor tendon

Figure 7   The muscles, tendons and ligaments of the hind-limb

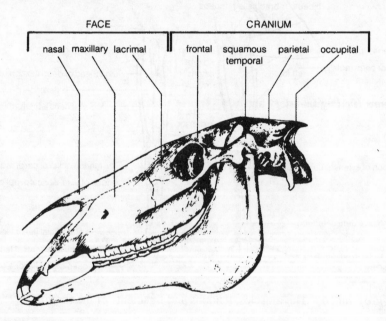

FACE

nasal   maxillary   lacrimal

CRANIUM

frontal   squamous   parietal   occipital
temporal

Figure 8   The skull

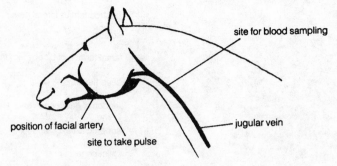

Figure 9   Jugular and site of pulse

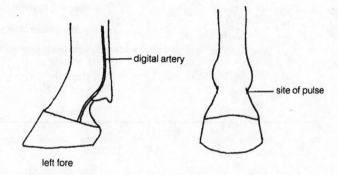

Figure 10 Digital artery and site of pulse

INTRODUCTION

With the arrival of the new millennium, *Veterinary Notes for Horse Owners* by Horace Hayes entered its third century in the Gregorian calendar. After 125 years in print it is regarded within the publishing profession as a phenomenon somewhat along the lines of Shakespeare and the Bible. Indeed, one famous member of the horse racing world, on being interviewed for the BBC programme *Desert Island Discs*, chose this Hayes volume as the one book to be allowed on the island in addition to those two other, more widely circulated, works. Is one to suppose that the desert island in question has a horse population, or is reading about the well-being of horses sufficient in itself?

I first became involved with the literary estate of Horace Hayes in 1975 when my step-father Frank Pyett, nephew of Horace's wife Alice, and by then the sole trustee, asked me to help him find a literary agent to replace the much respected and sorely missed Margaret Sanders. She had looked after the estate for many years, but had just died. Before this search was complete, Frank Pyett asked me if I would take on the role of agent, and after appropriately thorough deliberation, I agreed.

So things continued until 1982, when Frank Pyett died. As a result, my sister Pamela Sitch and I became joint trustees of the literary estate. I continued to act as agent.

It was in discussion with the publishers in the year 2000 that the decision was taken to produce a new edition – the 18th. Dr. Peter Rossdale, the editor of the 17th edition, kindly agreed to give advice and provide continuity between the editions. He was unable to take on the role of editor because of the pressure of his other work, and so I find myself in that role, seeking to follow his well-chosen path.

Much has changed in the world since the first edition of *Veterinary Notes for Horse Owners* was published in 1877, but not everything. On a trivial level, this introduction to the 18th edition is being written at Horace Hayes' own writing desk, and the chimes that sound in the background come from the same long-case clock that Alice grew up with – some of their personal effects have been passed down through the family.

On a more important and relevant level, the aims of this book in its 18th edition remain precisely the same as those set out by Hayes in his introduction to the first edition. To quote his words:

> This work is the result of an attempt to produce a treatise on the pathology and treatment of the more frequent diseases of horses.
>
> Whilst specially addressing non-professional readers, my object has been to indicate a rational method of treatment, and not to furnish them with any vaunted nostrums or specifics which constitute the stock-in-trade of the quack and empiric.
>
> Though I heartily deprecate amateur interference in case of illness when the aid of a veterinary surgeon can be procured, still I am convinced that the better the principles of veterinary pathology are understood, the more ready will horse owners be to avail themselves of professional experience and ability when disease appears in the stable; and the more attention will they bestow at other times on the health and comfort of their dumb servants.

We can perhaps overlook the present day connotations of those last two words in view of the commendable contents of the quotation as a whole ...

From the first edition, Hayes, himself an esteemed horseman and veterinary surgeon, enlisted the help of other highly qualified and experienced experts in assembling his book. This practice has continued and extended as specialisms have developed. By the time of the 16th edition in 1968, some, but little, of Hayes' original text remained, and by the next edition the need had arisen to revise even that. Today the book consists entirely of contributions by contemporary experts in the various fields. These are listed in a section that follows, and I am delighted to acknowledge the authoritative and enthusiastic contributions they have made. Particular thanks are due to our overseas contributors for not letting distance and nationality inhibit their participation.

Editors of this book in the past who have played a particularly significant part in keeping it in the forefront of its field, and to whom it is a pleasure to express sincere appreciation, are the late J. F. Donald Tutt, and Dr. Peter Rossdale. Donald Tutt steered the book through many years in the middle of the 20th century, and Peter Rossdale introduced the excellent new format in 1987 which will surely stay with all future editions of the title. He is to be thanked additionally for providing the continuity between the 17th and 18th editions as referred to above.

Another dedicated contributor to the success of the book in earlier times was the late Miss Margaret Sanders, previously mentioned, who worked tirelessly over more than 45 years as literary agent for this and ten other books written by Hayes. Her vital contribution is gratefully acknowledged.

As for the astoundingly energetic Horace Hayes himself, who through this book has brought comfort and relief to thousands of horses and their owners over generations, little has previously been said within the book itself, or indeed elsewhere. With the publication of the first edition of the new millennium, it seems appropriate to take the opportunity to rectify this, and so a biographical sketch follows this introduction.

The vital role of the publisher has yet to be very gratefully acknowledged. The name on the spine of the book changes from time to time as acquisitions within the publishing industry take place. However the enthusiasm and co-operation of the actual publishing staff in continuing the life of this unique book remain the same throughout, and are much appreciated. In particular Matthew Parker of Ebury Press has been helpful far beyond the call of duty.

Thanks are due also to the many individuals approached who gave help willingly and cheerfully, and made contacting them a pleasure. They include:

within libraries, the staff of the reference sections of the Dereham and the Norwich public libraries, the British Library, and the Royal College of Veterinary Surgeons library;

in researching the history of Horace Hayes, Lady Jean Mann of the Veterinary History Society, Mike Bulmer at R. E. & G. B. Way, antiquarian booksellers of Newmarket, Norman Comben, Sherwin Hall, and Dr. Christopher Stray of the University of Wales in Swansea;

in locating authors and expediting responses from them, Brigitte Heard and Nick Kelly of Rossdale and Partners;

in providing additional illustrations, Mr John Fuller;

in giving permission to reproduce copyright material, the journal *Horse & Hound*, and the Horserace Betting Levy Board;

in providing moral support and practical help, my sister Pamela and her husband Barry Sitch.

Finally, for helping with this, as with all things, my partner Judith Jane Mitchell.

To all these contributors I give my sincere thanks.

Roy Knightbridge,
North Elmham,
Norfolk
June 200

CAPTAIN M. HORACE HAYES

Biographical Sketch

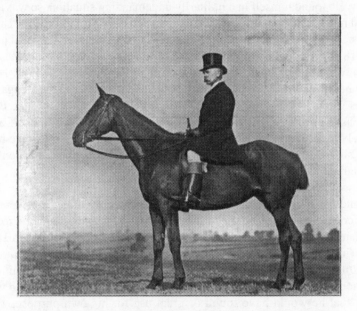

Horace Hayes was born in 1842 of an Irish father and a Scottish mother, in the county of Cork – 'a very horsey part of the world', as Hayes himself put it somewhat later.

His father was a flour miller who had horses, but they were a miscellaneous lot used for cart work, and he took so little interest in them that he was never able to recognise any of his own. He was not a good businessman and money was always a difficulty within the family.

His mother was broad-minded, charitable and of refined and educated tastes, which did not include horses and hunting.

Horace used to ride every horse that came his way. When he was twelve, the family moved from the country to the suburbs of Cork, where he was obliged to spend more time on running, rowing, boxing and other athletic sports than on horses. The people of Cork were so devoted to amusement that, as a boy, Horace made little progress in study. Because a career as a military officer was by then his objective, he went to Dublin to cram for the necessary examinations.

He worked hard and passed 'fairly well up on the list' for entrance to the Royal Military Academy at Woolwich for a three-year course. Before starting this he went for a year to the continent, where he added gymnastics and fencing to his sporting activities, and French and German to his existing knowledge of Latin and Greek. Later he was to add Hindi and Urdu. At the end of his military course he obtained a commission in the Royal Artillery.

Within six months he was posted to India. This gave him the opportunity to increase his involvement with horses, because they were used there so extensively. He found himself in a militarily undemanding situation, so was able to spend much time on training racehorses and chasers. At this time, in 1869, he also started writing on the subject of horses, with articles in the local press.

In 1874 he brought out his first book, *Training and Horse Management in India*, which quickly became the standard authority on the subject. He was enjoying life in India so much that he obtained a transfer to the Bengal Staff Corps. There he remained for nine years, followed by one year in the Buffs – the East Kent Regiment. Throughout this time he devoted himself almost entirely to racehorse training, and had his own stable of ten to twelve horses. He also became very active in the field of horse dealing, and this continued throughout the rest of his life.

Although he had acquired a great knowledge of horses through years of practice and listening, he felt greatly handicapped by his ignorance of veterinary science. He therefore obtained a year's furlough and attended Professor William's Veterinary College in Edinburgh, obtaining his diploma in 1883.

Having thus gained the knowledge he required, he wrote *Veterinary Notes for Horse Owners*, first published in 1877. He felt that he had obtained the solutions to a sufficiently large number of questions to enable him to write a book that he would have found of great use for his own purposes twelve months previously. He also wrote as 'a man who had not had time to forget how ignorant' he had been. He said somewhat modestly of the first edition, 'The only bit of originality about it was that it had been written by a confessedly ignorant man for others who were more ignorant than himself'. He later conceded that, with each new edition, it became the repository of all the useful veterinary information that he had ever acquired.

Anticipating that the surplus of officers in the army would lead to enforced early retirement, Hayes resigned his commission and returned to London in 1880. There he wrote several more books which received good reviews and sold well.

Hayes' liking for new experiences led him into the educational field. Using his military background, he coached classes of young men for the entrance examination to the military college that he had attended some twenty years previously. He also wrote a manual for students on the course.

After three years in these activities, his love of horses took over again. He moved to Newmarket and there began to work on *Points of the Horse*, a major work, which was ultimately published in 1893. Over the same period he broadened his interests to include horse breaking.

For the next ten years Hayes travelled extensively abroad, teaching and giving performances to demonstrate the effectiveness of his horse breaking methods. The places he visited included Gibraltar, Malta, Egypt, Ceylon, Singapore, the Straits Settlements, China, Japan, Burma, India again, Russia (three times) and South Africa (twice). He was by this time married, and his wife Alice shared most of these travels with him, taking an active part in his demonstrations. The money he earned abroad was spent in England on his greatest love – riding and hunting, particularly in Leicestershire.

Hayes was a very gregarious man, especially in sporting circles. A book in which he allowed himself gossip – *Among Men and Horses* – mentions over three hundred friends and associates. Numbered amongst these were Rudyard Kipling, who featured Hayes in one of his *Tales from the Hills*, and David Livingstone, the explorer. Many of these friends were made on his extensive travels, particularly on the sea voyages. These were not always in the comparatively speedy steamships by then in service on some routes – he made three voyages round the Cape of Good Hope in sailing ships.

His exceptionally active life ended in 1904 when he died in Southsea, England, at the age of 62 years. In his lifetime he had written twelve books, eleven of them about horses.

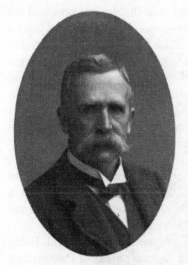

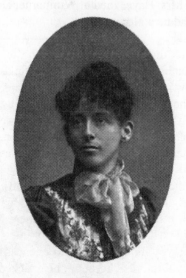

Captain M. H. HAYES

Mrs HAYES
(Photo by Wallery)

MRS ALICE HAYES

Horace Hayes' wife, Alice, played such a large part in his life that it is appropriate to make a mention of her.

She was the daughter of William Pyett of Esher, Surrey, which appropriately is the home of Sandown Park racecourse. Twenty years younger than her husband, she was described by him as 'musical, a clever actress, and born to shine in society'. This gives the impression of delicacy, yet she was a fearless rider, and often rode the fiercest horses that the toughest men rejected at her husband's demonstrations of horse-breaking. She was also an author, writing *The Horsewoman* in 1893, a book which is now sought-after because of a resurgence of interest in side-saddle riding.

In her travels with her husband in badly deprived areas she took a keen and active interest in the plight of women, and particularly those in leper hospitals. She wrote articles and a book to bring them to public attention, befriended them and made regular visits to see them. All the royalties from her book were donated to a leper fund in Calcutta. One result of her actions was that the Indian Government undertook to make special provision in the future for the neglected victims she had discovered. A contemporary correspondent in Calcutta referred to her as 'our brave young citizen, Mrs. Alice Hayes, whose kindness and courage are certainly unequalled in India'.

Mrs. Hayes died at Wimborne, Dorset, in 1913 at the age of 50 years. She had no children.

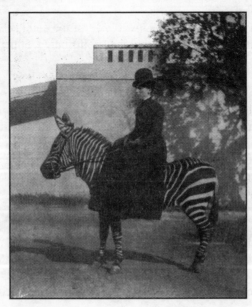

THE AUTHORS OF THE EIGHTEENTH EDITION

Books are as good as their authors, and in this respect the Trustees of the Horace Hayes Literary Estate have been most fortunate.

Where the authors from the 17th edition were still in a position to contribute, they were invited to up-date their previous work. In the remaining cases a new author was approached, based on recommendations made by Dr. Peter Rossdale, whose knowledge of the literary sector of the veterinary profession is unsurpassed. As a result the contributors listed below were commissioned, each a recognised specialist in the field being covered. The outcome is a team that it would be very difficult to strengthen.

The 43 authors involved, listed here in alphabetical order, bring with them totals of over 300 person-years of university study and research and over 1000 person-years of professional practice.

Brief Curricula Vitae are given below for all of the authors, together with the number or numbers of the chapters they contributed, either as sole or as joint author.

Janet Anderson (Chapter 55)
Involvement with the thoroughbred racing and breeding industry began at Cheveley Park Stud in Newmarket, when this was acquired by family friends. From the age of 11 to 18, every weekend and holiday was spent at the stables. Has spent most of her working life in Newmarket, firstly with Peter Rossdale and the Equine Veterinary Journal, and subsequently nine years as secretary to racehorse trainer Sir Michael Stoute. Is currently in fifth year as secretary and general administrator with the trainer James Fanshawe at Pegasus Stables.

Professor K. P. Baker, MA MSc PhD DVD FTCD FRCVS MRCVS (Chapter 7)
Initially in mixed practice in southern England; subsequently lecturing and research in Trinity College, Dublin. Diplomas in Veterinary Dermatology in 1982 and 1987. Professor & Head of Dept. of Clinical Veterinary Medicine, University

of West Indies 1989. Currently Professor Emeritus, University College, Dublin. 100 publications, joint author of one book and various book chapters.

Annalisa Barrelet, BVetMed MS CertESM MRCVS (Chapter 5)
Rotary Foundation Scholarship to study at University of California. Thesis on radiological and pathological changes in carpal bones of racehorses. Returned to England to join Rossdale and Partners in 1988, where she is still working. Particular interests are stud medicine and clinical pathology/diagnostics.

Frederic E. Barrelet, DipVMS(Berne) DrMedVet(Berne) MRCVS (Chapter 22)
Swiss Federal Stud Farm, Avenches. Dept. of Internal Equine Medicine, University of Berne. Working in Equine Practice in Switzerland. Joined Rossdale & Partners in 1991 where he is now a partner.

Peter Calver, BVMS MRCVS (Chapters 39 & 51)
Graduated Glasgow 1960. Founder member of BEVA. Has held licence to train under Jockey Club Rules for 20 years. Currently retained by British Bloodstock Agency. Veterinary consultant to Racehorse Owners Association. On Jockey Club Veterinary Committee. On Animal Health Trust Industry Committee.

Deidre M. Carson, BVSc MRCVS (Chapters 23, 24, 34 to 36 & 41)
Graduated Sydney University 1982. In mixed practice until joining Rossdale & Partners in 1983. Became partner in 1996. Special interest in neonatal and older foal medicine, equine gynaecology and obstetrics, developmental problems and soft tissue surgery.

Dr. C. M. Colles, BVetMed PhD MRCVS (Chapter 20)
Recognised RCVS Specialist in Equine Orthopaedics. Graduated Royal Veterinary College, London, 1971. Worked in mixed and equine practice before joining Equine Clinical Department of the Animal Health Trust in 1975. Appointed Head of Dept. in 1984. Research primarily into disorders of the foot, including effects of shoeing on hoof function and gait. Returned to equine practice in 1989. Elected Honorary Fellow of Worshipful Company of Farriers in 2000 for research into shoeing and foot disorders. Published and lectured widely in UK, Europe & USA.

Dr. J. E. Cox, BSc BVetMed PhD FRCVS (Chapter 21)
Qualified from Royal Veterinary College 1965. Worked with Prof. G.H. Arthur as lecturer in Veterinary Obstetrics from 1966 to 1971. Moved to Liverpool University where he is now Senior Lecturer in Equine Studies. Developed a blood test for equine cryptorchidism and wrote text book on surgery of the reproductive tract, as well as numerous papers on reproductive tract surgery and seasonal adaptions (endocrine, behaviour, metabolism) in horses. Elected

Fellow of RCVS in 1987 for Meritorious Contributions to Learning.

The Late H. W. Dawes, CBE FRCVS (Chapter 45)
Howard Dawes qualified from London in 1913 after a brilliant academic career. After service with the Royal Army Veterinary Corps in France, he joined his father's horse practice in West Bromwich. Elected to the Council of the RCVS in 1934, developing a special interest in veterinary education. Elected President of the RCVS in 1946. For 47 years was a veterinary officer for the Royal Show, latterly as Chief Veterinary Officer. Was regarded as one of the great veterinary practitioners of the 20th century, and it was felt that with his passing in 1977 an era within the annals of the profession had ended.

Nicholas J. Wingfield Digby, BVSc MRCVS (Chapters 39 & 51)
Qualified as a veterinary surgeon at the University of Bristol in 1972. Post graduate work fostered a love and commitment to equine stud medicine. After working in Iran and Australia, returned to the U.K. where he is a partner with Rossdale and Partners. He is involved in veterinary work in the racing stables and on the stud farm. Particular interests are in mare fertility, growth problems in foals and yearlings, and their sale and purchase as yearlings.

Dr. Sue Dyson, MA VetMB PhD DEO FRCVS (Chapters 11 to 18 & 43)
Qualified from Cambridge 1980. Awarded a Thouron Scholarship to the University of Pennsylvania and completed an Internship in Equine Medicine & Surgery at New Bolton. Spent a year in private equine practice in Pennsylvania. Returned to England to join the Centre for Equine Studies of the Animal Health Trust, specialising in orthopaedics and diagnostic imaging, and is a Recognised Specialist of the RCVS. Has published extensively and lectured worldwide. Past President of BEVA

David R. Ellis, BVetMed DEO FRCVS (Chapter 19)
Son of a veterinary surgeon, graduated from RVC London in 1967. Following two years in practice in Hampshire, has since stayed with the same equine specialists, Greenwood, Ellis & Partners, which employs 16 other veterinary surgeons in Newmarket. From BEVA received the Richard Hartley Clinical Prize and the Sir Frederick Hobday Memorial Medal, and was BEVA President in 1991. Regularly contributes to its courses, congresses and meetings. Director of the Veterinary Defence Society Ltd., and acts as adviser to Tattersalls and the Thoroughbred Breeders Association. Associate Lecturer of Cambridge University. Author of several papers and chapters. RCVS Recognised Specialist.

Rachel Flynn, BAHons (Dunelm) (Chapter 52)
Qualified as a solicitor in 1994, she has specialised in bloodstock and equestrian law, and is in practice with Taylor Vinters in Cambridge. A regular

speaker on equine topics, including at the prestigious US National Annual Equine Law Conference in Lexington Kentucky. A regular contributor to bloodstock and equine journals and a member of the Thoroughbred Breeders Association and the Amateur Jockeys Association. Is a successful amateur rider on the flat.

Professor David L. Frape, BSc Dip Agric (Cantab) PhD FRCPath CBiol FIBiol RNutr **(Chapter 38)**

MAF Scholarship to Emmanuel College, Cambridge. American Scholarship to USA and post-doctoral fellowship. Phi Kappa Phi Scholastic Honorary (1st Class Honours). Numerous appointments, directorships and consultancies, e.g. Head of Research Dept. of Large Animal Nutrition and Laboratory Animal Nutrition and Toxicology. Chief Scientist, Clinical Science Research International Ltd., Hinchingbrooke Hospital. Advisor to the Government of the Hashemite Kingdom of Jordon. Visiting Professor, International Livestock School, San Antonio. Membership of numerous committees. Various editorial responsibilities, membership of 12 scientific societies, author of books on equine nutrition, and 107 papers on nutrition, toxicology and diet related diseases.

Linda Galpin, BSC (Hons) Diploma in Equine Science **(Appendix 1)**

Graduated in Applied Biological Sciences from Bristol Polytechnic in 1991, spending placement year with the Department of Comparative Physiology (muscle metabolism) in the Animal Health Trust. Obtained diploma in Equine Science at Aberystwyth University in 1993. Worked for two years at the Animal Health Trust, being Yard Manager during part of the FEI Atlanta Olympic Study of 1996. Spent four years at the Newmarket racehorse stables of W. Haggas before joining Rossdale & Partners as veterinary pharmacist in January 2000. Is currently in the second year of a pharmacy technicians' course at Chelmsford College, having achieved distinction for the first year.

Dr. Ian Gill, BSc PhD FLS **(Chapter 46)**

At present retired but Senior Fellow, University of Liverpool. Vice-Chairman of Rare Breeds Survival Trust. 1997 – retired as Senior Lecturer in Genetics at University of Liverpool, but still teaches genetics to BVSc course. Wrote Equine Breeding and Genetics course for the International Equine Institute, University of Limerick 1999-2000. Presentations at World Conferences on Gene Conservation and Rare Breeds Survival in Britain 1989, Hungary 1991 (keynote lecture) Canada 1994 and Nepal 1998. Publications on chromosomal evolution, chromosomes and infertility, chromosome studies in equines, genetic conservation and DNA technology.

Timothy R. C. Greet, BVMS MVM CertEO DESTS DECVS FRCVS **(Chapters 1, 2 & 10)**

Graduated University of Glasgow in 1976. Horserace Betting Levy Board

Scholarship leading to Master's Degree 1977. Equine Research Station, Newmarket, working with Professor Bob Cook on equine ENT disease. In 1982 joined private equine practice of Dr. Peter Rossdale, becoming a partner in 1984, since when he has been responsible for the surgery department. Instrumental with his partners in developing a large purpose-built equine hospital near Newmarket. Has won the Centenary Award of the British Veterinary Association, and the Richard Hartley Clinical Prize of the British Equine Veterinary Association. Has lectured around the world on a variety of equine topics. Has published various papers and contributed a number of chapters to veterinary textbooks. Was the President of BEVA in 2000.

Dr. Francoise E. Hess-Dudan, Dr MedVet (Appendix 2)
Graduated in Veterinary Medicine from the Veterinary College of Berne University in 1978, and received Doctorate in 1983. Four years as Assistant in the Horse Clinic of the Veterinary College of Berne University. Seven years in positions as clinician, researcher, post-doctoral fellow and instructor in England, France, USA (Cornell University, Ithaca, and Lexington) and in Switzerland (University of Berne). Last ten years in own private practice. Accessory duties: sampling of horses at international shows for the Medication Control Programme of the FEI. A member of GST GZST SVPM BEVA AAEP ISVP.

Professor Harold F. Hintz, BS DPhil (Chapter 44)
Professor Hintz received his BS from The Ohio State University, and his PhD from Cornell University. He is currently Professor of Animal Nutrition in the Department of Animal Sciences at Cornell University, where he has been a faculty member since 1967. As a member of the equine nutrition team at the College of Veterinary Medicine, he conducted research on energy, mineral and protein requirements of the horse.

Richard D. Jones, MA VetMB CertEP MRCVS (Appendix 1)
Graduated from Cambridge University in 1966. Worked as House Surgeon at the Cambridge University Veterinary School before entering general practice. Has worked primarily in equine field since the mid 1970s. In 1989 started a solely equine practice, Bell Equine Veterinary Clinic, at Mereworth, West Kent, and is now senior partner of a nine person equine practice with full clinic and surgical veterinary facilities. Past Examiner, and for three years Chairman of Examiners, for the RCVS. Served on the Council of BEVA for five years, being President in 1995. Member of the BVA Ethics Committee and past member of the BEVA Medicines Select Committee. Founder Member and Secretary General of FEEVA. This body belongs to the UEVP, a section of the Federation of Veterinarians of Europe.

Dr. David Lloyd, BVMS MRCVS (Chapters 8, 13, 14, 15 & 18)
Dr. Lloyd qualified from the University of Glasgow Veterinary School in 1994.

After two years in mixed practice he worked in a busy equine practice before undertaking a two year scholarship at the Weipers Centre for Equine Welfare at the Veterinary School in Glasgow. In 1999 he took the post of Resident in Equine Surgery at Rossdale and Partners in Newmarket. He spends the majority of his working time dealing with referral surgical and lameness cases at Beaufort Cottage Equine Hospital.

Dr. Sheelagh Lloyd, MVB PhD MRCVS (Chapters 32 & 33)
Qualified from the University of Cambridge in 1969. Has taught and carried out research in parasitology in the USA and the UK, and is currently with the Division of Animal Pathology of the University of Cambridge. Interests have included post-immunological responses to parasites and the epidemiology and control of infections. In addition to being previously an equestrian, she has worked on parasites of horses, cattle, sheep and dogs, with emphasis on some of the zoonoses.

Dr. S. G. Long, BVMS PhD DipECAR MRCVS (Chapter 46)
Graduated from Glasgow University Veterinary School, and obtained a PhD from the same university. Is a Diplomate of the European College of Animal Reproduction, and currently lectures on that subject at the University of Bristol. Research interest is domestic animal cytogenics. Teaching responsibilities include genetics (to veterinary and veterinary nursing undergraduates) and clinical reproduction (to veterinary undergraduates).

The Late Dr. Mary E. Mackintosh, BSc MSc PhD (Chapter 29)
Sadly, we have heard that Dr. Mackintosh, who contributed to the 17th edition of *Veterinary Notes for Horse Owners*, died a year ago. Her CV was not included in the 17th edition and so details are not available to reproduce here.

Dr. Tim S. Mair, BVSc PhD DEIM MRCVS (Chapters 4 & 28)
Graduated from the University of Bristol in 1980. After two years in general practice he returned to the University to undertake research into the immune system of the equine respiratory tract, for which he was awarded a PhD in 1986. He stayed at Bristol as lecturer in equine internal medicine. Returned to practice in 1989 and is currently a partner at the Bell Equine Veterinary Clinic in Kent. He has particular interest in equine internal medicine, gastroenterology and soft tissue surgery. Is an RCVS recognised specialist in equine internal medicine. Is currently editor of *Equine Veterinary Education* and assistant editor of *Equine Veterinary Journal*.

Dr. David John Marlin, BSc(Hons) PhD (Chapters 49 & 50)
Graduated University of Stirling 1983. Doctoral Research 1984 -1988, investigating high-density exercise, training and performance in the thoroughbred racehorse, and various aspects of equine nutrition in relation to performance.

1988-1990 Consultant Exercise Physiologist to Luca Cumani, Newmarket, with 180 horses in training. Development and application of field and treadmill based tests of ability and fitness. 1991 to date, Cardiorespiratory Section of the Dept. of Physiology at the Animal Health Trust, Newmarket. During 1993-1996 was Leader of the Atlanta Project to investigate problems of transport and climate for horses competing at the 1996 Atlanta Olympic Games. Has organised several conferences, and lectures at De Montford University, University of Wales, Hartpury College, University of Bristol and British Horse Society. Has published over 100 technical papers throughout the world.

Bonny M. Millar, CVT(USA) VN EVN (Chapter 53)
Graduated from Harcum College in Pennsylvania, USA, in 1984, with an Honours Degree in Animal Health Technology. Pennsylvania Certified Technician from 1984 to present. 1984-1989 Medical Charge Nurse at the New Bolton Centre at University of Pennsylvania. Specialities included teaching, neonatology, supervising the isolation unit, managing the plasma bank and performing plasmapheresis, as well as critical care nurse. 1989-1991 Toxicology Technician at Rhone-Poulenc Rorer Pharmaceuticals in the Drug Safety Division, USA. 1991, moved to England and became Head Nurse at Rossdale and Partners, responsible for managing the nursing team, all aspects of patient care and ensuring that the newly-built equine hospital is equipped for a 24 hour service. Involved with the implementation of an equine nursing certificate in conjunction with the RCVS, BEVA and BVNA. Enrolled in the first group of candidates to take the exam for the certificate in 2000.

William G. N. Morgan (Chapter 48)
Educated at Radley and Corpus Christi, Cambridge, as a classicist, graduating as MA. Gained Diplomas from the National Stud of the U.K. and Ireland. 1983 to date, Manager of the Limestone Stud in Lincolnshire. Has hunted a great deal and ridden winners under National Hunt rules.

Dr. Jenny A. Mumford, BSc(Hons) PhD (Chapter 31)
Obtained BSc with 1st Class Honours in Biological Sciences at Nottingham University in 1968. Gained PhD in Microbiology at Sheffield University in 1972. Post Doctoral Research with The Lister Institute of Preventive Medicine, Elstree, working on the development of Cholera vaccines. 1974 Post Doctoral Research at The Royal Veterinary College, London, working on equine respiratory viruses and immunity to equine herpesviruses (funding by Horserace Betting Levy Board). 1980 Head of Equine Virology Unit at the Animal Health Trust. 1988 Head of Dept. of Infectious Diseases, Animal Health Trust. 1996 Head of Centre for Preventive Medicine, Animal Health Trust. 1999 to date, Director of Science, Animal Health Trust. Member of ten professional societies and committees. Equestrian Award for Outstanding Scientific

Achievement, 1994. Dubai Award for Equine Research at 8th International Conference on Equine Infectious Diseases, 1998. Honorary Associateship of Royal College of Veterinary Surgeons, 1998. Personally the recipient of 12 scientific grants for research.

Dr. Graham Munroe, BVSc PhD CertEO DESM DipECVS FRCVS **(Chapter 6)**
Graduated with Honours from the University of Bristol Veterinary School in 1979, then spent eight years in mixed and equine practices in Wendover, Newmarket, Arundel, New Zealand and Wokingham. In 1987 became lecturer in Equine Surgery and Reproduction at the Glasgow Veterinary School, at the same time running the Equine Surgical Hospital and conducted research into neonatal equine ophthalmology leading to his PhD. 1994 moved to the Royal (Dick) School of Veterinary Studies at the University of Edinburgh where he became senior lecturer in large animal surgery. 1997, Diplomate of the European College of Veterinary Surgeons. Since 1998 has been running Flanders Veterinary Services, a specialist equine consultancy practice in Duns, Berwickshire.

John Parker, MA VetMB FRCVS **(Chapter 9)**
Qualified with distinction from Cambridge University in 1963. Worked as assistant in Yorkshire until starting own practice in 1965. In 1995 retired from the practice, which by then had ten veterinary surgeons, but remained as Consultant in the equine field. He also provides second and expert opinions for other practices, and for insurance and legal bodies. Served for 15 years on the Council of BEVA, including as President and as Treasurer. Has lectuured on BEVA and other courses on many occasions, and published many papers and articles. Awarded Fellowship of the RCVS in 1995, and at present is an elected Council Member. A member of the Veterinary Advisory Committee to the Horserace Betting Levy Board since 1991. He chairs the Codes of Practice and serves on the Education Sub-Committees of that body.

Professor Jan Philipsson, PhD **(Chapter 47)**
Head of the Dept. of Animal Breeding and Genetics at the Swedish University of Agricultural Sciences (SLU), Uppsala, Sweden. Has carried out internationally recognised research in areas of horse and cattle breeding, contributing to modern breeding programmes in both species. Since 1983, Secretary of Interbull, an international organisation for the international genetic evaluation of dairy cattle. Is initiating similar work in horse breeding through the working group Interstallion in collaboration with the World Breeding Federation of Sport Horses.

Major John D. Reilly, RAVC BSc(Hons) BVSc PhD MRCVS **(Chapter 16)**
1985 Graduated BSc(Hons) Agriculture from Seale Hayne College, Devon. 1990 Graduated BVSc from University of Bristol. Awarded Nat West Prize for Animal Health and James Rowland Award for thesis. 2001 Awarded PhD

Veterinary Science, Edinburgh University. Worked in two-man mixed
practice in the West Country, leading to Partnership, 1990 - 1992. For the next
two years studied horse hoof horn at Edinburgh University, sponsored by
Horserace Betting Levy Board. 1994 to date, Officer in the Royal Army
Veterinary Corps, and Honorary Research Fellow at De Montford University,
Leicester. Has published numerous technical papers, and is Supplement Editor
and Referee for the *Equine Veterinary Journal*. Is committed to improving
animal welfare by seeking through research nutritional and material science
solutions to hoof horn, nail, hair and skin maladies.

Professer Sidney W. Ricketts, LVO BSc BVSc DESM FRCVS (Chapter 41)
Graduated as a veterinary surgeon at Bristol in 1971. Was an intern in equine
medicine and surgery at the University of Pennsylvania, as a Thouron Fellow.
In 1972 joined the equine practice of Rossdale and Partners in Newmarket.
Became a partner in 1975 and is now managing partner. Awarded the honour
Lieutenant of the Royal Victorian Order by Her Majesty the Queen in 1998
for services to the Royal Studs. Has been responsible for developing the
internationally acclaimed Beaufort Cottage Laboratories. Awarded Honorary
membership of BEVA in 1997. Has been a member of the Horserace Betting
Levy Board's advisory committee for their Code of Practice on Equine
Venereal Diseases since 1990. He is joint author of a textbook on equine
studfarm medicine, and has contributed to a number of multi-author books.
He has also published widely in international journals, and has lectured at all
the UK university veterinary schools. Has recently been appointed Visiting
Professor of Equine Studies at the University of Bristol.

Dr. Colin A. Roberts, BVSc PhD FRCVS (Chapter 50)
Graduated 1978 with BVSc from University of Bristol. Spent eight years
in equine practice in Kent. In 1987 joined the Animal Health Trust, and
until recently was currently a Senior Scientist there. In 1993 became a
RCVS Recognised Specialist in Equine Internal Medicine. His main areas
of professional interest are equine respiratory disorders, and performance-
related problems. He has extensive teaching experience at both
undergraduate and post-graduate levels. Is Chairman of the Pet Allergy
Association and a member of the Executive Committee of the National
Equine Welfare Council. In late 2001, joined the Department of Clinical
Veterinary Medicine at the University of Cambridge.

**Professor Malcolm Clive Roberts, BVSc PhD MPH FRCVS FACVSc
(Chapter 29)**
Graduated 1967 with BVSc from University of Liverpool. 1972, PhD in the
Faculty of Medicine at the University of Bristol. 1967, Member of the RCVS;
1982, Fellow of the RCVS, researching equine gastrointestinal disorders.

1976, Member of the Australian CVSc; 1978, Fellow of the same college. Returned to Bristol and held positions of Post Doctoral Fellow, and Lecturer. Following two years with a specialist equine practice in Buckinghamshire, held the post of Senior Lecturer in Equine Medicine in the University of Queensland, Australia. 1980, Visiting Professor at New York State College of Veterinary Medicine, Cornell University, and Adjunct Professor of Equine Medicine at North Carolina State University. From 1981 to date, Professor of Equine Medicine at North Carolina State University. Has carried out numerous projects on supported or funded research, published over 80 technical papers, and contributed over 30 book chapters, and 20 abstracts.

Dr. Peter D. Rossdale, OBE MA PhD Drmedvet(Berne) FACVSc FRCVS (Chapters 3 to 5, 8, 22 to 27 & 41)

Dr. Rossdale is in veterinary practice in Newmarket, providing surgical and medical services to local and referral clients. There are some 20 veterinary surgeons in the practice, which he established in 1959. Besides his practice duties he has played an active role in research, having published over 150 papers in peer reviewed journals, and has served on the Scientific Advisory Committees of the Wellcome Trust, the Horserace Betting Levy Board and the Animal Health Trust. He has written a number of text books for lay and professional readership. In 1987 he was responsible, as Editor, for establishing the present format for Horace Hayes' *Veterinary Notes for Horse Owners*. In 1996 he was awarded an OBE for services to equine veterinary science.

Donald H. Steven, MA VetMB FRCVS (Chapter 24)

Graduated King's College, Cambridge, 1960. Assistant in mixed practice in Upton-on-Severn, Worcestershire. Lecturer in Veterinary Anatomy, Cambridge Veterinary School. Editor and part author of *Comparative Placentation*. Director of Veterinary Anatomy, University of Cambridge, 1980-1990. Fellow of Churchill College, Cambridge, 1975.

W. Neil Steven, BVMS MRCVS (Chapters 36 & 39)

Graduated in 1974 from Glasgow University Veterinary School. For many years has been a partner in Rossdale & Partners in Newmarket.

Dr. Jill Thomson, BVSc PhD DipECVP MRCVS (Chapter 2)

Graduated as veterinary surgeon from the University of Pretoria, South Africa. Started riding at an early age and progressed to competing in dressage, three-day eventing, show jumping and pentathlon, at both junior and senior levels. Joined an equine practice in Johannesburg, working primarily with racehorses. A desire to travel brought her to the UK where she joined the Department of Large Animal Medicine at the University of Edinburgh. Here she pursued her interest in equine medicine, especially respiratory medicine. She was awarded a PhD for her work on chronic obstructive pulmonary disease. Since then she has specialised in laboratory-based diagnostic work, including pathology, cytology and microbiology. She retains both a professional and recreational love and respect for horses.

Professor A. Simon Turner, BVSc MS (Chapter 19)
Graduated with Honours at University of Melbourne, 1972. Post-Graduate training at Ohio State University, followed by award of MS Degree, and acceptance as Diplomate of the American College of Veterinary Surgeons. Held posts as Assistant Professor of Surgery at Saskatchewan and Colorado. Sabbatical appointment to Laboratory for Experimental Surgery in Davos, Switzerland. Currently Professor, Department of Clinical Sciences, Colorado State University. Has been a member of numerous college and university committees, and has delivered technical papers at over 180 conferences and courses throughout the USA, Western Europe and in Australia. Has published over 180 technical papers, nine books and sections of another seven books.

The Late J. F. Donald Tutt, FRCVS (Chapter 53)
Donald Tutt qualified from the Royal Veterinary College in 1914. After war service in the Royal Veterinary Corps, he joined his father in the family practice in Winchester, where he stayed for the rest of his life. He became senior partner in 1942 and retired in 1970. He served as a Member of the Council of the Royal College of Veterinary Surgeons from 1936 to 1966, and was Vice-President for one year. He had sincere and strong views, and was a very active member. In his role as principal of a first class practice, he had great experience with horses, including those in thoroughbred studs and training stables. His clients owed much to his progressive work, and the veterinary profession owes much to him for his outstanding contribution to advancement in its status. In 1968 he edited the 16th edition of Horace Hayes' *Veterinary Notes for Horse Owners*, and subsequently revised it on two occasions.

Dr. Lesley Young, BVSc DVA DVC DipECVA PhD MRCVS (Chapter 3)
Dr. Lesley Young qualified in 1987 from Liverpool University, where she also obtained her Royal College Diploma in Veterinary Anaesthesia. In 1992 she moved to Edinburgh University where she began to use ultrasound to study the effects of general anaesthesia on the equine heart, and was awarded a PhD in 1995. During this period she developed her interest in equine cardiology and is currently Equine Cardiologist at the Animal Health Trust. For some years her research interests have been focused on the effects of athletic training on the equine heart. She was awarded the Royal College Diploma of Veterinary Cardiology in 2000. At the Trust she provides a specialist referral service for horses with heart problems, and is currently involved in a large research project funded by the Horserace Betting Levy Board, evaluating the effects of cardiac valve regurgitation on athletic performance.

Abbreviations Used in the Authors' Curricula Vitae.

BAHons	Bachelor of Arts with Honours
BS	Bachelor of Science (United States of America)
BSc	Bachelor of Science (United Kingdom)
BVetMed	Bachelor of Veterinary Medicine (Berne)
BVMS	Bachelor of Veterinary Medicine and Surgery
BVSc	Bachelor of Veterinary Science
CBE	Companion of the Order of the British Empire
CBiol	Chartered Biologist
CertEO	Certificate in Equine Orthopaedics
CertEP	Certificate in Equine Practice
CertESM	Certificate in Equine Stud Medicine
CVT	Certified Veterinary Technician (United States of America)
DECVS	Diplomate of the European College of Veterinary Surgeons
DEIM	Diploma in Equine Internal Medicine
DEO	Diploma in Equine Orthopaedics
DESM	Diploma in Equine Stud Medicine
DESTS	Diploma in Equine Soft Tissue Surgery
DipAgric	Diploma in Agriculture
DipECAR	Diploma of the European College of Animal Reproduction
DipECVA	Diploma of the European College of Veterinary Anaesthesia
DipECVP	Diploma of the European College of Pathologists
DipECVS	Diploma of the European College of Veterinary Surgeons
DipVMS	Diploma in Veterinary Medical Science
DPhil	Doctor of Philosophy (United States of America)
DrMedVet	Doctor of Veterinary Medicine (Berne)
DVA	Diploma of Veterinary Anaesthesia
DVC	Diploma of Veterinary Cardiology
DVD	Diploma in Veterinary Dermatology
EVN	Equine Veterinary Nurse
FACVSc	Fellow of the Australian College of Veterinary Scientists
FIBiol	Fellow of the Institute of Biology
FLS	Fellow of the Linnaean Society
FRCPath	Fellow of the Royal College of Pathologists
FRCVS	Fellow of the Royal College of Veterinary Surgeons
FTCD	Fellow Emeritus of Trinity College, Dublin
LVO	Lieutenant of the Royal Victorian Order
MA	Master of Arts
MPH	Master of Public Health
MRCVS	Member of the Royal College of Veterinary Surgeons
MS	Master of Science (United States of America)
MSc	Master of Science (United Kingdom)
MVB	Bachelor of Veterinary Medicine
MVM	Master of Veterinary Medicine
OBE	Officer of the Order of the British Empire
PhD	Doctor of Philosophy
RAVC	Royal Army Veterinary Corps
RNutr	Registered Nutritionist
VetMB	Bachelor of Veterinary Medicine
VN	Veterinary Nurse

The Organ Systems

The life of any individual, man or animal, depends upon the functions of the organs of the body. In this section the organ systems are described in terms of their functions. They comprise:

*   The digestive system, which consists of a tube running from the mouth to the anus along which food is propelled. Included are the glands, such as the liver, pancreas and salivary glands, which are involved in the digestive process either by secreting substances that break down food into more simple compounds for use by the body, or which, as in the liver, receive the products of digestion and deal with them so as to make the constituents of the food useful to the body in terms of energy for body-building processes.

*   The respiratory system, which has, for the sake of description, been divided into the upper and lower parts, i.e. the airways of the head and neck, and those of the lungs.

*   The heart and blood circulation, the blood and the lymphatic system, which form part of the means of transporting substances and gases around the body. These are described separately, but they are interrelated systems, although, apart from the heart, they may not fit exactly the description of an organ.

*   The urinary system, which is responsible for filtering the blood to divest it of noxious substances which would otherwise accumulate in the body. The kidneys are the organs which help to maintain a proper fluid and electrolyte balance in the body.

* The skin, which is not generally regarded as an organ but it is nonetheless a collection of cells with a specialised function: namely to protect the body against outside influences such as injury, friction and the entry of microbes, while at the same time helping to maintain the integrity of the internal medium on which life depends. Skin represents the frontier between life outside and inside the body.

* Hormones, which, like the heart and blood circulation, are a means of transport. The glands that produce the hormones, together with the nervous system and neuroendocrine system, enable one part of the body to control another, as for example, the pituitary controlling the oestrous cycle of the mare. The nervous system contains not only the means of communicating action – for example, forces required to deliver a kick by the hind leg – but also the sensory pathways – for example, sensation of the prick of a needle which causes the horse to deliver the kick.

* The eye and the ear, special organs of sense that communicate much of the sensory input by which an individual is made aware of its surroundings in terms of sight and hearing.

1

THE DIGESTIVE SYSTEM

The horse has a completely herbivorous (vegetable) diet and its digestive system has evolved to deal with this type of food material. For example, the large intestine contains a population of microbes which break down the vegetable cellulose. This chapter presents a brief outline of the functional anatomy of the digestive system and describes some of the more common problems affecting it.

FUNCTIONAL ANATOMY

Mouth
The mouth is specialised to enable a horse to grasp grasses and other vegetation and to grind them into a digestible pulp. The adult horse has forty or forty-two teeth (see Figure 1) (compared with twenty-four temporary teeth in the foal). These are classified into incisors (twelve), which grasp and shear the grass just above its roots, and premolars and molars (twenty-four), which are the specialised grinding teeth. The canine (rushes) and wolf (first premolar) teeth appear to have no function in the modern horse and are vestiges of a more primitive ancestor.

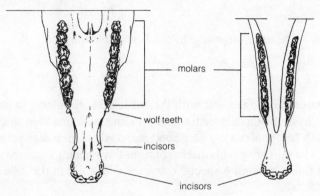

Figure 1   Grinding surfaces – the upper and lower jaw

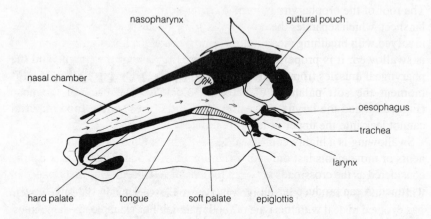

Figure 2   The upper airway when breathing

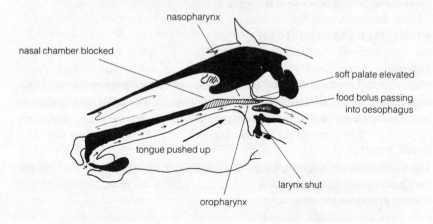

Figure 3   The upper digestive tract when swallowing

The muscular tongue acts with the hard and soft palates to propel food material from the incisor teeth to the grinding teeth and then to the back of the mouth (oropharynx), where food material accumulates prior to swallowing. The salivary glands discharge from tiny openings into the mouth and provide fluid containing special enzymes which aid in the degradation of food material.

Oropharynx (back of the mouth)

The oropharynx is a muscular compartment which is continuous with the back of the mouth, and it is here that food material is stored prior to swallowing. The roof of the oropharynx is formed by the soft palate, a horizontal muscular sheet, which separates the oropharynx from the nasopharynx, which is only involved with breathing (see Figures 2 and 3). When a bolus of food material is swallowed, it is propelled backwards by the base of the tongue and the pharyngeal muscles from the oropharynx into the oesophagus (gullet). At this moment the soft palate is elevated to block off the back of the nose (Figure 3), and the larynx moves forward and closes so that food material cannot leak into the upper or lower respiratory tracts.

Swallowing is a highly coordinated activity in which the individual components or movements last only for a fraction of a second. The pharynx can be considered as the crossroads between food material and air. Any disturbance in its function can produce serious difficulties in swallowing and/or breathing.

Oesophagus (gullet) and stomach

The muscular tube of the gullet transfers food material by means of wavelike movements which squeeze food in the direction of the stomach.

Food material enters the stomach through a one-way muscular valve which prevents regurgitation of food material back up the oesophagus except under the most extreme conditions (for example, when the stomach is massively distended). Consequently a horse cannot vomit. The stomach lining is partly glandular and partly non-glandular. The glandular portion provides enzymes and acids which help to digest the food material. From the stomach ingesta pass through a valve into the small intestine (Figure 4).

Small intestine

The small intestine is a long muscular tube with a glandular lining. In the upper part enzymatic fluids secreted by the liver and pancreas, along with the enzymes produced by the intestinal glands, help to break down the ingesta into their basic constituents. These constituents – fats, proteins and carbohydrates are absorbed and transported by the blood stream to be utilised by the body to produce energy and materials for growth. The small intestine lies in coils in the left side of the abdomen and is connected to the large intestine (caecum and colon) by another muscular valve (ileocaecal). Food material is transported by muscular wave movement.

Caecum and large colon (large intestine)

Ingesta are passed through the ileocaecal valve into the caecum and large colon, where the resident microbial population breaks down cellulose into its basic constituents. The muscular contractions of the caecum and large colon are rather complex, but these structures, the largest in the equine abdomen, are responsible for the absorption of a considerable amount of water from the ingesta.

The muscular coat of the caecum and large colon is complicated, having bands and sacculations, but ingesta are still moved by waves as in the simpler oesophagus and small intestine. The large colon is folded on itself and narrows at one of the bends (the pelvic flexure), predisposing this site to blockage. The large colon is continuous with the transverse colon and the small colon.

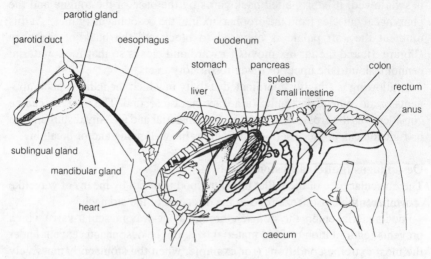

Figure 4   The digestive system and its accessory glands

Small colon, rectum and anus

The small colon continues the process of electrolyte and water absorption, its muscular structure having bands and sacculations similar to the large colon and caecum. It transfers the ingesta to the rectum, a simple muscular tube through which faecal material (dung) passes to the external environment. The anus is a muscular valve which regulates defaecation.

Conditions of the Digestive System

THE TEETH (see also Chapter 54)

Overshot jaws (**parrot mouth**) are relatively common, whereas undershot jaws (**sow mouth**) are extremely rare. Horses affected with both types of incisor **malocclusion** cope well with grazing and mastication and rarely lose condition. There is a variety of other congenital abnormalities of the mouth which involve malocclusion of the teeth. One of the more commonly encountered of these is absence of cheek teeth. This appears most frequently in ponies and usually involves the absence of one or two cheek teeth on each side of the lower jaw. This results in relative overgrowth of the teeth in the upper jaw, which develop very sharp points, which can cause oral discomfort and quidding of food.

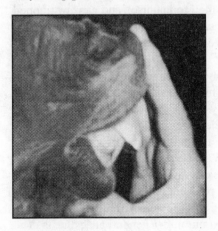

Figure 5
A parrot mouth

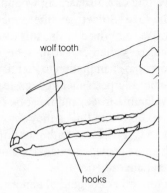

Figure 6
Part of the skull, showing the sharp hooks of the first upper molar and last lower molar

In the normal horse the upper cheek teeth are located more widely apart than the lower cheek teeth, and this results in the development of sharp points on the outside of the upper teeth and on the inside of the lower teeth. These can be smoothed by regular rasping. Dental irregularities also develop because of the manner in which the horse masticates. Thus a sharp point or hook forms on the first upper cheek tooth and the last lower cheek tooth on each side. Although regular rasping of the teeth will remove these, the sixth tooth on the lower jaw is more difficult to rasp. Eventually, in older horses, a sharp point develops which may cause discomfort during eating.

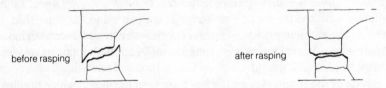

Figures 7 and 8
Teeth edges before and after rasping

The temporary or milk teeth (both incisors and cheek teeth) are usually shed without difficulty. However, occasionally a temporary cheek tooth may become wedged between the adjoining teeth and this can result in difficulty with chewing, often producing a foul smell to the breath because of trapped food. Any horse which appears to salivate and drop food should be examined by a veterinarian who will remove the wedged tooth with a pair of forceps.

Dental disease in the horse is relatively uncommon and it is surprising how, when a genuine dental problem occurs, many horses appear to carry on eating without difficulty. The sign which usually attracts the owner's attention is either a swelling or a discharging wound on the lower jaw or a swelling on the side of the face. Sometimes there may be a foul-smelling discharge from one nostril, as described in sinusitis (see p. 57). If any of these signs develop, a vet should be called and it may be necessary to carry out a radiographic or endoscopic examination to identify the problem.

Removing permanent cheek teeth of a horse is a difficult job, requiring considerable force, and must be carried out under general anaesthesia. The one exception to this is the removal of wolf teeth, which may be indicated if there is a problem with mouthing the bit. These vestigial teeth are small, with short roots, and usually can be removed relatively easily without a general anaesthetic.

Rarely other congenital abnormalities of teeth may be noticed. The commonest of these is the so-called **dentigenous cyst**. Affected horses usually have a discharging sinus at the base of the ear which produces a honey-like or waxy substance. Sometimes this discharge may be associated with a tooth developing on the side of the skull at this point. This tooth cannot be seen by the naked eye but is visible on a radiograph. Removal of the tooth and the cystic lining can be carried out, usually under general anaesthesia, by a vet.

THE MOUTH

Other conditions which affect the mouth include **paralysis of the face**, which is usually the result of an injury to the side of the face in which the nerve supply to the facial muscles is damaged. Affected horses have a droopy lower lip on the affected side and the muzzle and nostrils are twisted to the other side. In most cases the problem gradually resolves without treatment over a period of six months to a year. During that time the affected horse can have some difficulty in masticating food.

Paralysis of the tongue is rare but has been seen in some cases of botulism (see p. 477) or following nerve damage after fungal infection of the guttural pouch (see p. 67).

THE PHARYNX

Pharyngeal diseases are relatively uncommon in horses but almost always produce some difficulty in swallowing. The usual signs of this are coughing during swallowing and a nasal discharge containing food material. In severe cases aspiration of food material can produce a gangrenous pneumonia with foul-smelling breath and usually considerable loss of bodyweight.

The commonest cause of pharyngeal disease is **paralysis of the pharyngeal muscles** after fungal infection of the guttural pouch (see p. 64). **Pharyngeal abscesses** may form in the wall in strangles infection (see p. 474). Foreign bodies may also lodge in the pharynx, typically if a horse swallows a hawthorn twig in hay. In such cases there is usually severe coughing.

Foals with a **cleft palate** usually discharge milk down their nostrils while suckling (see p. 65). Swallowing can be impaired in diseases which produce distension of the guttural pouch (i.e. infections producing accumulations of pus in the guttural pouch or, in foals, distension of the guttural pouch by air – see p. 65).

If a horse has difficulty in swallowing it is important to alert your vet immediately because this may be the first indication of a serious problem, such as fungal infection of the guttural pouch. In such cases early recognition is important if loss of life is to be prevented. It is quite common for vets to carry out an endoscopic or radiographic examination to try to identify the cause of pharyngeal disease; in particular the flexible fibre-optic endoscope has proved to be an invaluable tool for identifying the cause of pharyngeal obstruction.

OESOPHAGUS (GULLET)

The commonest condition affecting the oesophagus is **obstruction by impacted food material (choke)**, the most usual being dried sugar-beet pulp. An affected horse usually stands with its head and neck extended in a rather uncomfortable position and food material and saliva pour from both nostrils. **Recurrent oesophagal obstruction** may result in chronic dilatation of the oesophagus, which predisposes the horse to further bouts of blockage. In cases of oesophagal obstruction a vet must be called. He/she may choose to treat the horse conservatively with relaxant or sedative drugs, allowing the obstruction to clear itself; alternatively, he/she may free the obstruction by passing a stomach tube. Rarely, foreign bodies may become lodged in the oesophagus and require surgical removal under general anaesthetic.

Rupture of the oesophagus occurs rarely, sometimes following a kick in the neck. Usually there is a wound which discharges food and saliva. Veterinary attention should be sought immediately in such a case, as a delay in treatment may have serious consequences.

Both fibre-optic endoscopy and radiography can be of immense help in examining the oesophagus.

COLIC

Colic is the general term given to abdominal pain which may be caused by a variety of different conditions affecting different organs in the abdominal cavity. This section refers only to those causes of colic resulting from diseases of the digestive system. Abdominal pain may occur in a variety of different degrees, but in all cases it should be recognised by the owner as a cause for concern and veterinary advice sought immediately.

The most frequent cause of abdominal pain is spasm of the muscular wall of the intestine; hence the name **spasmodic colic**. There are many causes for this; for example, damage to the intestinal wall by migrating parasitic larvae or feeding too soon after fast exercise. There are other less well-recognised causes and often the cause cannot be determined. Affected horses are usually moderately distressed, show signs of sweating and constantly lie down and get up; they may look frequently at their flanks, kick at their abdomen and roll; they may even become cast in the box. They usually pass few droppings, but the condition may come and go quite rapidly. In some cases there may be sounds of intestinal movement; in other cases these sounds may not be heard. Treatment with a relaxant (spasmolytic) drug usually alleviates the problem rapidly.

The next most common type of colic, **impactive colic**, is caused by impaction of food material in the large intestine. Most frequently this occurs in the large colon at the pelvic flexure, which is a relatively narrow point in the intestinal system. It occurs for a variety of reasons, often when a horse has eaten a large quantity of straw bedding. Affected horses are usually in less pain than those with spasmodic colic and tend to lie down or look off colour without signs of violent abdominal pain. They may get up and down in rather an uncomfortable manner, roll or look at their flanks. A vet will usually be able to identify the site of impaction by manual examination via the rectum (i.e. by feeling inside the horse's abdomen). Administration of large volumes of liquid paraffin, salt water and some agent to stimulate gut movement through a stomach tube is the usual method of treatment. It is also frequently necessary for painkilling drugs to be given to keep the horse out of discomfort while the impaction is being cleared.

A more unusual form of colic results from **gaseous distension (tympany) of the intestines**. There are several causes of this type of colic, which is usually particularly painful. Affected horses may show signs of severe abdominal pain, with sweating and violent rolling. Areas of gaseous distension may occur in front of an impaction, but there are other reasons for the development of gas in the intestine. The most common of these is a major obstruction to the flow of the material caused by the intestines becoming twisted (see below). Gaseous distension of the stomach and intestines also occurs if food material ferments within the intestines; this occurs, for example, when brewer's grain has been used as a feed. In such cases veterinary attention must be sought immediately. The pain associated with the condition can usually be relieved only when a tube is inserted into the stomach to allow gaseous release. In some cases it may be necessary to carry out general anaesthesia and laparotomy (opening the abdomen) to relieve gas-filled intestines.

The final major category of colic, and usually the most dramatic in presentation, is that of **intestinal catastrophy** (or what is popularly known as **twisted gut**). This includes twisting (volvulus) of the intestines, intussus-ception (one piece of intestine becomes telescoped into the following piece) or rotation of the intestine about its mesentary which produces obstruction of the blood supply. In most of these cases the clinical signs are very dramatic and affected horses usually show severe pain or agony and sweating; they are often uncontrollably violent in their behaviour. Collapse, shock and death are the usual result if the condition is allowed to progress. As with other types of colic, immediate veterinary attention should be requested. In many cases a diagnosis can be made fairly rapidly because of the severity of clinical signs. Sometimes it is not possible to carry out any form of treatment and humane destruction should be performed as quickly as possible. However, in recent years considerable advances have been made in abdominal surgery in the horse and it is now possible for some cases to be saved if they can be referred quickly to a centre with the appropriate expertise. Despite improved techniques, a considerable number of cases still die or are destroyed humanely because of problems associated with surgical treatment.

ENTERITIS

This means literally 'inflammation of the intestines' and the usual presenting sign is that of **diarrhoea**. This can occur in any age or type of horse and there are many possible causes. The most frequent causes of diarrhoea are those produced by nutrition, such as overfeeding with highly proteinaceous food materials. Other causes include parasitic infestations (for example, **Strongyloides** species) in foals (see p. 536) and intestinal infections with bacteria and viruses (see Chapters 30 and 31).

Recognition of the nutritional causes of diarrhoea and their correction usually result in a resolution of the problem. Probably the simplest method of treatment is to feed affected horses with hay and water only for a few days. However, if the diarrhoea is profuse or if it continues for more than twenty-four hours, it is essential to call a vet so that further investigation can be carried out. This usually involves collecting samples of dung for parasitic analysis or identification of pathogenic bacteria which may have caused the problem.

Appropriate treatment with anthelmintics can usually eliminate parasitic causes of diarrhoea but bacterial causes can be more difficult to treat. In particular the diarrhoea produced by **Salmonella** bacteria (see p. 479) has potentially serious public health risks, but a vet will be able to advise on the isolation of affected horses and the appropriate treatment in such cases.

In severe cases of enteritis it may be necessary for the horse to receive fluid intravenously and other forms of supportive therapy as recommended by the vet. Antibiotics may or may not be effective in treating bacterial causes of diarrhoea. A number of cases of diarrhoea appear to have no specific cause; some of these can be treated quite effectively with drugs. However, despite some advances in methods of treatment, enteritis remains one of the most difficult problems to manage in veterinary practice.

WEIGHT LOSS

There are many causes of weight loss, some of which involve diseases of the digestive system. Obviously any horse which is unable to eat or swallow will lose weight. Similarly horses with persistent diarrhoea will eventually lose bodily condition. Some horses are unable to absorb the nutrients from their feed although they may show no signs other than weight loss. Such horses may suffer from cancerous thickening and destruction of the intestinal lining or merely chronic inflammation of the intestines; occasionally no cause can be found for the problem. Undoubtedly the commonest cause of unthriftiness or weight loss is severe intestinal parasitism or its after-effects. Subacute or chronic grass sickness (see below) may also produce dramatic loss of bodily condition.

GRASS SICKNESS

Grass sickness is a relatively common disease which affects horses and ponies at grass. The cause of the disease is unknown and symptoms are variable. However, the most usual presenting feature, and the one which draws the attention of the owner, is colic. Affected horses have constipation, usually associated with impaction of the colon. They may also show other signs, such as patchy sweating or trembling of the muscles of the shoulder, quarters or neck. Some horses may die rapidly (acute type), often after rupture of the stomach; in fact, some horses are found dead (peracute type). It is more usual for signs of colic and distress to be seen, followed by rapid loss of condition (subacute type). There is also a more chronic form of the disease in which the horse wastes away without showing signs of colic or the other typical features.

Although most horses which contract the disease die or are humanely destroyed, it appears that a few animals may show clinical signs and recover. It is important that a vet be contacted early. Treatment will usually be aimed at alleviating the impaction of the colon and relieving gastric distension by passing a stomach tube.

MISCELLANEOUS ABDOMINAL CONDITIONS

There are a number of relatively uncommon conditions which can affect the abdomen of the horse and produce signs of digestive disturbance or abdominal pain.

Peritonitis (inflammation of the lining of the abdominal cavity) is fortunately very rare in horses but can occur as a sequel to colic, parasitic larval migration, enteritis or surgical treatment for any abdominal condition. Affected horses usually show moderate abdominal pain not typical of colic; they stand depressed, are reluctant to move, and are very tender to being touched around the flanks. They usually turn rather stiffly, preferring to stand dejectedly in one position. A vet can usually confirm the presence of peritonitis by collecting a sample of peritoneal fluid (the fluid which lubricates the interior of the abdominal cavity) for laboratory analysis. Treatment is prolonged at best (antibiotics and anti-inflammatory or painkilling drugs) and many cases do not recover.

In young animals **lymphosarcoma** (see p. 661) of the intestines (usually occurring as a tumour of the bowel wall) can occur and affected horses may show diarrhoea or loss of condition. Occasionally **malignant tumours** of the stomach may cause signs of peritonitis and weight loss; usually these are associated with abdominal discomfort. In older horses **lipomas** (tumours of fat) occasionally twist round the intestine, producing the clinical signs of twisted gut. Such cases can be diagnosed by exploratory surgery and, in some animals, resection of the affected piece of intestine can result in complete recovery.

Abdominal abscesses which may or may not be associated with the intestines can produce clinical signs of colic. They are most usually seen in young foals but can occur in horses of any age. Diagnosis can be very difficult but a vet can attempt to ascertain the cause of the problem by collecting peritoneal fluid and a blood sample. Foals with abdominal abscesses usually do not thrive very well and have increased body temperature which may fluctuate. Treatment is by a prolonged course of antibiotics and this may resolve the milder cases, but a number of horses succumb to the problem.

Rupture of the stomach occurs occasionally in horses, usually as the end result of intestinal blockage. It most commonly occurs in association with intestinal twists or following grass sickness. Horses which have shown signs of violent abdominal pain and suddenly become quiet usually have just suffered rupture of the stomach. Signs of shock precede death, which is usually fairly rapid.

Rupture of the diaphragm is very uncommon in horses but may occur in brood mares following foaling or in horses after major accidents. It is a very difficult condition to diagnose, but affected horses may present with abdominal pain. Usually an exploratory operation is required for a diagnosis to be made, but the prognosis is usually poor.

A **hernia** is the passage of a loop of intestine or even of the fat associated with the abdomen through a natural or acquired hole in the body wall. The two most common sites are at the navel or through the inguinal ring into the groin. Any horse or foal found with a swelling in these regions should be examined by a vet as soon as possible in case a piece of intestine becomes entrapped through the hernia. This cuts off the blood supply to that piece of intestine, producing severe colic, and requires an emergency operation (see Chapter 40).

Small pieces of intestine can also herniate through other sites within the abdomen, but these can only be diagnosed by a vet by an internal examination or an exploratory operation.

Prolapse of the rectum occurs rarely in horses and its cause is uncertain. The prolapse protrudes through the anal sphincter and immediate veterinary attention must be sought before serious damage is done to the wall of the intestine, as this can result in the death of the horse.

Accessory Glands of the Digestive System

The accessory glands of the digestive system comprise the liver, the pancreas and the salivary glands.

THE LIVER

The liver is a large organ, red-brown in colour and, in an adult horse, weighs about 10 lb (5 kg). It is found in the abdominal cavity sandwiched between the diaphragm, the stomach and the intestines. It has right, middle and left lobes and is attached by ligaments to the diaphragm and the abdominal wall. It is covered by a capsule and represents the largest gland in the body.

The liver is supplied by arteries, veins, nerves and lymph channels. In addition it possesses a duct which carries bile into the duodenum. Unlike other mammals, the horse has no gall bladder, a fact which has proved a trap to many a veterinary student during professional examinations.

About 75% of the blood passing through the liver enters from the portal vein, which contains blood coming from the intestines. The liver thus receives the products of digested food which have been absorbed through the wall of the gut. The other 25% of blood is carried into the liver by the hepatic artery and nourishes the liver cells.

After passing through the liver, blood flows out into the large veins leading to the heart. The organ is therefore strategically placed to act as a filter for the digestive processes that start in the gut.

The liver of the newborn foal is relatively large, weighing about 3 lb and the ratio of liver to bodyweight is about 1 to 5; in the adult the ratio is 1 to 100.

In foetal life the foal's liver receives blood from the umbilical vein, which carries blood from the placenta. All the blood from the placenta has to pass through the liver. This is in contrast to other species, in which a duct (the ductus venosus) allows a substantial proportion of the blood flow to bypass the liver. There is no ductus venosus in the horse.

Following foaling and severance of the umbilical cord the vein has no further function and it shrivels, leaving a cord known by anatomists as the round ligament of the liver.

The liver cleanses the blood of noxious substances, such as drugs and poisons, and forms part of the defence mechanism against microbes. It is capable of over a hundred different functions. These may be classed as (a) excretory to the exterior, as in the excretion of bile into the intestines; (b) excretory into the blood; (c) metabolic processes such as those concerned with the storage of sugar and the regulation of blood levels of carbohydrates, protein and fat.

The minute structure of the liver is composed of cells arranged in sheets between which blood circulates freely. Between adjacent sheets of liver cells there are tiny canals into which bile is secreted. The canals join together and eventually deliver bile into the common bile duct. Each liver cell has, therefore, a passage containing blood on one side, into which secretory products of the cells can pass, and a system of bile canals on the other side.

Under the microscope a section of liver reveals cells arranged in lobules which form columns radiating from a central vein. The vein thus receives blood that has passed between the sheets of liver cells. The central veins collect together and carry blood to the great veins passing to the heart. On the periphery of the lobule strands of fibrous tissue act as scaffolding. These contain the portal vein and bile canals.

A fine network of special cells is present in liver. These cells are responsible for taking up bacteria and other unwanted particles. This system is similar to that in other parts of the body and is known as the reticulo-endothelial (RE) system.

Some functions of the liver
Storage
Liver cells take up sugar and convert it into glycogen. In this form it is suitable for storage and can be converted to sugar when required for metabolism.

The liver converts amino acids into protein, which can be stored or utilised in various parts of the body for growth or converted into sugar for energy. The liver also stores fat and vitamins.

Regulating blood content
The liver helps to regulate the concentration of fat, sugar and amino acids in the bloodstream. According to the amount present in the blood received by the liver, the cells take up these substances or deliver them back into the blood-stream as required.

Converting substances and metabolism
The liver can transform various substances into simple compounds or convert them into more complex ones. Thus they can protect the body against poisons by changing them into harmless substances. For example, the liver prevents the accumulation of ammonia, a toxic substance formed by the breakdown of amino acids, by converting it to urea. Urea is a relatively non-toxic substance eliminated from the bloodstream by the kidneys, which could not deal effectively with ammonia.

The liver also detoxicates drugs so that their concentrations in the bloodstream fall from the time of administration. For example, phenylbutazone (bute) is converted by the liver into oxyphenbutazone before it can be excreted in the urine.

The same principle applies to nutritional matter absorbed from the gut; the liver deals with this material so that it can be useful to the body cells. For example, protein is changed into carbohydrate, and fat is combined with choline and phosphorus to form the valuable phospholipids, essential components of cell membranes.

Liver also forms the blood proteins albumin and globulin, which give the blood its viscosity (thickness), and fibrinogen and other substances necessary for clotting (see p. 109).

Bile secretion
An adult horse's liver produces about 10 litres of bile a day. Bile contains pigment (bilirubin), salts, protein, cholesterol and certain crystalline substances formed from the breakdown of haemoglobin. Bile pigment is a waste product, but bile starts are useful substances which help in the digestion of fat. Bile also contains many of the hormones produced by the adrenal cortex and the sex gland. The liver alters these hormones so that they are excreted in an inactive form, although some may be excreted unchanged and reabsorbed from the intestines back into the bloodstream.

The horse is a herbivore and, in the natural state, eats continuously, in contrast to carnivores and man, who eat occasionally. For this reason bile passes continually so that there is no reason for an organ of storage, i.e. a gall bladder.

Conditions of the Liver

There are few diseases of the horse's liver which have a primary origin. Most conditions are the indirect result of infections, toxins or poisons which are absorbed from the gut or arrive, as in focuses of infection, from other parts of the body.

However, because the organ has so many functions it has a corresponding part to play in many disease processes. For example, in the newborn foal suffering from lack of oxygen due to problems of lung function, the liver cells may become damaged and the function of the organ seriously or even fatally compromised.

The diagnosis of liver disease is made on the basis of symptoms and confirmed by tests on blood samples and liver biopsy. Symptoms include jaundice, wasting, diarrhoea and neurological signs such as aimless walking, staggering and running into objects. Oedema of the chest, abdomen and legs may also be present due to disturbances in fluid balances.

Symptoms are the result of liver dysfunction, such as the inability to deal with bilirubin or with the products of digestion.

In severe liver disease blood albumin concentrations fall and globulin rises. Blood enzymes such as sorbitol dehydrogenase (SDH) and aspartate amino-transferase (AST) increase.

Liver function may be tested by injecting a dye, such as bromosulphthalein, and measuring its rate of disappearance from the bloodstream. This will be abnormally slow if the liver cells are damaged.

Liver may be observed directly by obtaining a small piece with a biopsy needle. This specimen is then processed in the laboratory and various features of pathology may be examined.

Pathology of liver disease
A similar pattern of cellular damage is found on microscopic examination whatever the agent causing liver damage. First the cell swells and the nucleus starts to break up. This is followed by cellular death and the laying down of fat. The damaged cells are then replaced by fibrous (scar) tissue. The last phase of fibrosis is also known as cirrhosis of the liver and is a particular feature of poisoning by alcohol and plants, such as ragwort.

Fortunately the liver has remarkable powers of regrowth and it replaces damaged areas by growing new cells. The undamaged parts can take over the function of destroyed areas, and it is only when the damage is widespread that the healthy areas cannot perform the minimal requirements. When this occurs symptoms develop. Symptoms of liver disease are closely associated with the pathology. The following diseases and conditions are predominantly liver-orientated.

THEILER'S DISEASE (SERUM HEPATITIS)

This disease was described first by Theiler in South Africa following the administration of anti-serum against African horse sickness. The condition may also follow the use of any anti-sera. More recently it has been identified in horses that have not received any serum. It is characterised by degeneration of the liver cells and the appearance of jaundice.

Other symptoms include depression, inappetence and an unsteady gait, pressing the head against a wall, sleepiness and violent nervous reactions.

It is not clear whether the condition is caused by a virus or is an allergic response to foreign material, such as that contained in serum.

EQUID HERPESVIRUS 1 (EHV-1, RHINOPNEUMONITIS)

The foetus and newborn foal may suffer liver disease from El-IV-1 infection. The virus damages the liver cells, resulting in minute abscess-like areas in the liver (focal necrosis). The disease is not confined to the liver and the virus also affects the lungs, brain and other organs. The cumulative effect is foetal death followed by abortion or, if near to full term, the birth of a foal showing symptoms of jaundice, convulsions and other behavioural abnormalities.

For a detailed account, see p. 397.

PARASCARIS EQUORUM INFECTION

The liver of young horses may be damaged by the migration of roundworm larvae as they pass from the intestine to the lungs through the peritoneum and diaphragm.

For a detailed account, see p. 531.

JAUNDICE

Contrary to popular belief, jaundice is a symptom not a disease in itself. The yellowness of the skin, sclera of the eye and mucous membranes of the mouth, vagina and eyelids is due to the accumulation of bile pigment which the liver normally excretes into the intestines.

If the liver is prevented from clearing the bloodstream of this pigment, its concentration increases until it finally spills into the tissues to stain not only the skin but the muscles, brain and other organs.

There are three types of jaundice: haemolytic, obstructive and that caused by liver damage (hepatitis).

HAEMOLYTIC JAUNDICE

This results from destruction of red cells, i.e. haemolysis. The membrane of the red blood cell ruptures and haemoglobin escapes. Special cells lining the blood channels in the spleen, bone marrow and liver take up the haemoglobin and split it into two parts, globin (containing the iron radical) and bilirubin (the yellow pigment).

This process normally takes place continuously throughout the lifespan of the individual. However, the rate of breakdown of red cells is low; it is only when the breakdown is excessive that we speak of haemolysis and jaundice.

Normally the body retains the iron for the resynthesis of haemoglobin in the bone marrow. It is only the bile pigment that is excreted by the liver.

In haemolytic disease the destruction of red cells is increased to such an extent that the bone marrow fails to keep pace with replacement cells and, importantly so far as the jaundice is concerned, the liver cannot deal with the great quantities of bile pigment.

Haemolytic disease of the newborn foal is an obvious example of jaundice caused in this way. In this case antibodies, absorbed from the colostrum of the mare, destroy the foal's red cells (see p. 453). There is a dramatic fall in the number of circulating red cells from the normal 9 x 109 per litre to sometimes less than 2x109 per litre, and a corresponding fall in haemoglobin and haematocrit.

Destruction of red cells on this scale results in severe anaemia, the urine turns red due to haemoglobin passing through the kidneys, and, if left untreated, the foal dies from a shortage of red cells and a consequent insufficiency in the oxygen-carrying capacity of the blood.

Haemolytic disease may also be caused by bacteria, virus or parasites. In these instances the red blood cells are destroyed by the microbes or their toxins. This occurs in conditions such as equine infectious anaemia (see p. 497), leptospirosis (see p. 483) and piroplasmosis (see p. 504). However, jaundice is only caused when the breakdown of red cells is so excessive and rapid that the liver cannot perform its normal function of clearing the blood of bile pigment.

OBSTRUCTIVE JAUNDICE (HEPATIC JAUNDICE)

Jaundice develops when the flow of bile from the liver to the duodenum is obstructed. Pressure in the bile duct rises. This causes a backflow and bile pigment finds its way back to the blood. Its concentration in the bloodstream then increases until it becomes deposited in the tissues and the symptoms of jaundice are seen.

Obstructive jaundice may be caused by inflammation of the duodenum, by bot larvae entering the bile duct or as a result of roundworm (*Parascaris equorum*) migration through the liver. It may also be caused by tumours or be associated with certain conditions of the gut involving obstruction of the large or small intestines (stoppage or impaction).

LIVER DAMAGE (HEPATITIS)

Any process which disrupts the liver cells themselves may lead to jaundice by allowing bile pigment to enter directly into the lymph stream from where it is returned to the blood. It is not always possible to distinguish accurately between obstructive jaundice and that caused by hepatitis. The two conditions often coexist.

The cells may be injured by plant toxins or noxious chemicals. Chemicals include lead, phosphorus, arsenic, copper and carbon tetrachloride. Plants which contain poisons that injure liver cells, include buckthorn, ragwort (*Senecio jacobaea*) and wild pea. The poisonous principles in these plants are alkaloids, some of which, such as morphine, strychnine and hyacine, have medical properties; others are harmful. For further details, see Chapter 38.

Viruses and bacteria causing inflammation of the liver cells result in jaundice, for example, the virus causing equine infectious anaemia (see p. 497).

THE PANCREAS

The pancreas is an important gland which lies in the abdomen, nestling against the duodenum and the spleen. It has a dual function both as an exocrine and as an endocrine gland, that is, it produces secretions which pass in ducts to the gut and others which pass directly into the bloodstream in which they are carried to other parts of the body.

The exocrine secretion is collected and delivered by a duct system into the second part of the duodenum. The secretion is alkaline and helps to neutralise the acid stomach contents. It also contains special substances (enzymes) concerned with the digestion of proteins, carbohydrates and fat. The enzymes are not active until they reach the intestine, where they are rendered potent. They help to break down protein into amino acids which can be absorbed through the gut wall. The pancreatic juices contain enzymes that break down starches to sugars or emulsify fat.

The endocrine secretions of the pancreas are formed by cells known as the Islets of Langerhans. These cells are responsible for producing insulin, the hormone that controls levels of blood sugar.

There is increasing interest in conditions in the horse, such as hyperlipaemia (see below), which are associated with the action of insulin.

Metabolic Conditions

DIABETES MELLITUS

This condition is rare in the horse. The symptoms are associated with a lack of insulin production by the pancreas. This results in the body cells being unable to take up glucose from the blood so that an excessive blood glucose level (hyperglycaemia) develops. The excess glucose spills over into the urine, making it smell sweet. The glucosuria (glucose in the urine) is abnormal and takes with it large volumes of water. Consequently the affected horse is seen to drink and urinate more than usual. Weight loss occurs as the animal is unable to utilise absorbed glucose and must rely on the breakdown of body tissue for energy. Metabolic changes occur as a result of this and the animal becomes weak; neurological signs may develop in the long term. Diagnosis is based on demonstration of excessive levels of blood glucose and glucosuria.

DIABETES INSIPIDUS

This is another cause of excessive drinking and urination in the horse. Unlike diabetes mellitus, the urine is very dilute and contains no glucose. This condition is caused by a deficiency in antidiuretic hormone, one of the hormones produced by the posterior pituitary gland and, in the horse, this is usually due to a tumour in the pituitary gland. It is characterised by the excretion of large volumes of pale, thin urine, excessive thirst, weight loss, weakness and exercise intolerance. Confirmation of the diagnosis is made by demonstrating a temporary response to injections of pitressin.

Treatment, if undertaken, involves administration of pitressin, but this is often not practical.

HYPERLIPAEMIA

This condition, caused by an excess of blood lipid (fats), is most often seen in horses with reduced food intake, the consequent breakdown in adipose tissue leading to a build-up of an excessive amount of lipid in the blood. Pony mares are also susceptible. Clinical signs include inappetence, moderate to severe depression, weakness, muscle fasiculation (involuntary twitching) and ataxia. The tongue may have a greyish-white coating and the breath may be malodorous. Mares with a foal at foot may stop producing milk. Most cases can be avoided by ensuring that a horse or pony has an adequate food intake (see Chapter 44). In certain cases the administration of insulin and glucose or heparin may be beneficial.

THE SALIVARY GLANDS

There are three glands that produce saliva: the parotid, the submandibular and the sublingual. These glands are paired, one lying on either side of the midline. Saliva contains some cells, but is mainly a thin watery-viscous fluid varying in composition according to the type of stimulus initiating its secretion. It is made up of 99.5% water and 5% salts and organic material consisting of enzymes and mucin.

Saliva provides lubrication and moistens the mouth and lips. It is continuously produced but in much greater quantities when food is taken into the mouth. It aids the process of swallowing and provides a means whereby the mouth is washed clear of debris which might otherwise provide a culture medium for bacteria.

Saliva moistens the food and transforms it to a semi-solid or liquid mass so that it may be swallowed easily. An adult horse secretes over 50 litres of saliva daily.

Salivary enzymes help to break down starch to maltose, and the secretion or lack of secretion of saliva may indirectly aid in the control of water balance in the body.

The parotid glands are found in the space between the back of the lower jaw and the base of the ear. They are well defined with a strong fibrous capsule and each has a duct which opens in the region of the second upper molar tooth.

The submandibular glands lie on the inner surface of the lower jaw and their ducts open into the floor of the mouth. They also have a well-defined capsule.

The sublingual glands do not have a capsule. They are found near the midline below the mucous membrane of the floor of the mouth. Their secretions empty by several ducts.

2
THE RESPIRATORY (BREATHING) SYSTEM

It is convenient for descriptive purposes to divide the upper from the lower respiratory tract. However, the reader should not lose sight of the fact that the two parts of the breathing system are confluent and from a biological point of view they should be considered as one.

In this chapter the term 'respiratory' is used in the sense of breathing rather than to refer to the entire biological system of respiration, namely, the exchange of oxygen and carbon dioxide between the tissues (muscles, organs, etc.) and the air outside the body. The total system consists of the action of the lungs and bloodstream pumped by the action of the heart. These functions are described in Chapters 3, 4 and 5.

P.D.R.

THE UPPER RESPIRATORY TRACT

Functional anatomy

The equine upper respiratory tract is a complicated arrangement of mucous-membrane-lined compartments which have the main function of allowing efficient passage of air from the nostrils to the lower respiratory tract.

The nostrils are continuous with the nasal passages, each a rather complicated structure consisting of air channels and delicate bone surrounded by mucous membrane with a rich blood supply (turbinates). The nostrils and nasal passages are divided into two by a partly cartilaginous and partly bony septum.

Beyond the nasal passages is the pharynx, a single muscular cavity separated from the back of the mouth by a horizontal muscular sheet, the soft palate. This sheet divides the nasal part of the pharynx (nasopharynx) from the back of the mouth (oropharynx). It is through a hole in this muscular sheet that the passages of the voicebox or larynx protrude; thus the pharynx is continuous directly with the larynx and trachea (windpipe) and the lower respiratory tract.

Other air-filled cavities communicate with the main airway. The sinuses are a series of intercommunicating air-filled compartments, closely associated with the roots of certain cheek teeth in the upper jaw and other important anatomical structures. The paired guttural pouches are air-filled sacs which sit between the roof of the nasopharynx and the floor of the cranial vault (the bony box which contains the brain). They are outpouchings of the Eustachian tubes connecting the middle ear to the nasopharynx and are only found in the equine species.

The pouches are closed by cartilaginous flaps on either side of the pharangeal wall and are opened only during swallowing (hence the relief of middle-ear pressure noted by people on aeroplanes). Several important arteries and nerves travel around the walls and roof of these sacs, and diseases affecting the guttural pouch may have profound effects on these structures.

The internal anatomy of the upper respiratory tract varies depending on whether the horse is breathing quietly, galloping or swallowing. The nostrils are extremely distensible and act to funnel air into the nasal passages when the horse is travelling at speed. Similarly the nasal passages become more stream-lined by shrinkage of the vascular turbinates and nasal mucous membrane.

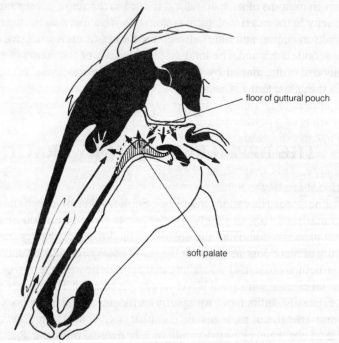

floor of guttural pouch

soft palate

Figure 1 Soft tissue structures of the throat which may produce an abnormal noise or respiratory obstruction with excessive poll flexion

The larynx can be considered as a biological valve which, when opened fully, allows the maximum flow of air to the lower respiratory tract during galloping. It also acts to prevent the aspiration of food material during swallowing, when the laryngeal opening is completely closed. During resting respiration, the valve is open in an intermediate position.

The other significant alteration in upper respiratory architecture occurs during swallowing. At the exact moment of swallowing the muscular soft palate is elevated to block off the back of the nose, and the larynx moves forward and becomes closed (see Figures 2 and 3 in previous chapter). This allows the passage of food material from the back of the mouth into the oesophagus (gullet) without leakage into the respiratory tract.

Thus the upper respiratory tract is a marvellously designed aerodynamic system which permits the passage of large volumes of air to the lower respiratory tract during fast exercise. The horse is frequently used as a competitive animal and it is obvious that diseases which result in the narrowing of any part of the upper airway can produce serious impairment of airflow and therefore of performance.

Methods of examining the upper respiratory tract
Diseases of the upper airway have been recognised for hundreds of years. The clinical symptoms of such diseases have been recorded since the beginning of veterinary literature. However, the recent introduction of more advanced radiographic techniques and fibre-optic endoscopy (using a flexible telescope) has revolutionised our understanding of the anatomy and physiology of the upper airway and of the diseases which affect the respiratory system.

It is important that a horse owner is observant, taking careful notice of even what appear to be rather unimportant details, for it is the recognition of the early signs of a disease which can provide the vet with vital information to help in early diagnosis.

The most common sign of upper airway disease is the presence of a nasal discharge. This may contain mucus, pus, blood or even food material. Identification of the nature of the discharge and of whether it comes from one or both nostrils can provide essential information in the localisation of its source.

Similarly, if a horse has a nosebleed, it is important to know whether the quantity of blood loss was large or small, whether the nosebleed occurred down one or both nostrils, and whether it was associated with exercise.

The other common sign of upper airway disease is obstruction to the airflow (see Figure 1). In its most severe form this may produce severe respiratory embarrassment, but more usually it results in reduced tolerance of exercise and/or an abnormal respiratory noise during exercise. There may also be other important signs such as inappetence, raised body temperature, difficulty in swallowing and enlargement of local lymph glands.

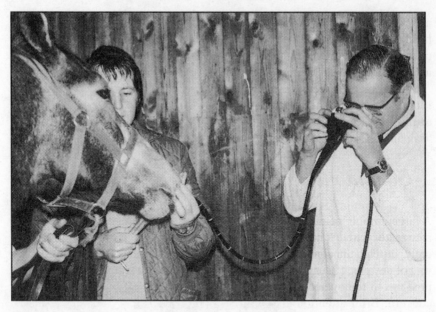

Figure 2   Carrying out an endoscopic examination

The observant owner should be aware of many of these features as they will aid in the rapid diagnosis of the problem. When a vet is called in it is important to supply accurate information about the horse. In particular it is important to divulge whether other animals are affected, whether the horse was kept in or out of doors and its state of fitness.

In addition to carrying out a clinical examination, many vets carry out an endoscopic examination in an attempt to locate the source of a discharge or haemorrhage or to identify the nature of respiratory obstruction.

The modern endoscope is a flexible telescope which, like many other fibre-optic instruments used today, works on the principle of total internal reflection of light. In simple terms this means that light is transmitted from a source down fine glass fibres to the end of the telescope, illuminating even the darkest and most inaccessible regions of the respiratory system. Thus a clear view of the internal anatomy of these areas is transmitted back up optical fibres to the eyepiece.

Most endoscopes flush air and water to keep the distal lens clear of mucus and other debris which are present in the respiratory tract. Although a nasal twitch is usually applied to permit passage of the tube up the nose, the procedure is seldom resented and in most cases can be carried out safely and without complications.

The radiography machine can also be used effectively to investigate the respiratory tract. In many cases the examination is carried out with the patient conscious, but it may be necessary to sedate the horse or to carry out general anaesthesia to obtain special views of certain regions. Although the horse's head is large and bony, the many air-filled cavities inside provide excellent radiographic contrast to the relatively dense structures, such as bone and tooth, and to soft tissues in the throat region.

Nuclear medical technology is developing rapidly and in the not too distant future such techniques as chest scanning will become accepted routine in equine practice.

Conditions of the Upper Respiratory Tract

A large number of diseases related to the upper respiratory tract have been recognized and it is not the purpose of this chapter to catalogue them individually. Instead, the common presenting signs of upper respiratory tract disease will be described because these are usually the symptoms which first bring the problem to the owner's attention and are usually the immediate cause for concern. Brief attention also will be given to veterinary therapy of these conditions, but some mention will be made of appropriate management to be employed by owners in each circumstance.

NASAL DISCHARGE

All normal horses produce a small quantity of mucus which may be seen to discharge from both nostrils on occasions, particularly after exercise. The quantity of this discharge may vary from animal to animal but should not be a cause for concern. The commonest type of abnormal discharge is mucus and pus from both nostrils and this is frequently associated with a cough. A frequent misconception is that the discharge has originated from the sinuses whereas in fact in the vast majority of such cases the horse is affected by chronic obstructive pulmonary (lung) disease (see p. 82).

Sinusitis usually produces a fairly typical discharge of thick pus from one nostril. Often there is a foul smell to the discharge, particularly if a dental problem is involved or if the condition has become chronic. There may be some obstruction to airflow through the affected nostril, and in advanced cases there may be severe blockage with facial swelling. Such horses usually produce a snoring respiratory noise. The lymph gland under the jaw is often swollen on the affected side and occasionally there may be facial pain. A slight discharge from the eye on the affected side may develop.

Under any of these circumstances veterinary attention should be sought immediately. An endoscopic examination may confirm that the nasal discharge has originated from the sinus region and radiographic views may show the presence of pus in the sinuses or even a dental abnormality.

In mild cases antibiotic therapy may be enough to alleviate the problem but in more advanced cases surgical drainage of the sinus is necessary and this is usually carried out under general anaesthesia. At this time the presence of an abnormal tooth can be identified and if necessary removed. (Dental abnormalities are dealt with on p. 42.)

Post-operative treatment involves flushing the sinus and this must be done on a daily basis. Sometimes this procedure is entrusted to the owner or groom but will be carried out under veterinary advice. As a general rule regular post-operative exercise is also recommended.

A discharge down one nostril also follows infections of the nasal passages, the commonest of these being a **fungal infection of the turbinates**. These usually produce a scanty, foul-smelling discharge which may sometimes be associated with a nosebleed. In such cases veterinary treatment is required and an antifungal drug is usually administered via a facial catheter (a tube for administering drugs or fluids).

Bacterial infections of the nasal passages may be treated by appropriate antibiotic therapy, and the collection of a nasal swab for bacteriological culture to find out which organism is involved and to test its antibiotic sensitivity (that is, to find out which antibiotic will destroy the bacteria) is often of value. Affected horses are not usually ill and there is little reason to suspend normal riding activities.

There are other less common causes of a nasal discharge. **Cystic swellings** associated with the nasal passages and sinuses (for example, **maxillary cysts**) occur, usually in foals and young horses, but they are occasionally seen in older animals. There is often marked facial swelling and nasal obstruction and mucus may be discharged down one nostril. Surgical removal of the cyst is carried out under general anaesthesia.

Nasal tumours (cancer) are relatively uncommon in horses. However, they may be responsible in older animals for a discharge down one nostril which in almost all cases is associated with nasal haemorrhage. The discharge may have a foul smell and frequently there is facial pain and swelling. In advanced cases there may be blindness or other ocular abnormalities. Treatment is only effective if the problem is recognised early enough and comprises radical surgical removal of the growth. This is always carried out under general anaesthesia. In many cases the prognosis is unfavourable.

Rarely **foreign bodies** (usually twigs) may become lodged in the nasal passages, resulting in nasal discharge, haemorrhage and acute headshyness. Removal by a vet usually requires general anaesthesia.

Discharges from both nostrils (bilateral) originate from farther back in the respiratory tract than the nasal septum, that is, in the pharynx or lungs. **Infections of the guttural pouch** usually produce a bilateral discharge, but often this is more profuse down the nostril on the side of the affected pouch.

Fungal infections of the guttural pouch are most common in this country. Affected horses usually have severe nosebleeds and there is frequently a foul-smelling nasal discharge. Horses with major nosebleeds should be investigated immediately as fungal infections of the guttural pouch can produce a fatal haemorrhage (see p. 56). In such cases the internal carotid artery may be tied off and the fungal infection treated topically; such treatment may be life-saving.

Abscesses in the throat sometimes burst into a guttural pouch (**guttural pouch empyema**), which then becomes full of pus, and this is usually discharged from both nostrils (sometimes intermittently). There is also swelling of the throat and frequently difficulty in swallowing or breathing. Sometimes the discharge may be foul-smelling. Occasionally horses are very ill, reluctant to raise their heads and display total inappetence. The vet should be consulted immediately; clinical impressions can be confirmed by endoscopic or radiographic examination.

Treatment is usually by flushing the affected pouch using an indwelling catheter. This usually produces fairly rapid relief from symptoms, but affected animals may be sent home for further treatment, which usually involves irrigation of the pouch under veterinary supervision. Nasal swabs may be collected for bacteriological culture and antibiotic sensitivity testing to determine the appropriate antibiotics.

A similar swelling of the guttural pouch is seen in young foals when the pouch becomes distended with air (**guttural pouch tympany**). Affected foals may have difficulty in breathing and sometimes a snoring respiratory noise can be heard. Usually the condition requires surgical treatment. Tympanitic pouches may become secondarily infected and require treatment in the manner described for guttural pouch empyema.

In general, nasal discharges originating from the guttural pouch require irrigation of the affected pouch, but drainage can be encouraged by feeding the horse from the floor or turning it out of doors. The guttural pouch orifice opens during swallowing and if this occurs with the head lowered (as with grazing) efficient drainage of inflammatory exudates is facilitated.

NASAL DISCHARGE OF FOOD

Sometimes a nasal discharge contains food material and such horses may discharge food or water from the nose when they swallow. There are many possible causes for this problem.

In young foals milk may run from both nostrils from birth when there is a defect such as a **cleft of the hard or soft palate**. Such cases usually develop **aspiration pneumonia**. Surgical treatment of the cleft is ineffective and humane destruction should therefore be carried out as soon as diagnosis has been confirmed by clinical or endoscopic examination.

Obstructive problems of the throat, such as guttural pouch empyema or tympany, may produce difficulty in swallowing and nasal return of food material. This may be encountered if abscesses (e.g. strangles – see p. 474) or tumours are present in the pharyngeal region.

Pharyngeal abscesses require immediate veterinary attention otherwise affected horses may suffer from severe respiratory obstruction. However, the condition is generally resolved by appropriate antibiotic therapy.

In younger animals **pharyngeal cysts** may cause difficulty in swallowing and lead to nasal return of food material. These can be diagnosed endoscopically and removed surgically.

One of the most serious causes of nasal return of food material is that of **pharyngeal paralysis** following fungal infection of the guttural pouch. This condition is usually associated with nasal haemorrhage, but some cases only show nasal return of food material and coughing.

Horses with such signs should be examined immediately by a vet and antifungal treatment carried out via an indwelling catheter in the guttural pouch. Antiinflammatory drugs may also be given. The prognosis is sometimes unfavourable because some cases develop aspiration pneumonia, which necessitates humane destruction.

Probably the commonest cause of the nasal return of food material is choke or oesophagal obstruction. This and other problems associated with the digestive system are described in Chapter 1.

NASAL HAEMORRHAGE (EPISTAXIS)

Nasal haemorrhage is surprisingly common in horses. Some of the simple laws which apply to nasal discharge also apply to nasal haemorrhage, namely, if a horse bleeds from one nostril only, the most likely source of the nasal haemorrhage is in the nasal passages on that side. Conversely, horses that bleed from both nostrils usually have a problem in the nasopharynx, the guttural pouches or in the lower respiratory tract. In some horses small nosebleeds from one nostril may or may not be associated with exercise and no other clinical signs are noted.

Endoscopic examination may reveal the haemorrhage to have originated in the nasal passages, but in many cases it is impossible to identify the source of haemorrhage accurately. Such haemorrhages usually resolve without the need for treatment. Some cases of acute sinusitis may have slight nasal haemorrhage but this is always associated with a nasal discharge of pus.

Nasal tumours almost invariably induce nasal haemorrhage (usually from one nostril). An endoscopic examination is the most reliable means of confirming this diagnosis. In advanced cases other symptoms, particularly a foul-smelling nasal discharge, may develop. In such cases veterinary attention must be sought and treatment is by radical surgical removal.

Rarely **foreign bodies** may be trapped in the nasal passages, producing epistaxis. These can usually be removed under general anaesthesia. Horses which have bled from one nostril should be examined as soon as possible by a vet; in some cases treatment is unnecessary, but it always important to eliminate more serious causes of the problem.

The commonest cause of bilateral nosebleed is **haemorrhage from the lungs** which occurs, to some extent, in almost all horses at fast exercise (see p. 86).

Horses with a disease affecting both sides of the nasal passages can produce bilateral nosebleeds, but the most important cause of this condition not associated with exercise is **fungal infection of the guttural pouch**. Fungal infection of the guttural pouch can produce a foul-smelling nasal discharge and difficulty in swallowing. However, the most frequent presenting sign is nasal haemorrhage. This may vary in quantity but can be massive and even fatal. Any horse which has a bilateral nasal haemorrhage unassociated with exercise requires immediate veterinary investigation.

Other features of fungal infection of the guttural pouch are pain under the base of the ear, swelling in the throat region, neck stiffness, colic or patchy sweating and, rarely, signs of eye disease. The most useful way of confirming fungal infection of the guttural pouch is by endoscopic examination.

Once the diagnosis has been confirmed an emergency operation should be carried out to tie off the artery producing the haemorrhage. The outlook for horses which cannot swallow is not good, although many cases eventually recover.

There are other causes of bilateral nosebleeds but these are much less common. They include pharyngeal foreign bodies, which are usually associated with paroxysmal coughing and difficulty in swallowing. **Fractures of the skull** usually follow trauma such as a horse rearing over backwards and may be associated with swelling of the head and other signs of facial damage or nervous impairment. In cases in which skull fractures are suspected a radiographic examination is the diagnostic method of choice.

RESPIRATORY OBSTRUCTION

At rest

Many of the conditions described in previous sections will cause some degree of respiratory obstruction at rest. These include sinusitis (p. 63), nasal tumour (p. 64), maxillary cyst (p. 64), guttural pouch tympany and empyema (p. 64), pharyngeal abscess (p. 66) and pharangeal tumour. In most of these cases there are other signs accompanying respiratory obstruction. For obstructions of the trachea (windpipe), see p. 70.

At exercise

The conditions described under this heading are those that will not usually cause obstruction at paces slower than the trot. Most of them do not cause significant obstruction until a horse canters or gallops. The most common of these is the condition which affects young horses, particularly young race-horses, and results from obstruction to airflow in the pharynx by **enlarged tonsular tissue**.

The tonsular tissue of a horse is very much more diffusely located than in man or other domestic animals. In all young horses there are aggregations of lymphatic (tonsular) tissue (**lymphoid hyperplasia**) in the roof of the nasopharynx and these can be readily identified using an endoscope. In the vast majority of cases the condition causes no problem and the tonsils gradually reduce in size as the horse matures. It is thought that they enlarge in response to exposure to infectious agents and allergens in the environment.

In a few horses the lymphatic tissue becomes enlarged to such an extent that it causes obstruction to airflow during exercise. This produces an abnormal inspiratory sound at exercise which may be likened to a whistle or a roar. The problem is exacerbated in unfit animals and will usually disappear as the horse becomes more mature. If such a noise is heard a vet should be asked to examine the horse and to carry out an endoscopic examination in order to eliminate this problem from other more serious complaints. Usually no treatment is necessary.

As mentioned previously, cystic structures occasionally develop in the pharynx of foals and young horses and these may produce signs of respiratory obstruction during exercise. An endoscopic diagnosis is required and treatment is by surgical removal of the cyst.

Another problem occurring most commonly in racehorses, but also in eventers and some hunters, is that of **choking up**; it is also sometimes known as **soft palate disease** or **tongue swallowing**. The condition usually occurs at the end of a race when a horse is apparently galloping easily and the jockey asks it for a last effort. Suddenly there is a rather terrifying gurgling noise and the horse stops within a few strides as if shot. It is then usually able to regain its breath and continue the race, but will have lost all chance of winning. By the time the horse is pulled up and a veterinary examination is requested there are usually no symptoms of respiratory disease.

The problem is thought to be related to a disruption in the anatomical relationship between the larynx and the soft palate. In the normal horse the larynx fits snugly through a hole in the soft palate, forming an air-tight and food-tight seal, and this junction is only disrupted during swallowing.

It is thought that during racing the junction between the larynx and the soft palate is disrupted, breaking the seal and allowing the normally nasal-breathing horse to breathe through its mouth. Thus air passes both above and below the soft palate, producing an effect similar to a sail flapping in the breeze, with considerable turbulence (therefore noise) and severe airway obstruction. The situation is rapidly corrected when the horse swallows and the soft palate and the larynx return to their normal respiratory position.

It is usual when such a noise is identified to ask a veterinarian to carry out a detailed investigation. This is mainly to eliminate other causes of respiratory obstruction. Some abnormalities of the heart may produce similar clinical signs and it is thought that a number of respiratory problems may manifest themselves in the same manner (e.g. **lung disease** or **laryngeal hemiplegia** - see below).

In a significant proportion of horses no primary cause can be found for choking up and under these circumstances surgical treatment is usually advocated. However, a number of managemental aids can be used to help the problem. These include using a dropped noseband in order to keep the mouth closed, tying the tongue forward with a tongue strap, and using a milder bit. Surgical treatment is usually only recommended after trying these aids. The results of surgical treatment are rather variable and if the operation is unsuccessful it may be necessary to insert a tube into the trachea (windpipe) to allow the horse to breathe by bypassing the obstruction (tracheostomy).

Conditions of the Larynx

The larynx (voicebox) is a biological valve which permits an adequate flow of air to the lower respiratory tract during galloping and prevents aspiration of food material during swallowing. Diseases of the larynx, therefore, have considerable importance in relation to the function of the upper respiratory tract. Since the introduction of fibre-optic endoscopy, the larynx is an organ which has received much attention and now a number of different laryngeal problems have been recognized.

The most commonly encountered disease is **laryngeal hemiplegia** (also known as **whistling** or **roaring**): in 90% of cases the left side of the larynx is paralysed, either completely or partly. The cause is a degeneration of the nerve that supplies the muscles which open and close the larynx. Affected horses make abnormal inspiratory noises at exercise, typically a whistle or a roar. The diagnosis can be confirmed endoscopically. Many horses perform satisfactorily without the need for treatment, but if a horse is suffering from exercise intolerance, several types of operation can be performed, including that popularised in this country by Sir Frederick Hobday. In fact, for horses with advanced disease more recent operations – for example, tying back the paralysed side of the larynx c have superseded hobdaying.

Alternatively a tube can be inserted into the trachea, thus bypassing the obstruction and allowing the horse to breathe more freely. Such tubes have to be removed and cleaned at least daily and involve careful management by the owner or trainer. Horses with an unguarded hole in their trachea are prone to inhaling debris and must be kept well away from water (i.e. rivers, lakes or the sea) for obvious reasons.

Several other types of laryngeal obstruction have been recognized since endoscopy has been regularly used and can now be readily differentiated even though their clinical signs are similar to laryngeal hermplegia. Most of these cases can be treated by surgical means.

Conditions of the Trachea (Windpipe)

Diseases affecting the trachea which produce narrowing, such as **congenital collapse**, development of an **abscess** or other **compressive lesions** or **severe trauma**, will result in obstruction to airflow, an abnormal noise during exercise and severe exercise intolerance. Apart from treatment of infections or excision of accessible masses, the only other method of treatment is to insert a tracheostomy tube below the obstruction. Unfortunately, with a collapsed trachea, this is impossible, as it is with masses at the front of the chest which compress the trachea.

THE LOWER RESPIRATORY TRACT

Functional anatomy
The equine chest is the second largest of the body cavities and is roughly cone-shaped, being narrow and deep anteriorly but wide and flat posteriorly. The shape of the chest is maintained by the ribs, which are well sprung and form the side walls. The posterior wall consists of the diaphragm, which is very oblique and convex. There is a thin membrane running from the top to the bottom of the chest which divides the cavity medially into two halves.

The lungs occupy a large percentage of the chest space, with the heart situated anteriorly and to the left. A number of other important structures are also found within the chest. These include major blood vessels, the oesophagus (foodpipe), lymph glands and tubes carrying lymph. All these organs fit tightly within the chest and the shape of the lungs conforms to them (Figure 3).

Air is conducted to the lungs by means of the trachea (windpipe), which has an average length of 75–80 cm and is approximately 5–6 cm in diameter. The windpipe is situated in the lower aspect of the horse's neck and is held open by rigid C-shaped rings of cartilage.

The trachea divides to form the two bronchi, which enter the lungs and in turn subdivide into numerous smaller tubes which branch throughout the lung tissue. The larger tubes are supported by plates of cartilage which become smaller as the tubes diminish in size. Cartilage is absent in tubes of about one mm diameter and these open into regular, roughly circular air cells (alveoli). This meshwork of air cells gives the lungs a soft, spongy consistency.

The function of the respiratory system is to conduct air to and from the air cells of the lungs and to bring about gas exchange, allowing the body to absorb oxygen into the bloodstream and to give off carbon dioxide into the exhaled air. Oxygen is required in order to maintain many of the normal body functions such as the metabolism of food and muscle activity. Carbon dioxide is given off as one of the waste products and has to be removed from the body.

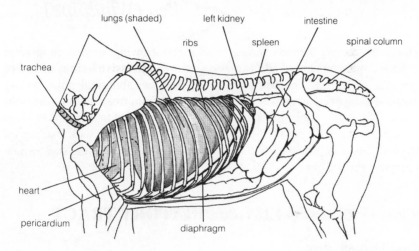

Figure 3   The lower respiratory tract

The mechanics of breathing are complex. Essentially, contraction of the muscle fibres in the diaphragm and in-between the ribs causes the chest cavity to expand and air to be drawn into the lungs. Relaxation of these muscles has the opposite effect and air is exhaled.

Capillary blood vessels are situated in very close association with the air cells in the lungs and, in the normal horse, gas exchange occurs readily across the membranes separating these structures (Figure 4). Blood pumped to the lungs from the heart is rich in carbon dioxide, which is given off into the air cells; in exchange, oxygen is absorbed into the blood, which then returns to the heart to be circulated around the body.

In the normal horse the airways are lined by a thin film of mucus, which is constantly being moved up the airways towards the throat. This is done by minute hairlike projections (cilia), which also line the airways and which beat anteriorly in a wavelike motion, causing the mucus to move over them. Dust particles and any other foreign material become trapped in the mucus and are removed from the airways in this way. Once reaching the throat this material is swallowed by the horse. In the lining of the airways and alveoli there are many cells whose function is to neutralise and remove any harmful agents which may have penetrated the mucus and gained access to the membrane. These are the basic mechanisms which prevent infections from developing in the lung.

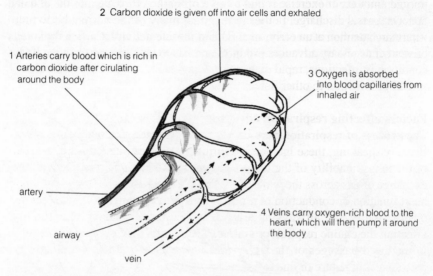

2 Carbon dioxide is given off into air cells and exhaled

1 Arteries carry blood which is rich in carbon dioxide after cirulating around the body

3 Oxygen is absorbed into blood capillaries from inhaled air

artery

4 Veins carry oxygen-rich blood to the heart, which will then pump it around the body

airway

vein

Figure 4   The process of gas exchanges in the lung

Healthy respiration
In the normal resting horse respiration is a quiet, relaxed process, with inhalation and exhalation of air occurring in a regular, rhythmical fashion. The nostrils are relaxed and clean, although a slight watery nasal discharge is quite normal. There should be no abnormal respiratory sounds such as coughing or wheezing.

The normal respiratory rate of the horse is ten to fourteen breaths per minute and can be counted by watching the breathing movements of the flanks or the nostrils. There are several factors unrelated to disease which can lead to an increase in respiratory rate. These include excitement, exercise, high altitude, high environmental temperature or humidity, and obesity.

The rhythm of respiration is important. In the normal resting horse inspiration and expiration are followed by a pause. The period of expiration is usually slightly longer than that of inspiration, and the length of the pause becomes shorter if the horse is excited or has been exercised preceding examination, or if it has a respiratory problem. The normal horse should be able to undertake exercise in keeping with its degree of fitness and should recover from exertion in five to ten minutes.

Signs of respiration malfunction

In addition to general signs of ill health, conditions which warrant veterinary attention include: (a) coughing or other abnormal respiratory sounds at rest or exercise; (b) increased respiratory rate or deep or laboured breathing in a quiet, resting horse; (c) irregular breathing – that is, spells when a horse appears to stop breathing followed by a spell of rapid breathing; (d) inability to carry out normal amounts of exercise followed by a prolonged recovery period; and (e) abnormal nasal discharge. In the event of any such signs it is advisable to seek veterinary attention at an early stage. This will minimize suffering for the horse, prevent unnecessary advancement of the condition, and hasten recovery. If the condition is infectious, rapid diagnosis, isolation and treatment will minimize spread of infection to other horses.

Factors affecting respiration adversely

The process of respiration may be adversely affected in a number of ways. Broadly speaking, these include interference to the passage of air in and out of the lungs, inability of the lungs to expand normally, interference with the exchange of gas across the walls of the air cells or blood capillaries, abnormal heart function or conduction of blood to and from the lungs. Of these factors, obstruction of the airways appears to be the most common abnormality affecting the equine respiratory system. Obstruction may occur at any level – in the nasal passages or throat, or in the windpipe or lungs – and may be mechanical in nature or due to a disease process.

Narrowing of the airways may occur due to pressure being exerted from outside the airway, for example, by a growth or abscess. Spontaneous collapse of the cartilaginous rings supporting the airways may also occur in rare instances, resulting in reduced airway diameter. Narrowing, which in some instances leads to blockage of the airways, may occur in a number of other ways. These include contraction of the muscle layers in the walls, inflammation of the membrane lining the airways, or an increased amount of mucus in the airways. These latter processes are particularly important in the very small airways where such changes may give rise to significant airway obstruction, particularly if the changes are widespread.

At birth the lungs of a foal are collapsed and contain no air, but soon thereafter the foal starts breathing and the lungs become distended with air. In some instances incomplete distention occurs and this gives rise to marked respiratory difficulty in newborn foals. In older foals and adult horses infection may give rise to excess fluid material accumulating in the narrow space between the lungs and the chest wall. This prevents the lungs from expanding to their normal limits and may even compress them. On occasions severe injury to the chest wall may result in the thoracic cavity being penetrated. This allows air to be drawn into the chest cavity, which is normally under negative pressure, resulting in the collapse of a lung.

Any mechanical or chemical irritation to the lower respiratory tract will result in coughing – a highly coordinated reflex action designed to remove such irritants. Sensitive nerve endings or receptors are situated under the lining of the respiratory passages from the throat down to the tiniest airways. Thus, irritation at any level will result in coughing. The processes described here and the ways in which they affect horses will be discussed in more detail under the individual conditions.

Methods of examining the lower respiratory tract
The onset of a respiratory problem may be sudden or gradual. The severity may range from mild, with the occasional cough and slightly reduced exercise tolerance, to severe, with the horse coughing frequently and appearing breathless when standing at rest.

Observations made by a groom or owner can be very helpful to a veterinarian. In addition to the rate of onset and effect of exercise, questions will be asked about recent events which may have some bearing on the horse's respiratory problem, such as contact with other horses, either within the stable yard or away from the premises, for example, at competitive events. Inquiries will be made into the health of other horses in the yard, whether there have been any visiting horses, the horse's vaccination status and any previous illness that the horse has had. The circumstances in which the horse developed the respiratory problem may be explored: for example, whether the horse was kept outdoors or stabled and, if the latter, the type and quality of the bedding and forage. More detailed questions will be asked about the horse's wellbeing, such as appetite, thirst and evidence of nasal discharge (amount, colour, consistency, one nostril or both).

When examining a horse with a respiratory problem a veterinarian initially carries out a general examination. Thereafter a visual assessment of the horse's respiratory movements will be made at rest in order to establish the rate, rhythm and depth of breathing. Abnormal respiratory sounds such as wheezing will also be noted. A true reflection will only be gained if the horse is relaxed; thus quiet surroundings and a calm, patient person holding the horse are of utmost importance.

The inspiratory and expiratory effort can be assessed by watching the horse's flanks and nostrils during breathing. Expiration occurs in two phases - a passive relaxation of the chest muscles followed by slight contraction of the flank muscles. In some conditions the latter phase is accentuated in order to force air out of the lungs and contraction of the abdominal muscles is increased. This is sometimes referred to as a double lift or heave (Figure 5). In normal horses the amount of flank movement varies depending on the type of horse and its bodily condition. This is usually considered in conjunction with breathing sounds in the windpipe and chest.

Using a stethoscope, the vet will listen for abnormal respiratory sounds, whether they are present in one or both lungs and, within a lung, whether they are localised or widespread. This provides an indication of the nature of changes within the lung but will rarely establish the cause with any certainty. Another test which may be performed by a veterinarian is percussion. This is the process of tapping the chest in horizontal and vertical directions by means of a percussion hammer or the fingers. This is done in order to establish the area of chest resonance, that is, the extent of the lungs, and to try to locate areas of consolidation. In the horse this technique is generally considered to be of limited value as many deep-seated lesions cannot be detected by this method because of the volume of the chest.

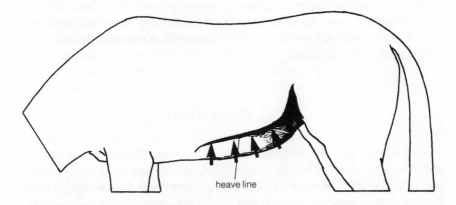

heave line

Figure 5   Location of the heave line

An examination of the heart will be carried out in the resting horse. The vet may then ask for the horse to be exercised in order to assess the effects on the heart and lungs.

The diagnosis of respiratory conditions is complex and a vet may wish to take samples for laboratory analysis. These might include samples of blood or, swabs taken from the throat area via the nose. The vet may wish to examine the horse's windpipe using a fibre-optic endoscope. This will enable him or her to visualise any changes, particularly the amount and consistency of mucus, and even to collect a sample of mucus if appropriate.

More specialised examinations involving expensive equipment are usually confined to veterinary schools or specialised research centres. They include radiographic examination of the chest and more detailed lung function testing, descriptions of which are beyond the scope of this book.

Conditions of the Lower Respiratory Tract

Lower respiratory conditions may arise due to infectious micro-organisms (viruses and bacteria), parasites (lungworm), hypersensitivity to possible allergens in the environment, and mechanical irritants or abnormalities.

The first signs of lower respiratory malfunction are an increase in respiratory rate (more than fifteen breaths per minute), coughing and reduced exercise tolerance. The signs may increase in severity to include an increase in the depth of respiration up to a state of severe respiratory distress. Clinical signs that warrant veterinary attention are described in more detail on p. 73.

The most common conditions affecting the lower respiratory system fall into five categories: (a) virus infections; (b) bacterial infections; (c) parasitic infections; (d) allergies such as chronic obstructive pulmonary disease; and (e) pulmonary haemorrhage.

Virus Infections

Virus infections are common causes of respiratory illness in horses. The viruses spread rapidly where horses are grouped together in close proximity, for example, in stable yards, and the transporting of horses over long distances may lead to the rapid spread of infections over a wide area. Some outbreaks of respiratory disease are due to mixed infections involving more than one agent, but the majority involve either an influenza virus or a herpesvirus.

EQUINE INFLUENZA (FLU)

Equine influenza is a severe virus respiratory infection which is sudden in onset. The main clinical signs are a high temperature and coughing, with a watery nasal discharge. Most cases recover in two to three weeks but a period of convalescence is desirable. Influenza is prevented by comprehensive vaccination programmes.

For a detailed account, see p. 485.

EQUID HERPESVIRUS 1 (SNOTTY NOSE, STABLE COUGH, VIRUS ABORTION, RHINOPNEUMONITIS)

Equine herpesvirus is a respiratory infection giving rise to outbreaks of illness.

Other strains of the virus cause abortion in mares (see p. 394). The clinical signs are a high temperature and increased respiratory rate with listlessness and inappetence. The condition is prevalent in young horses.

For a detailed account, see p. 490.

EQUINE RHINOVIRUS AND ADENOVIRUS (COLD VIRUSES)

These are widespread viruses causing little or no clinical illness. For a more detailed account of the various cold viruses, see p. 496.

Bacterial Infections

Bacteria may enter the body in a number of ways; by mouth, by inhalation, through wounds and, in young foals, via the navel. Bacteria are commonly found in the respiratory passages of healthy horses and, in many instances, will only give rise to disease under conditions of stress or secondary to another illness such as a respiratory virus infection. However, certain bacteria may be the primary cause of respiratory disease, for example, strangles (*Streptococcus equi* - see p. 474). Bacterial infections may affect both upper and lower respiratory tracts and vary in severity according to the type of infection, the age and immune status of the animal. The most severe infections involve the lungs and result in pneumonia.

PNEUMONIA, BRONCHOPNEUMONIA

Pneumonia is a severe respiratory condition in which there is inflammation of the lung tissue caused by infectious organisms or foreign materials in the lungs. Bronchopneumonia is a more extensive condition, affecting the airways of the lungs in addition to the lung tissue.

The bacterial organisms which cause pneumonia in the horse most commonly are the *Streptococcus* species. Other organisms, including *Actinobacillus equuli*, *Bordetella bronchiseptica* and *Pasteurella* species, may be involved occasionally. Foreign material such as drenches that have gone down the wrong way, viruses and parasites may also give rise to pneumonia.

Clinical signs
Foals and horses with pneumonia are dull, listless, inappetent, have an increased respiratory rate and a high temperature. Animals cough and may

have a purulent nasal discharge. The condition may increase in severity, indicated by an increase in the depth of breathing and a worsening in the general condition. In a state of severe respiratory distress horses will have flared nostrils, very laboured breathing and a distinct double expiratory effort or heave (Figure 5).

Course of the condition

Bacterial respiratory conditions resulting in pneumonia are contagious. Horses become infected through contact with horses carrying the organisms or with infected nasal discharges or sputum which has been expelled during coughing. Usually infections are acquired by inhalation; however, in newborn foals bacteria may enter the body via the navel, circulate in the blood and, in this way, reach many parts of the body, including the lungs.

Once in the lungs, bacteria multiply and rapidly reach large numbers while continuing to invade the lung tissue. The body's response to infection results in severe inflammation and the formation of pus in the air cells and airways. In addition, abscesses can develop and these may involve large areas of lung tissue, take many months to resolve and can result in permanent lung damage.

Pneumonia is a very serious condition and to a certain extent the outcome depends on the body's ability to fight infection. The condition may progress rapidly and prove fatal. In view of this it is imperative that veterinary attention is sought early in the course of the illness.

Adult horses may also suffer from bacterial infections of the respiratory passages without the development of pneumonia. Such cases may have increased respiratory rate, an intermittent cough and poor work performance but a normal appetite and body temperature. These infections may persist for long periods or recur at intervals if untreated.

Diagnosis

A diagnosis of pneumonia or bronchopneumonia can be made on clinical examination. A sample of mucus may be taken from the airways in order to try to identify the organisms involved and to test their sensitivity to antibiotics. This gives an indication of the drug(s) of choice for treating the infection.

Treatment

A course of antibiotics is required to kill or inhibit the growth of bacteria. Expectorant drugs which assist the removal of mucus and pus from the airways are advisable. Bronchodilating agents facilitate breathing and the removal of mucus from the lungs by widening the air passages. Horses which are very ill will benefit from treatment for pain and may require intravenous fluid treatment and oxygen administration.

Nursing is very important. The horse should be kept warm and comfortable on a deep layer of clean bedding and be supported to lie upright rather than flat out. Small, easy-to-eat feeds such as mashes should be offered frequently and water should be available at all times.

Horses with chronic low-grade respiratory infections should be rested, treated with antibiotics, expectorant drugs and/or proprietary cough mixtures.

Prevention
Horses with respiratory infections should be isolated; care should be taken not to spread infection via personnel, tack or utensils to other horses.

PLEURITIS (PLEURISY)

Pleuritis is a severe respiratory condition in which there is inflammation of the membranes lining the chest cavity and covering the lungs. The name of this membrane is the pleura, hence the name pleuritis.

It is usually caused by a bacterial infection and may be secondary to pneumonia. It may also occur following severe stress such as being transported over long distances or experiencing marked temperature changes when moving from a hot to a cold climate or vice versa. Infection may enter the chest cavity by means of penetration wounds.

Clinical signs
In the early stages horses will have increased respiratory rate, shallow breathing, elevated temperature, poor appetite and look generally off colour. As the condition progresses respiration becomes increasingly more difficult and severe cases will be in a state of respiratory distress.

Course of the condition
When certain bacteria gain access to the pleura and multiply, the membrane becomes inflamed and pus is formed. As the chest is an enclosed cavity, the pus accumulates and forms a pool at the bottom of the cavity due to gravity. The amount of pus may increase to such an extent that normal lung expansion during inhalation is impaired and breathing becomes laboured in an attempt to overcome the shortage of oxygen. Toxins from the pus are absorbed and circulate in the bloodstream, causing a deterioration in the horse's general condition. This is a very serious, painful disease and may prove fatal; thus veterinary attention should be sought at an early stage.

As a horse recovers from this condition fibrous strings (adhesions) may form between the lung surface and the chest wall. These are permanent and impair normal collapse of the affected parts of the lung during exhalation, thus interfering with function.

Diagnosis

Pleuritis can be diagnosed on clinical examination, part of which involves percussion of the chest in order to ascertain the extent of the accumulation of pus. If fluid of any type has accumulated at the bottom of the chest cavity, this can be detected as an area of dullness with a horizontal top line or 'fluid line'. Radiographic examination will confirm this. A vet may also take a sample of pus from the chest cavity in an attempt to find out what bacterial organisms are involved and their antibiotic sensitivity pattern.

Treatment

As this is a very serious condition horses are usually hospitalised for intensive care. If much pus and fluid are present in the chest cavity, the vet will draw this material out by means of a needle and syringe and may insert a drain so that this procedure can be carried out as often as required. This will allow the horse to breathe more easily and also help to remove toxins. Antibiotics are needed in order to overcome the infection, and treatment for pain is advisable. Depending on the severity of the condition, intravenous fluids and oxygen administration may be required.

As in the case of pneumonia, good nursing is imperative. The horse should be kept warm and comfortable, in clean surroundings, on light, regular feeds, with water available at all times.

Prevention

As severe stress is a major contributory factor, efforts should be made to avoid or minimize this.

RHODOCOCCUS EQUI INFECTION (SUMMER PNEUMONIA, RATTLES)

This bacterial infection causes pneumonia and abscessation of the lungs, primarily in foals up to the age of six months. For a detailed account, see p. 478.

Parasitic Conditions

LUNGWORM INFECTION

This is a chronic respiratory infection of donkeys and horses caused by lungworm larvae living in the air passages of the lungs. Donkeys seldom show clinical signs of infection, but horses develop intermittent coughing which

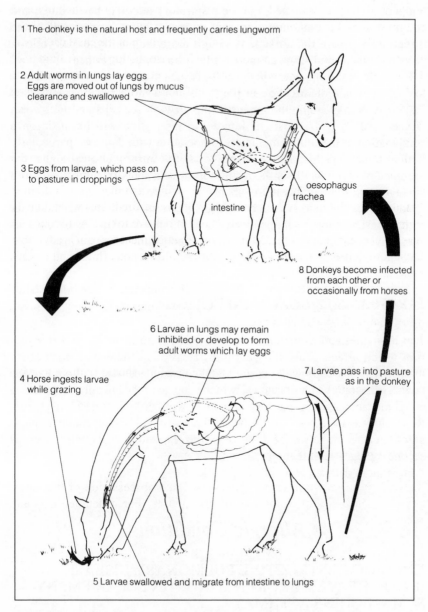

Figure 6 The lifecycle of lungworm

may persist for many months. General body condition, appetite and temperature are not affected, but the respiratory rate may be elevated, and coughing may become more apparent when the horse is exercised. If the infection is severe the horse may cough more frequently, expel yellow-coloured mucus and show an increased expiratory effort or heave.

The cycle of the lungworm in the horse is such that it is not always possible to find evidence of infection in the dung and a more reliable method of diagnosis is to examine the mucus in the airways for cells and lungworm larvae. Usually a diagnosis of lungworm infestation will be made on a combination of the following factors: association with donkeys, particularly if the donkeys yield positive faecal tests, the horse's clinical signs, the presence of certain cells in the respiratory mucus, and, retrospectively, if a horse responds favourably to treatment.

Both horses and donkeys can be treated successfully with ivermectin. Other anthelmintics, such as fenbendazole and thiabendazole, can be used as alternatives at higher doses than those required for intestinal worms.

For a more detailed account, see p. 534.

PARASCARIS EQUORUM INFECTION

This is an intestinal worm infestation caused by the parasite *Parascaris equorum* which affects foals and yearlings. Heavy intestinal infections cause marked loss of weight with possibly fatal consequences due to rupture of the bowel. Respiratory signs occur early in the course of the infection and include coughing, increased respiratory rate and a whitish-yellow nasal discharge. Respiratory signs may persist for two to three weeks. The temperature remains within normal range for the duration of the respiratory signs unless there is secondary bacterial infection.

For a more detailed account, see p. 531.

Allergic Conditions

CHRONIC OBSTRUCTIVE PULMONARY DISEASE (COPD, HEAVES, BROKEN WIND, ALVEOLAR EMPHY-SEMA, EQUINE ASTHMA)

This is a chronic respiratory condition due to the horse developing pulmonary hypersensitivity to organic dust antigens in the environment. It is probably the most common cause of chronic coughing in horses in the temperate parts of the northern hemisphere.

The condition is seen most frequently in stabled horses and is associated with a dusty atmosphere and mould in hay and straw. *Micropolyspora faeni* (which causes farmer's lung in man and cattle) and *Aspergillus fumigatus* (a fungus) appear to be the most predominant causative agents in northern Britain, but the principle antigens may vary in different parts of the world. Extremely large numbers of such organisms occur in hay and straw with visible spoilage. Baling fodder with a high moisture content results in heat being generated within the bale, which creates optimum conditions for multiplication of these heat-loving organisms.

The problem may be encountered when horses are out of doors during summer months. These cases are thought to be associated with pollen from grass or trees. It is common for horses to show hypersensitivity to more than one agent.

The reason for this hypersensitivity in certain horses is not clear, although a respiratory allergy seems the most likely cause.

Clinical signs
The disease affects horses of two years old and above, becoming more common as horses get older. The clinical signs vary according to the severity of the condition. Early cases of the disease, or horses which are mildly affected, have an intermittent cough, slight increase in respiratory rate and expiratory effort, and a reduced capacity for exercise. Horses which are more severely affected cough frequently and may cough up thick yellow-coloured mucus. The respiratory rate exceeds twenty breaths per minute and the horse exhibits forceful abdominal respiratory movements with a marked double expiratory effort which gives rise to the so-called heave line (Figure 5). The horse may appear dull and breathless, with flared nostrils. Wheezing can be heard at the nostrils of severely affected cases.

COPD-affected horses have a normal temperature. Appetite is not usually affected unless a horse is suffering severe respiratory embarrassment.

Course of the condition
Initially the onset of the condition is gradual; however, once established, a horse can suffer attacks which develop rapidly. In this respect the disease has been likened to human bronchial asthma. An affected horse may show signs as rapidly as a half to one hour after first being exposed to the causative agent, but usually signs become noticeable from five to ten hours thereafter. Once a horse is showing signs, they may persist at approximately the same severity for the duration of the exposure to the antigen. Alternatively the signs can become progressively worse, with the horse becoming increasingly breathless. Removal of the offending material allows most cases to improve gradually over the course of a few days.

In affected horses exposure to the causative agent brings about widespread changes in the lungs. These include inflammation of the very small airways (less than 2 mm diameter), production of excessive, thick mucus, and spasm of the muscle in the walls of the airways. These changes cause narrowing of the internal diameter of the airways; thus the horse has to make considerably more effort in order to breath its usual volume of air.

The pressure exerted when a horse with this condition exhales causes the small airways to become even narrower, and some collapse completely. This makes exhalation difficult and an increased volume of air is retained in the alveoli. Because these changes are widespread, the lungs have an overinflated appearance which, for many years, was thought to be the result of irreversible emphysema; hence the term 'broken wind'. However, relatively recent studies have shown that the vast majority of alveoli do not undergo destructive changes. Instead there is a ballooning effect, with the alveoli deflating back to their original size with the remission of clinical signs. The lung changes which occur in affected horses lead to a reduction in the change of air in the alveoli with each breath, and less oxygen is absorbed into the blood, resulting in a general shortage of oxygen in the body.

Changes in the respiratory pattern appear to be reversible in the majority of cases if suitable managemental changes are introduced. If care is taken to maintain these measures a horse can remain free of clinical signs of the disease (asymptomatic) for long periods. However, once a horse becomes affected with COPD, it appears to retain its hypersensitivity for many years, if not for life, and exposure to the antigen at any time will cause the onset of clinical signs.

Diagnosis

If horses are showing distinct clinical signs of COPD, a veterinary surgeon can make a diagnosis on these grounds. In addition, an injection of a bronchodilating agent brings about a marked though temporary improvement in the horse's condition. The diagnosis can be confirmed retrospectively by assessing the horse's response to a change in the environment.

If horses are asymptomatic or in the early stages of developing the disease, the diagnosis can be very difficult. The veterinary surgeon takes account of the horse's past history of respiratory disease and the clinical signs, and may attempt either to exacerbate or to improve the condition through environmental changes. Such cases may be referred to veterinary schools or equine research centres for assistance with diagnosis.

Treatment and prevention

The most important aspect of treating COPD-affected animals is to introduce environmental control measures (a so-called minimal-dust environment), which can be used in conjunction with drug therapy.

As most cases of COPD are associated with stabling and exposure to hay and straw, the most favourable long-term method of controlling the disease is to use substitutes for hay and straw. Any of the following forms of stable bedding are suitable: shredded paper, hardwood shavings or peat, with soiled material being removed on a daily basis rather than the horse being deep-littered. The horse should be fed on a complete cubed diet and no hay or, alternatively, vacuum-packed hay in combination with a type of cube appropriate to the horse's energy needs. The stable should preferably be at least 50 metres to the windward side of the hay store, according to the direction of the prevailing wind. Dust should be removed from ledges, beams and fitments at regular intervals while the stable is vacated, and time allowed for airing before the horse is brought in. However, it is futile to take these precautions for an individual horse if it is going to be exposed to dust and antigens from the stables of neighbouring horses (via half walls or in barn-type accommodation). All animals sharing airspace with the affected horse should be subject to the same environment-control measures.

The alternative method of environmental control is to keep affected horses at grass, provided that they are not hypersensitive to pollen or, if so, that the grasses and trees are not in flower. No supplementary hay should be fed and grazing areas should not be adjacent to hay or straw stores. Simply being out of doors does not alleviate the condition if affected horses are fed hay regularly. Any supplementary feeding should be in the form of a cubed diet.

Even good-quality hay and straw contain large amounts of fungal spores; thus attempts at controlling COPD by using only the 'best' hay and straw will invariably fail. Feeding hay which has been soaked for hours in water is not universally successful. This may be because dust generated in handling the hay (for example, when filling hay nets) blows into the vicinity of the horse, or it may be that wetting the hay does not prevent the effects of exposure to the antigens.

It is never possible to eliminate fungal spores completely from the environment because they can be airborne for many hundreds of miles. However, using environment-control measures, it is possible to reduce the levels of the antigens to below a threshold required to cause clinical disease. Applying these measures allows most COPD-affected horses to become asymptomatic in one to two weeks. However, severely affected horses, in which the illness has been of long duration, may take considerably longer to attain a satisfactory improvement.

There are two approaches to drug therapy of COPD: (a) treatment of horses showing clinical signs of the disease; and (b) preventive medication of asymptomatic horses in anticipation of exposure to the antigens.

When COPD-affected horses are in severe respiratory distress, bronchodilator drugs help to alleviate their condition. In addition drugs which assist in the removal of thick mucus from the airways can be used in the treatment of symptomatic horses. The resulting improvement lasts only for the duration of the treatment; for this reason permanent environment-control measures should be introduced as well. The use of these drugs has no place in the long-term treatment of equine COPD as a substitute for environmental control.

If unavoidable exposure to the antigens is anticipated, horses can be treated with a drug called sodium cromoglycate in an attempt to prevent the onset of clinical signs. Horses should be asymptomatic before treatment commences as it is not intended as a therapy for patients showing clinical signs of disease. A short course of treatment may be useful when there is short-term risk of exposure (for example, a horse stabled away from home for a few days). Alternatively, long-term intermittent sodium cromoglycate treatment could facilitate the management of horses kept at livery or in large stable yards where providing special environmental control measures for a single horse can be difficult.

EXERCISE-INDUCED PULMONARY HAEMORRHAGE (EIPH, LUNG HAEMORRHAGE, EPISTAXIS, NOSEBLEED)

Exercise-induced pulmonary haemorrhage (EIPH) is a condition in which haemorrhage occurs in part of the lungs as a consequence of moderate to strenuous exercise.

The cause(s) are not fully understood but it is considered to be an athletic injury. It is related primarily to mechanical stress in the lungs which occurs with forceful breathing during exertion. This causes the delicate walls of the air cells to rupture, resulting in haemorrhage. It happens in many horses with otherwise normal lungs, but any pre-existing respiratory conditions are believed to increase the risk of EIPH. Any breed or type of horse may be affected and it is recognized worldwide. There is no apparent association with climate, altitude, type of housing, or feeding or bedding materials. Thoroughbreds in training first experience EIPH as two-year-olds with the start of fast work. It can occur in horses of any age.

The amount of haemorrhage varies considerably between horses and episodes. In most cases the quantity is small, and although evidence of haemorrhage can be found on endoscopic examination of the airways, no blood is seen at the nostrils. In more severe cases blood loss will occur from the nostrils in varying quantities and performance can be severely impaired. Haemorrhage occurs in the uppermost posterior part of the lungs and can be seen as an area of increased density on radiographic examination. These changes may resolve within ten days in some cases, but in others it can take months, depending on the degree of the initial changes, repeated exertion with further haemorrhage in the area and subsequent bacterial infection with possible abscess formation in the damaged tissue.

A wide range of drugs has been used in attempts to prevent EIPH, but to date none has proved universally successful. Further studies and a better understanding of the cause(s) of EIPH are required if successful prophylactic measures are to be found.

3
THE HEART AND CIRCULATION

Blood, as discussed in Chapter 5, is the medium that carries vital nutrients and hormones around the body and facilitates exchange of respiratory gases. It is ideally adapted for this role, but it cannot perform any of its life sustaining functions if it is not continuously circulated around the body by the heart and circulation.

Blood travels from the heart via a system of branching vessels known as arteries, capillaries and veins that are discussed in more detail later in the chapter. The heart is basically an 'intelligent pump' able to fulfil its obligation to supply blood to the tissues under all conditions; during sleep, rest and at peak exercise.

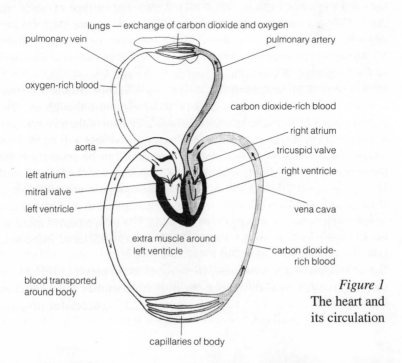

Figure 1
The heart and
its circulation

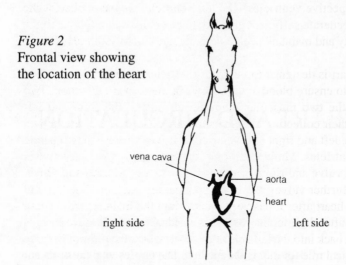

Figure 2
Frontal view showing
the location of the heart

vena cava

aorta

heart

right side   left side

BASIC ANATOMY AND PRINCIPLES

The equine heart is a large muscular organ that lies slightly to the left of midline in the chest (Figure 1). It can be located by placing the flat of the left hand on the horse's chest behind his elbow. In this position rhythmic contraction of the left heart can be felt in all but the fattest or hairiest of horses and ponies. With the palm in this position, a thud will be detected every time the heart beats. This 'thud' is known as the **apex beat** and is produced from vibrations caused by the heart contracting. The average weight of the heart of a fit Thoroughbred racehorse is 5kg, although in the horse population as a whole, there is great variation in heart size and weight with breed, fitness and body size.

To circulate blood efficiently, the heart is divided into two discrete sides: the **left** side is supplied with oxygenated blood from the lungs and pumps it to the muscles and vital organs such as the brain, gut, muscles and kidney. The deoxygenated blood then returns to the **right** side of the heart to be pumped to the lungs, where it is replenished with oxygen and carbon dioxide is expelled (Figure 2). Each side has a muscular pumping chamber, or **ventricle**, and a collecting chamber, or **atrium**.

With each beat, a typical adult horse pumps approximately one litre of blood out of each side of his heart, this is the **stroke volume**. With a resting heart rate of 30 beats per minute, this means the total blood pumped in one minute, the horse's **cardiac output**, is 30 litres. Contrast this to man with an average output of 5 litres per minute and it becomes apparent why the horse is a much better athlete.

The muscular walls of both collecting chambers are thin compared with those of their respective ventricles. The left ventricle has the thickest walls of all, as it must generate sufficient pressure to eject blood throughout all the arteries in the body and maintain peak blood pressures up to 200mmHg during heavy exercise.

Because the heart is designed to work most efficiently, it is also equipped with four valves to ensure blood always flows in the forward direction. Two **valves** separate the two muscular pumping chambers, the right and left ventricles, from their collecting chambers, or atria. These valves are known collectively as the left and right atrioventricular valves because they separate atria from the ventricles. More commonly the left atrioventricular valve is called the **mitral valve** and right atrioventricular valve the **tricuspid valve**. In addition, two further valves prevent blood leaking back into the left and right sides of the heart after it has been ejected into the main arteries. These valves are named after the arteries where they reside. The **aortic valve** ensures blood cannot leak back into the left side of the heart whilst the **pulmonic valve** performs an identical role for the right ventricle. The four heart valves prevent back-flow of blood, making sure the maximum amount of blood is pumped with every beat. Normally the muscles of the heart chambers contract in a rhythmic and orderly manner, so that blood returning from the veins is squeezed through the chambers of the heart into the arteries. Efficient forward movement of blood would not occur without the valves. Imagine what would happen if an attempt was made to squeeze toothpaste onto a toothbrush from the middle of a tube of toothpaste that is open at both ends. Despite the most vigorous efforts a disappointing amount of toothpaste finds its way onto the brush. The situation is similar in the heart, if a valve becomes severely defective; very little blood appears in the arteries despite frantic muscular efforts by the ventricles.

To recap the full anatomy of the heart, we will follow the progress of a red blood cell through the heart and circulation starting from one of the body's large central veins such as, the **vena cava.** Our cell travels with the flow of blood and then enters the right heart collecting chamber, the right atrium. As the walls of this chamber contract, the cell is propelled through the open tricuspid valve, so called because it is made up of three cusps, into the right ventricle. As this chamber contracts a short time later, the cell is ejected through the pulmonary valve into the pulmonary artery. It travels through the lungs, entering the capillaries and then leaving the lungs in one of the pulmonary veins. These veins take it back to the heart, but this time our cell enters the left collecting chamber. From here it passes through open mitral (two-cusped) valve, into the left ventricle. From the left ventricle it is pumped through the open aortic valve into the aorta. From here the blood cell will travel down the branching arteries into the capillaries of the tissues. Once out of the capillaries, the cell begins its journey back to the heart through veins of everincreasing diameters until it reaches the vena cava, ready to begin the cycle again.

CONTROL OF HEART RATE AND RHYTHM

The heart is instructed to beat by an electrical impulse that originates from a group of specialised cells, **the sinus node**, situated high in the wall of the right atrium. This pulse of electricity travels quickly through the walls of both collecting chambers and causes them to contract, pushing any remaining blood into the ventricles. For maximum efficiency, it makes sense for the ventricles to delay their contraction until the collecting chambers have completely emptied, and that is exactly what happens. Instead of travelling directly into the ventricles the electrical impulse reaches a special area in the muscle between the left and right sides of the heart, **the atrioventricular node**. Here the signal is delayed for almost half a second before it continues its journey into the pumping chambers. This electrical activity can be recorded at the body surface as an electrocardiogram, or ECG. The ECG is a map of the journey of the electrical impulse through the heart.

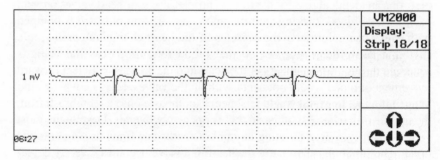

Figure 2

The first small upward 'p' wave comes from the two collecting chambers and often, as in this example, it is m-shaped, reflecting the journey through first the right atrium, then the left. Then the line goes flat, as the impulse is held up at the atrioventricular node allowing the atria to empty. The large downward pointing signal, 'r' wave, is the rapid journey of the impulse around the muscle of the pumping chambers. As the impulse passes through each muscle cell, their electrical charge is reversed and the final 't' wave represents the muscle returning itself back to normal in readiness for the next heart cycle. Notice that the line is flat between heart beats

Normal Heart Rhythm

The electrical impulses fire off repeatedly from the right atrium providing a regular rhythm. As a horse becomes fitter the rate of firing is damped down because his larger more muscular heart needs not to beat so frequently. In human athletes this damping occurs at the source of the impulse in the right atrium, so overall pulse rate slows down. In horses this damping is most likely to occur further down the impulse's journey, where it is delayed between the chambers at the atrioventricular node. This is why a normal horse will regularly miss beats at rest. In fact, the collecting chambers do contract, but the electrical signal is blocked before the pumps can be activated. This is called atrioventricular block because the impulse stops between the atria and ventricles at the atrioventricular node. An example of this can be seen below (Figure 3), when the second 'p' wave is not accompanied by an 'r' or 't' wave.

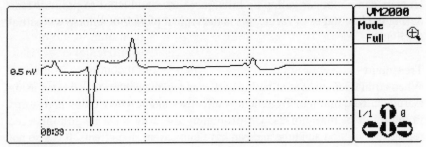

Figure 3

Occasionally the heart rhythm can go wrong and the most common example occurs in the condition called atrial fibrillation.

What happens in atrial fibrillation?
In atrial fibrillation the electrical activity of the collecting chambers is completely deranged. As a result, instead of beating regularly in a coordinated pumping motion, the atria beat completely out of synch. In fact, to the naked eye a fibrillating atrium looks just like a 'bag of worms'. The uncontrolled chaotic electrical activity of the atria is visible on an ECG as a constant irregular wavy baseline, instead of regular neat little 'p' waves. Meanwhile, the ventricles are being bombarded by electrical nonsense from their control centres. They do their best, but there is no longer a regular heart rhythm with the odd missed beat, instead there is a chaotic irregular rhythm which the vet can recognise by taking a pulse, or listening with a stethoscope.

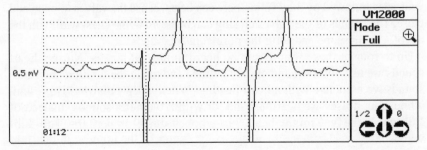

Figure 4

What happens to the horse?
Affected horses usually appear normal at rest, however at all levels of exercise the heart must beat faster to make up for the reduction in efficiency. In horses that work well below their maximum cardiac capacity, the rider may still be unaware of the problem. Examples might include horses used for draught, dressage, hacking and showjumping. It is in the disciplines that require all of the heart's capacity that atrial fibrillation becomes obvious. Hunters can no longer gallop up hills, racehorses and point-to-pointers fade during the late stages of races; this is the typical picture of a horse with atrial fibrillation.

Treatment
When atrial fibrillation is affecting performance, the condition is treated using a drug called quinidine. Treatment is effective and normal rhythm is restored in eight out of nine horses. Unfortunately the drug must be administered repeatedly via stomach tube and can have unpleasant side-effects. It is also not without risks, death, though rare, can occur in healthy horses. As a result, when the rhythm is not affecting performance the vet may decide to leave well alone. In racehorses or hunters though, treatment is a worthwhile option in the first instance. Unfortunately the problem can recur, but it may be years after the first incident, and treatment is simply repeated. The treatment is not 100% successful and for every eight horses returned to normal rhythm one will remain in atrial fibrillation. When treatment fails, horses can continue successfully in a less demanding sporting discipline, so failure may still not mark the end of a working life.

On occasion other abnormalities of heart rhythm can also result in poor performance or symptoms of lethargy and collapse. Such abnormal rhythms can arise as a result of severe cardiac valve regurgitation (see below), poisonings or due to other serious medical conditions affecting other body systems. In general though, these conditions are rare.

What are the normal heart sounds?
The normal events of each heart cycle, i.e. contraction of the muscular ventricles followed by their filling between beats, cause the valves to open and close. The sounds of the valves closing can be heard at the chest wall with the aid of a stethoscope and form the normal heart sounds.

Up to four of these sounds can be heard in normal horses. Normal heart sounds are usually short and clearly defined and make the familiar 'lub-dub' sounds we associate with a heart beating. When a heart murmur is present, whooshing noises are heard around, or within the heart sounds. Instead of 'lub-dup', the vet might hear 'lub-whoosh-dup', or perhaps 'lub-dub-whoosh'.

HEART MURMURS

These abnormal noises between the normal heart sounds occur very commonly in performance horses, in fact in a group of race fit Thoroughbreds only 1 in 10 didn't have a heart murmur of some description. In humans and dogs the presence of a murmur may mean that one of the heart valves is leaking, however in horses this is not always the case. The horse's heart is large and a large stroke volume enters and leaves each side of the heart with each beat. These factors, coupled with the horse's thin skin, low heart rate and large stroke volume, mean that the vibrations caused by normal blood flow travel easily to the chest wall. As a result, a veterinary surgeon can sometimes hear blood entering and leaving the heart. These noises are called **flow** murmurs and they are completely normal. The "whooshing" sound made by blood leaving the heart can be quite loud, especially if a horse is particularly excited, or stressed by other diseases such as colic. It can sometimes be hard for veterinary surgeons to decide if a loud murmur on the left side of the chest is caused by normal blood flow, or a serious leak on the left atrioventricular (mitral) valve. Often flow murmurs come and go depending on the horse's state of excitement. They may also appear, disappear or change after exercise. If the veterinary surgeon is sure that the murmur he hears is a normal flow murmur, no matter how loud it is, the horse can be passed without question at a veterinary examination, the heart is completely normal.

What happens if the vet hears a murmur that suggests that one of the heart valves is leaking?
Obviously this depends on how bad is the leak and which valve is affected. In most, but not all, cases the louder the murmur, the bigger the leak. Sometimes, in the worst cases, the vet can feel the vibrations caused by the back-flow of blood by placing his hand on the chest wall over the leak; a stethoscope isn't required. On such occasions the backflow may be so severe the heart is unable to cope. An affected horse will be reluctant to exercise and slow to recover after any exertion. Resting heart rate increases to over 50 beats per minute, as the heart is forced to beat faster to compensate for the blood flowing backwards through the leaking valve. However, this picture is an unusual exception rather than the rule. Diagnosis of a heart murmur in a performance horse is not usually such bad news. Smaller leaks are often very well tolerated and do not affect athletic performance, especially in horses performing less demanding roles. Quiet murmurs associated with small leaks on the left (mitral) and right (tricuspid) valves are present in excess of 25% of Thoroughbreds in training. In fact, by looking at racehorses before and after training we know that after training murmurs are present in a greater proportion of horses than before and that the loudness of any murmurs present usually increases. As we now know that the heart gets bigger with training – that's what makes the horse fit – it seems likely that this process also increases any tendency of the valves to leak.

So how does the vet decide when a murmur is a problem?
First the vet must decide whether a murmur is caused by normal blood flow, or whether a heart valve is leaking. If a valve is leaking, the valve must then be identified. A murmur can usually be identified by considering whereabouts on the chest wall the murmur is most obvious. The timing and character of the murmur often also provide useful clues to its origin. In nine out of ten cases a stethoscope is all that is required to give an accurate diagnosis. If a murmur is caused by a valve leaking, the vet must then try to gauge its significance and decide whether the leak is likely to worsen with time. The vet uses the loudness of the murmur, exercise history and the horse's resting heart rate to try to make this decision. In the scenario of a pre-purchase examination this decision can be difficult and the vet may suggest the horse undergo further evaluation at a specialist centre where the heart and valves can be visualised with ultrasound.

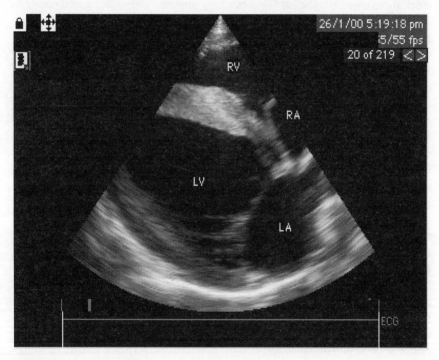

Figure 5   Ultrasound image of the heart of a normal horse, (LA left atrium, LV left ventricle, RA right atrium, RV right ventricle)

In this image the heart is tilted onto its side. The black areas are blood-filled. The image is obtained by holding a small probe behind the horse's elbow. By moving the probe slightly, each chamber and valve of the heart can be visualised and the dimensions accurately measured. Heart function can be assessed and the most advanced equipment allows blood flow through the heart valves to be visualised. This allows detailed assessment of valve regurgitation. Because of their size, horses are poor subjects for thoracic radiography and X-rays are all but useless for assessment of heart size. Cardiac ultrasound however, has revolutionised equine cardiology and greatly improved our understanding of heart problems in horses.

Blood flow through the heart can also be examined using a technique called Colour Flow Doppler echocardiography, allowing the actual leaks to be seen and quantified. This investigation is coupled with measurement of heart chamber size by conventional ultrasound and assessment of heart rate and rhythm during fast exercise. These tests allow the vet to determine whether a horse will be able to continue in its chosen discipline. In the vast majority of cases, diagnosis of a cardiac murmur certainly does not mean the end of a horse's working career.

In most cases, heart murmurs in horses require no treatment, and most horses cope well with mild and moderate leaks. They are usually able to continue in their work and are rarely limited by their heart condition. With most horses the leak worsens slowly, if at all, so that the horse usually retires from active life before its ability to perform is hampered by the heart condition.

Occasionally a heart valve leak may suddenly worsen, so to be absolutely sure that the horse remains well and able to do fast exercise, the vet should regularly monitor the heart valve leak with his stethoscope. Occasionally more specialised examinations may be needed periodically. The owner can also keep weekly records of resting heart rate. If the rider feels the horse begins to tire more easily, or blows excessively after exercise, the heart must be checked immediately. Only on the very rare occasions that the heart begins to fail is any treatment given. Valve replacement as would occur in a human patient is not practical for the horse, so the failing heart is supported using drugs to help it to contract and to improve its rate and rhythm. In additions diuretics are given to reduce any water retention.

Once the heart fails, the horse's outlook is poor and any treatment is aimed at maintaining quality of life only. The onset of heart failure marks the end of the horse's working life even if response to that treatment is good.

HOW DOES THE HEART ADAPT TO EXERCISE?

There are two main types of adaptation to exercise. The first group occur rapidly in the short term and are irrespective of fitness. The second occur over a much longer period of weeks to months when repeated exercise is performed. The process of repeated exercise bouts leading to these longer-term adaptations is more popularly known as **athletic training**.

SHORT TERM ADAPTATIONS

As we have said the heart is an 'intelligent' pump, but it has a fairly limited range of options to increase its output to meet the increasing demands of exercise.

1: Increase the amount of blood pumped with each beat; increase stroke volume

When the heart beats, it does not empty completely, instead a proportion of blood remains in the left heart chamber. When exercise begins, circulating adrenaline makes the contraction of the heart muscle more forceful, so more blood is ejected from the ventricle with each beat. Additionally, the huge muscles of locomotion contract and squeeze more blood back to the heart increasing the amount of blood available in the circulation and further increasing stroke volume.

2: Increase heart rate:

Resting heart rate is between 28 and 36 beats per minute in Thoroughbred horses. Maximum heart rate during peak exercise in the Thoroughbred is between 225 and 240 per minute. The huge range of heart rate is the most important mechanism for increasing cardiac output during exercise, especially as work intensity increases. Heart rates above 200 beats per minute ensure that cardiac output increases from 35 litres per minute at rest to above 200 litres per minute during maximal exercise.

LONG TERM ADAPTATIONS

Just as the muscles of locomotion become stronger and better able to do their job efficiently, so too does the heart muscle. Using ultrasound, (Figure 5), we are now able to measure cardiac dimensions very accurately and assess how efficiently the organ works. We can also monitor what happens as the horse goes through its training programme. By scanning large numbers of Thoroughbreds in various training yards, we know that the amount of heart muscle, and the width and area of the left heart chamber increase dramatically with training. Increased heart volume allows the heart to hold more blood at rest and during exercise, whilst increased muscle also allows the more powerful 'fit' heart to eject more of this blood with each beat.

How heart rate is measured:

At rest:

Using a stethoscope on the left side of the horse's chest behind the elbow:
Undoubtedly the most accurate method. The heart rate can be easily counted

and should be measured over one minute after the horse becomes accustomed to the stethoscope.

Using palpation of the apex beat: In absence of a stethoscope, the next best method is to place the flat of the left hand on the horse's chest behind the elbow. You will feel a thump every time the heart beats. This thump is known as the **apex beat** and is produced from vibrations caused by the heart contracting. The apex beat should also be counted over one minute to obtain heart rate.

Using palpation of a peripheral pulse: Arterial pulses in horses can be detected as the facial artery crosses the lower jaw. It is possible to count the pulse to measure heart rate. In horses, the technique is less reliable, as they often refuse to keep their head still long enough to obtain a true estimate of the resting heart rate.

During exercise:
Heart rate monitors: These monitors detect the electrical signals that instruct the heart to beat. As each electrical signal is accompanied by a physical contraction of the heart, they are accurate monitors of heart rate. The horse wears flat electrodes and a transmitter device under the saddle. The heart rate is transmitted to a watch monitor worn by the rider. These monitors can be of varying degrees of complexity and expense. All of them give an instantaneous heart rate; the most expensive units allow accumulated heart rate information from one or more training sessions to be downloaded into a personal computer.

Radiotelemetric ECG (electrocardiograph) recorders: Similar to heart rate monitors, as the electrical signals from the heart are recorded and transmitted via radio to a distant monitor. These units transmit the whole ECG, so heart rhythm as well as rate can be checked. This sophisticated equipment is very expensive and tends to be restricted to specialised veterinary clinics, where it is used to investigate horses with suspected cardiovascular problems. More recently a system capable of storing two hours of ECG data has been developed specifically for horses. This system can be used at rest and during all types of fast exercise, including high intensity work over fences. This type of equipment allows the vet to assess abnormalities when they are most important, during the demands of exercise.

An example of such a recording is shown below

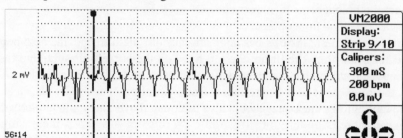

Figure 6   ECG from a seven-year-old NH chaser schooling over fences. Heart rate 200 beats per minute. Heart rhythm normal. Horse had had atrial fibrillation diagnosed after fading in a recent race. ECG recorded at the trainers request during normal work to determine suitability for racing four days later. Heart rate and rhythm is normal. The horse ran in the race and won.

What can my horse's heart rate tell me?

At rest
Increased stroke volume caused by training means that the athlete's heart beats less frequently at all times, including during periods of rest. Because of the greater volume ejected from the 'fit' heart with each beat, cardiac output remains the same as in the untrained state, although the heart beats less often. So it should be possible to see a difference in your horse's heart rate at rest, before and after training. Indeed, the true resting heart rates of conditioned racehorses are often at, or even below, 30 beats per minute. In human athletes the effect of training on resting heart rate is marked. For example, the average heart rate of the competitors in the Tour de France cycle race was below 40 beats per minute compared to the average for a normal man of 75 per minute. In horses, with a much lower resting heart rate to start, not only is the effect much less marked, but their character often masks our ability to detect it. In horses, heart rate is greatly influenced by stress and anxiety. The very act of measuring heart rate is often sufficient to increase it by 3-4 beats per minute, enough to mask any changes induced by training.

During exercise
Heart rate during exercise is an invaluable monitor of the cardiovascular system, fitness and performance. The speed at which heart rate recovers after work also reflects cardiovascular fitness. During any exercise session the heart rate can be used to determine when the horse is sufficiently recovered to gallop or canter again. Heart rate monitoring also allows us to train specifically for endurance or speed. This is the basis of **interval training**, a technique that has

been adopted almost universally in human athletics. Since the advent of interval training, records in every human track event have been smashed, as athletes benefited from optimal cardiovascular conditioning. When any horse's heart rate reaches 225 beats per minute and approaches maximum, the horse will fatigue within a short time. No matter how much he is urged the horse cannot give any more.

The table shows the average heart rate and respiratory rates of conditioned Thoroughbreds undergoing treadmill exercise at gradually increasing speed. You can see how heart rate increases as the workload goes up to the next speed.

Gait/Speed	Average Heart Rate (b.p.m.)
Rest	35
Walk	75
Trot	127
Canter @ 7m/s (16 mph)	170
Canter @ 8m/s (18 mph)	182
Canter @ 10m/s (22 mph)	201
Canter @ 11m/s (25 mph)	219
Canter @ 12m/s (27 mph)	224
Walk – 1 min recovery	106
Walk – 2 min recovery	89

When an individual's heart rate is monitored over time and over a standard piece of work, the trainer knows exactly how hard the horse is working on any given day. When the workload is standardised, individual horses can be compared with each other to assess their fitness and ability. In every sport, serious athletes and trainers use heart rate during exercise to devise training plans and monitor progress.

CONCLUSIONS

The purpose in this chapter has been to provide the reader with a general account of various aspects of the heart, how it functions, and how apparent defects occur and may be interpreted. The point has been made that the equine heart is an amazingly adaptable organ and that its function is to pump blood. A diseased heart is not necessarily incapable of achieving its function, although it may not be able to do so when called upon for maximum performance during peak exercise. With advances in technology we are now better able to assess the heart during exercise, and our ability to monitor horses with heart problems has greatly improved with the availability of advanced ultrasound equipment. As a result, many horses with heart defects can continue in their work for many years, and horses that might previously have been written-off continue to compete successfully in all types of equestrian sport.

4
THE LYMPHATIC SYSTEM

The lymphatic system consists of a network of fine tubes or vessels which ramify throughout the body in a similar manner to blood vessels. However, the difference is that the lymph fluid they contain is not driven by a pump, as the heart pumps the blood. The movement of fluid is effected by massage from the extremities as the limbs and their muscles move.

The tubes have blind ends where lymph fluid forms, and these join up with one another to form increasingly larger channels on their way towards the chest. This is identical to the branches of arteries ending as capillaries in the tissues. The difference is that the smallest lymph tubes have blind ends instead of connecting with veins, as is the case with the arteries. For this reason the lymph fluid in the vessels does not circulate in the same way as blood is pumped through the system by the heart.

Lymph drains towards the heart, carried on its way by the massaging action of the movement of muscles and tendons. The flow is aided by valves situated at intervals throughout the system of tubes. These valves prevent backflow and thereby ensure that lymph drains in one direction only. The smaller tubes drain into larger tubes, until eventually the main drainage channel of the lymphatic system discharges into the bloodstream close to the heart.

The lymph vessels have very fine walls, so water can pass easily through them. The channels are thus in close communication with the interstitial fluid, that is, the fluid which bathes the cells of the body tissues such as muscles.

The main function of the lymphatic system is to drain off excess fluid from all parts of the body. The pressure in the blood vessels is greatest in the lower parts of the limbs due to the effect of gravity. The role of the lymphatic system is to facilitate the drainage of fluid from the tissues of the limbs so that they do not become waterlogged.

If the free flow of water into the lymph system is impeded, the tissues become waterlogged and the area becomes swollen or oedematous. The oedema (filling) can be recognised by swellings which pit when firm pressure is applied by the fingers.

Normally there is a balance between water in the bloodstream, in the tissue spaces between the cells and in the lymph stream. This balance depends on the concentration of salts and proteins in the bloodstream on one side of the capillary wall and in the tissue spaces in the other. Any factor which upsets this balance may produce waterlogging of the part unless the lymph can drain away the excess fluid.

More water than normal may pass out of the blood vessels because their walls are affected by toxins or inflammation. In these instances not only fluid but protein may pass into the interstitial tissues, thus drawing additional water with it. The blood is thinned by the loss of protein and this lowers the osmotic pull across the membrane of the blood capillary walls.

Excess feeding and too little exercise leads to waterlogging because the richness of the food disturbs the delicate protein and electrolyte balance, and the lymph system is unable to carry away the waste material and excess fluid. This occurs in the dependant parts of the limbs because of the particular difficulty of returning water up the limbs against the pull of gravity. If the horse is not exercised, this accentuates the problem due to the fact that movement is necessary to massage the lymph flow back towards the heart.

Lymph also contains lymphocytes and a small number of other white cells. It plays an important role in the defence of the body against infection. Thus at various points along the course of the system there are glands (lymph glands) which filter off noxious substances and microbes. The glands also play a part in the production of antibody. This is formed by certain cells (plasma cells) in the gland and released into the bloodstream to help combat infection.

Conditions of the Lymphatic System

In practice we are not normally aware of the lymphatic system because we cannot recognise the vessels in the same way as we can see veins and arteries. Further, the glands of the system are too small to feel. However, when the system is disturbed, its presence becomes obvious in a number of ways.

The flow of lymph may be reduced by lack of movement as described above. Drainage is then restricted so that water collects and the part becomes filled (**filled leg**). This is an example of **humour** in the horse's limbs which disappears when the individual is exercised and the flow of lymph is increased by the massaging action of the muscles and tendons.

The legs may become filled when the walls of the blood and lymph vessels are damaged by toxins or inflammation, so that water passes into the tissue spaces at an abnormal rate. The causes of this condition may be an allergy following the eating of substances to which the horse is allergic, the injection of drugs or it may occur as a direct result of a viral or bacterial infection. Diets high in protein may aggravate the swellings due to the nutritional element adding to the problem of drainage; lack of exercise may play a further role.

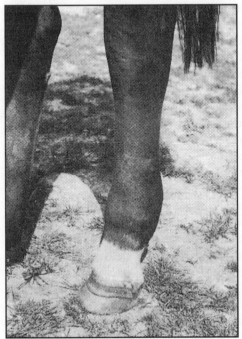

Figure 1   A horse with lymphangitis

The lymph glands may themselves become swollen due to toxins and microbes carried to them in the lymph stream. One such example of the swellings, occurring between the angles of the lower jaw, is the mandibular gland. This occurs in young horses as a consequence of microbes passing from the lining of the airways of the head into the lymph channels that drain the tissues of the head.

Some bacteria, particularly *Streptococcus equi* (the cause of strangles – see p. 474) and other species of streptococcus, may cause pus to form in the glands. An abscess develops which eventually bursts through to the outside, discharging pus. These glands may also become infected as the result of bacteria entering the lymph stream from the tissues around newly erupting molar teeth.

The lymphatic system plays an essential role in the repair of injuries by removing debris and excess fluid in the tissues, brought to the area as a result of inflammation (see Chapter 37). If a wound becomes infected, this may spread to the lymphatic vessels and they too become inflamed.

This results in a condition known as *lymphangitis* (Figure 1). In contrast to the ordinary filled legs, in which excess fluid is quickly removed once the cause has been eliminated and proper drainage restored, lymphangitis may lead to a permanently enlarged limb.

In severe cases the inflammation spreads to the tissues surrounding the lymph vessels and drainage becomes so disturbed that excess fluid escapes by breaking through the skin in ulcer-like eruptions.

The hind limbs are most often affected by lymphangitis, as they are by oedematous swellings, by virtue of the increased distance from the heart occupied by the hind compared with the front limbs.

Problems may also arise because of the anatomy of the lymphatic system in the hind limb. As the lymphatic vessels pass over the inside of the hock they are very prone to blockage. It is probable that some cases of lymphangitis are caused by emboli (small clots) lodging in the channels at certain key points as they pass over the bony structures of the hock. This virtually cuts off the drainage of lymph from the lower part of the limb, causing it to become very swollen, hot and painful.

Pain is a feature in lymphangitis. It has the effect of causing the horse to refrain from placing weight on the limb or moving it at all. This accentuates the problem of drainage and creates a vicious circle of fluid and products from damaged tissue, microbes and other matter accumulating to cause further pain from lack of drainage.

Treatment is aimed at combating any infection by the administration of antibiotics and/or other anti-microbial substances, together with pain-relieving drugs such as phenylbutazone or anti-prostaglandins. If the pain can be controlled, the horse starts to put weight on the leg and can then be induced to walk, which helps to restore the circulation of lymph. However, in some cases the tissues under the skin become chronically enlarged and replaced by permanent fibrous tissue.

It is not only the limbs which are affected by oedema due to poor lymphatic drainage. Swellings may appear on the belly of a pregnant mare as the lymphatic vessels become overburdened due to excessive activity associated with mammary development in preparation for the birth of the foal. This oedema usually quickly disperses after foaling.

Oedematous fluid may also accumulate along the belly in horses affected by low blood protein levels secondary to liver disease or gut disease (e.g. colitis and malabsorption syndromes). Generalised oedematous swellings may occur as a result of congestive heart failure or widespread neoplasia of the lymphatic system (lymphosarcoma).

5
THE BLOOD

Blood is the red fluid pumped by the heart through the arteries and veins, forming the circulation. It is carried to every part and acts thereby as a transportation system carrying nourishment, vital substances, gases and waste material. Among its many functions it carries oxygen from the lungs to the muscles and other tissues, transports digested food from the gut to the liver and from this organ to all other tissues. It carries the hormones, regulates the water and electrolyte balance, and acts in the defence of the body against infection by mobilising the body's resources against noxious agents such as microbes, poisons and foreign proteins.

Blood is composed of cells suspended in a fluid known as plasma. There are two types of cell: red and white, and small cellular bodies called platelets

Plasma

Plasma consists of water in which certain proteins and mineral salts are dissolved. It is normally straw-coloured with a slightly yellowish tinge. This can be appreciated when blood is allowed to stand and the red and white cells sediment out, leaving the plasma lying above. This may also be appreciated when the blood is centrifuged. The reading of the percentage by volume of plasma to cells is known as the haematocrit or packed-cell volume (PCV). This is normally 35-45% of the total blood. PCV is quite variable between types of horses, and should be interpreted in the light of the type and level of fitness. A Thoroughbred (especially a sprinter) in work should have considerably higher red cell count, PCV and haemoglobin concentration in the blood, than a warm blood-type horse or pony. The percentage is lower in cases of anaemia (see p. 122). It is higher after exercise because red cells contained in the spleen are discharged into the circulation in large quantities when a horse is exerted. The percentage is also higher in horses suffering from dehydration, for example, as a result of prolonged exercise or in cases of severe diarrhoea.

The plasma contains about 93% water and about 6% protein. Minerals and salts such as sodium, potassium, calcium, magnesium, chlorides, bicarbonates and organic acids comprise the other 1%. The water content passes readily through the capillary walls in either direction. It can thereby enter or leave the tissues of the muscles and organs, and this exchange plays a vital part in fluid balance.

The protein is made up of various components, the majority of which are albumin and globulin. The proteins have different sized molecules. The albumin molecules do not normally pass out of the bloodstream through the capillary membrane into the tissues due to their large size. They provide the blood with its osmotic gradient, that is, the biological process which pulls water through membranes from an area of lower concentration to that of a higher concentration, until equilibrium is established on both sides.

The protein globulins are divided into alpha, beta and gamma globulins and fibrinogen. The total concentration of the blood proteins is about 60g/litre of plasma. In the laboratory proteins are usually measured from the serum, which is the yellow gel formed when blood clots.

The difference between plasma and serum is that plasma contains fibrinogen, which is part of the clotting mechanism that prevents excessive bleeding. The fibrinogen is not activated until exposed to air, which is why, when collecting plasma for analysis, we have to add anti-clotting substances. For further discussion of the clotting mechanism, see below.

The role of plasma proteins is varied. Clotting has already been mentioned. The globulins also contain the immune protective substances known as antibodies or gamma globulins. Proteins are also associated with hormones, enzymes and vitamins. Without sufficient protein in the bloodstream, water seeps through the blood vessels into the tissue spaces, a condition known as oedema and recognised in horses as filled legs or soft swelling beneath the skin, especially on the ventral abdomen (lower aspect of the body wall) where it collects under the influence of gravity. In a male horse, the sheath will also appear enlarged. This may occur because the proteins leak through blood vessels, the walls of which have been damaged by toxins or other noxious substances. Protein may also be lost by leakage through the intestines (e.g. damage from worms), or through diseased kidneys. Albumin is made in the liver, and liver disease can result in lower production of albumin, which will lead to a lower level in the blood.

The smaller molecules of salts also act in the equation of equilibrium on either side of the capillary membrane. Sodium and potassium are particularly involved in this process and their levels are regulated by the kidneys. The kidneys, as we shall see later (see Chapter 6), play a major role in conserving required and eliminating unwanted material from the body.

The acidity of the blood is represented by its pH. The pH is the measure of hydrogen ions associated with organic acids. If there are too many, the blood becomes more acid; if too few, it becomes too alkaline.

Normally blood has a pH of about 7.4 units. The balance between acidity and alkalinity is referred to as base status and is measured in terms of bicarbonate. Bicarbonate acts as a buffer, giving up hydrogen ions when the blood becomes alkaline and absorbing them when it becomes acid.

Bicarbonate levels are usually in the region of 28 mmol/litre of blood. Mmol is a chemical unit by which scientists measure the content of salts dissolved in fluid.

The blood becomes too acid (acidosis, acidemia) in states such as diarrhoea, in which large amounts of alkali are lost in the faeces. A normal acid state develops after exercise when lactic acid is produced in the muscles and passes into the bloodstream. However, this state is only temporary and the mechanisms of balance soon neutralise the lactic acid and restore the base acidity balance to normal. Excessive build up of lactic acid in the muscles causes muscle fatigue or tiring, which is performance-limiting.

Excess alkalinity rarely occurs. It may develop when the horse over-breathes at rest. This is because the gas carbon dioxide is then eliminated from the lungs. Carbon dioxide is one of the radicals of organic acids and its elimination leaves an alkaline balance, which is soon restored when the horse stops overbreathing.

The lungs form part of the system of conserving acid, and the kidneys conserve alkaline material. The gut plays a part in regulating both acid and alkaline substances. These organs respond to acidity or alkalinity in the appropriate manner by eliminating acid radicals or, to a lesser extent, alkaline radicals according to the acidity of the blood at any given time.

Blood cells

Red cells (erythrocytes) The red cells give blood its colour. They are also known as erythrocytes. They consist of a cell membrane or envelope containing a red pigment called haemoglobin. They are extremely small cells whose special characteristic is that they do not have a nucleus, as have all other cells in the body.

Horses have about 7-9 million red cells per cubic millimetre of blood. The modern measurement is the number of cells per litre and this is expressed as x 10^{12}/litre. In illustrative terms this means there are about 3200 million red cells per teaspoonful of blood. Red cells, which outnumber white cells by about 1000 to 1, have a characteristic disc shape and are concave on both sides. This shape acts to provide the greatest surface area for gas diffusion per volume of the cell. They consist of about 60% water and 33% haemoglobin.

Red cells carry the gas oxygen. This is essential to life. The blood receives this in the lungs, where it comes into close contact in the capillaries of that organ. The oxygen does not dissolve to any great extent in plasma and, without the red cells, it would therefore not be carried in quantities nearly sufficient to satisfy the body's needs. The haemoglobin in the cells has a much greater affinity for oxygen and also the peculiar property of being able to combine with oxygen when exposed to high concentrations in the lungs. It then forms a product called oxyhaemoglobin.

The blood then passes from the lungs through the heart to the tissues, such as the muscles, and here it is surrounded by tissues containing much less oxygen. In these circumstances the haemoglobin gives up oxygen and becomes what is known as reduced haemoglobin. The muscles are then able to take up the oxygen and use it for burning carbohydrate (sugar) to produce energy. The blood then returns to the lungs, where the reduced haemoglobin takes up oxygen and is again converted to oxyhaemoglobin.

When there is more oxyhaemoglobin than reduced haemoglobin, the blood is bright red; when the reverse is the case, the blood becomes dark or even blue.

Haemoglobin is confined in the red cells and escapes into the plasma only when the cells are destroyed in large quantities (haemolysis). This condition occasionally occurs in newborn foals as a result of incompatibility between antibodies ingested in the colostrum and foal red blood cells (see p. 453). Haemoglobin is released in large amounts into the plasma and causes jaundice, staining the tissues of the membranes of the mouth, eyes and vagina. It also causes the skin to go yellow but, of course, in animals with hair this cannot be seen as easily as it can in humans. In severe cases the red cell count plummets to fatally low levels and death can only be prevented by whole blood transfusion.

Red cells have a limited life of approximately 120 days and there is thus a turnover in the population present at any given time. Red cells are produced in the bone marrow. These replace the ones which are old and destroyed in the spleen and liver. The rate of replacement and destruction is normally in balance, so that numbers remain the same. If more cells are eliminated than are produced, anaemia results. This may occur if the rate of destruction is normal but the production in the bone marrow is reduced by disease.

The iron-containing component of haemoglobin is retained in the body when the old red cells are destroyed. The waste content of pigment is excreted in the bile. If the liver is damaged, the bile does not escape and is resorbed into the blood. This may also occur if the channels through which bile is excreted into the gut become blocked. Pigment then accumulates in large quantities in the plasma, a condition called hepatic or obstructive jaundice (see p. 55). In this condition, in contrast to haemolytic jaundice, the individual is not suffering from haemolysis of red cells and the number of red cells in the bloodstream remains normal. In haemolytic jaundice the red cell count may plummet to less than 4×10^{12}/litre.

Red cells also carry the gas carbon dioxide from the tissues to the lungs. Carbon dioxide is produced as a waste gas in the metabolism of sugar for energy. The red cells can easily absorb and release large quantities of carbon dioxide because of their relatively enormous surface area.

The red cell has no nucleus and therefore the whole of its interior is available for haemoglobin. A further attribute is that the cells have rounded edges, which helps them to pass easily through the minute lumen of the capillaries. Further, they have considerable ability to change shape, so that they can squeeze past obstructions or through vessels with narrow diameters.

White cells (leucocytes) There are five kinds of white blood cells or leucocytes. These fall into one of two groups according to whether or not they contain granules. The granules are identified in the laboratory by special staining techniques.

The granular white cells are eosinophils, which take up the red stain because they are acid; basophils, which take up the blue stain because they are alkaline; or neutrophils, which take up neither blue nor red because they are neutral.

The neutrophils are also called polymorphonuclear (PMN) because of the many different shapes of the lobed nuclei, which change as they mature. Neutrophils can engulf microbes and foreign particles.

Two types of white cells which do not contain granules are lymphocytes and monocytes. There are also plasma cells, which may be regarded as modified lymphocytes. Plasma cells are not found in the circulation in health. They are found in tissues, where they are important in the production of antibodies to infectious agents. All these cells play a fundamental role in the immunity of the body. Monocytes are able to engulf particles. They are the largest of the white cells and gather in large numbers wherever there is chronic infection, such as in lungs affected by pneumonia. Monocytes act as scavenger cells for infection and foreign particles. They are also involved in presentation of the infectious agent to lymphocytes for antibody production.

White cells have many functions. Neutrophils and other white cells migrate from the bloodstream whenever tissues are damaged by infection, wounds or foreign bodies such as splinters of wood. They play a fundamental part in the inflammatory process (see Chapter 37).

Blood clotting

Blood has the remarkable power of remaining fluid in the blood vessels but clotting as soon as it is shed. This is essential, because although the blood must be fluid to perform its main function of transport and circulation, the risk of excessive bleeding when a vessel breaks is always present.

When blood clots it forms a jelly which, under a microscope, can be seen to consist of a network of gelatinous threads radiating from clumps of disintegrating platelets. The platelets are special blood cells which contain a substance called thrombokinase. Entangled in the threads are red and white cells. After an hour or two the clot gradually separates into a red mass containing cells and a straw-coloured fluid, serum.

By clotting, blood blocks any rents in the blood-vessel wall and thereby prevents further bleeding. The exception is when a break occurs in a large artery. In these cases the blood pressure prevents a clot forming or remaining in position to prevent blood loss (haemorrhage). Arterial bleeding is, therefore, much more dangerous than bleeding from veins, where blood pressure is much lower. Bleeding from an artery may cease only if the elastic wall of the artery contracts to seal off the vessel and/or if the bleeding is so severe that blood pressure falls sufficiently to allow a clot to form and stay in position.

Internal bleeding from an artery may eventually stop if the tissues around the broken vessel became sufficiently engorged so as to prevent further blood escaping. This occurs when the pressure formed by the lost blood counteracts that in the artery. However, this may not happen in the case of an artery rupturing in the broad ligament of the uterus at foaling, for example (see p. 442).

Clotting of blood is a result of a series of events, each of which represents a key which must be turned before the next stage can proceed. First, tissue is damaged and platelets release thrombokinase. This reacts with the substance prothrombin to give thrombin. Calcium is required in this step from prothrombin to thrombin. Thrombin acts on fibrinogen, one of the proteins already described as being present in plasma. Fibrinogen is formed by the liver under the influence of vitamin K. The reaction of thrombin and fibrinogen is to form fibrin, which are the threads that can be seen in a clot under the microscope.

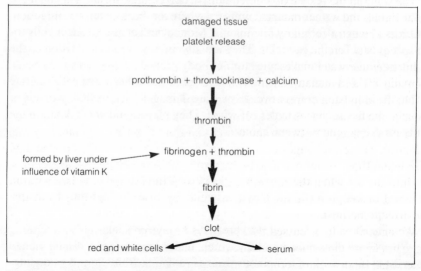

Figure 1   The stages of the clotting process

To prevent clotting we may use anticoagulants, that is, anti-clotting agents. These include substances which precipitate calcium and prevent the step from prothrombin to thrombin occurring.

The essential element in clots is fibrin. This is carried in the inert form fibrinogen in the bloodstream; otherwise the blood would clot in the vessels. Because thrombin is required to convert fibrinogen to fibrin, thrombin is present in the bloodstream only in its inactive form prothrombin. The enzyme thrombokinase, which converts prothrombin to thrombin, is present in the platelets but is locked in unless liberated when tissues become damaged.

There is a further substance, heparin, which is produced by special cells, known as mast cells, distributed throughout the body. It is only present in such quantities as to exert a modifying effect on clotting. When local damage occurs, this overwhelms the heparin present in the bloodstream. However, heparin may be used as an anti-clotting agent in treating heart disease and for keeping blood samples from clotting.

Blood-fluid balance
The fluid balance of the body is a property of the bloodstream and the water it contains. Water is the largest single constituent of the body and makes up about 70% of its total weight. A horse weighing 500 kg (1100 lb) contains about 350 litres of water. This water is distributed evenly throughout the body with the exception of bone, which contains only about 20%, and the hoof, the various parts of which contain between 23 and 40%.

The water in the body exists essentially in two compartments. The intracellular fluid is the water contained within the cell; the extra-cellular fluid is that outside. The extra-cellular water may be in the bloodstream, i.e. in plasma, or in spaces between the cells. These are usually referred to as the tissue spaces.

Intra-cellular water makes up about 70% of total body water, whereas plasma contains 8% and interstitial fluid (fluid between the cells) about 2%.

The fluid in each compartment is interchangeable. It can thus pass from cells to the tissue spaces to the blood, or in the reverse direction. Water may also be exchanged between the blood and the intestines regulated by the kidneys. These exchanges occur according to the needs of the body at any particular time. Water can also be lost from the skin when the horse sweats or into the air when the horse breathes out. This last process is a natural method of keeping the air moist in the long air tubes leading from the nostrils to the lungs.

We have already discussed the role played by protein, especially albumin, in maintaining the osmotic pressure of the blood within normal limits. In the interstitial fluid, sodium forms the major constituent which maintains the concentration, and therefore the osmotic pressure of interstitial fluid, in balance with the fluid in cells and in the blood. If, for example, there were too little sodium, water would pass abnormally out of the interstitial fluid and this compartment would shrink. It would pass into the blood or into the cells. In the latter event the cells would swell abnormally.

Water in the cells is maintained by the normal concentration of potassium. Thus the osmotic pressure of the cell is influenced by the amount of potassium it contains. Again, if there is too little of this substance, water will pass out of the cell into the interstitial fluid and the cells will shrink.

There are complex mechanisms whereby potassium and sodium are moved into and out of cells in order to maintain the osmotic pressure and thereby the fluid balance of the body.

Examining the blood

Blood is often examined to help diagnose disease, because it is simple to obtain by inserting a small-size needle into a vein. The sample may be collected using a syringe or a vacutainer (vacuum test tube).

The examination of blood in the laboratory helps to establish the health status of many parts of the body and to identify abnormal happenings as a result of the indirect changes that occur. We know the normal composition, and if we establish the significance of change we can, with experience, relate our findings to events taking place in various parts of the body. We might liken this approach to recording a sample of traffic using a main road. Using this analogy, we might observe that there are a large number of fire engines on the road and from this we might deduce that there is a fire. Similarly, if we observe an abnormally large number of neutrophils in the bloodstream, we may be sure that this is a response to infection or to stress. If, however, we find the eosinophils in large numbers, we can deduce that a state of allergy or infection with parasites is present. When there is damage to an organ (e.g. liver muscle), cells are disrupted and this results in the release of their specific enzymes into the blood in abnormally high concentrations. Thus a blood sample showing high muscle enzymes indicates muscle damage. Additionally, the kidney is involved in the removal of waste products from the blood, and an increase in these products indicates poor kidney function.

Of course, we do not rely on these signs alone but read them in conjunction with other signs of clinical and laboratory examination.

Conditions of the Blood

Apart from haemolytic disease of the newborn foal (see p. 453), there are few specific diseases of the blood in the horse. The examination of blood which is so frequently carried out on normal and sick horses is undertaken because changes in the normal constituents of the blood reflect changes in the organs and tissues which may themselves be abnormal. The clotting process may be abnormally activated inside blood vessels in cases of severe underlying disease such as severe colic, systemic infection, and neoplasia. This condition is called DIC (disseminated intravascular coagulation) and may have very serious consequences, as blood clots may starve vital organs of their blood supply.

Haemophilia is a rare inherited disease of horses. In this condition Factor VIII, which forms part of the clotting mechanism, is missing.

Horses may become anaemic due to infection, for example, equine infectious anaemia (see p. 497). However, this is not really a disease of the blood but a generalised infection by a virus.

Piroplasmosis is a specific disease of blood caused by a parasitic protozoan called Babesia (see p. 501).

6
THE URINARY SYSTEM

Functional anatomy

The urinary system consists of the kidneys, ureters, urinary bladder and urethra (Figure 1a and b).

In the horse the right kidney lies under the cover of the last three ribs, whereas the left is slightly farther back, just opposite the last rib. Both are tightly held up under the lumbar part of the spine. Each kidney is connected via the ureter to the bladder, which lies on the floor of the pelvis when empty. As it fills it expands forwards onto the wall of the ventral abdomen. In the adult the bladder can accommodate 3-4 litres of urine before micturition is stimulated. The bladder empties to the outside via the urethra. In the male the urethra passes through the penis (Figure 3) and is very long (75-90 cms). In the female it is short (2-3 cms) it exits into the distal vagina with urine being voided via the vagina (Figures 1b and 2).

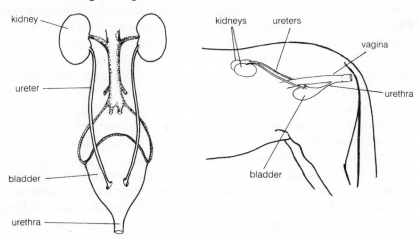

Figure 1 a and b   The urinary system

The function of the urinary system is to maintain water and electrolyte balance within the body, and to excrete from it certain waste products of metabolism, particularly urea (and other nitrogenous and organic substances). The kidneys also secrete certain hormones, including those responsible for controlling red blood cell production and calcium levels in the body (vitamin D_3).

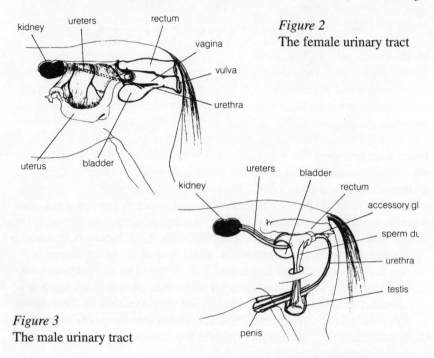

Figure 2
The female urinary tract

Figure 3
The male urinary tract

Symptoms of urinary system disease vary according to which part is affected. Diseases involving the kidneys often upset this organ's control of water and electrolyte balance in the body, as well as decreasing the excretion of waste products. These changes in levels can lead to multiple symptoms, often remote from the urinary system, involving the heart and blood vessels, and the digestive and nervous systems.

Diseases of the lower urinary tract (the bladder and urethra) present mainly as disturbances in the normal flow of urine to the outside (micturition). It is most important to be familiar with the normal act of micturition in order that these disturbances can be observed early on.

Horses usually urinate only at rest, especially when a straw bed is laid down or when they are placed in their stall box. The posture normally adopted by both males and females is with the hind legs separated, the animal leaning slightly forward, and with obvious contraction of the abdominal wall and elevation of the tail. Very often horses grunt and groan and, occasionally, the penis is protruded in the male.

In individual animals bouts of urination may be remarkably regular. The mare in oestrus shows changes in behaviour, including continual winking of the clitoris often associated with frequent squirts of urine, which may be thicker and darker-coloured than usual. Adult horses urinate 4-11 times a day (foals urinate hourly), producing between 2 and 16 litres per day depending on water intake, diet, ambient temperature, exercise and lactation. The urine character varies and it can be viscous and cloudy.

Methods of assessing function

Careful observation and external examination of the horse provides valuable information about the urinary system. Early recognition of abnormal signs by the owner or attendant allows prompt investigation by the veterinary surgeon and limits the possible effects and complications of urinary disease. For example, the presence of dried urine on the tail, vulva and legs of a mare may indicate urinary incontinence. The most common presenting complaints for horses with urinary tract disease are weight loss and abnormal urination.

The act of micturition should be observed and the following assessed:

(a) Normality of position and whether there are continual attempts at adopting this stance. The inability of the horse to adopt the correct position, e.g. as in a recumbent animal, can lead to urine retention.

(b) Frequency of urination and the volume passed at each bout. This will decrease if the horse is unable to drink normally or if fluid intake is restricted.

(c) The nature of the urine passed and, if possible, a sample collected in a clean receptacle.

(d) Signs of pain associated with micturition, i.e. continual straining, excessive grunting and discomfort, and tensing of the abdominal wall muscles. It is important to differentiate these symptoms from those due to colic in other systems. This may require more sophisticated judgements or techniques only available to the veterinarian.

To make a diagnosis in urinary conditions requires an accurate history of the patient, including general information such as the age of the animal, its use, its diet and any previous problems, as well as more specific questions based on the list described above. The approximate daily water consumption is also valuable in evaluating the urinary system. The adult horse consumes an average of 20-35 litres of water per day depending on environmental conditions, diet (especially salt content) and exercise/sweating. Water intake can be determined over 24 hours by removing all other sources except a measured supply via a bucket. Having ascertained the history, the following regime may be adopted.

In the mare the external entrance of the urethra can be palpated easily or visualised directly with a vaginal speculum. In the male it is often necessary to tranquillise the animal before the same area can be examined. In foals the umbilicus can be palpated and the abdomen balloted to detect the presence of excess fluid.

Following examination the veterinary surgeon may decide to catheterise the bladder. This involves passing a lubricated flexible rubber or plastic tube up the urethra into the bladder. This technique provides information, including whether the urethra is blocked (for example, by a stone), and allows the collection of a urine sample. It can also be used to introduce treatment.

Passage of a flexible fibre-optic instrument (endoscope) up the urethra into the bladder is an extremely useful diagnostic aid particularly when the complaint is abnormal urination. In either sex it is possible to pass the instrument up the urethra in the sedated animal. Previous drainage of the bladder via a catheter allows the internal surfaces to be examined and samples taken. Not every veterinary surgeon may have access to a suitable endoscope.

Rectal palpation (insertion of the hand and arm into the rectum) is a useful technique for examination of the urinary system in the adult horse. In the majority of average-sized horses the left kidney is the only one palpable, although the right may be felt if enlarged. Enlargement and pain may be present in acute kidney disease whereas shrinkage and firmness may be felt in chronic cases. In the male the bladder is easy to feel and its size and position identified. In the female the state of the uterus (womb) (i.e. whether the mare is pregnant or not) will affect palpation of the bladder.

Radiography (X-rays) is of little use in investigating urinary tract disease in the adult horse but can be helpful in foals. Plain and contrast radiographs can be used to investigate bladder and urethral/ureteral problems.

The urinary tract can be examined using ultrasonography. The kidneys can be visualised by placing the probe of the machine on the abdominal skin, whereas the bladder and distal urinary tract are best examined with the probe placed up the rectum. The use of ultrasonography has been a major adjunct to the diagnostic capabilities of the equine veterinary surgeon and this is certainly true for the urinary tract. Acute and chronic renal disease can be distinguished and the presence of kidney cysts, urinary calculi (stones), tumours and defects detected.

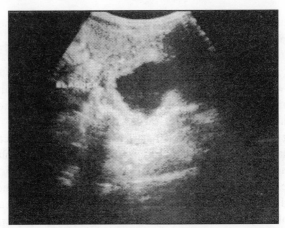

Figure 4   An abdominal ultrasound picture of the intact bladder of a young foal which had previously been repaired for a ruptured urachus

Following the physical examination, the veterinary surgeon may decide to take various samples in order to further identify the nature of the problem. Urine can be collected either as it passes from the animal or by catheter. Normal equine urine varies in colour from light yellow to amber and may darken on standing. It can be clear or cloudy, the latter being especially obvious in horses receiving large quantities of calcium in their diet. The pH and specific gravity of the urine vary with diet and environment.

Microscopic and biochemical analysis of urine can be helpful. The presence of blood, as red blood cells or as haemoglobin, may indicate haemorrhage in the urinary system or damage to blood cells elsewhere in the body. Proteins and glucose may also be discovered, the latter increasing in diabetes mellitus. Sediment in urine can be examined for the presence of crystals, blood cells and damaged urinary tract tissue (casts). The specific gravity or concentration of the urine may also be measured and is helpful in assessing animals that are drinking and/or urinating excessively.

Circulatory blood may be analysed usefully in several ways. Most importantly, concentrations of urea and creatinine (waste products) are looked at. These rise in the bloodstream if the kidney filtering system is affected by disease. Other substances in the blood increase or decrease with urinary disease. The creatinine clearance test involves taking a simultaneous urine and blood sample and examining the creatinine, phosphate, sodium and potassium content of each. The results of this test provide useful information about kidney function and some metabolic processes, such as those associated with bone.

Other specialised diagnostic techniques are available and include ultrasonically guided renal biopsy via a skin incision. This is only warranted if the additional information gained will be vital in determining treatment, as there are significant risks that haemorrhage can occur.

Conditions of the Urinary System

Diseases of the urinary system, particularly of the kidney, are uncommon in the horse. To some extent this situation is brought about by the kidney's ability to function even when considerably damaged (up to 75%). Despite this remarkable ability of the kidney to compensate, urinary tract diseases are serious, require prompt veterinary attention and, in some cases, are life-threatening.

Conditions of the Kidney

Damage to the kidney, if severe enough, leads to a situation known as renal failure and this can be separated into two categories: acute and chronic. It is not always true that chronic renal failure follows acute damage, because the onset of renal failure may indicate the sudden failure of chronically diseased kidneys.

ACUTE RENAL FAILURE

Rapid deterioration in kidney function has multiple causes. These can be divided into three basic groups: prerenal, in which the blood supply to the kidney is affected; renal, due to intrinsic failure of the kidney; postrenal, in which there is physical obstruction of urine flow somewhere in the urinary tract. The first two types are more common in the horse.

Prerenal causes include decreased blood pressure due to severe dehydration or blood loss (haemorrhage) and defects in the circulation such as occur in shock or heart failure. Certain substances also directly damage the kidney tissue (nephrotoxins), including some plants (oak trees, onions, oxalate-containing species), heavy metals (e.g. mercury, lead), and drugs (e.g. some antibiotics such as gentamicin and sulphonamides, non-steroidal anti-inflammatory drugs including phenylbutazone). Myoglobin, the pigment from muscle, can also cause renal damage when released in large quantities after an attack of setfast or azoturia (seep. 278)

In the young foal renal disease is usually associated with systemic infections (septicaemia). These occur particularly in the colostrum-deprived foal and are caused by a variety of bacteria (see p. 282)

Postrenal forms of acute renal failure are caused by obstruction of the bladder neck or urethra by calculi (stones) and by rupture of the bladder but this complication of these conditions is rare in the horse.

Clinical Signs

Symptoms of acute renal failure are similar, whatever the cause, but may be complicated by other symptoms derived from the primary cause. The onset of signs may take up to twenty-four hours to occur. Animals are uraemic and, therefore, depressed and off their food, whilst severe cases may exhibit a range of neurological signs. There may be a decrease in the production of urine which becomes concentrated. The kidneys may become swollen and painful which may be appreciated on rectal palpation, and enlarged on ultrasonographic examination. Some cases have mild colic, a temperature or even laminitis.

If the animal survives the initial phase, the quantity of urine passed increases dramatically (diuresis) and it becomes very dilute. This may persist for several weeks. Urine and blood samples confirm the diagnosis and also help the vet arrive at a prognosis.

The urine may contain increased protein cells, casts and some blood. The concentration of the urine varies with the stage of the disease. The blood picture varies, depending on other coexisting disease, but will often show increases in blood urea and creatinine. Electrolyte levels in the blood are often distorted.

Treatment

Treatment of any predisposing disease and removal of any suspected toxic substance should be the first priority. During the initial phase, when little urine is being passed, treatment is aimed at correcting fluid and electrolyte imbalances (oral and intravenous fluids) by the administration of diuretics and general supportive therapy. If the horse survives the early stages, then it will enter the phase of increased urine production, when measures to maintain the fluid/electrolyte intake and to decrease the nitrogen content of food (grass, hay) are taken. The animal may now be eating and drinking normally, in which case water and salt licks should be available at all times.

Prognosis

The recovery rate for horses suffering from acute renal failure depends largely on the cause and severity of the condition. Laminitis is a possible complication and can be difficult to treat in these animals. The mortality rate can be as high as 50% in some renal failures due to toxic chemicals (oxalates), but diuresis following little urine production is a good sign.

CHRONIC RENAL FAILURE

It was originally thought that this was a rare condition in the horse but now it is considered a significant cause of weight loss and loss of appetite in the horse.

The most frequent cause is chronic glomerulonephritis (damage to the tubes and filtering mechanism) due to self-attack by antibodies or the laying down of immune complexes in the kidneys. Other causes include chronic infections in the kidney, changes subsequent to acute renal failure, tumours (rare) and congenital problems.

Clinical Signs
These vary depending on the cause but include loss of weight and appetite, depression, dehydration, excess drinking and/or urination, swelling of legs and ventral abdomen and, occasionally, mouth ulcers.

Rectal and ultrasonographic examinations may reveal shrunken, firm kidneys. Biopsies of these kidneys often reveal extensive damage of an irreversible nature. Blood and urine samples are helpful in reaching a diagnosis and assessing the degree of failure. Blood changes include anaemia, increases in white cells and BUN/creatinine, electrolyte changes and protein loss. Urine samples may contain pus, blood and protein.

Treatment
Chronic renal failure is a progressive condition and resolution is not possible. Prolonging the animal's life is the primary aim. Treatment should involve supplementation of electrolytes and diet, restriction of protein, encouragement of appetite or supplemental feeding, anabolic steroids and, where appropriate, corticosteroids and antibiotics.

Prognosis
The long-term prognosis is poor in chronic renal disease cases due to the irreversible and progressive nature of the pathology. In the short term some cases may fair better, particularly if the weight loss can be counteracted.

UPPER URINARY TRACT INFECTIONS

Bacterial infections of the upper urinary tract (kidneys and ureter) are uncommon in the horse and, as in other species, are usually due to infection ascending up the urinary system from the urethra and/or bladder. Problems that interfere with the normal function of the ureter emptying into the bladder will increase the risk of upper urinary tract infections, e.g. ectopic ureter, bladder distention and paralysis, urinary tract obstruction or pregnancy. Septic nephritis may also be a consequence of septicaemia (blood-borne infection) especially in young foals. Female horses are at a higher risk than male horses because of their shorter urethra decreasing the resistance to ascending infections.

Clinical Signs

Unless the amount of kidney involved is extensive, the infection may go undetected and may later lead to the development of kidney stones or chronic renal failure months or even years later.

In the more severe cases clinical signs will include difficulty in urination, with blood or pus in the urine, fever, weight loss, loss of appetite and depression. The upper urinary tract infection may also be accompanied by stone formation in the kidney or passage of them down the ureter. The latter may lead to signs of colic and constant straining to urinate without production of urine.

Diagnosis is dependent on careful clinical examination of the horse including a rectal palpation and ultrasound examination. An enlarged kidney and/or ureters may be palpable in acute cases and stones may be visible on the ultrasound scan. Analysis of urine samples and bacteriological culture are very important in identifying the bacteria involved and choosing the most suitable antibiotic. Blood samples will allow the veterinary surgeon to assess the general inflammatory response to the infection and its affect on the function of the kidneys. Endoscopy of the bladder and catheterisation of the ureters is possible to assist in collection of relevant samples.

Treatment and Prognosis

Treatment of upper urinary tract infections includes a prolonged course of appropriate antibiotics and supportive therapy such as good nursing and management, fluids, electrolytes and diet. In select cases involving only one kidney and/or ureter, surgical removal of these structures can be performed but the cost and surgical expertise required to carry this out mean that it is rarely undertaken.

Unfortunately, successful treatment of upper urinary tract infections is rare, especially if both kidneys are involved, and euthanasia may be necessary. The poor prognosis is related to the failure to detect and diagnose the condition until relatively late in the course of the disease and the irreversible nature of the damage leading to chronic renal failure.

Conditions of the Bladder

CYSTITIS (INFLAMMATION OF THE BLADDER)

Cystitis is uncommon in the horse. The problem can arise as an ascending bacterial infection up the urethra or secondary to diseases resulting in in complete emptying of the bladder (e.g. bladder paralysis, urethral calculi) or bladder irritation (e.g. by cystic calculi – bladder stones). These predisposing conditions affect the bladder's ability to protect itself and to prevent multiplication of bacteria, of which it is normally free.

As in the human, the condition is more common in females than in males, for two reasons. First, the female urethra opens into the vagina, which can act as a source of infection in cases of metritis (Inflammation of the uterus). Secondly, the urethra in the male is much longer and narrower, and therefore less liable to be a route of ascending infection.

Clinical signs
Acute Cystitis occurs rarely and presents as abdominal pain (colic) associated with straining and frequent attempts at passing urine, usually only in small amounts. More often the condition is chronic, with clinical signs which include frequent urination with straining and sometimes urine dribbling, caking of the vulval lips with sediment in the female and urine scalding. In the male the penis may be protruded and sediment accumulates on the front of the hindlimbs. The urine can be discoloured by blood and is more turbid than normal.

Diagnosis
The diagnosis of cystitis is not difficult from the symptoms but has to be confirmed by examination of a urine sample. It is important to suggest a cause for the disease. The urine can be cultured for bacteria and examined microscopically. In a cystitis sample bacterial cells, mineral crystals and red and white blood cells may be present. A rectal examination allows evaluation of the bladder for calculi, paralysis or pain. Endoscopy of the bladder can be used to assess the bladder lining and to take samples.

Treatment
Treatment of cystitis involves the removal of any predisposing causes and the administration of antibiotics for a considerable period of time based on culture results. Flushing the bladder with antibiotic solutions is not necessary, but using an antibiotic excreted at high levels in the urine is important. The horse is rarely very ill, but full nursing and supportive management are important, including maintaining water intake, keeping the patient warm with rugs and bandages, rest, and preventing urine scalding by applying Vaseline.

CYSTIC CALCULI

Urinary calculi or stones may form in any part of the equine urinary tract, but the most common site is the bladder (cystic). Urolithiasis (or formation of calculi) is the most common cause of obstruction of the urinary tract, especially distally. Two basic forms of calculi are found but both are primarily composed of calcium carbonate (Figure 5). Factors that may contribute to the formation of calculi include the increased concentration of salts in the urine, increased times for the transit of urine and reduction in the natural inhibition of crystal growth in the urine. The concentration may increase when the horse is deprived of water or loses water excessively (sweat, diarrhoea, etc.). Diets/water high in mineral content will increase salt concentration. Diet changes will also affect the urine pH (acidity/alkalinity) and subsequent crystal formation.

Calculi are formed by salts in the urine being precipitated around a collection of cells (bladder, red or white blood cells) and, therefore, any condition leading to urinary tract damage and shedding of cells will predispose to calculi formation. In addition to the calculi the horse has been recorded as accumulating a crystalloid sludge in its bladder (sabulous urolithiasis), particularly in conditions where there is decreased bladder emptying, e.g. bladder paralysis.

Clinical Signs

All breeds and ages are equally likely to develop calculi. Both sexes develop calculi but their apparent incidence is higher in males, especially geldings, because small stones are easily passed out via the short, distensible urethra in the mare.

The symptoms of cystic calculi are similar to those seen in cystitis (which may be present concurrently). Affected animals may urinate, or posture to urinate, more frequently, with straining and dribbling of urine, which may contain pus or blood. Males often protrude their penis and mares may wink their clitoris leading to confusion with oestrus behaviour. Other less common signs include urine scalding, irritability, recurrent bouts of colic and loss of weight. Passage of a calculus into the urethra may lead to an obstruction.

Diagnosis

Veterinary help should always be sought in cases in which there is difficulty in the passage of urine. Calculi can occur at a number of sites in the urinary tract and, therefore, thorough evaluation of the whole system is warranted. Cystic calculi can be diagnosed on rectal palpation of the bladder in some cases, preferably after emptying of the bladder naturally or by catheterisation. The latter confirms patency of the lower tract and allows collection of urine for analysis and culture.

Blood samples are useful in determining the presence of infection or metabolic derangement. Endoscopy of the bladder can help to identify calculi and the severity of lining mucosal damage. Sediment and calculi are both visible on ultrasonography of the bladder per rectum.

Treatment

Surgical removal of the calculus is the only effective method of treatment. The approach and type of surgery is determined by the size of the stone and the sex of the patient. Following surgical removal, systemic antibiotics are usually administered for a minimum of seven days.

Some cases may also require treatment for concurrent cystitis.

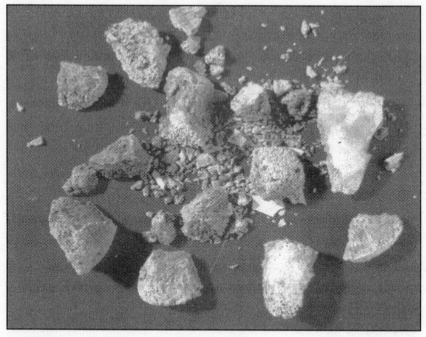

Figure 5
These are the remnants of a large cystic calculus removed from the bladder of a mare by crushing the stone in the bladder with an instrument passed up the urethra. The fragments were subsequently removed using fine forceps

Prognosis
Prognosis for cases treated successfully by surgery is guarded because the affected horse may remain predisposed to chronic cystitis and calculus formation. Preventive measures are limited to correct dietary management, particularly in regard to mineral and concentrate proportions, adequate sources of drinking water and prompt veterinary attention to any case of suspected cystitis.

LOSS OF CONTROL OF BLADDER FUNCTION

This condition occurs in horses in which there is damage to or disease of the sacral (pelvic) segment of the spinal cord or to local spinal nerves. It also occurs in problems associated with other areas of the nervous system, including injuries to the sacrum, fractures of the vertebrae, infections of the spinal cord (EHV-1 – see p. 490), spinal abscesses and tumours, poisoning (see Chapter 38), and neuritis of the cauda equina (the end of the spinal cord in the sacral and coccygeal regions).

Clinical signs
Symptoms vary according to the cause of the neurological problem. Normal emptying of the bladder does not occur and the collecting of urine distends and stretches it. Eventually the bladder fills to its maximum capacity, and the horse becomes incontinent. The continuous release of urine leads to scalding of the back of the thighs in the mare and some inflammation of the vulva. A secondary cystitis may develop. On rectal examination the bladder will be very distended and displaced ventrally into the abdomen.

Treatment
Treatment of bladder paralysis is designed to control the secondary cystitis and keep the bladder emptied by catheterisation and manual palpation. The success of this supportive care and likely prognosis depend on the actual cause of the paralysis.

BLADDER TUMOURS

These are very unusual in horses and present in a similar way to cystitis and cystic calculi. They may be distinguished by rectal palpation and/or endoscopy of the bladder. Treatment by surgery is possible but spread to other areas may have already occurred.

UROPERITONEUM

The accumulation of urine in the abdominal cavity can accompany a number of urinary tract disorders involving disruption of its physical integrity. The most common cause in the horse is the rupture of the bladder or urachus seen in young foals (see below). Other less common causes include: various ureteral or bladder congenital defects; bladder rupture in mares at foaling or following obstruction of urine flow by stones, especially in males.

RUPTURED BLADDER / URACHAL TEARS

Rupture of the bladder wall or tears in the urachus are a fairly common cause of uroperitoneum in the young foal. The classical ruptured bladder is seen mainly in colt foals (long urethra decreases chances of pressure release) and is due to increased external pressure on a full bladder during delivery. The bladder can rupture anywhere, but in these cases it is usually at its widest point on the dorsal surface. It is, however, seen in other foals where there is infection of the urachus leading to urachal leakage or tearing.

Clinical signs

Symptoms can be quite subtle and, as in all foal diseases, require careful observation over a period of time to detect them. Foaling is usually unremarkable and the foal appears normal for the first twenty-four to forty-eight hours. At this stage it may become lethargic and depressed, suck less and show a distended abdomen.

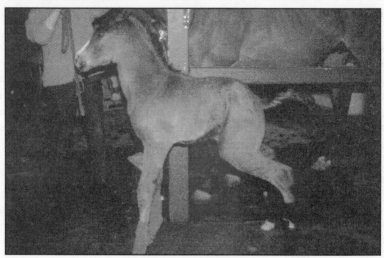

Figure 6   A two-day-old Thoroughbred foal with a ruptured bladder showing the classical posture adopted by these foals whilst straining to pass urine

Symptoms of urination are quite variable, but often there will be an increase in the frequency and a decrease in the amount of urine passed. There is often straining and signs of mild colic, which can lead to confusion with meconium colic. The two conditions can be differentiated by observing the position the foal adopts while straining. With a ruptured bladder the foal stands with its back hollowed out, head raised and legs extended out backwards; whereas the foal with meconium impaction tends to have a more humped-up appearance, with tall raised, and occasionally walks backwards. As the condition worsens, more urine collects in the abdomen, leading to difficulties in breathing, an increase in heart rate and greater depression. Those cases involving infections of the umbilicus and urachus may present with symptoms related to spread of infection elsewhere.

Diagnosis

This condition is life-threatening and early recognition of abnormal signs is important. Diagnosis involves several techniques. If ballottement of the abdomen suggests fluid is present, then a needle is placed through the abdominal wall to collect a sample which can be analysed to determine whether it is urine.

Blood samples show increase in blood urea and creatinine content as well as changes in electrolyte levels and blood pH. Other diagnostic techniques include radiography using radio-dense dyes inserted into the bladder by catheter, or retrieving dyes placed in the bladder from the abdomen by needle puncture. Ultrasound examination of the abdomen is very useful in confirming the presence and amount/type of fluid present, assessing the integrity of the urinary tract and detecting infections of the umbilicus/urachus.

Treatment
Treatment is surgical repair of the rupture as soon as possible. First, urine is drained from the abdomen to decrease complications during anaesthesia and intravenous fluids given to correct any metabolic/electrolyte alterations. After surgery the foal requires continuous observation, monitoring of its condition, nursing and appropriate therapy. If an abdominal drain and/or urethral catheter is fitted it requires regular attention.

Prognosis
Prognosis for recovery is good if the diagnosis is made early, but on occasions repair to the bladder or abdominal wall may break down, necessitating further surgery.

PATENT URACHUS

The urachus is the tube connecting the bladder of the unborn foal via the umbilicus to the allantois (see p. 390). Normally the urachus closes at the time of birth and the umbilicus shrivels within hours. When the urachus does not close (i.e. when it becomes patent or pervious), then urine continues to leak from the umbilicus. The urachus may fail to close or may re-open due to excessive traction on the umbilicus at birth, infection of umbilical cord remnants and pronounced abdominal straining (meconium retention).

The degree of patency varies considerably, ranging from that which allows an occasional drip and a moist navel, to streams of urine appearing from both the umbilicus and the urethra when the foal urinates. Either sex may be affected. The umbilical area becomes scalded and/or infected, causing local abscesses. The infection may spread further up into the bladder (cystitis), or into the bloodstream and via this to the joints (joint ill – see p. 230. It may also be associated with leakage of urine into the peritoneal cavity (see above).

Clinical signs and diagnosis
Diagnosis is based on clinical signs and umbilical ultrasonography to check for any evidence of infection in the umbilical cord and urachal remnants.

Treatment

A patent urachus may close spontaneously but, in most cases, treatment is necessary. The foal is given antibiotics to reduce the chance of the spread of infection and a barrier cream is applied around the navel to decrease scalding. A cauterising agent (iodine, formalin or phenol soaked in cotton swab) or silver nitrate styptic may be applied for several days. This produces a localised inflammation within the tube and gradually this closes it. The foal will need to be carefully restrained, manually or chemically, for these procedures. Cautery is contraindicated in the presence of umbilical infection. If the urachus fails to close spontaneously or following cautery, or where sepsis is present, then surgical removal of the umbilicus and urachal remnants under general anaesthesia is indicated.

Conditions of the Urethra

The urethra is only occasionally affected by disease and almost exclusively in the male.

URETHRAL OBSTRUCTION

The urethra can be obstructed anywhere in its length from diseases within and exterior to it. The main causes include urethral calculi and injuries to or tumours of the penis. Urethral calculi are much less common than their bladder counterparts but their source is almost certainly the same. The calculus is usually trapped at the point where the urethra passes around the posterior part of the pelvis or at the end of the penis (where there is a slight narrowing of the diameter). Even if the stone passes on, the trauma caused to the urethra can cause obstruction.

One way in which the urethra can be obstructed from external sources is following an acute case of paraphymosis (the penis becomes trapped outside the sheath in an erect or semi-erect state).

Clinical signs and diagnosis

Symptoms of urethral obstruction are very similar to those seen in diseases of the bladder and include mild colic, straining and difficulty in passing urine, prolapse of the penis, dribbling of urine and sometimes passage of blood.

The diagnosis of urethral disease is based on a complete physical examination, including palpation of the penis in the male and the distal vagina (vestibule) in the female. Palpation of the penis may reveal repeated urethral contractions and a firm mass in the urethra. Rectal palpation may detect a tight, distended bladder. Bladder rupture may occur secondarily leading to depression, loss of appetite and severe metabolic abnormalities. The diagnosis is confirmed by passage of a catheter or endoscope up the urethra to the level of the obstruction.

Treatment
Treatment of urethral calculi depends on where they become lodged. If lodged in the distal urethra they can often be removed in the sedated horse by gentle crushing by hand or with a forcep. If it is lodged higher up or cannot be removed from the distal part of the tract then surgical removal via an incision into the urethra is necessary. This often requires general anaesthesia. The urethra may be closed or allowed to heal by granulation tissue. Trauma to the urethra often resolves without consequence but strictures can form. Antibiotics and anti-inflammatory agents are given post-operatively.

The prognosis for these cases is guarded since there are a number of potential complications of the surgery and the disease.

URETHRITIS

Damage and inflammation to the urethral lining usually occurs in male horses (long urethra) and can follow the passage of a urethral calculus, repeated or traumatic catheterisations, penile injury or ascending bacterial infections.

Clinical Signs and Diagnosis
Symptoms will depend on the primary case but include blood in the urine and semen (stallions), straining and difficulty in urination and other signs very similar to urethral obstruction. In stallions this condition can cause pain during covering of a mare with a reluctance to thrust and ejaculate. Contamination of the semen may lead to lowered fertility levels.

Diagnosis involves examination for any predisposing condition including problems of the penis, prepuce and accessory sex glands, examination of the urethra by endoscopy and the taking of urine/semen samples for cytology and culture.

Treatment
Stallions should be stopped from mating until resolution has occurred and any specific cause treated. Applications of topical antibiotic and anti-inflammatory drugs are often supplemented by systemic versions.

Tumours of the Urinary Tract

Tumours are rare in the horse urinary tract but all levels can be affected. Kidney tumours can vary but the most common is benign and can be treated by surgical removal of the affected kidney. Renal tumours may be detected as enlargements on rectal palpation or by changes on ultrasound examinations. The bladder and urethra are affected by a number of different tumours, the most common being the squamous cell carcinoma which is locally invasive and often ulcerative. Bladder tumours can present in similar ways to cystitis and cystic calculi, but may be distinguished by rectal palpation, ultrasound and endoscopy. Surgical removal is possible, but complete excision and, therefore, total resolution are difficult to achieve.

7

THE SKIN AND ITS DISEASES

The skin is the only visible organ of the body and yet it is much more than an inert sheath. Its efficient functioning is essential for health.

It protects against the sun's actinic radiation, prevents trauma and the entry of micro-organisms and is part of the body's immune system. It prevents dehydration, has an excretory function, plays an important part in the control of body temperature, carries sensory nerves for the appreciation of temperature variation, pressure and pain, has a social function in interrelation with other horses, synthesises vitamin D for subsequent absorption and provides the hooves, which are composed of modified skin on a skeletal framework.

The mammary glands are modified sweat glands of the skin adapted for nourishing the foal, while the eyes (excluding the retina) are also derived from the skin.

The body, in simple terms, can be considered to be encased in a three-layered structure (Figure 1). The outermost layer (the hair) is lifeless and is composed of pure protein (hard keratin) and assists in regulating body temperature. Beneath it is the epidermis, which itself is composed of several layers. The outermost layer of the epidermis (the stratum corneum) is soft keratin and is also lifeless. Thus, all that we see when looking at a horse is a sheath of lifeless hard and soft keratin.

The skin varies in thickness over different parts of the body: it is thickest over the dorsal trunk and thin on the ventral abdomen, lower neck and face. In temperate and cold climates long hair is produced for added insulation during the winter months. The hair follicles then pass into a resting phase. As the duration of daylight increases in springtime, they are stimulated into activity again, and new hairs are produced which grow up through the follicles, dislodging the old hairs.

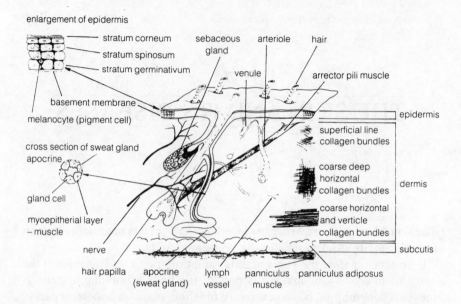

enlargement of epidermis

stratum corneum
stratum spinosum
stratum germinativum
basement membrane
melanocyte (pigment cell)
cross section of sweat gland
apocrine
gland cell
myoepitherial layer
– muscle
nerve
hair papilla
apocrine
(sweat gland)
lymph
vessel

sebaceous
gland
venule

arteriole

hair

arrector pili muscle

superficial line
collagen bundles
coarse deep
horizontal
collagen bundles
coarse horizontal
and verticle
collagen bundles

epidermis

dermis

subcutis

panniculus
muscle
panniculus adiposus

Figure 1   Anatomy of the skin

The epidermis may be greatly modified in various regions for functional adaptations. It rests upon a basement membrane. The first layer of cells resting on the basement membrane is the stratum germinativurn where the cells of the epidermis are produced by division.

With time, each cell produced by the stratum germinativum is pushed up to the surface, becoming keratinized and receiving pigment as it does so. It eventually dies and is sloughed off as a dander or scale from the outermost layer of the epidermis, the stratum corneum.

Horses have several different types of hair. Sinus hairs are thick, short hairs found on the muzzle and lips. The base of each sinus hair is surrounded by cavities containing blood , which transmit pressure stimuli to the sensory nerves wrapped around the base of the follicle. This arrangement makes the sinus hair an exquisite organ for passing on information of the surroundings. The body hair is of variable length and diameter. The emulsion which results from the mixing of the secretions of the glands of the skin and the skin itself flows along the hair and assists it in insulating the body. Body hair is replaced yearly. The hair of the mane is thicker and longer and has a longer life. This is particularly so for tail hair, which may continue growing for many months.

Observation of the coat will reveal the flow of hair which follows the lines of tension in the skin. The hair flow pattern is characteristic for each horse and may be used for identification. Whorls of hair will be noticed, and linear patterns or feathers may be present. Their presence and position should be recorded with the horse's identification certificate.

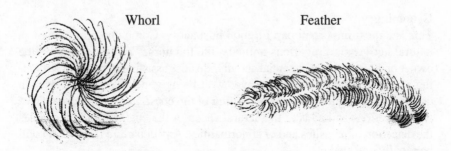

Whorl   Feather

Figure 2   Whorl/Feather patterns in hair

The hair follicles are formed *in utero* from downgrowths of the epidermis. They in turn produce the skin glands, sebaceous and apocrine. The epidermis rests upon the much thicker dermis, which consists of a mass of interwoven collagenous fibres and comparatively few cells. It contains vessels and nerves.

Beneath the dermis is the subcutis, a layer of fatty connective tissue to which the skin is usually loosely attached for its mobility. It contains a sheet of muscle, the panniculus muscle, the function of which is to move the skin to dislodge parasites and to generate heat by persistent contraction (shivering).

The skin is intimately affected by environmental factors and also by systemic factors. Generalised malignancy, liver disease, starvation, dehydration, and heavy parasitic worm burdens, for example, may all have profound effects on the skin. Systemic disease may produce itchiness, loss of hair, decreased elasticity (hidebound), increased scaliness of the skin or photosensitization. Thus an apparent change in the skin condition may not be due to local factors.

Diseases localised to the skin are most usually infectious in origin, the signs presented depending upon the pathogen. Ringworm primarily attacks dead keratin of the hair and epidermis; hair loss results, an allergic reaction may develop and changes in the dermis and epidermis then become apparent.

Skin mites live on or in the epidermis; their activity provokes much itchiness with marked self-excoriation of a particular area. Lice may suck blood or live on skin scale and may also provoke an allergic response; they too are often accompanied by severe excoriation of the body.

Bacterial infections of the skin are not common in the horse: usually they result from poor husbandry, badly fitting and/or dirty tack. Therefore they may be seen on those parts of the body in contact with tack; frank pus with an associated loss of hair may occur.

Breeding may bring together harmful traits which result in imperfect formation of the skin which may be apparent at birth or become obvious shortly afterwards. Areas of ulceration or comparative hairlessness may be seen, as in epitheliogenesis imperfecta.

Grooming

This is a most important part of good husbandry. Communal grooming is a natural activity in gregarious animals like the horse, and grooming by the owner or attendant is an essential activity. Besides assisting in bonding, grooming stimulates the skin and improves well-being generally. It removes skin debris and falling hair, it prevents felting of the coast, assists in the spread of skin secretions and adds to the natural sheen of the coat. Grooming enables the detection of parasites and of abnormalities. Any departure from health will be rapidly detected.

Examination and diagnostic aids

The veterinarian will seek to determine the previous history of the case before or while making a clinical examination. This will be a general examination to determine if the present skin symptoms are primary to the skin or secondary to a systemic reaction.

The general examination will be followed by a particular examination of the skin. Brushes and combs may be used to isolate any larger parasites; a hand lens may be used during this examination. Fine forceps may be used to pluck hair for detailed examination in the practice laboratory and possible outline for ringworm. Swabs may be collected for microscopic examination and/or culture for bacterial examination. Small pieces of skin may be removed for detailed examination of the tissue after processing and staining at higher magnification under the microscope. Specimens of blood may be collected in various tubes for examination of the haematology, blood enzymes and electrolytes.

Many skin diseases are easily transmitted by contact, though cleaning of tack minimises the risk. It is foolish to share tack between horses or use clothing belonging to other riders. Pathogens can survive for long periods on clothing and tack.

Conditions of the Skin

VIRAL PAPILLOMATA (WARTS)

These are caused by a virus similar to that causing warts in man, though cross-infectivity rarely occurs. Transmission is often from the dam, the foal being affected during suckling, with slow development over a number of months. Transmission often occurs between foals or from contact with infected material or woodwork.

The disease is almost always confined to young horses less than eighteen months of age. Warts are usually multiple and are most usually found on the relatively hairless parts of the body – the muzzle, nostrils, eyelids and often the front legs, less often elsewhere. They are small, grey, often cauliflower-shaped and firm. They may be very extensive if about the mouth. They may be subject to trauma and bleed or become secondarily infected. The diagnosis is made on the clinical appearance, with confirmation if necessary by biopsy examination.

Treatment
Local therapy is unsatisfactory in unskilled hands. The veterinarian may produce an autogenous vaccine. The warts are self-limiting and regression occurs within four months. If secondary infection occurs, regular antisepsis is advisable, with mild soap and water and an antiseptic dusting powder.

Transmission between young horses easily occurs, therefore affected animals should be isolated from others of the same age group.

EQUINE SARCOID

This is the most common skin tumour of the horse and is viral in origin. Unlike viral papillomata (which is caused by a different virus), it affects adult horses. Sarcoids can be one of three types: verrucae (wartlike), fibroplastic or mixed.

The different characteristics of the warts are determined by histopathological examination. Each type may be squat or stalked. Sarcoids are most often found on the limbs or head – sites commonly subjected to trauma.

The diagnosis of sarcoid is based on the clinical history and clinical signs; it may be confirmed by histopathological examination. They do not regress with age and may return after excision.

Treatment
Treatment should be by surgical excision (many recur after excision) or cryosurgery (see p. 633) or by the application of a cytotoxic agent. The latter should always be applied with the surrounding area of unaffected skin protected by lanoline ointment. Although sarcoids do not spread widely through the body, they are generally locally invasive.

ACNE (SADDLE BOILS, HEAT RASH)

Staphylococcus areus is the microbe most commonly associated with acne. It is a common normal resident on the skin surface where it causes no harm. It may enter the skin to provoke a pustular reaction where the skin is abraded and dirty, where there is poor husbandry or lack of grooming. The presence of ectoparasites, dirty or ill-fitting tack and soiled saddle clothing are predisposing factors. Acne is predominantly seen in mild wet winters.

The lesions resemble somewhat those seen in acne in man, though they are not usually pustular in appearance. They are small, multiple, painful raised pimples or boils up to 1cm in diameter in the saddle, girth or loin region. Occasionally there may be considerable swelling.

The diagnosis is made after a consideration of the history and a clinical examination, with an examination of a skin scrape of a lesion.

Treatment

Acne is caused by poor husbandry and self-abrasion. Standards of husbandry and hygiene must be improved to prevent recurrence. During treatment animals should not be worked. The affected area should be clipped if necessary to ensure adequate cleaning with a mild antiseptic wash. An antibiotic cream or ointment may be prescribed.

DERMATOPHILOSIS (STREPTOTHRICOSIS, MYCOTIC DERMATITIS, RAIN SCALD, MUD FEVER, GREASY HEEL)

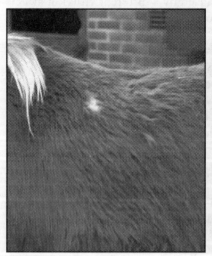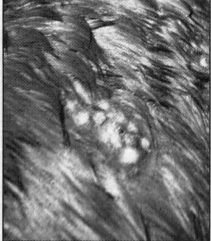

Figure 3 Dermatophilosis. The affected area has tufted hair
Figure 4 Dermatophilosis. The exposed dermis upon removal of the tufts

The causative organism is *Dermatophilus congolensis* which gains entry into the skin when it is saturated by prolonged rain and self-excoriated due to ectoparasites. It is predominantly seen in mild wet winters. Poor husbandry is a predisposing factor. Lesions are seen on the back, belly and lower limbs.

Horses in poor condition and badly cared for at pasture are at risk and show signs of the condition along the dorsal midline. The hair appears matted and tufted. With gentle pulling some tufts will lift off, revealing grey-green pus stuck to the lower ends. Affected areas may be quite extensive.

Horses kept in small muddy paddocks in prolonged wet weather may develop dermatophilus of the lower limbs and sometimes of the abdomen. Horses with shaggy coats or with feather are particularly at risk. Older texts refer to 'greasy heel'. This is a chronic inflammatory condition with weeping and matting of the hair. It has a number of causes, one of which is dermatophilus infection.

Diagnosis is based on the appearance of the lesions and the isolation and microscopic examination of the stained filamentous organisms.

Treatment
The cause of the condition should be considered in treatment. It is favoured by prolonged moisture and poor hygiene; therefore dry conditions and improved hygiene should be the first step in therapy. Affected animals must be housed. Long hair shielding the lesions must be removed by clipping (sterilising the blades after use). Astringent lotions are beneficial and a systemic antibiotic may be given when the lesions are severe. Fissuring and cracking of the skin may require prolonged careful treatment.

Remove long hair and wash with mild soap and tepid water. Areas must be kept dry after initial washing. Dressing with an antibiotic ointment is helpful. Rest in a dry area for several weeks will be essential.

Prevention is better than cure. The moral therefore is to practise good husbandry, prevent prolonged wetting by providing some shelter, examine regularly for ectoparasites, and *never* subject a horse or groups of horses to confinement in small muddy paddocks without shelter.

STRANGLES (*STREPTOCOCCUS EQUI* INFECTION)

The clinical signs and treatment are discussed elsewhere (see p. 474).

Strangles is a highly infectious disease, predominantly of young horses. It is not primarily a skin infection. However, the skin overlying infected lymph glands may become inflamed too, with swelling, heat, loss of hair and ulceration, particularly in the angle of the lower jaw and upper neck. The abscessed glands rupture and discharge a thick yellow sticky pus. The affected area should be bathed three times a day with warm saline solution and dried with an antibiotic powder. Affected animals must be isolated and care taken to prevent transfer of infected material. Visitors should be discouraged. The location of the abscesses permits easy transfer of the tacky pus to the stable door and thence to visitors' clothing. Normal animals are then at risk when viewed over their stable door. A later sequel to strangles may be the urticarial plaques of purpura haemorrhagica (see p. 474).

PASTERN FOLLICUTLITIS

This is an inflammation of the hair follicles of the lower limb or limbs. The infectious agent is usually a *Staphylococcus* species. Skin disease of this region is common and may be due to a variety of infectious agents. The generic term 'grease' or 'greasy heel' may also be used. The predisposing factor common to all is poor management and lack of hygiene. Any horse that is persistently exposed to wet, muddy conditions in the absence of grooming or attention is predisposed to diseases in this region, particularly those horses with 'feathered' patterns.

The inflammation is usually limited to the posterior aspect of the pastern(s) or bulbs of the heel(s). The initial sign is a small group of papules which progress to pustules. These will be overlooked in the ungroomed horse; neglect permits spread. Swelling and ulceration may develop and lameness result. There may be extensive dermatitis with suppurative exudation and matting of the hair. This is a painful condition and close examination will be resented; sedation may be necessary. Isolation of the pathogen(s) is necessary to determine the appropriate antibiotic. Thorough cleaning of the affected area(s) is the first essential. This can be accomplished by clipping. Thereafter the inflamed areas should be soaked at least once daily in chlorhexidine or povidone iodine diluted to antiseptic strength, then dried and the indicated antibiotic ointment applied. Whilst the disease does not usually become systemic, it may be obstinate of cure. Severe cases may warrant systemic antibiotic therapy. Unless the underlying predisposing factors are removed, treatment will not be successful.

BACTERIAL GRANULOMA

The former name for this condition is botryomycosis, literally from the Greek meaning a bunch of grape-like swellings believed to be of fungal origin. In fact it is a chronic deep staphylococcal infection resulting from a penetreating injury. With induration and multiple abscess formation in the deeper layers of the skin and subcutis, there may be pustular discharge on the surface. It is seen on the parts of the body subject to injury. It may follow surgery when the wound has become infected. It may also occur at sites of ill-fitting tack. Surgical removal is advisable.

GLANDERS

See p. 464. This has long been eradicated from the British Isles.

RINGWORM (GIRTH ITCH, JOCKEY ITCH)

Ringworm of horses in the British Isles is caused by members of two groups of pathogenic fungi, *Trichophyton* and *Microsporum*.

Ringworm fungi are able to survive for at least a year in the crevices of buildings housing horses, in transporting vehicles and in wooden fences. Horses rub themselves on stanchions and woodwork and pick up infected hairs.

Horses may also be infected by other animals, for example, cattle and cats, and by contaminated tack or grooming utensils. Young horses are particularly at risk and may contract infection during transportation, at shows or in sale rings. It is common for such animals to develop the initial signs of ringworm within two weeks of such events.

Symptoms
Young horses are particularly at risk but horses of all ages may be affected, although the disease is less common in older horses for immunity develops with increasing age.

The lesions are mainly seen on areas subjected to trauma from tack, clothing and riding boots. The term 'ringworm' is unfortunate: the lesions are rarely ringlike and the disease is not caused by a worm.

The early sign is one or more circular tufted areas (about 1-2cm in diameter) with a little scale; the hair shortly falls out revealing the scaly skin. These may be abraded and become infected, with pus formation. Itchiness is rarely encountered; scraping a scaly area over with a fingernail may, however, provoke signs of irritation. In foals there may be large, extensive lesions covered by thick grey scale.

Treatment
After isolation, the affected area is clipped with scissors to remove the hair and the lesions treated with a fungicidal dressing for seven days. An antimycotic agent may be prescribed for oral administration.

An attempt should be made to trace the source of the infection. Contaminated woodwork should be cleaned by pressure hosing. All tack that has come into contact with the patient must be treated, first by scrubbing with mild soap and water and then disinfected, preferably by formalin gas. This is a skilled procedure and should be undertaken only under the direction of the veterinarian.

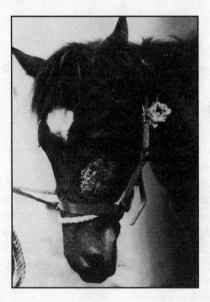

Figure 5
Ringworm

LOUSINESS

Two species of lice parasitize horses: one (the larger) is a blood-sucking parasite, *Haemtoapinus asini*; the smaller is a biting louse, *Damalinia equi*. Lice are small (1.5-3mm in length), slow-moving, and easily overlooked. They spend their entire life cycle on the host, their eggs (nits) being attached individually to hairs, for there the first immature stage (appearing like a miniature adult) develops. The life cycle is complete within three weeks.

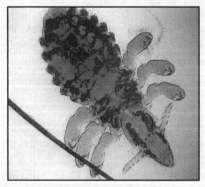

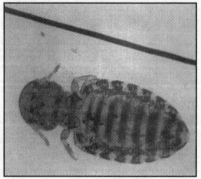

Figure 6
Haematopinus eurysternus, the larva of equine sucking louse attached to hair

Figure 7
Damalinia equi, adult of equine biting louse

Louse infestation is particularly common in the winter months. Numbers increasing greatly from the end of autumn, with a precipitate numerical decline in the spring. Horse lice may cause a transient itchiness on the skin of humans.

Younger animals are most often infested, but older, debilitated animals may also carry heavy burdens.

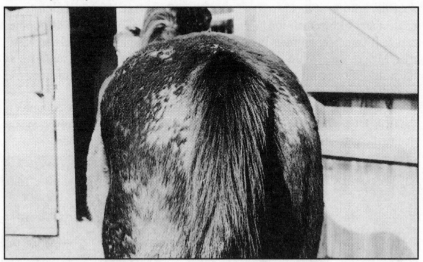

Figure 8   Lice

Symptoms

Lice are found particularly on the neck, shoulders and on areas where there are opposing skin surfaces, for example, under the base of the tail. However, in heavy infestation the entire body may be parasitised. In young animals louse infestation is associated with marked itchiness. Itchiness provokes self-excoriation with associated hair breakage and loss, so that the body may develop a motheaten appearance. The skin may become thickened; persistent itchiness may cause restlessness and debility. Close inspection by parting the hair and examining with a hand lens (though the lice are invisible to the naked eye) reveals the stationary or slow-moving dorsal, ventrally flattened parasites, which are grey-yellow in colour. Nits may be seen too, several being stuck to individual hairs along their length.

Treatment

Several proprietary preparations with an active principle of organophosphorus or synthetic pyrethrolds are available as sprays or washes or concentrated pour-on solutions. Therapy should be repeated at least twice. Contact horses should also be treated.

Animals which are regularly inspected and groomed should never be troubled by these parasites. Lice do not survive for long on the host but there is a distinct danger that infestation may be transferred if rugs are shared between horses.

ACARIASIS (MANGE, SCAB, ITCH)

An early edition of this textbook stated that 'Prevalence bears relationship to neglect and filthy conditions – mange is not common in the stabled, groomed and well-cared-for animals in civilian or military employ.' This advice is still true. Mange was common when horses were employed in large numbers by the army. Close confinement in horse lines during wartime or manoeuvres permitted rapid spread.

Sarcoptic mange – scabies, a notifiable disease – was once very common in the British Isles but has now been eradicated for many years. However, mange due to the parasitic mite *Chorioptes equi* is still relatively common.

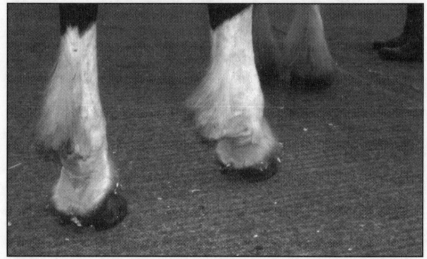

Figure 9   Chorioptic mange, infestation with the mite *Chorioptes equi*

The mite is small (less than 1mm in length), active, but barely visible to the naked eye. All stages are parasitic. It lives on the surface of the skin where its burrowing activities promote intense itchiness with consequent self-excoriation.

Symptoms
It is most common in stabled horses during winter. Initially the mite produces irritation on the lower hind limbs, but from there may be spread to the upper limb, inguinal areas, belly and forelimbs. The horse nibbles constantly at these areas, which may be denuded of hair, excoriated and exudative. There will be stamping and restlessness. If neglected, the skin may become thickened and ridged.

The disease should be distinguished from infestation with the harvest mite (see below) which occurs in grazing horses during the summer and autumn.

Diagnosis is confirmed by examination of a skin scraping under the microscope. After isolation, the affected areas are clipped and treated with a parasiticide; the dressing is repeated a week later.

A member of the genus *Chorioptes* may live in the ear canal, where it may incite waxy exudation and head shaking (ear mange). Handling of the head may be resented. If suspected, veterinary advice should be sought. The mite can be killed using ear drops containing a parasiticide; the treatment should be repeated a week later.

Forage mites (non-parasitic) can cause extensive skin irritation in horses. Failure to keep mangers clean or allowing fallen food to accumulate may permit massive increase in numbers of non-parasitic mites, which usually are harmless, in confined spaces. However, migration over the body may occur with irritation, loss of hair and self-excoriation. The examination of material taken from affected areas using a fine-tooth comb and subsequent examination under the microscope will reveal forage mites. A parasiticide wash will remove them but the original cause should be dealt with.

NEOTROMBICULOSIS (BERRY BUG, TROMBICULOSIS, HARVEST MITE, HEEL BUG)

Harvest mites, *Neotrombicula autumnalis*, are parasitic only as larvae. Most of the life cycle is spent in the soil. The larvae emerge from the soil from May to late October and are particularly active in warm weather. They are less than 0.5mm in length. They clamber up herbage and their hooked legs enable them to affix themselves to any passing animal or bird. Horses may therefore pick them up on their legs or about the muzzle. The larvae produce a feeding tube which enables them to feed on tissue fluid. When replete in two to three days they fall off to complete their life cycle.

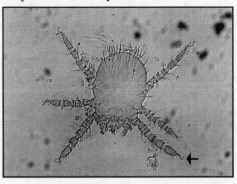

Figure 10   *Neotrombicular autumnalis*, larva of a harvest mite.
The arrow indicates the claws used for attachment

Symptoms

Close inspection of the skin reveals small mites 3mm in diameter attached to the skin; a group may crowd together to form an orange patch. Feeding mites cause local irritation, so that there may be shifting of the feet and nibbling of the limbs. Infestation may be suspected when horses at grass show lower-limb irritation (there may be a papular response) or when there is pedal irritation in stabled horses fed fresh hay in mild dry weather during summer.

Treatment

Local antiparasitic dressing is usually sufficient. Control is difficult because of the life cycle of the parasite and the wide availability of potential hosts.

TICK INFESTATION

Ixodes ricinus – the sheep tick – is the only potential tick parasitising horses in the British Isles. Usually only very small numbers are observed firmly attached to the finer skin of the ventral abdomen.

The sheep tick is easily visible with the naked eye at all stages of its life cycle. The feeding apparatus (hypostome) is armed with backward-pointing barbs. If an attempt is made to remove the tick without making it relax, this is pulled off and a septic focus may result.

Ticks should therefore be removed by applying a pledget of cottonwool soaked in spirit, ether or chloroform to them, waiting a few moments, and then applying gentle traction. The tick can then be pulled off and the triangular hypostome will be seen attached to the tick.

SWEET ITCH
(SUMMER SEASONAL RECURRENT DERMATITIS)

This is an allergic reaction to the bites of flies of the genus *Culicoides* – the midges. Horses of all types are affected, particularly ponies. Sweet itch is a common seasonal problem and occurs in all ages other than the first year of life. Midges are active from April to early November, particularly on calm humid days, mostly biting at daybreak and nightfall. Only the females of the genus are bloodsuckers. Moist decaying vegetation is required for development of the immature stages, so that the midges are more common in well-wooded areas, particularly by watercourses and lakes.

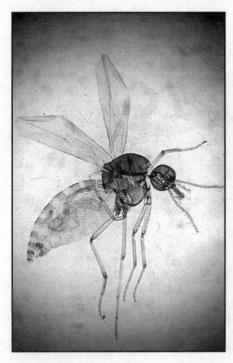

Figure 11
Culicoides, a parasitic midge,
the cause of sweet itch

Symptoms

The disease is an intensely irritant dermatitis, the lesions of which have a characteristic distribution. They are found along the dorsal midline, mostly in and at the junction of long hair and short hair, forelock, mane, saddle region, trunk and tail base. With time they become more extensive, extending laterally. With continued self-excoriation the hair, particularly of the mane and tail, is broken and lost and the skin thickened and ridged. Severely affected horses are unworkable. The disease recurs during the warmer months of each year throughout the remainder of the animal's life.

Diagnosis

A recurring summer seasonal dermatitis of the dorsal midline with marked self-excoriation is characteristic. The only other diseases which might be confirmable are infestation with the bowel worm *Oxyuris equi* (pinworm) and mange.

With *Oxyuris equi* the female deposits large numbers of creamy-coloured eggs in masses about the anus. There is marked perineal irritation with rubbing of the buttocks against fixed objects. This causes redness of the area and the long tail hairs are broken, making it rat-tailed in appearance. Oxyuris infestation is not seasonal, only the buttocks are irritated, and investigation will reveal the eggs, which can be identified by the veterinarian under the microscope.

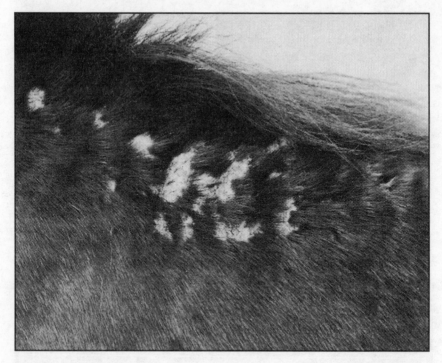

Figure 12 Sweet itch

Mange is also irritant. The causal mites can be found in combings and skin scrapings. No mites are isolated from the lesions of sweet itch.

Treatment
Severely abraded areas may be treated with mild astringent lotion (2% zinc sulphate). The availability of pour-on synthetic pyrethroids means that prevention of biting is now possible. These should be diluted according to the manufacturer's instructions and applied at six-day intervals along the animal's dorsal midline. In wet weather this should be more frequent. As midges are particularly active on mild, humid, still days and, at daybreak and nightfall, affected animals should then be housed.

FACE FLIES

A number of flies resembling house flies are attracted to the secretions produced by the orifices of the body. The eyes and mouth may be particularly attractive and horses may be severely tormented by the attentions of these pests. Some control of the life cycle is possible if the breeding sites (manure piles) are restricted and cleared regularly.

Synthetic pyrethroid-impregnated tags are available which can be attached to the headcollar. Alternatively the head can be swabbed at weekly intervals with synthetic pyrethroid diluted according to the manufacturer's instructions.

EAR PLAQUES

Raised whitish thickened areas sometimes several centimetres in diameter are very occasionally found on the inner aspects of the ear of adult horses. They may be singular or several in number. The cause is not known. Viruses, mites and biting flies have all been considered but there is no evidence to incriminate either. They apparently cause no pain or irritation. No treatment is necessary.

NODULAR NECROBIOSIS (BUMPS)

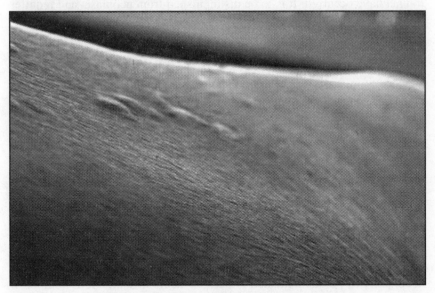

Figure 13   Nodular necrobiosis, saddle area of show jumper

A number of conditions can cause nodules (bumps) in the skin. A common cause is an inflammatory reaction to the bites of horse flies, which are seen in some horses. These are usually seen in groups, and are palpable as thickenings beneath the skin, particularly in the saddle region where they may cause discomfort when the horse is ridden.

AURAL PLAQUES (WARTS)

These are raised white/grey thickened areas which may become several centimetres in diameter to completely cover the inner aspect of the earflap of adult horses. They are now believed to be caused by a papilloma virus. They do not usually cause pain or irritation, although they may be attractive to black flies (*Simulium* spp.) Some affected animals may resent having their ears touched or having a head collar put on, however there may be other reasons for such behaviour which may require attention. There is no age immunity and the lesion(s) persist throughout life. There is no treatment.

NEOPLASIA (TUMOURS) (see also Chapter 42)

Neoplasms induced by viruses – warts and sarcoids – have been referred to earlier. Exuberant granulation tissue (proud flesh) is an excessive production of normal repair tissue and is relatively common on the limbs where cuts and trauma have occurred. It is to be distinguished from neoplasia and requires veterinary attention.

The aetiology of tumour development is not understood. Some tumours are initiated by viruses, while actinic sunlight may provoke tumours of the skin in relatively unprotected areas. Thus squamous cell carcinomas are more common on the eyelids and in the skin of light-coloured horses. This is so in humans too and emphasises the dangers of excessive sunbathing. Tumours of pigment cells melanomas – are common in grey-skinned horses. Sarcoids are commonest on areas subject to trauma – the limbs, head and neck.

Growths should be reported for veterinary examination as soon as they are discovered. Failure to do so may permit them to increase in size, making subsequent removal difficult or impossible, or allowing spread to other organs – a most dangerous development. Early excision is advised for all tumours. Advice about possible recurrence should be sought.

'Neoplasm' literally means new growth in the skin. By definition a neoplasm is uncontrolled cell division in tissue(s) which serves no useful purpose. The result is a visible change in conformation of the skin. Not all such growths are neoplastic: to be distinguished is nodular necrobiosis. Here a number of non-painful nodules, usually ovoid, about 2cm in diameter and slightly elevated, are found in the saddle area of yearlings and older horses. The hair over them is undamaged. Their cause is not known but they may regress with time. Surgical removal may be advised; topical therapy is of no value.

URTICARIA
(ALLERGIC REACTIONS, HIVES, NETTLE RASH)

The natural response of the skin to allergic reactions may be the sudden appearance of variable-sized elevations. Allergic dermatitis may follow insect bites, ingestion of substances to which a hypersensitivity has been developed (food, drugs), injection of foreign substances (vaccines, drugs), contact with allergens or following some infections (strangles, for example).

In each case prior exposure to the sensitising allergen must have occurred at least once. The resulting reaction causes the release of fluid into the dermis and elsewhere, the nature of the response being variable according to the allergen. Allergic reactions to certain midges produce the clinical signs of sweet itch, allergic reaction to the stable fly (*Stomoxys calcitrans*) results in the appearance of flat elevations 1-2cm in diameter scattered over the trunk.

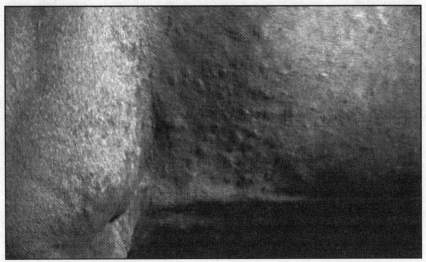

Figure 14   Papular urticaria

A fairly common allergic reaction is to animal proteins in concentrates and fresh grass proteins. This is particularly seen in young adults. Numerous papules (small firm elevations) 0.5cm in diameter appear, scattered over the trunk. There may be severe itchiness and loss of appetite. Earlier texts refer to this condition as surfeit (excessive feeding).

Reactions to injection of foreign substances (earlier vaccines, drugs) may be severe (anaphylaxis), with widespread swelling (oedema). There may be oedema of the eyelids and elsewhere, while released fluid in or about the respiratory tract may cause respiratory distress. The sudden appearance of extensive oedema should be regarded with concern and veterinary advice sought immediately.

When contact dermatitis occurs in the horse, it is most usually of irritant origin, though sometimes allergy is the cause. It may be a reaction to tack or clothing, soaps or shampoos. Allergic contact dermatitis is characterised by the elapse of a period of time from the initial period of exposure until the development of the allergic reaction. In contrast irritants act immediately on contact.

PRESSURE SORES (BED SORES (DECUBITUS ULCERATION), SITFASTS, SADDLE GALLS, SADDLE SORES)

Long-lasting pressure in the recumbent animal may result in death of skin tissue (at pressure points) and severe ulceration, while persistent rubbing or pressure (even though light) may cause loss of hair, swelling, thickness of the skin, depigmentation and even ulceration. Common sites for the latter are in the saddle and bridle area and at points of contact with badly fitting harnesses on prominences.

Pressure sores are preventable. Recumbent animals should be regularly turned and well bedded. Their pressure points require gentle massage and washing regularly with soap and water. After drying they should be treated with a silicone cream. Contact points beneath tack should be frequently inspected for early evidence of unnatural pressure, heat, loss of hair and swelling, and the correct adjustments made while the tack itself should also be inspected regularly for wear.

PITYRIASIS (DANDRUFF)

Early texts refer to pityriasis as a disease but this is not correct; it is not a disease but a clinical sign which may occur in several diseases. It may occur in extensive ectoparasitism and in chronically sick or severely debilitated horses. Extensive exfoliative dermatitis with marked pityriasis is a feature of the rare auto-immune disease *periphigus foliaceous*. Mild dandruff may accumulate in neglected, ungroomed, stabled animals on poorly balanced diets.

The cause of pityriasis should be investigated and the primary aetiological factor treated if this is possible.

LEUKODERMA

This is whitening of the previously pigmented skin or hair. Vitiligo is not recorded in the British Isles, but loss of pigmentation of the skin occurs in tropical countries. Acquired leukoderma is a result of trauma to the skin by badly fitting harness or saddlery, the resulting destruction of the pigment cells is permanent with the production of white hairs (adventitial mark).

Loss of pigmentation about the commissures of the mouth may follow the usage of rubber bits. Leukoderma is permanent and there is no treatment. Adventitial marks must be recorded on identification charts (see Chapter 54).

PHOTOSENSITISATION (BLUE NOSE)

Photosensitization results from ingestion of agents which sensitise the skin to actinic rays in sunlight. It can also result from liver damage with subsequent imperfect excretion of the breakdown products of chlorophyll (the green colouring in plants), which in turn sensitise the skin to actinic rays. It may occur in both young and old horses and fortunately is uncommon.

Symptoms
Because the action of the rays is more intense on relatively uncreased skin, the signs are seen in relatively hairless parts of the body – the muzzle and nostrils (particularly if unpigmented) and the tips of the ears. In extensive damage large white-haired areas may be affected. The condition occurs in summer during bright, sunny weather. The first sign may be increased sensitivity – flicking of ears, rubbing of the body. Within a few hours there is reddening and then purplish discoloration and oedema of the underlying skin. The skin of these areas may slough off several days later to reveal the red moist dermis.

Prognosis and treatment
The prognosis for photosensitization must be guarded: if it is due to extensive liver damage, the outcome may be poor to hopeless. However, if it is the result of the ingestion of a photosensitising plant such as St John's wort (*Hypericum perforatum*), the chances of recovery are quite good. Affected horses should be removed immediately from exposure to bright sunlight and housed in dim light. In the early stages an intravenous injection of an antihistamine may be beneficial. There may be extensive sloughing of the skin, particularly on light-coloured areas and on the extremities. These parts should be lightly dusted with an antiseptic drying powder and regularly inspected for deposited blowfly eggs.

AUTOIMMUNE DISEASES

These are a group of diseases which may not be confined to the skin in which the immune system becomes programmed to react to the animal's own tissue with resulting damage. There is an apparent genetic component, some may follow the use of particular drugs, and infections may play a part.

They are characterised by scaliness, redness of the skin and patchy loss of hair, giving a moth-eaten appearance. In some, there may be local loss of pigment, whilst there may be ulceration of the skin and also the mucous membranes. All are uncommon. Most are responsive to anti-inflammatory therapy but may require life-long medication.

8
SYSTEMS OF COMMUNICATION

The reader has arrived at this page through a series of actions often taken for granted. The recognition of the book, opening the pages, reading and understanding the print, and the decision as to whether or not to proceed with reading it in the context of the time available and motivation are conscious actions. But, awake or asleep, other forms of communication take place in order that the respiratory and metabolic processes of the body are regulated in such a way that we live in comfort with our environment. For example, when the environment is hot the body produces less heat; when we exert ourselves we breathe more deeply and accelerate the circulation of the blood in order to meet the increased oxygen demands. All of these processes depend on communication between one part of the body and another.

In health we are unaware of these processes; it is only in disease when the systems are disordered that recognisable symptoms appear.

If we analyse the systems upon which communication depends, we find that they may be separated roughly into two categories: (a) appreciation of external stimuli and happenings and (b) response. It is possible therefore to recognise an input (i.e. a stimulus) and an appropriate action initiated by the input stimulus (i.e. a response). The means of communication between the input and the response are the messages upon which the body depends for its communication. For example, the stimulus of pinprick causes us to hurriedly withdraw the part pricked. The response to the prick depends on the messages relayed from the skin through the central nervous system to the muscles, which respond by pulling away the affected part in an effort to diminish or avoid the painful stimulus. There is thus an afferent (towards) pathway along which the messages are transmitted to the brain and an efferent (away) pathway along which messages are carried from the brain to the muscles instructing them to withdraw the part from pain.

In essence all systems of communication within the body are based on these afferent and efferent pathways carrying messages. However, although this analogy is readily understood with regard to nerves, which work in the same way as telephone messages, passed through a central exchange from one house to another. The same applies to messages in the form of hormones which issue from glands and carry chemical messengers to organs, evoking an appropriate response.

These messages are relayed by the following body systems: the central and peripheral nervous systems, the autonomic nervous system, the endocrine (hormonal) system, the neuroendocrine (hormonal) system, and the special senses of sight, hearing and smell. The sensations of touch, pain, heat, cold, etc., will be considered under the central and peripheral nervous systems.

THE CENTRAL AND PERIPHERAL NERVOUS SYSTEMS

The nervous system, as its name implies, is composed of nerve cells and their fibres. The fibres conduct electrical impulses (messages) and are responsible for feeling, consciousness and action. The cells and their fibres are grouped together in the brain and spinal cord. The fibres extend to the periphery, e.g. the skin and muscles, so that the whole system may be likened to the links of a telephone system.

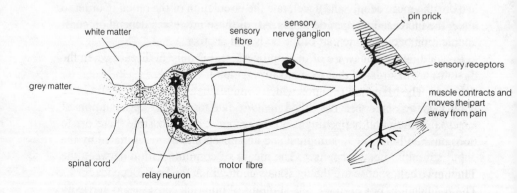

Figure 1　The reflex arc

The nerve endings in the skin, for example, have special properties of being sensitive to pain and touch, pressure and temperature, etc.. When these physical stimuli are applied to the skin they set off messages that are conducted along the pathways of the nerves to the cells in the spinal cord. These relay the messages to other cells and their fibres which conduct outward-bound messages to the muscles if the sensation is painful. This reflex arc is illustrated in Figure 1.

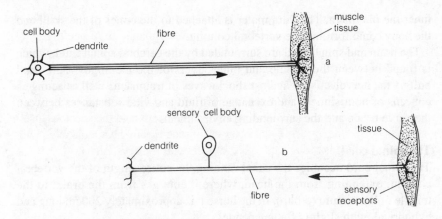

Figure 2 Nerve cells: a) a motor neuron, b) a sensory neuron

The brain is made aware of this nervous activity through nerve fibres that conduct the information up the spinal cord to the brain. In this way the individual has a conscious capacity to modify any action or response and to be aware of what is taking place in the environment.

The response of a nerve cell (Figure 2) is always the same. It conducts a wave of excitation (nervous impulse or message) from one end of the cell to the other. The cell's fibre may be several metres long and can conduct impulses at a very fast rate of up to 100 m/s.

Nervous tissue extends to almost every part of the body, but each segment is connected to form a whole system. This might be likened to the wires and cables of a telephone system connected to the exchange and branching in all directions. The greatest concentration of nervous tissue is in the skull, that is, the brain. The brain and spinal cord are known as the *central nervous system* (CNS) whereas other nervous tissue of the body is described as the *peripheral nervous system* (PNS). Higher functions depend on the CNS and basic functions on the PNS.

The nerve cell

The basic unit of the nervous system is the nerve cell or neuron. Many cells and their fibres are collected together, forming bundles. To the naked eye the nerve fibres appear white and the cell bodies brownish-grey tinged with pink. Nerve tissue is therefore described as white or grey matter. Ganglia (bunches of nerve tissue) are composed of grey matter and are situated on the efferent (sensory) nerve trunks (Figure 2). The nerve trunks are classed according to their connection with the central nervous system as cerebral (cranial), spinal or sympathetic.

The brain and spinal cord are enclosed in three membranes or meninges. The outermost is called the dura mater, the middle the arachnoid mater and the inner the pia mater. The dura mater is attached to the bones of the skull and the bony canal forming the vertebral column.

The brain and spinal cord are surrounded by the cerebral spinal fluid, which is found between the middle and inner layers of the meninges. This fluid buffers the nervous tissue against shockwaves of trauma, as well as acting as a means of nourishment and exchange of fluid and vital substances between the nerve tissue and the surrounding environment.

The spinal cord

The spinal cord occupies the canal running the entire length of the vertebral column, extending from the head, where it emerges from the brain, to the middle of the sacrum (croup). In the horse it is approximately 200cm long and cylindrical, with slightly flattened sides.

Forty-two pairs of spinal nerves emerge from the cord at intervals between each vertebra. There are eight neck or cervical nerves, eighteen chest or thoracic, six back or lumbar, five croup (sacral) and five tail (coccygeal) nerves. The arrangement of white and grey substance in the cord and the way in which the nerves emerge is illustrated in Figure 3.

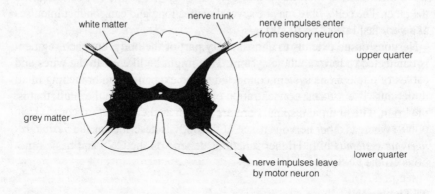

Figure 3   Cross-section of the spinal cord (based on a radiograph)

The brain

The brain is that part of the central nervous system contained in the skull. It weighs about 650g in an adult horse and forms 1% of the bodyweight. It is composed of various parts, containing white and grey matter and fluid-filled cavities (ventricles) which connect with the space surrounding the spinal cord that contains the cerebral spinal fluid.

The brain has three primary segments – the hind, the mid- and the forebrain – each associated with specialised functions. The hind brain is formed by the brain stem and contains the centres that regulate breathing. It also contains the pons, which controls emotions and other behavioural activity, and the cerebellum, which controls movement. The midbrain is responsible for sensations of sight and smell and the control of lower centres in the hind brain, e.g. the voluntary control of breathing, behavioural patterns and movement. The forebrain is connected to the pituitary gland and modifies its hormonal secretions (see p. 170).

There are twelve nerves that leave the brain and pass to various parts of the body. Each is responsible for sensory (feeling) or motor activity. These nerves are numbered as follows: I olfactory, II optic, III ocular motor, IV trochlear, V trigeminal, VI abducens, VII facial, VIII acoustic, IX glossopharangeal, X vagus, XI spinal accessory, XII hypoglossal. All these nerves except X and XI are concerned with feeling or with muscular movement of the head.

Conditions of the Central and Peripheral Nervous Systems

Diseases and conditions of the nervous system occur when impulses normally passing through the fibres are disturbed. If the impulses are slowed or prevented from passing, this may cause loss of feeling if the nerves affected are sensory or paralysis if they serve motor functions.

Because the central nervous system is concerned with coordination, interference with the passage of nervous impulses may lead to incoordination (ataxia).

If the nervous impulses are speeded up or increased in number, they may result in convulsions or hyperirritability, causing spasm, as in lockjaw (see p. 475).

The cause of these conditions may be damage, viral infection, bacterial toxins, haemorrhage or trauma causing disturbance of the pathways.

In the diagnosis of lameness we take advantage of our knowledge of the nerve trunks to cause numbness in certain parts. This technique is known as nerve blocking (see p. 197).

PARALYSIS

Paralysis is usually a sign of an injured nerve which prevents impulses passing from the central nervous system to the muscles. This prevents the horse from using the muscles supplied by the affected nerve. For example, the facial nerve is particularly vulnerable to injury as it passes across the back of the angle of the lower jaw. This nerve supplies the muscles of the lips, nostrils, cheeks, eyelids and ears.

Symptoms of **facial paralysis** are a drooping eyelid and ear, a partially collapsed nostril and sagging upper and lower lips. Usually only one side is affected and the upper lip tends to be pulled towards the side away from the affected area because the muscles on the opposite side still have normal nervous control.

It is usual to give the paralysis the name of the damaged nerve, e.g. facial paralysis. **Obdurator** is another common form of paralysis in which, following foaling, the obdurator nerve becomes pinched, causing partial paralysis of the hind leg.

Another commonly affected nerve is the suprascapular nerve, which emerges from the chest underneath the shoulder and supplies the muscles of the shoulder. Injury results in wasting of the muscles on the outside of the shoulderblade because of damage to their nerve supply (see Figure 2, p. 288). This condition is known as **sweeny**. It sometimes causes an abnormal gait, best observed when the individual is walked slowly towards the observer.

Radial paralysis can occur following collisions occasionally it is seen when the horse has to lie on the leg for long surgery under general anaesthesia. The radial nerve emerges from the chest wall underneath the shoulderblade. It supplies the muscles which advance the leg when the horse moves forward. The muscles also hold the elbow joint in position. Symptoms of radial paralysis therefore include a dropped elbow and difficulty in moving the leg forward (see Figure 4, p. 282).

Paralysis is also experienced in conditions caused by equid herpesvirus (see p. 490) and other viral infections. In the human the most well-known example is poliomyelitis. Symptoms displayed by horses suffering from viral infections vary with the nature of the virus and the particular damage that it causes to the central nervous system.

INFECTIONS (see also Chapters 29-33)

Infection may affect the lining of the brain and spinal cord (**meningitis**) or the substance of the brain (**encephalitis**). It may also affect peripheral nerves, causing neuritis.

Conditions of nervous disease in horses are Eastern, Western and Venezuelan encephalomyelitis (see p. 498), the nervous form of equid herpesvirus 1 (rhinopneumonitis) infection (see p. 488), rabies (see p. 499) and lockjaw (see p. 475).

LOSS OF SENSATION (see also Chapter 19)

Damage to sensory nerves, that is, those taking messages from the periphery to the central nervous system, causes loss of sensation or numbness. Crushing of the spinal cord, as in a broken neck or back, causes loss of sensation to large areas of the hindquarters. Because motor nerves are also affected there is associated paralysis.

The loss of sensation may be diagnosed by pricking the skin with a needle or drawing a sharp instrument over the surface of the skin. This normally causes the horse to move the skin or underlying part. However, if the muscles are also paralysed, it may be impossible to be certain that there is also loss of feeling.

Injury to the optic nerve, which conveys messages from the eye to the brain, causes blindness. This is often the result of an injury to the head causing haemorrhage and pressure on the nerve. Depending on the severity of the damage, sight may return as the blood clot contracts.

Head injuries may likewise cause paralysis or loss of sensation in any part of the body. Horses suffering from concussion or a fractured skull may show incoordination, staggering and convulsions. Mild cases recover, but frequently the damage cannot be repaired and the horse dies or has to be destroyed on humane grounds.

LARYNGEAL HEMIPLEGIA (ROARING, WHISTLING)

This condition results from a paralysis of the muscles which control the movement of the larynx. In almost all cases it is the left side that is affected. The muscles are supplied by the recurrent laryngeal nerve and it is damage to this nerve that results in the paralysis.

Paralysis of the movement of the larynx causes the vocal cords and arytenold cartilage to hang in the airstream when the horse breathes in, and this results in an abnormal sound; hence the popular name of whistling or roaring.

For treatment, see p. 69.

WOBBLER SYNDROME

The wobbler syndrome results from damage to the nerve trunks passing along the spinal cord in the neck. This is usually the result of injury to the bony canal through which the spinal cord passes on its way to the brain. The nerve trunks involved are those carrying messages that enable the horse to be aware of where its limbs are, at a particular moment. This sense of proprioception is important in the coordination of movement. If the sense is impaired the affected individual suffers an unusual incoordinated gait. The condition is described in detail on p. 326.

SHIVERING AND STRINGHALT

Symptoms in these conditions are, as their names imply, unusual shivering movements of the hind legs as they are lowered to the ground from a flexed position. Their cause is poorly understood. However, it is probable that they are the result of damage to the nerves at some point in their course from the muscles that control the hind limbs to the higher centre of the brain. For further details, see pp. 309-10.

CEREBELLAR HYPOPLASIA (CEREBELLAR DEGENERATION)

This occurs in Arab horses and is characterised by tremors of the head, incoordination of the legs and a faulty blink response when the eye is, challenged'. A fine head tremor is usually the first sign and this develops before a foal is four months old. It consists of nodding movements which become more obvious when a purposeful movement is made. In some instances the animal is unable to stand, and in others it lurches or sways when it tries to walk.

There is no treatment. As the disease is thought to be genetically based on a recessive gene, action should be taken to diminish the risk by avoidance of breeding from mares and stallions known to be carriers.

EQUINE MOTOR NEURONE DISEASE

This occurs rarely in most areas of the world but is most common in north-east America. The precise cause is unknown but commonly horses or ponies have little access to fresh forage and a lack of Vitamin E or Selenium has been implicated with the individual affected showing lower serum levels than their counterparts. Dysfunction of the nerves causes weakness but not incoordination. Weight loss, lying down, poor muscle tone, sweating and low carriage of the head are common signs; there are alterations in gait and there may be a characteristic tail lift. Diagnosis can be difficult unless characteristic signs are present and may be made by elimination of other causes of weakness and weight loss. It is possible to perform muscle or nerve biopsies. Treatment with access to fresh forage and supplementation may help stabilise the condition but it is usually slowly progressive. Stabilised cases rarely improve to return to normal.

THE AUTONOMIC NERVOUS SYSTEM

The autonomic nervous system can be divided into two parts: the sympathetic and the parasympathetic. The sympathetic nervous system carries impulses to the muscles of the heart and gut and to the secretory glands. It also conducts impulses from the various organs of the chest and abdomen to the central nervous system and thereby serves to control involuntary activity, such as movement of the alimentary tract (peristalsis) and the secretion of the salivary and other glands. It regulates the size of blood vessels by acting on their muscular coat, causing them to constrict or relax and thus influencing the resistance to bloodflow and blood pressure.

The action of the sympathetic system is roughly opposed to that of the parasympathetic system, the nerves of which are carried mainly in the Xth cranial (vagus) nerve. This system decreases gut movement, slows the heart and decreases or changes the character of glandular secretions.

One of the conditions of the autonomic nervous system is grass sickness (see p. 48).

THE ENDOCRINE (HORMONAL) SYSTEM

Hormones are the chemical messengers of the body. They are substances produced by glands, and are carried in the bloodstream to control organs at a distance from their source of secretion. For example, the pituitary gland, which is situated just below the brain, secretes the hormone FSH. This is carried in the bloodstream to the ovaries, where it causes follicles to develop.

The hormones of the body, the glands which secrete them, the organs they affect and their action are shown in Table 1.

Measurement of hormones
The reader will probably be more familiar with the subject of hormones in terms of phrases such as 'hormonal imbalance', which is often used of mares that are difficult to get in foal. 'Adrenal exhaustion' is another phrase sometimes used when horses in training perform poorly. These phrases are imprecise and best avoided; they have little relevance to the actual hormonal status of the individual.

Such terms were used in the past, when our knowledge was far from complete. More recently, sensitive methods of measuring hormones in the bloodstream have been developed. These have been used to identify the true hormonal status of individuals for diagnostic purposes. However, before describing their application to horses, it is necessary to explain some of the limits of these methods.

The most obvious limitation is that the measurement of the level of a hormone in the blood reflects only its level in transit. It does not necessarily reflect its power of action on the organ which it controls.

There are two main implications behind this statement. First, the hormone being measured in high concentrations in the bloodstream may fail to have a corresponding powerful action because the target organ has a reduced capacity to respond.

For example, ACTH, the hormone stimulating the adrenal cortex to produce cortisone, can only have an effect if the cortex is responsive to the action of ACTH. This action depends on the presence of structures known as receptors.

To put it at its simplest, this means that the ability of ACTH to cause release of cortisone is related to the number of receptors present. The number of receptors varies according to factors which need not concern us here. However, if the number of receptors is small, a large amount of ACTH in the bloodstream will not cause a corresponding increase in secretion. Indeed, the reverse may be true; a large number of receptors will cause a relatively large output despite the presence of only a small amount of ACTH in the bloodstream.

This example reflects the position with regard to all hormones. It also demonstrates the need to be cautious about interpreting the levels of hormones present in the bloodstream at any given time.

The second reason why blood levels do not necessarily reflect the degree of activity resulting from the presence of a hormone is that many hormones are balanced by the action of others. For example, progesterone and oestrogen have contradictory actions and it is the balance of the two that controls uterine contractions at birth.

Notwithstanding the above cautionary remarks, there exists sufficient experience in employing modern methods of measurement for us to comment on selected hormones.

Steroid hormones

Steroid hormones include progesterone, oestrogen, testosterone and cortisone. They have a chemical structure of four carbon rings and are therefore closely related to one another. The simplest form is cholesterol. The body is able to change one steroid hormone into another.

Progesterone   Progesterone in the non-pregnant mare is secreted by the yellow body of the ovary. Its presence in the bloodstream at levels over 1 ng/ml is diagnostic of an active yellow body in one or other of the two ovaries. A detectable level of progesterone in the bloodstream may therefore be taken as a diagnostic sign of dioestrus, that is, the mare is not in heat.

This helps us to confirm the sexual state of the individual as shown when the mare is teased. The test distinguishes between sexual states of heat (oestrus), not in heat (dioestrus), anoestrus (sexually inactive) and prolonged dioestrus.

Table 1 Some Main Hormones of the Body, Their Source and Action

Gland	Hormone	Target organ	Action
Pituitary			
Anterior	FSH	Ovary	Stimulates follicle development
	LH	Ovary	Causes ovulation and yellow body function
	Prolactin	Mammary glands	Causes milk secretion
	GH (growth)	General action on metabolism	Promotes increase in protein, fat, sugar and water in body
	TSH	Thyroid	Causes thyroxine secretion
	ACTH	Adrenal cortex	Causes cortisol secretion
Posterior	Vasopressin, oxytocin	Smooth muscle in arteries and uterus	Raises blood pressure, contracts uterine muscle
Pancreas	Insulin	General	Controls level of sugar in blood and tissues
Thyroid	Thyroxine	General	Controls general metabolic rate
Adrenal cortex	Cortisone	General	Controls salt, sugar and water content of blood and tissues
Adrenal medulla	Adrenaline		Affects sweating, increases blood flow to muscles
Ovary	Progesterone	Uterus and genital tract	Changes of dioestrus and pregnancy
Yellow body			
Follicle	Oestrogen	Uterus and genital tract	Causes oestrous behaviour and lubricates genital tract
Uterus	Prostaglandin	Yellow body of ovary	Stops yellow body secreting progesterone
	PMSG	Probably ovary	May protect yellow body of pregnancy and has immune suppressing role
Brain	Releasing factors	Pituitary	Hormones that cause pituitary to release its own hormones such as FSH, LH, ACTH

Pregnant mares have relatively high levels of progesterone for about 120 days after conception. Progesterone is the hormone which maintains pregnancy and it is produced by the ovaries up to this time. From then until the end of pregnancy it is produced by the placenta and does not appear in any quantity in the mare's bloodstream.

Up to 120 days we would expect a pregnant mare to have varying levels over 4 ng/ml. The actual amount is not related to the pregnancy as such but to the activity of the yellow body. We cannot therefore use progesterone as an indication of pregnancy, except in the negative sense that if the value is below 4 ng/ml the mare is unlikely to be pregnant. If it is above 4 ng/ml the mare may be pregnant or merely in a state of dioestrus.

There are divided opinions as to whether progesterone therapy prevents mares from aborting. The problem, as with so many clinical situations, is the absence of objective studies. The facts are that progesterone is indeed required for continuing pregnancy. However, the quantity of progesterone in the bloodstream does not necessarily indicate the effectiveness of the hormone at the target site, i.e. the uterus. For reasons explained above, a small amount of hormone may have a marked effect. Further, because the placenta is producing progesterone from about day 50 of the pregnancy, the hormone may be adequate at the level of the interface between the placenta and uterus, even though there are low levels in the mare's bloodstream.

If the level of progesterone in the blood is less than 4 ng/ml, we may assume that the individual is suffering from a deficiency of progesterone, at least up to day 120. After this time we expect very low levels because the progesterone is being produced entirely by the placenta and not by the mare's ovaries. The progesterone does not pass from the placenta into the mare's bloodstream except in very small amounts and the levels of progesterone in the last two thirds of pregnancy is often below 4 ng/ml.

In most cases of abortion progesterone levels fall because and not as a cause of the abortion. Most of the claims for the successful use of progesterone as a preventive measure are based on cases in which the drug was given and the mare did not abort, and on mares which were not given progesterone therapy but which did lose their pregnancy. Unfortunately there have been no properly conducted trials using sufficient numbers and containing matched controls, that is, mares given progesterone and those not given progesterone being of identical status with regard to their likelihood of aborting.

It requires 2000 mg of progesterone injected every six days to maintain levels of 4 ng/ml in a mare's bloodstream. This dose rate is far in excess of what is generally administered (and often claimed to be successful). This is a further argument used by those who believe that progesterone therapy is ineffective or, at least, has unproven efficacy.

Progesterone, if given daily, suppresses the output of pituitary hormones (see

p. 385) and may be used as a treatment of anoestrus. In these instances the pituitary hormones (FSH and LH – see below) are being produced in insufficient quantity by the pituitary to develop follicles which ovulate. Therefore these individuals are not cycling (see p. 382). The progesterone, by preventing release of FSH and LH from the pituitary, ensures that these hormones are stored. When the progesterone therapy is stopped, the hormones are released in substantial quantities and thus start the mare cycling. This therapy requires daily injections. More recently, the availability of a powerful progesterone-type drug (allyl trenbolone) which can be fed or administered by mouth daily has simplified the approach. However, this therapy will only work in certain individuals that are truly anoestrus and is more likely to be successful if spring follicles are present in the ovaries. The treatment should therefore be given only on veterinary advice, otherwise there may be disappointment and waste of costly drugs.

Oestrogens   Oestrogens are hormones secreted by the lining of the follicles in the ovaries. They are also formed by the placenta from special substances produced by the ovaries of the foetus. They enter the mare's bloodstream and are excreted from her body in the urine. They can be used, therefore, as a means of pregnancy diagnosis from about 120 days of pregnancy until full term. This test is named Cuboni after the scientist who developed the means of analysis.

Oestrogens is a collective term for substances which have varying degrees of activity: oestradiol, oestrone sulphate and oestrone. In the pregnant mare there are two other substances, equenin and equilinin, which are unique to the horse family.

Oestrogens are responsible for signs of heat (oestrus) and for feminine characteristics, and they are essential for the growth and wellbeing of the foetus. At birth they make the uterus more susceptible to the action of oxytocin and prostaglandins, which cause the muscular contractions of uterus.

Various synthetic compounds are available for therapy, the most well known of which is stilboestrol; another that is often employed is oestradiol benzoate. Oestrogens are used to accentuate signs of heat in mares which, although technically in a state of oestrus, may not otherwise accept the stallion.

They are also used as an adjunct to therapy in infections of the uterus in that they improve the blood supply to the mucosal lining and mobilize the action of the white cells (leucocytes) which play a part in the defence against infection.

They may also be used as an adjunct to oxytocin therapy and also at the time of induced foaling in order to soften and relax the cervix.

Therapy should always be applied under veterinary supervision because oestrogen therapy can have adverse side effects if not used at a suitable dosage rate or for appropriate conditions in any particular individual.

Testosterone	Testosterone is the male sex hormone. It is secreted by the testes and is responsible for male sexual characteristics. Levels rise when mares are teased or become sexually excited. It is also responsible for engorgement of the penis with blood and the sexual quality or strength known as libido, in which the male mounts the mare and ejaculates.

Testosterone has an anabolic effect, that is, it promotes the development of muscle and the retention of nitrogen in the body. There are similar steroid substances, known as anabolic steroids, which have a similar effect but without the obvious masculinizing features. For this purpose they are nowadays usually employed in preference to testosterone. They may be used because of their supposed benefit on performance but are consequently banned under Jockey Club Rules for racehorses.

Testosterone may be administered to stallions and young colts with poor libido. However, any beneficial effect is temporary and the hormone may, if used over a long period, have a counter-productive effect because it suppresses the individual's own output of testosterone. The use of LH (see below) is therefore preferred.

Cortisone	Cortisone is produced by the cortex (outer lining) of the adrenal gland. There are a number of related compounds, some naturally and some synthetically produced. Cortisol (hydrocortisone) is a compound released naturally; cortisone and hydrocortisone are also produced synthetically, as are dexamethasone and betamethasone.

Cortisone stimulates metabolism and is a hormone which prepares for and sustains the individual in athletic performance. It is released when the trophic hormone ACTH is secreted by the pituitary. This is in response to fright or to meet the need for exertion and exercise. High levels in the blood occur when a foal is attempting to get to its feet for the first time. The exception is premature foals, which do not have the ability to secrete cortisone, although they are able to achieve high levels of ACTH; the adrenal cortex in premature foals is unresponsive to the action of ACTH.

Preparations of cortisone are used in therapy in order to enhance the body's response to inflammation and to counter the effects of shock. In general terms cortisone reduces pain and swelling. It is therefore an adjunct to treatment of inflammation due to trauma and, to a lesser extent, of infection.

The disadvantage of therapy in the presence of infection is that cortisone also reduces the response of the inflammatory process that is necessary in countering infection by bacteria. Cortisone may be used in joints and has a dramatic effect on relieving pain and promoting function. Unfortunately it also injures the joint surface and is no longer commonly used in the treatment of damaged joints in racehorses. In the control of inflammation the non-steroidal anti-inflammatory drugs (NSAID) such as phenylbutazone are usually preferred.

Follicle-stimulating hormone (FSH)   FSH is produced by the pituitary and stimulates the growth of follicles in the ovary and the secretion of oestrogen. It is also present in pregnant mare's blood from day 40 to about day 120, as pregnant mare's serum gonadotrophin (PMSG) (equine chorionic gonadotrophin or eCG), which is produced by cells in the lining of the mare's uterus (see below). FSH itself is not available as such, largely because it has not yet been synthesized artificially; its only source is the mare's pituitary. Drug therapy depends on the use of releasing factors, such as GnRH (see below).

Luteinizing hormone (LH)   LH is secreted by the pituitary gland and causes follicles in the ovary to ovulate. It subsequently promotes the formation of a yellow body in the ovary which secr~tes progesterone.

LH is produced by the placenta in pregnant women and excreted in urine. Pregnant women's urine can be purified and a drug extracted which contains a substance that acts in a manner similar to LH. This substance is known as human chorionic gonadotrophin (hCG). It is used extensively to cause ovulation in mares which are in oestrus and possess a mature follicle in the ovary. It is claimed to cause ovulation within forty-eight hours of administration.

The hormone is responsible for causing the interstitial cells of the testis to secrete testosterone. It may be used to improve the libido of stallions and young colts. This is a preferable therapy to the use of testosterone itself (see above) because it does not suppress the colt's own output of testosterone or LH.

Pregnant mare's serum gonadotrophin (PMSG)   As already indicated, PMSG contains both FSH and LH. It has been more recently termed equine chorionic gonadotrophin (eCG). The name PMSG is derived from the fact that the hormone is present in large quantities in the bloodstream of pregnant mares from day 40 to about day 120. The term eCG refers to the fact that its source is from cells that originate in the placenta (chorion) of mares.

Because it is present in mares' blood it has been used as the basis of a pregnancy test. Its function in the mare is not clearly established but it is thought to be involved in the protection of the foetus against the immune response which would otherwise be mounted by the mare's uterus. It may also be responsible for causing follicles to ovulate in the ovary and for the maintenance of the yellow bodies of pregnancy.

During the last decade a major advance in our understanding of this hormone was provided by the work of Dr Allen and his colleagues in Cambridge. They showed that the hormone was actually produced by cells that migrated from the developing placenta on the 37th day after conception. At this time the placenta possesses a girdle of cells which comes into contact with the wall of the uterus at the junction of the horn and body (see p. 387). These cells transfer from the placenta and burrow into the wall of the uterus. The girdle thus forms rings of tissue known as the endometrial cups. Here they produce PMSG in large quantities. This forms a sticky secretion between the placenta and the uterine wall and is also absorbed into the mare's bloodstream.

After about 60 days (i.e. about 100 days of pregnancy) the mare mounts an immunological rejection of the cells and they cease to function. One must presume that by this time their function in maintaining pregnancy is at an end. This coincides, of course, with the cessation of activity in the mare's ovaries, and these become quiescent from this time until the foal is ready to be delivered.

PMSG may be harvested from the mare's blood and is available commercially as a drug. It is used extensively in promoting follicular development in sheep and cattle and even in women. However, it is a curious and somewhat frustrating phenomenon that the drug does not have any effect on mares' ovaries. The reason for this is not clear, but it is probably because the ovaries of non-pregnant mares are physiologically resistant to its action, having been exposed to its activity during foetal life.

In order to stimulate mares' ovaries we use GnRH (gonadotrophin releasing hormone).

Gonadotrophin releasing hormone (GnRH)   As described below, there are a number of hormones released in the brain which reach the pituitary and cause this gland to release specific hormones. Thus there is a releasing hormone – gonadotrophin releasing hormone or GnRH – for FSH and LH.

GnRH is available commercially in a synthetic form and has been used successfully for inducing oestrus cycles. However, it must be administered in pulsatile (i.e. several) rather than bolus (single) doses. It is therefore a drug which must be used under strict veterinary control.

Other hormones
Insulin, which regulates levels of sugar (carbohydrate) in the blood, may be used in cases of hyperlipaemia (see p. 57) in conjunction with glucose infusions. Otherwise this hormone does not form part of the equine veterinarian's armoury. Horses rarely suffer from diabetes mellitus (see p. 56) and treatment is not economic or justified on humane grounds.

Adrenaline is a hormone produced by the adrenal medulla (the central part of the gland surrounded by the cortex), which is part of the sympathetic nervous system (see p. 158). It may be used by veterinarians in tests but is not usually used in therapy. It was once used as a stimulant in cases of cardiac arrest but has now been replaced by drugs such as doxapram hydrochloride.

THE NEUROENDOCRINE SYSTEM

The two systems, nerves (pp. 154-60) and hormones (pp. 160-9), which regulate body functions have been known for a very long time. They may be likened to messengers carrying messages of control and feeling around the body. However, in recent years a newer concept has developed of a third system combining both nerves and hormones. This is called the neuroendocrine system.

This system provides a link between the environment and the mechanisms of internal control represented by the hormonal (endocrine) system. For example, it is the brain – the centre of the nervous system – that receives information about the length of daylight to which a mare is subjected. This information comes from the eye and is relayed to the nervous system by way of the pineal body, a collection of special cells within the brain.

The messages about daylight pass from the back of the eye (the retina), along the optic nerves, enter the brain, and cause the pituitary gland to release follicle-stimulating hormone (FSH) and luteinizing hormone (LH). It is these hormones which control sexual activity (see above). The information about increasing daylight hours in spring and summer is thus translated through the nervous system to the hormonal system, which in turn dictates whether or not a mare undergoes oestrus cycles.

Similarly, messages about changes in the outside world, e.g. hot, cold, danger, etc., are conveyed through the nervous system to the hormonal system and evoke an appropriate response.

We have seen that the basic unit of the nervous system is the neuron, i.e. the nerve cell from which nerve fibres originate. The basic unit of the endocrine or hormonal system is the secretory cell, that is, a cell which produces hormones in the hormonal glands.

The concept of the neuroendocrine system is that nerve and hormonal cells have much in common and that nerve cells, as well as possessing the capacity to transmit nerve impulses, can also secrete hormones.

What causes the pituitary gland to release ACTH?
Let us look at some examples to illustrate the subject, starting with ACTH, the hormone which stimulates the production of cortisone (see p. 166). If we address the question as to what causes the release of ACTH, we come to the answer that it is the production of another hormone secreted by nerve cells in the brain. This hormone is one of several releasing hormones (sometimes called releasing factors) which are secreted by cells in that part of the brain known as the hypothalamus.

There are corresponding releasing hormones for other hormones, e.g. for LH, FSH, prolactin, thyroid-stimulating hormone (TSH) and growth hormone (GH).

How do nerves produce hormones?

Nerve cells (neurons) form their own hormone product in the cell under the direction of their ribonucleic acid (RNA), which forms part of the genetic system of the cell. The product is packaged as granules and transported along nerve fibre to its end or terminal. Here the granules are released.

In the case of pituitary hormones, releasing factors are discharged into a special blood supply to the pituitary, thereby regulating the secretion of this gland. The distance is small but the secretion is termed a neurohormone because it enters the circulating blood.

However, similar secretions produced by cells at terminals cross to other cells and have a regulatory impact on these cells. These are termed neuromodulators, i.e. they modulate the activity of other nerve cells.

A third type of secretion from nerves of the hormone system is the hormones released by brain cells connected directly by nerve fibres to the posterior part of the pituitary gland. These cells release the hormones oxytocin (which causes the uterus to contract) and vasopressin (which raises the blood pressure by causing the blood vessels to constrict). Vasopressin is also referred to as antidiuretic hormone because it reduces the output of water from the kidneys.

These two hormones, oxytocin and vasopressin, are synthesized as prohormones in the neurons (nerve cells) in special parts of the brain. They are transported in vesicles (fluid bubbles) through the nerves' fibres to the pituitary, where they are stored. They are then released as hormones when the cells in which they are stored realise the need.

How does the neuroendocrine system function?

To understand how the neuroendocrine system functions, let us consider the example of vasopressin. The cells containing vasopressin are sensitive to changes in the osmolality of blood. Blood osmolality is the measurement of its concentration or thickness. Thus, if blood becomes too thick, antidiuretic hormone is released in order to prevent the kidneys from releasing water. In consequence the urine becomes concentrated and water is retained in the body. The blood is diluted sufficiently for the pituitary to recognise that it is now normal and the output of antidiuretic hormone is therefore decreased.

Similarly, when a foal goes to the udder of a mare, there is a nervous reflex transmitted from nerve endings in the udder. These are conducted through the spinal cord and up to the brain, where they release the hormone oxytocin. This causes contraction of the very small muscles in the udder, thereby releasing milk into the nipple for the foal to suck. This is known as the milk let-down reflex.

Oxytocin is also present when the uterus contracts during first-stage labour. This is the reason why there is a let down of milk at the time of foaling. Sometimes this happens before a mare foals. The stimulus for oxytocin release in these circumstances comes from the placenta and the foetus.

Why do we need to understand the neuroendocrine system?
The subject of endocrinology is complex, but it is necessary to advance the understanding of the subject so that those who are responsible for horses can adjust managerial and veterinary practice. In the past it has been necessary to comprehend the action of hormones such as FSH, LH and prostaglandins in order to grasp the logic of the control of the mare's oestrous cycle. The discovery of each of these hormones, at some time, has been a new development in our knowledge. It is only by such an understanding that we can extend the logic of hormone therapy and thereby our management of barren and foaling mares.

Peptides
Now let us take a further step in this story. I have already indicated that originally the nervous and the endocrine systems were considered to be entirely separate, each made up of their specific cells releasing different messengers.

Curiously, the first indication that this was not really the case came as long ago as 1931, when a discovery was made in horses that a substance known as Substance P could be extracted from the equine brain and gut. It was supposed, at the time, to come from the central nervous system and from cells lining the alimentary tract. It was not until the 1970s that this subject was advanced further. The reason for its advance was that techniques were developed for identifying Substance P in the tissues. This substance was identified as a peptide.

Peptides are substances of low molecular weight composed of organic acids (amino acids). It has been shown that Substance P occurs in nerves in the gut and also in a large number of organs.

The names given to these peptides are technical and some are included here only because the reader may hear them mentioned or read about them and will then be able to place them accordingly. They are vasoactive inhibitory protein (VIP), somatostatin, gastrin, motilin, renin, glucagon and gastrin.

Regulatory peptides are secreted by cells spread throughout the body. It is for this reason that they have not been previously studied in detail, as have organ systems such as nerves and hormone glands. These are so much easier to investigate because they can be removed experimentally to observe the effect. When the secretory cells are spread throughout the body this approach is not possible.

The discovery of these peptide hormones has given rise to the term 'peptidergic nervous system'. Changes in this system have been shown recently to be present in human gut disease and also in the condition of grass sickness (see p. 48). This is a new and expanding subject and we can expect some exciting developments in future knowledge about diseases affecting the gut, kidneys and other organs.

Another group of peptides which has come to light recently are the encephalins and endorphins, sometimes known as 'the brain's own opiates'. These powerful analgesics, similar in structure to the commonly used drugs pethidine and morphine, are secreted by the neuroendocrine cells in the brain in response to severe pain or stress. It is now believed that the sedating effect of applying a nose twitch to a horse occurs because of a release of these opiate-like drugs in response to the pain produced by this action.

9
THE OPTIC SYSTEM

The horse is a creature of the wide open spaces. With its few relatives, it has evolved on the great plains of the world. To escape natural enemies it has acquired the ability to move at great speed. In order to do so, it must be able to recognise its predators. To this end the horse has developed very sophisticated senses of sight, hearing and smell. In this chapter we are concerned with sight.

The eye

The eye of the horse is set high up on the head, towards the side rather than the front. The head in turn is on a long and flexible neck. These two attributes give remarkable all-round vision, even when the horse has its head down to graze. This vision can be both monocular or binocular, that is, the horse can see the same object with both eyes when looking forwards, but also can view a completely different picture on either side with each eye. This vision extends to behind the horse, and it has only to move its head slightly to achieve a complete circle of sight.

The eye lies in the orbit, a cavity formed in the skull. This cavity is encircled by bone which is of particular prominence and strength in front of and above the eye; here the bone is structured into a rigid arch which is called the supraorbital process. Forward of the eye lie the nasal bones and a bony prominence called the facial crest, and below the eye is the mass of the jaw muscles. These complete a circle which is very effective in protecting the eye from injury. Further to this, the orbit contains a large pad of fat. This lies behind the eye and can be felt from behind and above the supraorbital process, where there is an easily seen depression. This fat acts as a flexible, mobile cushion which allows any direct blows that reach the eyeball to be absorbed to a great extent. These, with the facts that the head is on a long neck and the horse has excellent reflexes, explains why the eyes are seldom injured.

Figure 1
Location of the eye

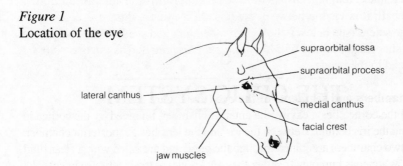

supraorbital fossa

supraorbital process

lateral canthus

medial canthus

facial crest

jaw muscles

The eyelids

The horse possesses two external eyelids and a third, inner, eyelid which arises from the medial canthus of the eye, that is, the lower inner angle between the external eyelids. This third eyelid is formed of mucous membrane and cartilage, and assists in the lubrication of the outside of the eyeball by spreading tears over the surface.

The external eyelids are composed of a sheet of cartilage covered with skin on the outside and the conjunctiva inside. The upper eyelid is the most movable, opening and closing the eye to the greater degree.

At the border, where the skin from the outside meets the membrane from the inside, are the eyelashes – the greater number being on the upper lid.

The tear ducts

The tears, which keep the eye moist, are secreted by the lacrimal gland, which lies beneath the supraorbital process. These tears are discharged onto the surface of the eye and are then collected into the two tear ducts in the inner corner of the eye. The tear ducts unite to run down beneath the bone and cartilage of the nasal bones, forming the naso-lacrimal duct, which eventually discharges on the floor of the nostrils. These openings are easily seen by looking into the nasal aperture while holding the nostril open with the finger. Should these ducts become obstructed, tears overflow the lower eyelid, run down the face and cause scalding with loss of hair.

The conjunctiva

This is a thin, pink, moist, mucous membrane on the inside of the eyelids and covering the third eyelid. From the inside of the eyelids it is turned back to lie over the surface of the eyeball, where it becomes the bulbar conjunctiva. This covers the front of the eye as a layer of transparent cells forming part of the cornea.

The cornea

This is a thick, tough, transparent tissue which forms the anterior portion of the eyeball; it is visible between the lids. At its outer edges it is continuous with the sclera (see below), the junction being called the limbus. The cornea is egg-shaped in outline, with the long axis running across the eye with the broad end to the inside.

The chambers and segments of the eye (See Figure 3)

Behind the cornea lies a cavity, the anterior chamber, bounded by the cornea in front and the iris behind. Between the iris and the lens lies the posterior chamber. These two chambers are joined through the pupil and are filled with a clear fluid known as aqueous humour. Together they are known as the anterior segment. The space between the lens and the retina is the posterior segment, and this is filled with a transparent, jelly-like material known as vitreous humour.

The iris is a pigmented muscular diaphragm situated in front of the lens and visible through the cornea. It contains a central aperture called the pupil, which varies in size and controls the amount of light entering the eye.

When light is bright, the pupil contracts to become narrow and elliptical, with its greatest length in the transverse (crosswise) direction. When dull, the pupil dilates to become more or less round.

The edges of the iris forming the pupil are not regular in outline, but are interrupted by pigmented projections called corpora nigra. These are much larger on the upper edge and may partially occlude (block) the pupil when it is contracted.

The lens is a transparent body, circular in outline, but biconvex when viewed from the side. The front surface is less curved than the back and is in partial contact with the iris. Around the circular periphery of the lens is a series of fine fibres which form the suspensory ligament of the lens, and which attach to the inner surface of the eyeball. The substance of the lens is made up of an outer elastic membrane called the capsule, which encloses layers of transparent tissue centred round a nucleus. These layers can sometimes be seen during examination, not unlike the structure of an onion.

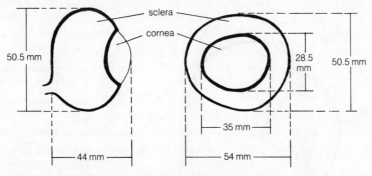

Figure 2   The dimensions of the eyeball and the cornea

The wall of the eyeball

This is made up of three basic layers: the sclera, the choroid and the retina. In the front of the eye the cornea fits into the sclera like a watchglass into a watch.

The sclera is the outside layer of the wall and is often known as the white of the eye as it is the portion showing between the eyelids. It extends all round the eyeball and is formed of thick, tough, white tissue. It gives shape and strength to the eyeball and is lined by the choroid layer.

The inner surface of the sclera, which is nearest to the lens and the iris, carries a pigmented thickening called the ciliary body. From this arise the iris and the lens attachments. It has a muscular component which, when it contracts or slackens, alters the convexity of the lens and thus the horse's ability to focus on objects at different distances. This mechanism is called accommodation.

The choroid is a thin membrane which lies between the sclera and the retina. In general it is pigmented and its inner surface is closely bound to the retina. It extends from the optic nerve to the ciliary body.

The retina is a thin, light-sensitive membrane lying on the inner surface of the choroid; it is in contact with the vitreous humour on its inside surface. It is complex in structure, containing a sophisticated arrangement of nerves and blood vessels. It is this part of the eye which receives the images of the objects seen by the horse and passes them on to the brain via the optic nerve.

The optic nerve

The optic nerve enters the back of the eye, passing through the sclera and the choroid and spreading out filaments to form the retina. It lies below the centre of the back of the eye and towards the outer side.

The anatomy of vision

The eye may be considered similar to a camera, by which small and inverted images are formed on the retina. Rays of light enter the eyeball and are bent by the cornea and lens to converge on the retina. This is called focusing. The lens shape can be altered, as described above, to make rays from objects

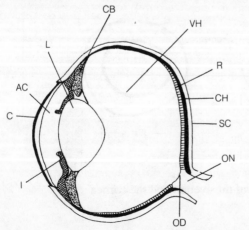

C – cornea
AC – anterior chamber
I – iris
L – lens
CB – ciliary body
VH – vitreous humour
OD – optic disc
R – retina
CH – choroid
SC – sclera
ON – optic nerve

Figure 3
Cross-section of the eye

located at varying distances focus on the retina. The amount of light entering the eye is regulated by the eyelids and the pupil. Light reaching the retina is transmitted as nervous impulses to the optic nerve and then to the brain, where they are translated into visual images.

Examination of the eye

This should be done in two parts. The first – the examination of the outside of the eye – should be done in bright light, preferably outside but otherwise inside with good lighting. The purpose of this is to establish the presence of obvious abnormalities such as tumours, injured eyelids, blocked tear ducts, discrepancies in the size of the eye, and the ability of the pupil to contract in bright light. Infections and injuries to the conjunctiva can be seen at this stage, but the eyelids may have to be opened with the fingers to obtain the best results. To make this examination, place the tips of the thumb and index finger closely together. Apply the tips, held together in this way to the eyelids, which will close when approached by the fingertips. See that the tip of the thumb rests on the lower lid near its margin, and the tip of the index finger on the upper lid. Press gently upon them and slowly draw apart the thumb and finger. This will separate and partly invert the eyelids, thus exposing the conjunctiva to view. Injuries to the cornea are often best seen in bright light.

The second part of the examination is done in the stable with a good pen torch and ophthalmoscope. This may reveal conditions, many of which were previously unknown and which are difficult to interpret; therefore the examination should only be carried out by a veterinarian. The horse should be stood quietly in the dark for several minutes before the examination takes place. The torch can be used to examine the surface of the eye, iris, pupil and anterior chamber, but the inside of the eye can only be examined with an ophthalmoscope, which enables the operator to focus on any part of the interior.

Sometimes, when the eye has a painful condition, the only way that the eye can be properly examined is for the veterinarian to use local anaesthetic to relieve the pain and other drugs to open the pupil, so that the interior of the eye can be seen.

When making a general examination of the eye the vet will note any growth, lumps or wounds to the outside of the eye and its associated structures and whether there is any discharge, either watery or purulent, which may run down the face. The vet observes the eyelids, whether they are free and properly open or closed or partly closed in spasm. The size of the eyeball can be estimated at this stage – sometimes one eye is smaller or deeper in its socket than the other. Some conditions of the head give a droop to the upper eyelid and the horse is unable to lift it in order to open the eye.

The conjunctiva should be pink and moist – not an angry, inflamed deep red colour – with no discharge, and no swelling or puffiness.

The surface of the cornea should be moist, bright and perfectly transparent. It should be free from grey or white spots or streaks or larger opacities, and should not have blood vessels or ulcers present.

The pupil should be regular in outline, and dilate in the dark and contract in bright light. The pupils of both eyes should behave similarly at all times and in all conditions of light.

There should be no deposits in the anterior chamber of the eye, and no strands of fibrous material or adhesions between the back of the cornea and the iris. The lens should be seen through the pupil only as a grey-blue area – cataracts can sometimes be seen as a white area filling the pupil. Occasionally, in certain lighting conditions, a bright fluorescent reflection is seen from the eye. This is a reflection from the back of the eye and is quite normal.

Conditions of the Eye

Some conditions are easily seen by the horse owner, but others can only be diagnosed by a veterinarian, who should always be consulted in any case of doubt or difficulty.

TUMOURS

There are two main tumours affecting the eyelids of the horse. Sarcoids (see Chapter 42) are raised, cauliflower-like growths arising usually above and to the side of the eye. These are difficult to treat or remove, and can become a nuisance to the horse because they tend to ulcerate and invade the eyelids. Carcinomas (see Chapter 42) occur on the eyelid margins or on the third eyelid. These cause profuse discharge to accumulate, make the eye very sore, and have to be removed surgically.

INJURIES TO THE EYELIDS

These are quite common: the eyelids may be torn by protruding nails, by the horse blundering into objects in the dark or by galloping into hedges or fences. They may become bruised or abraded from external injury such as a blow or a fall.

Whenever an eyelid is torn, seek advice immediately so that it can be repaired surgically. Repair must be carried out, as far as possible, so that healing takes place without contraction or distortion of the eyelid aperture.

ENTROPION

This condition occurs mostly in newborn foals. The eyelids, or one of them, are turned inwards so that the eyelashes and hairs on the outside are in contact with the cornea. This is very irritant, causing pain and discharge, and, if left unattended, the cornea may become inflamed or even ulcerated. Sometimes this condition can be overcome by repeatedly drawing the lid back and uncurling it from the surface of the eye. Often this is enough to make the eyelid regain its correct position, but if not the veterinarian should he asked to attend. He or she will suture the lid in place, or even remove an elliptical piece of skin at the lid margin so that when this heals it will cause sufficient contraction to keep the lid from curling inwards.

CONJUNCTIVITIS

Conjunctivitis is the name given to inflammation of the conjunctival membrane. It is caused by infection or irritation from foreign bodies or substances. It is recognized by a marked congestion of the membranes, which are swollen and turn an angry colour. There is discharge from the eye, often with pus present, and pain, which makes the horse unwilling to have the eye examined.

Treatment is best left to the veterinarian and will depend on the cause. If due to infection, an antibiotic ointment will be prescribed. Any foreign body, such as an oat husk or barley awn, will have to be removed with the help of local anaesthesia. As a first-aid measure, the eye can be washed with lukewarm saline solution made up by adding a teaspoonful of common salt to a pint of tepid water.

BLOCKED LACRIMAL DUCTS

These are indicated by the constant overflow of tears which run down the face. This discharge is clear and watery. The condition requires veterinary attention.

KERATITIS

Keratitis denotes inflammation of the cornea. It is a relatively common condition and may arise from conjunctivitis (see above) or may be due to direct injury or infection. The cornea is very sensitive and when it suffers from inflammatory changes the eyelids are always tightly closed, there is evidence of marked pain and a discharge of tears. This discharge may progress to become purulent after a day or two.

In mild cases the keratitis can settle down to a chronic state. This is when the eye, if examined closely in the light, has grey patches spread across the cornea. These are not always easily seen, but reduce the normal transparent lustre of the cornea and therefore impair vision.

In more severe and acute cases keratitis progresses until the whole of the cornea goes a grey-white colour and often has a fringe of blood vessels growing in from the edges. These appear like twigs and are an attempt by the body to speed the healing of the condition.

Sometimes the eyelids are so tightly closed that not much of this can be seen until local anaesthetic is introduced between the lids. When this is done, if the cause of the condition is injury rather than infection, a ragged ulcer will be seen on the front of the eye. Without proper treatment this can progress until the cornea is perforated and the aqueous humour escapes. Further to that, the iris may be drawn forward inside the eye to stick to the edges of the wound, or the eyeball may steadily collapse, with resultant loss of function and blindness.

If the ulcer is treated adequately, blood vessels will grow across it and it will slowly heal and the pain become less. The horse is best kept in a dark box at this time as light irritates the eye. When healing is complete often there is a small grey scar left on the cornea which can be seen when the eye is inspected closely.

EQUINE RECURRENT UVEITIS (PERIODIC OPHTHALMIA, MOON BLINDNESS)

This is a fairly uncommon disease, characterised by episodes of acute pain and inflammation in usually one or sometimes both eyes. There is apparent recovery after treatment, but the condition will commence again, sometimes in the same and sometimes in the other eye. The interval between these attacks can be as short as a few weeks – hence the old name periodic ophthalmia – or as long as years. There are a few cases in which there has been no apparent recurrence.

The signs of this disease are acute pain with the eye closed, discharge, and an unwillingness to expose the eye to light. There is no apparent reason for these symptoms. Horse owners often say that their animal has had a blow to the eye, but on close questioning it will he found that this is supposition and not fact. If the eye is examined at this stage, the cornea is cloudy and the anterior chamber has a deposit of white, or sometimes red, blood cells collecting in the bottom half. Detailed examination reveals a contracted pupil and deposits of inflammatory debris on the front of the lens. The microfilariae of *Onchocerca cervicalis* have been found in the eye and may be a cause (see p. 540).

After several days of treatment the cornea starts to clear, and the deposit in the anterior chamber becomes a denser white, then gradually becomes absorbed and eventually disappears. Sometimes the pupil will open and the eye return to normal, but occasionally it remains contracted and becomes stuck to the front of the lens, with an irregular and ragged outline instead of the normal smooth oval shape. The lens usually retains some of the debris on the front and examination with the ophthalmoscope often reveals a similar deposit at the back.

Subsequent attacks are similar, but after each one the residual damage to the eye is increased; it may shrink in size, and ultimately the horse is blind in one or both eyes.

Proper treatment modifies the course of the disease, especially if commenced early, and prolongs the horse's usefulness. It does not prevent recurrence and horses that have had one attack will almost invariably have another at some stage. It is important, therefore, to recognise the condition so that treatment can be started as soon as possible.

CATARACT

Any opacity of the lens or its capsule is by definition a cataract. These interfere with the passage of light, the degree of interference ranging from slight to complete obstruction. Therefore the horse's sight may be only slightly affected or it may be completely blind.

Cataracts may be developmental or degenerative. Developmental cataracts result from defects in the eye from birth, and these can vary from a small opacity in the middle of the lens to a total diffuse condition which involves the whole structure and in which the pupil appears as if it were filled with a white marble. It is unusual for congenital cataracts to be progressive.

Degenerative cataracts occur as a result of disease, injury or increasing age. These can be of any size or shape, although they usually radiate in lines out from a central focus, sometimes with a cobweb-like appearance. Often these progress to total dense cataracts and resultant blindness.

The detailed diagnosis of a cataract can only be done with an ophthalmoscope. In some horses layers of the lens reflect the light back to the observer's eye, which gives a fictitious appearance of opacity. Only the vet can really diagnose these cases. There is no effective treatment for cataract.

BLINDNESS

There are several conditions occurring at the back of the eye of which the outcome is usually a serious affect on vision. Such conditions are **inflammation and separation of the retina, degeneration of the vitreous humour** and **optic nerve atrophy**. These are only diagnosable by the veterinarian using specialist equipment. The horse owner will, however, realise that something is amiss with his animal and ask for advice. It is, therefore, necessary to have a working knowledge of how to assess vision.

First, the horse's behaviour and performance will be altered. The owner will notice apprehension when a normally placid horse is subjected to unexpected situations and challenges, such as being startled at the sudden appearance of traffic or not seeing objects that it normally should. If the animal is a performance horse, such as a showjumper, it may see objects on one circle but not on the other. This would indicate a one-sided eye defect. It may not pick up an obstacle which it normally had no difficulty with and so suddenly refuse to take a jump.

A menace response test can be tried: the horse is approached on each side and is suddenly lunged at with an open flat hand towards the eye. Care should be taken not to get too close, so as not to touch the eye or cause air currents that may be felt by the horse. A normal animal will blink and withdraw the head.

An obstacle course can be arranged. The horse is led quietly around an area with which it is familiar and, after one or two circuits, an upturned bucket or horizontal pole is put in its path. Brightly painted cones or drums, which the animal should have no difficulty in seeing, can be used. Obviously if it fails to negotiate them, defects in vision must be suspected.

Retinal degeneration is when patches of the back of the eye become ineffective and the images of the objects the horse is seeing are therefore incomplete. This can sometimes be more disturbing to a horse than complete blindness, which it may learn to accept.

The vitreous humour sometimes becomes affected with strands of inflammatory debris which float across the field of vision when the horse makes an eye movement. These can distort vision and disturb the horse by their sudden appearance.

The optic nerve may become injured or degenerate. This condition is called optic atrophy and results in complete and irreversible blindness.

CONGENITAL ABNORMALITIES

There are a number of rare congenital abnormalities which may be genetic in origin. These are listed in Chapter 46.

10
THE EAR

The ear consists of three parts – the outer, middle and inner ear – and is the organ of hearing. It is also of vital importance in maintaining balance; in particular the inner ear informs the brain of the position of the head.

Functional anatomy
The outer (external) car is what most of us are familiar with. It consists of an erect cartilaginous portion (pinna) which can be moved in all directions, enabling the horse to detect sounds from all sides. Each ear moves independently of the other. Thus a horse can scan the area for danger.

The pinna is attached to the head and at its base forms a delicately lined funnel which travels downwards and then makes a right-angled bend inwards until it meets the eardrum within the skull (Figure 1). The eardrum is a membrane which separates the outer from the middle ear and is connected to three small bones, the hammer (malleus), the anvil (incus) and the stirrup (stapes), so called because of their shape, which bridge the middle ear. The middle ear is lined by a mucous membrane and is connected to the pharynx (throat) by a tube (Eustachian tube) which allows equalisation of pressure between the middle ear and the atmosphere. The orifice into the pharynx is protected by cartilaginous flap which opens only during swallowing.

The horse has a remarkable structure called a guttural pouch which is a large outpouching of each Eustachian tube. These structures are peculiar to horses and donkeys (and a species of tree shrew) and consist of paired air sacs situated between the pharynx and the floor of the skull. These air sacs are closely associated with very important nerves and arteries, and these may be damaged by diseases affecting the guttural pouch (see Chapter 2).

The middle ear is separated from the inner ear by two membranous windows, one of which is attached to the stirrup-shaped bone, the stapes. Thus soundwaves reaching the eardrum are transmitted by the chain of small bones to the inner ear.

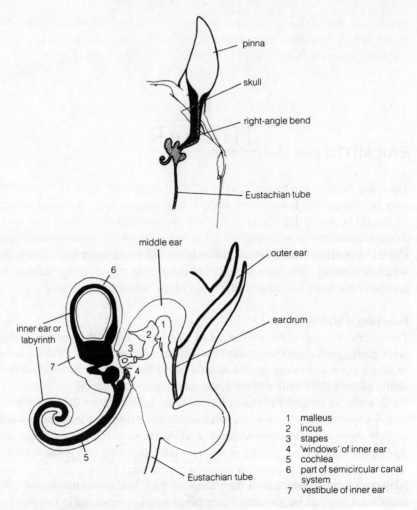

Figure 1   The external ear and its location in the skull
Figure 2   The internal ear middle ear

The inner ear consists of a series of membranous tubes which are filled with fluid called endolymph; many nerve endings are contained in the lining of the tubes. The inner ear is called the labyrinth because of its complex shape; it fits into cavities in the bone of the skull. The main cavity is called the vestibule. The complex anatomy of the inner ear can be simplified for descriptive purposes by considering it as two groups of tubular compartments. One, the cochlea, is somewhat like a snail's shell and is responsible for hearing. The other has three semicircular channels, each arranged at right angles to the rest. These semicircular canals are continuous with the main part of the inner ear or vestibule and thus share its endolymph circulation. It is by the movement of the fluid within these canals that positional changes of the head are relayed to the brain. Hearing occurs when the endolymph in the cochlea moves in response to waves transmitted via the small bones in the middle ear.

Conditions of the Ear

EAR MITES (see also p. 560)

Ear mites occur in horses and usually produce no clinical signs. However, they may be responsible for severe irritation, headshyness and an aural discharge (it should be noted that the normal horse ear contains thick, dark grey wax). Some affected horses will rub their ear or side of the head; rarely a haematoma (blood blister) is produced in the pinna as a result of such damage. Treatment with antiparasitic drugs is usually effective.

EAR CANAL INFECTION

Rarely infections may occur in the ear canals, often as a sequel to guttural pouch infections (see p. 54). An aural discharge and ear shyness are the usual clinical signs. If guttural pouch infection is the underlying reason for the aural discharge, there is often a concomitant nasal discharge and other signs.

TUMOURS

Malignant tumours of the pinna and canals of the external ear are rare, but when they occur they can be an extremely serious problem. Usually there is a visible growth and often a foul-smelling discharge which may be bloodstained; frequently such horses become extremely earshy. Much more commonly, however, small (often multiple) raised plaques of thickened white skin are visible on the inside of the pinna, but these do not produce clinical signs or require treatment. Other growths such as sarcoids (skin tumours) and dermoid cysts may develop in association with the ear. Usually these can be removed surgically.

DENTIGENOUS CYST

A discharging sinus at the base of the ear or from the edge of the pinna may be associated with a dentigenous cyst. This cyst is a congenital abnormality which may contain an aberrantly situated tooth and can be removed surgically.

NEURAL PARALYSIS

Damage to a branch of the facial nerve which controls movement of the external ear may result in paralysis of the ear, which can no longer be held in an erect position. This is usually associated with other signs of facial paralysis such as a drooping lower lip on the same side or the muzzle twisted away from the affected side.

SWOLLEN PAROTID GLAND

The parotid salivary gland is situated at the base of the ear and may occasionally become swollen when horses or ponies are at grass. Affected animals may look as if they are suffering from mumps. The cause is unknown but is usually considered to be an allergy. The condition spontaneously and rapidly resolves when the horse is brought indoors.

The parotid gland is also a common site for the development of a melanoma the black-pigmented tumours commonly seen in grey horses.

DEAFNESS

Little is known about deafness in the horse. Profound deafness of both ears is likely to be noticed, but it is difficult to recognise partial deafness or if only one ear is affected.

VERTIGO AND INCOORDINATION

Loss of balance (vertigo) and incoordination of the limbs may result from conditions affecting the inner ear. These fortunately are very rare in the horse. Some cases respond to corticosteroid therapy but in other cases no treatment is effective.

BLEEDING FROM THE EAR

Very rarely horses may bleed from the ear. This is usually caused by severe trauma, such as a fracture, to the skull but can also be caused by fungal infection of the guttural pouch (see p. 54).

The Musculoskeletal System

The musculoskeletal system derives its name from two features of the body concerned with form and movement. The skeleton comprises the bony scaffold to which muscle is attached. Without the skeletons, the body would have the flowing form of a jellyfish rather than the exact and circumscribed outline we recognise as a horse.

The skeleton is formed of bone, the hard substance of which individual bones are made. These individual bones form joints at one or both ends of their length. It is the joints which provide the supple nature of the skeleton and enable a horse to lie down, stand, trot, canter and gallop.

In the section that follows, chapters describe:

*   The anatomy of this system of bones and muscle;

*   The injuries and ailments that we recognise as stiffness, lameness and unsoundness;

*   Angular deformities of the limbs of foals;

*   Shoeing – the protection man gives the horse to prevent wear of the feet when it is being used for human purposes;

*   Some of the common problems of lameness and their possible causes, listed in tabular form.

11
LAMENESS: AN INTRODUCTION

Lameness is the abnormal movement and/or placement of a limb, due to pain and/or mechanical dysfunction. It is most readily assessed at walk and trot; only rarely will a horse appear lame at canter. Lameness may be sudden or gradual in onset and may affect one or more than one limb.

Normal paces

The normal horse takes equal-length strides with each forelimb and with each hind-limb and the feet are placed rhythmically to the ground in a definite sequence. At walk the sequence of foot falls is left hind, left fore, right hind, right fore and the rhythm is four-time. At trot the limbs are moved in a two-time rhythm in diagonal pairs, left hind and right fore together, followed by right hind and left fore together. Occasionally normal horses pace rather than trot, i.e. the left hind and the left fore move together, followed by the right hind

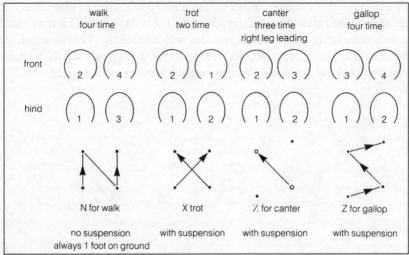

Figure 1   Sequence of limb placement

and right fore, in a two-time rhythm. The horse is said to be tracking up at either walk or trot if the hind foot is placed in or beyond the imprint of the forefoot on the same side.

Canter has a three-time rhythm. The sequence of footfalls for canter with the right foreleg leading is left hind followed by right hind and left fore together, and then the right fore. On a circle the horse usually canters with the inside foreleg leading. The sequence is reversed for left canter, i.e. right hind, left hind and right fore together, left fore. The horse is cantering on the wrong leg on a circle if the outside forelimb leads. If the horse changes the sequence of hind-limb movements while maintaining the correct lead in front it is said to be disunited. Some normal horses find it much more difficult to canter with one foreleg leading rather than the other and some tend to become disunited, especially if unbalanced.

Unlevelness
An alteration of the regular rhythmicity of a gait may occur if the horse is unbalanced, is hurrying or is finding a particular movement physically difficult, or it may reflect lameness. The term 'unlevelness' has been used to describe slight irregularities in rhythm. If there is consistent unlevelness, this probably reflects slight lameness. In the early stages of a lameness which is insidious in onset slight irregularities in rhythm may be detectable only when the horse is performing specific manoeuvres. With time these irregularities may become more obvious and frequent.

Gait abnormalities
Ideally the horse should move each leg straight, the left hind and left fore in one plane and the right hind and right fore in another plane. Many normal horses, with either good or faulty conformation, deviate one or more than one leg either to the inside or to the outside as the leg is advanced. This may result in the horse interfering, i.e. striking one leg with another leg. The horse brushes if it strikes the inside of one leg with the inside of the opposite leg. If the point of impact is above the mid-cannon region the horse is said to speedy-cut.

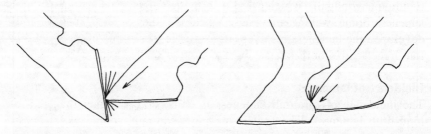

Figure 2   Forging   *Figure 3*   Overreach

A tread is an injury to the inside of the coronary band of one foot by the contralateral foot. Overreaching is the striking of the back of a forelimb with the toe of the hind foot on the same side and is usually due to asynchronous movement of the limbs because of tiredness, deep going or imbalance. Forging is the noise made by the striking of the hind shoe against the front shoe as the horse is trotting and occurs because the horse is tired or unbalanced or the hind feet are too long. Stumbling may be due to multiple causes including weakness, tiredness, unbalance, poor foot trimming, uneven ground and lameness. Some normal horses drag the toes of one or both hind limbs due to laziness, imbalance, overlong feet or tiredness, but toe dragging may also reflect lameness.

Deviations of limb flight of the forelimb occur more commonly than hind-limb gait abnormalities. However, some normal horses move very closely behind (plaiting), whereas others move very widely behind. When trotting in circles an unschooled or unfit horse will tend to cross the inside hind-limb under the body towards the outside forelimb, which makes the hindquarters tend to swing outwards. A well-schooled, balanced, fit horse is more able to flex the inside hind limb and advance it towards the inside forelimb. Many normal horses will appear stiffer when moving in circles to the left than to the right.

It is important to differentiate between gait abnormalities (variations of the normal) and lameness. In the early stages of insidious-onset lameness this may be difficult. In these circumstances it is helpful to know the horse in order to compare how it was with how it is now. This is particularly important in horses with problems which may affect both forelimbs (e.g. navicular syndrome) or both hind limbs (e.g. bone spavin). Initially these conditions cause a slight shortening of the stride or loss of freedom of stride without overt lameness being detectable.

Swellings and lameness

Although the onset of lameness may be associated with the development of an obvious swelling or an area of heat and pain, in many cases there are no detectable visible or palpable abnormalities. The fact that an area looks and feels normal does not preclude it from being the potential site of lameness. Many swellings, for example, distension of the digital flexor tendon sheath (tendinous windgall), which cause a cosmetic defect are unassociated with lameness. Some swellings may cause lameness as they develop, but when fully developed the lameness resolves (for example, periostitis of the second or fourth metacarpal or metatarsal bone, commonly called a splint).

Incidence of lameness

The incidence of forelimb lameness is considerably higher than that of hind-limb lameness. The foot is the most common source of lameness, especially in the forelimb. Lameness originating above the knee or hock is comparatively rare.

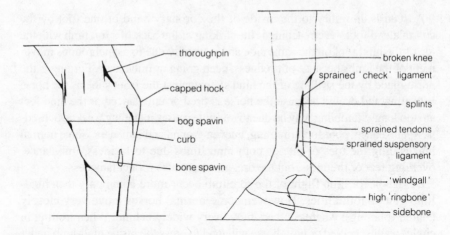

Figure 4   Sites of some common problems

The types of problem causing lameness vary considerably depending upon the age, breed, occupation and fitness of the horse. Chip fractures of the small bones of the knee occur not infrequently in Thoroughbred flat-race horses, but are otherwise an uncommon injury. Navicular syndrome is rarely seen in the young racehorse but is a common cause of lameness in the middle-aged riding horse.

Conformational abnormalities and the way in which a horse is trimmed and shod may predispose to lameness. The long-term prognosis for sustained recovery is influenced by the presence of conformational defects. Nevertheless, often it is not possible to detect an underlying cause of lameness.

There is minimal reliable information concerning heritability and lameness. There is a disproportionately high incidence of navicular syndrome in American Quarter horses. Osteochondrosis of the tibiotarsal joint of the hock has an unusually high incidence in the Shire horse. Intermittent upward fixation of the patella occurs not uncommonly in the Shetland pony. Thus there are strong indications that there is a heritability factor involved in some types of lameness in some breeds.

Lameness and performance
The fact that a horse is lame does not necessarily mean that the horse is unsuitable for work. Lameness implies pain or mechanical dysfunction. The level of pain which any horse can tolerate is extremely variable. Many horses are able to work satisfactorily despite low-grade lameness, especially hind-limb lameness. This depends not only on the temperament of the horse but also on its occupation. Lameness, however subtle, is unacceptable in the dressage horse. A jumping horse may be able to cope adequately with slight lameness. If a jumping horse starts to stop or to push off unevenly with the

hind legs as he takes off, these are indications that his performance is being compromised by the lameness.

Treatment

Treatment is usually aimed at returning the horse to full athletic function; an improvement without soundness is often unsatisfactory unless the horse is destined for breeding. Many kinds of lameness respond to rest. Enforcement of true rest in the horse is difficult. Turning a horse out is not true rest because the majority of horses are inclined to gallop sporadically. Despite this, for many lamenesses this type of rest is adequate. Sometimes it is necessary to confine the horse to a box; most horses adapt to this remarkably well although many owners find it psychologically unacceptable for the horse. Box rest can be combined with controlled exercise at walk and trot, which can provide valuable physiotherapy. With difficult horses it may be easier to ride the horse than lead it. Usually the weight of a rider will not affect the condition deleteriously.

Generally the earlier that a lameness is recognized and treatment is started the better. The quicker the horse starts to respond to treatment the more optimistic is the prognosis. Many slightly lame horses respond well to a few days' box rest and a true diagnosis is never achieved.

After an injury there is often pain, localised heat and swelling, and treatment is aimed at reducing these. Depending upon the age of the injury, local hot or cold treatment or alternating treatments may be beneficial. Local heat will increase the blood supply to the area. Cold treatment tends to reduce soft-tissue swelling, as do anti-inflammatory drugs such as corticosteroids. Many of the non-steroidal anti-inflammatory drugs, e.g. phenylbutazone, are also analgesics.

Local ultrasound treatment produces some heat and helps to dissipate soft-tissue swelling, but care must be taken to use the appropriate current strength and frequency to avoid causing additional damage.

Faradism is the use of an electrical current to produce controlled muscular contractions and is beneficial in the treatment of muscle strains. Electromagnetic therapy is in the embryo stages of development and, although it has potential, there are at present no clear guidelines for its use with horses. Firing is the application of red-hot iron to the skin. It has been widely used for the treatment of a variety of disorders. There is no scientific evidence to support its use, and the author considers it valueless and an unnecessary mutilation of the horse. Blisters are substances rubbed onto the skin which incite local inflammation of variable severity depending on the strength of the blister. The author considers that they have no beneficial effects.

Diagnosis of lameness

The aims of a lameness investigation are to identify the source or sources of pain and then the cause of pain. Only then can a rational treatment be offered and an accurate prognosis given. A systematic examination of the horse should ensure that nothing is overlooked. In many instances the detailed examination described below is unnecessary because the presence of heat, swelling and pain readily identify the site of the problem.

Examination at rest The horse is observed standing in the box or field. Most normal horses will rest intermittently one or both hind legs, perhaps favouring one more than the other. It is unusual for a horse not to bear full weight on both forelimbs. A horse with navicular syndrome or pain in the back part of a front foot may place one foot in front of the other, with or without the heel slightly raised and the fetlock slightly flexed (pointing). The horse may be observed to stack straw underneath the heels of the front feet. A pony or horse with laminitis of the forefeet tends to stand with the hind legs well underneath the body, with the forelimbs outstretched and its weight rocked back onto the heels.

The conformation of the horse is assessed because conformational abnormalities may have predisposed to the lameness and can influence the long-term prognosis. A racehorse with marked back-at-the-knee conformation is predisposed to small fractures of the carpal (knee) bones. The horse with a small foot relative to body size is predisposed to foot problems.

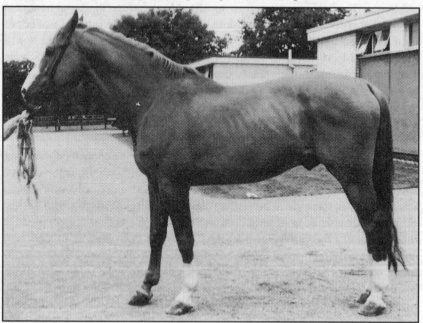

Figure 5   A horse pointing

The presence of any abnormal swellings is noted. With the horse standing squarely on a firm, level surface the symmetry of the muscles and bony structures is evaluated. Loss of muscle on one side compared to the other reflects disuse of the muscle but not necessarily injury to that area. For example, a degree of wastage of the muscles of one hindquarter may be associated with problems involving either the foot or the hip region.

The temperament of the horse should be assessed. A highly strung horse is likely to react to palpation much more than a stoical individual, making the identification of pain difficult.

The neck, back and legs are felt carefully, both weightbearing and non-weightbearing. The presence of swellings, unusual consistency of a structure (e.g. increased firmness of a digital flexor tendon), heat and pain on pressure are noted and compared with the contralateral leg. Each joint is flexed to find out whether it has a normal range of motion and if manipulation causes pain. The size and shape of the feet, the way in which they are trimmed and shod, and the wear of the shoes are assessed. Some normal horses have asymmetrically shaped front feet. If one foot is noticeably smaller than the other, it may reflect a current or a previous problem in the smaller foot, but may also be the result of lameness elsewhere in the leg. Hoof testers are used to apply pressure carefully all around the foot. Relatively gentle pressure is applied at first, and if there is no reaction the pressure is increased. A horse with a focus of infection in the foot will react to relatively light pressure applied to that area. Likewise pressure applied to a corn will cause pain. The sole and the hoof wall are also percussed.

Examination at exercise The horse is watched moving on a hard, level surface. On a hard surface the footfalls can be heard as well as seen. It is important that the horse should be moving freely without the head being restricted. It is necessary to watch the horse repeatedly, observing the whole horse first and then watching it from the front, side and back, focusing attention on the forelegs and then the hind legs. There are many things to observe in addition to detecting which is the lame leg. At walk the way in which each foot is placed to the ground should be noted. Is each foot placed to the ground squarely or does one side of the foot land first? If the horse lands consistently on one side of the foot first, this can predispose to problems or reflect a problem. A horse with navicular syndrome may place the foot to the ground toe first. The limb flight of the horse should be assessed. An abnormal limb flight such as swinging the leg outwards as it is advanced may be a reflection of lameness or a predisposing cause. The relative stride lengths of each forelimb and each hind limb should be compared. Subtle hind-limb lameness, when it is difficult to determine which is the lame leg, may be best assessed at walk. The affected leg may have a shorter stride length and bear weight for a shorter time, resulting in an irregular rhythm. The degree to which each fetlock sinks as the leg is weightbearing should be compared. If movement of a fetlock joint causes pain, then that joint may sink less than the contralateral joint. Turning the horse in small circles to right and left is useful to assess the flexibility of the neck and back and the ability to move each leg away from the body or towards the opposite leg. A horse with back pain may hold itself very stiffly when turned. A horse with a slight tendency to delayed release of the patella may hold the hindleg very stiffly and then move it rather jerkily. Pushing the horse backwards is also useful to detect odd limb placement as in shivering.

At trot the above observations should be repeated. In addition, the head carriage should be watched. If the horse has a forelimb lameness, then the head will nod as the sound leg hits the ground and will rise as the lame leg is lifted. If the lameness is severe, this will also be apparent at walk. The horse will land more heavily on the sound foreleg. The length of stride of the lame leg may be shorter than that of the sound leg. Watching the horse from the side and from the front is most useful. If the horse is lame on both forelegs, it may move with a short, pottery stride, occasionally taking lamer steps on one forelimb.

To determine which is the lame hind leg it is most useful to watch the horse from the side and from behind. The lame leg may have a shorter-length stride than the sound leg. This will result in an irregularity of rhythm which can be heard as well as seen. If the lameness involves the hock or upper hind limb, the horse may move the whole leg stiffly, resulting in a lower arc of flight of the foot, and perhaps may also drag the toe. The horse is unable to flex the hock without also flexing the stifle and hip joints. Therefore pain in any of these joints can cause similar stiff-limb flight and toe-drag. Hind-limb lameness will cause asymmetrical movement of the hindquarters. The hindquarter of the lame leg may appear both to rise and to sink more than the sound leg. This is best appreciated from behind. If the hind-limb lameness is severe, the horse may have a head nod as the forelimb on the same side as the lame leg hits the ground; this is because the lame leg is non-weightbearing. This can be confusing, which is why it is important to assess limb flight and stride length too.

Flexion tests Flexion tests can be useful. A joint is held partly flexed for approximately one minute and the horse is then trotted. Accentuation of lameness or production of lameness when the horse previously appeared sound can indicate pain originating from the stressed joint. It is often difficult to flex only one joint; the hock joint cannot be flexed without also flexing the stifle and hip joints, so the tests are nonspecific but can be very helpful. A normal horse may take two or three slightly lame steps, but sustained lameness is usually significant.

It is helpful to watch the horse move in circles on both soft and hard surfaces. Most horses move more freely on the lunge than when being led. The lameness should be compared on both reins. Although forelimb lameness is often accentuated when the affected leg is on the inside, occasionally it is more obvious when the leg is on the outside. Lameness due to corns may only be apparent when the horse is moving in the direction of the lame leg. If the horse has a short, pottery gait on the straight, obvious lameness may appear on the circle. Lameness associated with concussion, e.g. bruising, corns, etc., is often much worse on a hard than on a soft surface. Hind-limb lameness is sometimes worse with the affected leg on the inside and sometimes the outside. There are no firm rules.

Ridden exercise Lameness may be exaggerated when the horse is ridden, especially hind-limb lameness. This is sometimes most obvious when the rider is sitting on the diagonal of the affected leg. Bridle lameness is a term which has been used to describe an unlevelness only seen when the horse is ridden. This may be an evasion by the horse which is resisting going forward properly. Alternatively it may be induced by unsteadiness of the rider's hands. If there is doubt about whether a horse is genuinely lame, rather than bridle lame, it should be ridden by an experienced rider and driven forwards in a long, low outline to encourage it to step under more with its hind limbs (i.e. to improve hind-limb impulsion) and to swing its back more freely. If the horse is worked in this manner for several days many rhythm irregularities due to bridle lameness will disappear. Work on the lunge in a Chambon can also be helpful.

Local anaesthesia At this stage in the examination the lame leg or legs should have been identified and it might be possible to suggest where the pain originates. In many instances it is necessary to use local anaesthesia to define precisely the source of pain. This may be done in several ways. By injecting local anaesthetic over a nerve, transmission of nerve impulses is temporarily stopped and the area innervated by that nerve is desensitised. Therefore if pain originates in the desensitised area the horse should then be sound. This is called nerve blocking. Alternatively, local anaesthetic may be infiltrated around a suspect lesion, for example, a splint, and if the horse subsequently goes sound this proves that the splint is the cause of lameness. Pain originating in a joint can be relieved by injecting local anaesthetic directly into the joint. This is called intra-articular anaesthesia. The use of local anaesthesia is important because it allows precise identification of the source of pain. The area might appear normal on radiographic views (X-rays) despite the presence of a significant problem. Not all bony abnormalities which are seen on radiographic examination are necessarily of significance; in other words they do not all cause lameness.

Local anaesthesia may only improve lameness rather than eliminate it. This may indicate that there is more than one problem, or that the cause of the lameness is both painful and mechanical, or it may be due to an inability to desensitise totally the source of pain. In order to appreciate improvement in lameness it is necessary that the horse shows a reasonable degree of lameness initially. Therefore it may be necessary to work the horse to exaggerate a subtle lameness so that it can be investigated further. Although it may seem contraindicated to work a lame horse because it may exacerbate the problem, in most cases this will not alter the long-term prognosis and, unless the horse is lame enough to be investigated, a diagnosis may never be reached. It is usually impossible to diagnose the cause of a previous lameness unless the horse continues to be lame.

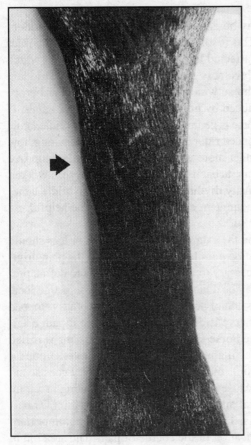

Figure 6   Craniocaudal view of the left metacarpal (cannon) region. There is a swelling on the medial aspect (arrow). Careful palpation reveals that this is an enlargement of the second metacarpal bone, a 'splint'

Radiography Having determined the source of pain, the area is then radiographed. A radiographic picture is a two-dimensional view of a three-dimensional object. It is necessary to obtain views of the object from more than one side to get a complete picture. It is important to recognise the limitations of radiographs and their ability to demonstrate abnormalities. Little information can be obtained about soft-tissue (muscle, tendon and ligament) problems. Abnormalities of bone are usually readily apparent, but cartilage cannot be seen on a radiographic examination, therefore a picture of a joint may appear normal despite the presence of cartilage damage (as in secondary joint disease or arthritis) unless there is major loss of cartilage with resultant narrowing of the joint space. Interpretation of radiographic views may be complicated by 'false' abnormalities. Dirt on the foot may be misinterpreted as a foreign body within the foot. Therefore interpretation of radiographic views requires a detailed knowledge of normal radiographic anatomy and its variations, which are manifold. 'Normal' abnormalities must be recognized.

Nuclear scintigraphy (bone scanning) (see also Chapter 12)

An alternative imaging technique for bone is nuclear scintigraphy or bone scanning. A radioactively labelled bone-seeking substance – for example, technetium – is injected into the jugular vein. After several hours the technetium is distributed in the bones. In the normal mature horse distribution is fairly uniform throughout the body, but if there is an area of increased bone activity or increased blood supply to the bone, technetium accumulates in that place, resulting in a 'hot spot'. This is detected using a gamma camera. The technique is more useful for acute cases of lameness than for chronic cases and is potentially more sensitive than radiography, enabling, for example, the detection of subtle fissure fractures before they can be seen radiographically. Nevertheless, it must be regarded as a complementary technique to radiography, not a substitute.

Muscle enzymes, faradism and ultrasound

Additional techniques are useful for evaluation of soft-tissue problems. Muscle cells contain two enzymes, aspartoamino transferase (AST) and creatine kinase (CK), which are released into the blood if the cells are damaged. An elevation in the concentration of these enzymes in the blood usually reflects muscle damage. Muscle strain may be identified by faradic stimulation. With experience, the type of contraction induced by the electrical stimulation of damaged muscle can be differentiated from that of normal muscle. The horse will usually show resentment of stimulation of damaged muscle. Diagnostic ultrasound is used to create images of soft-tissue structures and allows much better assessment of the structures involved in a soft-tissue swelling than can be detected by palpation (feeling) alone. Extremely subtle areas of damage within tendons and ligaments can be detected and adhesions within a tendon sheath may be identified. By sequential scanning the healing of an injury can be monitored.

Diagnostic medication It is sometimes useful to know whether or not a lameness responds to treatment with pain-relieving drugs such as phenyl butazone. It is necessary to treat the horse with an adequate dose relative to its bodyweight over a period in order to assess whether or not the drug is effective.

Surgical exploration Occasionally surgical exploration of an area is indicated to define the nature of the damage more precisely. Exploration of joints has been facilitated by the use of an arthroscope, a narrow viewing tube which is inserted into the joint via a small incision. This has been used in man for many years.

Some Common Problems and Their Causes
There are a number of clinical problems, such as swelling of the metacarpal (cannon) region, which have many different possible causes. The tables below aim to direct the reader towards the primary cause of some clinical complaints. The tables are not complete but include the most common causes.

'Filled leg'– swelling of the metacarpal or metatarsal (cannon) region
Bruising
Cellulitis (e.g. secondary to puncture wound)
Secondary infection following a cut
Subsolar abscess
Lymphangitis
Purpura haemorrhagica
Fractured splint bone
Cracked heels or mud fever
Enlarged blood vessels
Strained tendon or ligament (superficial digital flexor tendon, deep digital
    flexor tendon, accessory ligament of the deep digital flexor tendon,
    suspensory ligament)

Swelling of the carpus (knee)
Distension of the tendon sheath of extensor carpi radialis, common digital
    extensor tendon or lateral digital extensor tendon
Hygroma – false bursa
Enlarged joint capsule (antebrachiocarpal or intercarpal joint) due to
    degenerative joint disease, fracture or infection
Periarticular soft-tissue swelling due to trauma (bruising or sprain)
Cellulitis
Distension of the carpal canal

Swelling of the hock region
Thoroughpin
Bog spavin (idiopathic, secondary to osteochondrosis, degenerative joint
    disease, fracture or infection)
Periarticular swelling due to trauma (bruising or sprain)
Cellulitis
Curb
Fracture
Bone spavin

Swelling of the fetlock region
Suspensory ligament desmitis
Sprained fetlock
Enlarged joint capsule of the metacarpophalangeal joint due to degenerative
  joint disease, infection or fracture
Distension of tendon sheath (windgall) with or without constriction by the
  palmar annular ligament
Fracture of the metacarpal bone, proximal sesamoid bone or proximal phalanx
  Distal sesmoidean ligament strain
'Low' strain of the superficial or deep digital flexor tendons

Forelimb lameness with no obvious focus of pain or swelling
Foot pain (corns, navicular syndrome, degenerative joint disease of the distal
  interphalangeal joint, pedal osteitis, poor trimming and shoeing)
Early degenerative joint disease of the proximal interphalangeal joint
High suspensory desmitis
Desmitis of the accessory ligament of the deep digital flexor tendon
Subchondral bone cyst – any location
Osteochondrosis of the shoulder

Stumbling
Tiredness; bad riding; rough ground
Excessively long feet
Navicular syndrome
Ringbone
Incoordination

Hind-limb toe drag
Laziness; unfitness
Young, unbalanced horse
Excessively long toes
Hind-limb lameness (e.g. bone spavin)
Incoordination
Scirrhous cord (infection at castration site)

Hind-limb lameness with no obvious site of pain or swelling
Bone spavin
Subchondral bone cyst – any location (particularly the stifle)
High suspensory desmitis
Early degenerative joint disease of the proximal and distal interphalangeal
  joints

Very severe lameness
Joint infection (infectious arthritis)
Fracture
Subsolar abscess

Blood in joint (haemarthrosis)
Nerve damage resulting in inability to bear weight
Myopathy

Poor performance
Rider problem; sourness and/or overfacing
Bilateral forelimb lameness (e.g. navicular syndrome)
Bilateral hind-limb lameness (e.g. bone spavin)
Subclinical forelimb or hind-limb lameness
Excessive concussion ('jarred up')
Back pain
Medical problem (e.g. low-grade respiratory infection)
Temperamental problem (e.g. mareishness)

12
CONDITIONS OF BONE

Functional anatomy

Although the individual bones of the horse, such as the humerus, the radius and the metacarpal (cannon) bone, are different in shape, they all have the same basic structure. The long bones have a shaft which consists of a tubular structure with walls of dense, compact, cortical bone surrounding a central medullary (marrow) cavity. The extremities of the bone are cancellous bone, softer bone mixed with marrow, overlain by a thin layer of cortical bone. The cancellous bone is arranged in fine struts or trabeculae, which are orientated in a regular pattern along the lines of stress of the bone. The bone matrix consists of a collagen base in which are deposited bone salts, predominantly calcium phosphate. The matrix contains many bone cells (osteocytes) and is perforated by fine canals containing blood vessels and nerves. The main blood supply is via the nutrient artery of the bone, which enters the bone through the nutrient foramen, passes into the medullary cavity and then radiates to supply the cortical bone. The bone is covered throughout its length by a thin but tough membrane, the periosteum.

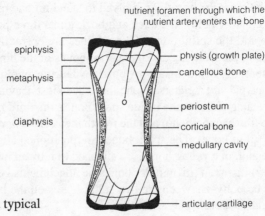

Figure 1
Structural anatomy of a typical
long bone

This is fibrous tissue overlying a layer of connective tissue which has a good blood supply and many cells which are capable of becoming active bone-forming cells or osteoblasts. Tendons and ligaments are attached to bone via the periosteum. At the site of attachment of a tendon specialized fibres called Sharpey's fibres penetrate into the bone, providing a strong link. Bone is not a static structure. It is constantly being replaced and, especially in the young animal, has a remarkable capacity to change shape and remodel according to the stresses placed upon it. Therefore if a bony lump develops as a result of trauma to the bone, it is likely that it will subsequently remodel, becoming smoother in outline and smaller. Some residual swelling is likely to persist.

Periostitis

Periostitis is either an inflammation of the periosteum resulting from a direct blow to the periosteum or a lifting of the periosteum away from the underlying bone. The osteoblasts in the connective tissue layer respond by producing new bone. On radiographic views periosteal new bone can be distinguished from cortical bone by its irregular and less opaque appearance. When inflammation has subsided the periosteal new bone remodels, resulting in a smoothly outlined bony lump or exostosis. Common sites of periostitis in the horse are the small metacarpal and metatarsal bones (so-called splints) and the large metacarpal and metatarsal (cannon) bones.

SPLINTS

Functional anatomy
Unlike man, the horse has evolved to stand on one rather than on five digits. Immediately below the knee and hock joints three bones persist, the cannon bone and the splint bones. These bones are correctly called the metacarpal bones in the front leg and metatarsal bones in the hind leg and are numbered sequentially from inside to outside. During evolution the first and fifth metacarpal and metatarsal bones have been lost, leaving the second metacarpal or metatarsal bone (the inside splint bone), the third metacarpal or metatarsal bone (the cannon bone) and the fourth metacarpal or metatarsal bone (the outside splint bone). The splint bones are positioned slightly behind the cannon bone and, in a young horse, are attached to it by an interosseous (between the bones) ligament. In an older horse the attachments become more fibrous and may be bony. Between the two splint bones on the back of the cannon bone lies the suspensory ligament.

In the front leg the splint and cannon bones articulate with the bottom row of bones in the knee, the second, third and fourth carpal bones. The splint bones provide some support to the cannon bone and forces are transmitted through them. The second metacarpal (inside splint) bone articulates with both the second and third carpal bones. This arrangement tends to result in very slight downward and backward movement of the second metacarpal bone when force is transmitted through the knee during weightbearing.

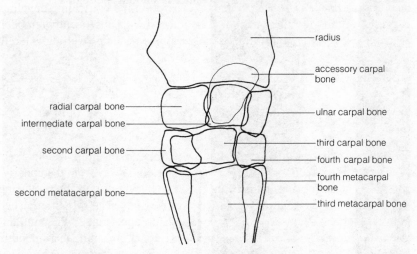

Figure 2 Dorsopalmar view of the left carpus. The accessory carpal bone is superimposed over the first row of carpal bones

This effect is exaggerated in a horse with bench-knee conformation (i.e. when the leg below the knee is set farther to the outside than usual). The fourth metacarpal (outside splint) bone articulates only with the fourth carpal bone and tends to be displaced only downwards during weightbearing. These functional anatomical differences are important when one considers that splints occur most frequently on the inside in a front leg.

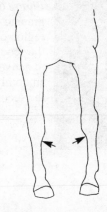

Figure 3
A bench knee

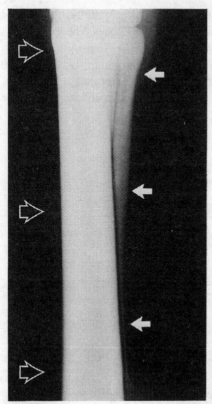

Figure 4 (left)   An oblique radiographic view of the metacarpal region of a normal horse showing the third metacarpal (cannon) bone (open arrows) and the second metacarpal (inside splint) bone (closed arrows). The outline of the latter is smooth and regular

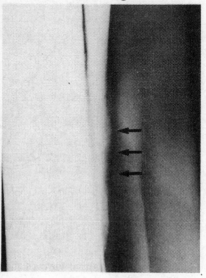

Figure 5 (above)   An oblique radiographic view of the metacarpal region of a horse with periostitis of the second metacarpal bone, i.e. an active splint. The middle third of the bone has a fuzzy irregular outline (arrows)

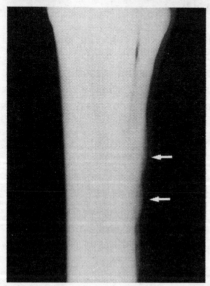

Figure 6 (left)   An oblique radiographic view of the metacarpal region of a horse after remodelling of the second metacarpal bone, a sequel to active periostitis. There is smoothly outlined new bone around the second metacarpal bone (arrows)

What are splints?
The term 'splint' is the colloquial name for a bony enlargement of one of the small metacarpal or metatarsal bones (see Chapter 11, Figure 6). A splint may develop for a variety of reasons. In the young horse it most frequently occurs as a sequel to slight tearing of the interosseous ligament between the splint bone and the cannon bone. This also results in lifting of the periosteum to which the interosseous ligament is attached. The damage to the interosseous ligament occurs because of relative movement between the splint and the cannon bones. Thus there is inflammation of the interosseous ligament and the periosteum (periostitis), causing pain and soft-tissue swelling. Some calcification in the interosseous ligament occurs and new bone is produced beneath the elevated periosteum, and ultimately a firmer union between the splint bone and the cannon bone develops. Poor conformation, such as bench knees, and improper trimming of the foot, resulting in the foot being placed to the ground unevenly rather than flatly, predispose to the development of splints. Incorrect proportions of phosphorus and calcium in the diet favour the formation of splints. A splint may also develop as a sequel to trauma to the bone such as a kick. If the horse moves very closely the damage may be self-inflicted, the narrow-chested horse which toes-in being particularly prone. Trauma to the bone results in haemorrhage beneath the periosteum, lifting it away from the bone surface. This stimulates new bone production. There will also be associated soft-tissue inflammation. Although splints occur in both front and hind limbs, the incidence in front limbs is much higher.

Clinical signs
The degree of lameness associated with a splint is variable. The horse usually bears weight fully on the affected leg at rest and is sound at walk. At trot there is mild to moderate lameness, which is most apparent on hard ground. The lameness does not improve with work and may deteriorate. The presence of severe lameness would suggest that there is a cause other than a splint. In the early stages of a splint, there is a variable amount of localised swelling, which is predominantly soft-tissue in origin. This swelling may be extremely subtle and may only be apparent by careful palpation of the leg and comparison with its pair. In the acute stages the swelling is usually soft and slight finger pressure may leave a temporary indentation. This is inflammatory oedema. In the later stages the swelling becomes considerably firmer. This swelling is partly bony and partly an overlying fibrous reaction.

Diagnosis
Careful digital palpation of the splint bone with the leg held semi-flexed off the ground usually reveals a focal area of pain. In some horses it is necessary to apply slight pressure on several aspects of the affected splint bone before a

painful area can be located. If the reaction appears to be equivocal, then a careful comparison with the other leg should be made.

Pain, and therefore lameness, usually persists until inflammation has fully subsided. Then a firm residual swelling persists. Thus the presence of a discrete swelling on or around a splint bone does not necessarily mean that it is the cause of lameness. It is only likely to be significant if pain can be elicited by palpation of the swelling. Especially in sensitive, hyper-reactive horses, it may be difficult to determine if the horse is really feeling pain; if there is some uncertainty, local anaesthetic may be infiltrated around the swelling. If the swelling is the cause of lameness, this procedure should eliminate the lameness.

Radiography

Radiographs are also useful to determine if a splint is active. The normal splint bone has a regular, smooth outline. It tapers from top to bottom. At the bottom is a slight enlargement, the so-called button of the splint bone. If the periosteum of the bone is inflamed, this will result in alteration of the contour of the bone and the edge will appear roughened rather than smooth. These bony changes take up to ten to fourteen days to occur; therefore at the time of onset of lameness there may be slight soft-tissue swelling but no bony change visible on the radiographs. Subsequent radiographs may demonstrate an active bony reaction. When the inflammation has subsided, when the splint is inactive, a bony lump persists which is smooth in outline. It may be necessary to obtain several radiographic views of the splint bone to identify the bony lesion, which may be localised to one side of the bone. Active new bone formation is most easily seen on an underexposed radiograph and the latter is also useful to eliminate the possibility of a fracture, especially if there was known trauma to the splint bone.

Treatment

The aims of treatment are to reduce inflammation and thus relieve pain. Rest, preferably box rest, is essential. Anti-inflammatory drugs may be of benefit, administered either by mouth (e.g. phenylbutazone) or at the site of the problem. Corticosteroids may be injected around the splint or dimethyl sulphoxide (DMSO) may be applied to the overlying skin and will be absorbed through it. Whether or not anti-inflammatory drugs are used, the horse must be given enough time, and this usually implies at least six weeks' rest; sometimes considerably longer is necessary. A premature resumption of work is likely to reaggravate the problem. Once the acute inflammation has subsided, daily massage may help to reduce the size of the swelling. The ultimate size of the swelling will depend upon the amount of new bone produced. The new bone tends to remodel and eventually decreases in size. One must remember that the visible swelling is not just bony. There is overlying fibrous tissue which contributes to the size of the swelling.

Some individuals seem prone to production of excessive amounts of new bone and occasionally the bony enlargement may interfere with the normal function of the suspensory ligament. In these circumstances surgical removal of the bony swelling may be indicated. It is sometimes desirable for cosmetic reasons to remove the bony swelling and, although this is a relatively straight-forward procedure, one must be aware that, however careful the surgeon is, occasionally new bone formation will recur spontaneously postoperatively. Thus a successful cosmetic outcome cannot be guaranteed.

BLIND SPLINTS

The term 'blind splint' is rather nebulous and has been used to describe inflammation of the interosseous ligament which unites the splint and cannon bones. There is no new bone formation visible on radiographs – hence the term 'blind splint'. The clinical signs are more subtle and a definitive diagnosis is usually only possible by infiltrating local anaesthetic into the suspected area. The treatment is identical and the prognosis, as for true splints, is generally good.

PERIOSTITIS OF THE THIRD METACARPAL OR METATARSAL (CANNON) BONES

The third metacarpal and metatarsal (cannon) bones are vulnerable to injury because they are protected by relatively little soft tissue. Above the knee and hock the bones are surrounded by large muscle masses; below the knee and hock only skin, tendons and ligaments surround the bones. A blunt blow to the metacarpal or metatarsal bones may incite inflammation of the periosteum and subsequent formation of periosteal new bone. In the acute stages there is usually overlying soft-tissue swelling. Although the area is painful to touch, this is often unassociated with lameness. The periosteal new bone will gradually remodel and be incorporated into the cortical bone, resulting in a residual thickening of the cortex.

SORE SHINS

Sore shins is a condition almost unique to the young Thoroughbred racehorse. It is poorly understood but results from a skeletally immature horse working on hard ground. The condition involves the forelimbs, is usually bilateral and causes a short, restricted, shuffly gait and/or lameness. There may be some swelling over the front of the bones, resulting in a more convex contour than usual. The exact cause of pain is not known. Pressure applied to the front aspect of the metacarpal bones causes pain. It is not usual in Great Britain to detect any abnormality of the bones, except remodelling of the cortex, on radiographs, although in America small fissure fractures (so-called saucer fractures) of the bone are sometimes seen. Saucer fractures are fatigue or stress fractures, the result of repetitive loading of the bone, and their higher occurrence in America is probably related to the different training and racing conditions. In Great Britain horses are trained predominantly in straight lines and gentle curves, and are both trained and raced on grass, whereas in America horses are trained and raced on oval-shaped, predominantly dirt, tracks, and run consistently anticlockwise. In Great Britain most horses respond well to rest. Additional treatment such as electromagnetic therapy has been tried but is of questionable benefit.

PERIOSTITIS SECONDARY TO MUSCLE OR LIGAMENT STRAIN

Muscles are attached to bones via tendons, which are fibrous structures which are less elastic than muscles. Ligaments are more fibrous and less elastic than tendons and are attached to bones at both ends. They usually cross a joint, their function being to provide support and stability. A strain of a muscle, tendon or ligament may involve its attachment to the bone and induce periostitis. At the site of attachment of the tendon or ligament the periosteum will be lifted and new bone production will be stimulated resulting in an exostosis (bony protuberance). The exostosis will not be seen on radiographs immediately after the injury but will take ten to fourteen days to develop. Lameness is associated with strain of muscles, ligaments and tendons and rest is usually the most efficacious treatment. It may take several months before repair is complete. A smoothly outlined exostosis may persist despite resolution of the lameness, but this is of no consequence.

Osteitis

Osteitis is inflammation of bone. The most common conditions in the horse which are described as osteitis are pedal osteitis and sesamoiditis.

PEDAL OSTEITIS

The distal (third) phalanx or pedal bone is the largest bone in the horse's foot and is supported in the foot by the laminae. The term pedal osteitis implies that there is current inflammation of the bone. This is difficult if not impossible to determine clinically and in the author's opinion the term is misused. The radiographic appearance of the third phalanx of normal horses is extremely variable. The bone may appear more or less porous and may have a relatively smooth or rough outline and narrow or wide vascular channels; it also may have a large or small notch (crena) at the toe. Thus, unless the radiographic appearance of the bone is very abnormal, it probably is a normal variation. A horse with large, flat feet and thin soles is predisposed to bruising, and severe bruising and/or repetitive bruising may incite inflammation of the pedal bone, but, except in a minority of horses, the radiographic appearance of the bone will be within the normal variation. The author believes that pedal osteitis is diagnosed much more frequently than it occurs. Bruising of the foot is discussed in the section on conditions of the foot (see p. 286). The following discussion on pedal osteitis relates to those horses in which major changes can be demonstrated radiographically.

Clinical signs

Both front feet are usually affected, although occasionally the condition is unilateral. The condition may develop secondarily to a distal interphalangeal joint flexural deformity (see p. 330). The horse moves with a shortened stride with or without obvious lameness, especially on hard ground. The horse may be lamer on a circle but not invariably so. In contrast to navicular syndrome, the horse does not point when at rest and there is less tendency to place the foot to the ground toe first. Although rest may improve the condition, lameness usually recurs when work is resumed and is worse on hard ground. It is necessary to desensitise the entire foot by a nerve block to improve the action.

Radiography

Radiographic changes include a marked increase in apparent porosity of the bone, it appears riddled with holes (seen in the dorsopalmar view) with or without an irregular roughened appearance of the front of the bone (seen in a lateral view).

Treatment

There is no effective treatment and prognosis for future soundness is guarded, although the horse may perform adequately on soft ground.

SESAMOIDITIS

Functional anatomy

The proximal sesamoid bones are two small bones on the back of the fetlock joint which form part of the suspensory apparatus. The suspensory ligament divides into two branches in the lower third of the metacarpal or metatarsal (cannon) region. The inside and outside branches attach to the top of the inside and outside sesamoid bones respectively. Attached to the bottom of the sesamoid bones are three pairs of ligaments – the deep, middle and superficial distal sesamoidean ligaments – which themselves insert on the proximal (first) and middle (second) phalanges (long and short pastern bones). An inter-sesamoidean ligament joins the two sesamoid bones. As the fetlock joint flexes and extends the sesamoid bones move up and down.

Sesamoiditis is a term loosely applied to several conditions involving the sesamoid bones, none of which occurs very frequently. There is limited knowledge of the exact nature of the pathology associated with changes identified on radiographs. Radiographic changes associated with the sesamoid bones include new bone growths on the sesamoid bones (the result of tearing of attachments of the suspensory ligament), variations in the radiopacity of the bone (coarse or mottled bone trabeculation and a change in the number, size and shape of the so-called vascular channels) and areas of mineralisation within the sesamoidean ligaments.

Predisposing causes
A long toe, resulting in a broken pastern–foot axis places abnormal stresses on the suspensory apparatus and predisposes to injury. The type of work the horse does influences the incidence of the disease. Injuries to the suspensory apparatus occur in horses racing at speed, especially over fences. Dressage horses and showjumpers place a lot of stress on the suspensory apparatus.

Clinical signs
Lameness is variable in severity and may be sudden or gradual in onset. Forelimb lameness may or may not be accentuated by flexion of the fetlock joint. There may be thickening of either or both of the branches of the suspensory ligaments above the sesamoid bones and pressure applied with the leg non-weightbearing may cause pain. In the acute early stage pressure applied to the sesamoid bone can cause pain if there has been tearing of the attachment of the suspensory ligament.

Diagnosis
Lameness is not affected by desensitisation of the foot, but is alleviated by desensitisation of the fetlock region. Oblique radiographic views of the fetlock are necessary to highlight the sesamoid bones. The identifiable bony changes have been described.

Treatment
Lameness which is associated with damage to either the suspensory ligament or the distal sesamoidean ligaments resulting in damage of the attachments to the sesamoid bones will resolve with rest, but there is a relatively high incidence of recurrence. Improvement in the pastern–foot axis by appropriate

trimming and shoeing is important. If bony abnormalities are present, lameness usually improves with rest but tends to recur with the resumption of hard work. There have been a few reports that isoxsuprine hydrochloride, which dilates peripheral blood vessels, is useful in the treatment of sesamoiditis, but results have been extremely variable.

Osteomyelitis

Osteomyelitis is infection of bone and, in the adult horse, occurs most commonly as a sequel to a deep wound on the metacarpal or metatarsal region. The metacarpal or metatarsal (cannon) bones are particularly susceptible because of their lack of protection by muscles.

Cause
Many different bacteria may infect bone. Infection usually occurs via an open wound but in the young foal may be blood-borne.

Clinical signs
There is soft-tissue swelling and a sinus (hole) through which pus exudes continuously or intermittently. Pressure applied to the area causes pain. The horse may or may not be lame.

Diagnosis
The history of a wound which either failed to heal satisfactorily or healed and then developed a sinus is suggestive of the presence of osteomyelitis or a foreign body. Diagnosis is confirmed by radiographs, with the infected bone having a characteristic fuzzy appearance. Sometimes a piece of bone dies and becomes surrounded by pus and granulation tissue, forming a sequestrum (dead bone) and involucrum (surrounding granulation tissue).

Treatment
Antibiotic treatment is often successful in eliminating infections, provided that there is no dead bone. It is useful to try to culture bacteria from the sinus and find out to which drugs they are sensitive, so that appropriate drugs are administered. If there is dead bone, it is often necessary to remove it surgically.

Prevention
Thorough cleaning of a wound is mandatory. The hair surrounding the wound should be clipped off. All dead and dying tissue should be removed. Hosing the wound is useful, followed by careful cleaning. If the wound is deep, veterinary advice should be sought.

Physitis

Physitis is the term applied to pain associated with abnormal activity in a growth plate (physis), usually the lower growth plate of the radius, just above the knee. It was formerly referred to as epiphysitis. The condition may be related to osteochondrosis (see p. 224).

Clinical signs

The condition occurs in rapidly growing young horses, and most commonly in yearlings. There is usually slight swelling and heat around the lower end of the radius, just above the knee. The horse is not always lame; it may be lame if only one leg is affected or may show a stiff stilted gait if both forelimbs are affected. Pressure applied to the area may cause pain.

Figure 7a and b   Bones of the fore- and hind-limbs

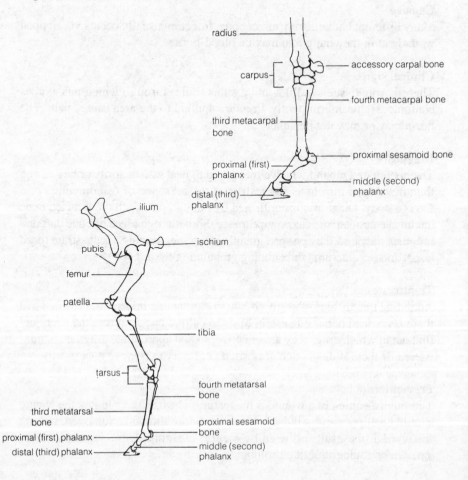

radius

carpus

accessory carpal bone

fourth metacarpal bone

third metacarpal bone

proximal sesamoid bone

proximal (first) phalanx

middle (second) phalanx

distal (third) phalanx

ilium

ischium

pubis

femur

patella

tibia

tarsus

fourth metatarsal bone

third metatarsal bone

proximal sesamoid bone

proximal (first) phalanx

middle (second) phalanx

distal (third) phalanx

Treatment and prognosis
The diet should be restricted and calcium–phosphorus ratios checked to ensure that there is not an imbalance. Dietary supplementation with minerals should only be undertaken with appropriate advice. If the horse is lame, it should be confined to a box or small paddock.

The prognosis is favourable. Given time, the swelling usually subsides.

Fractures

It has traditionally been thought that the majority of fractures in the horse are irreparable, but with improving techniques many fractures are potentially treatable either to return the horse to athletic function or to salvage it for breeding purposes. Prognosis depends on many factors, including which bone is involved, the configuration of the fracture, whether or not the overlying skin is damaged, when the fracture occurred, whether or not the fracture involves a joint and, finally but by no means less important, the size, age and temperament of the horse.

Classification
A simple fracture means that there is one fracture which breaks the bone into two pieces. A comminuted fracture has more than two pieces and is more serious. If the bone is not exposed the fracture is closed. If the skin is damaged, exposing the bone, the fracture is compound. The risk of infection is very high and the prognosis is poorer. If the fracture does not extend all the way through the bone, it is incomplete. If it does extend all the way through, it is complete. If the fracture fragments remain in their normal alignment, the fracture is nondisplaced. If the pieces have moved, the fracture is displaced and, depending on the degree of displacement, the pieces will usually require realignment if satisfactory healing is to occur. If the fracture does not involve a joint, it is non-articular. If the fracture extends into a joint it is articular and the prognosis is less good, because there is a significant risk of developing secondary joint disease (arthritis).

Diagnosis
A fracture may often be identified by a careful clinical examination. In some instances it is obvious – the leg is distorted and the fragments are readily felt, and movement between them (crepitus) can be detected, but this is not always the case. In some circumstances it is clear that it is highly unlikely that the fracture can be successfully repaired and the horse should be humanely destroyed. If the fracture is not readily identifiable or if there is a possibility of repair, then radiographs are mandatory. Several different views are necessary

to define the configuration of the fracture and the degree of displacement. If the fracture is only a fissure and there is no displacement, it may be extremely difficult to identify. Part of the normal healing process involves bone resorption (removal) along the fracture line, thus on subsequent radiographs the fracture line becomes wider and more readily identified. Therefore, if a fracture is suspected but cannot be seen on radiographs, the horse should be confined to a box and further radiographs taken seven to ten days later.

First aid

In many instances it is necessary to move the horse to suitable radiography facilities. Precautions must be taken to minimise the risks of making the fracture worse. Effective immobilisation of the upper forelimb and hind limb is impossible, but below the knee and hock a strong support bandage can be of great benefit. If possible, the joints above and below the fractured bone should be incorporated into the bandage. Sophisticated bandage material is unnecessary. although a proper plaster or synthetic cast is ideal if applied properly. Gamgee, two broomsticks, some pillows and plenty of crepe bandages will suffice in an emergency. Although it is important to provide adequate support, the bandages must not be applied too tightly since they may restrict the blood supply and damage the soft tissues. Plenty of padding (e.g. Gamgee and pillows) should reduce this risk. Although the horse may be in considerable pain, provided that it is not unduly distressed and unmanageable, painkilling drugs should not be administered because it is desirable that the horse should be discouraged from bearing weight on the limb. Most horses are quite adept at walking slowly on three legs. The incline of the ramp of the trailer or lorry should be as slight as possible. A loading bay or a slope against which the ramp is placed is useful. During transport the horse should be supported with straw bales if necessary. If the horse has fractured a forelimb, travelling the animal facing backwards reduces the risks of its inadvertently overloading the fractured limb if a sudden stop is necessary.

Fracture healing

Fracture healing requires adequate alignment and immobilisation of the fracture fragments. If the fracture fragments are widely separated or if there is constant movement at the fracture site, then healing will not occur or the pieces will be united by a fibrous rather than a bony union. If the fracture fragments are aligned and kept relatively still, then healing will occur by formation of a bony callus around the bone at the fracture site and direct union between the bone pieces. The more movement there is between the fracture fragments, the greater the amount of callus that will be formed. When healing is complete this callus will remodel and reduce in size to some extent.

In order to achieve adequate stability of the fracture fragments, either external support (a cast) or internal fixation (plates and/or screws) is necessary. Which method is used depends upon the severity of the fracture, its location, the intended use of the horse and financial considerations.

It may be possible to apply a cast with the horse standing, especially if a synthetic casting material which sets rapidly is used. This is satisfactory provided that the fracture fragments are not displaced and obviates the need for general anaesthesia. Major problems can arise during recovery from general anaesthesia: it is difficult to control the movement of a horse and it may take a mis-step while still not properly aware of how it is placing its limbs, resulting in refracture. However, if the fracture fragments are malpositioned, then they must be realigned, and this is only possible under general anaesthesia. Realignment may be achieved by applying traction to the leg. Sometimes it is necessary to expose the bone surgically and in these circumstances a bone plate and/or screws are usually applied. If a fracture fragment is small, surgical removal may be the treatment of choice, particularly if it is within a joint.

FRACTURES OF THE SCAPULA

Fractures of the scapula (shoulderblade) are comparatively rare and are usually the result of direct trauma. There is soft-tissue swelling and considerable pain. The horse is unwilling to move the leg or place weight upon it. The prognosis for most fractures is hopeless.

FRACTURES OF THE HUMERUS

Most fractures of the humerus are non-articular spiral fractures with or without comminution and displacement. There is considerable soft-tissue swelling. Prognosis in the adult horse is usually hopeless. Successful surgical repair has been achieved in foals.

FRACTURES OF THE RADIUS

Fractures of the radius occur in many configurations. There is usually a considerable amount of soft-tissue swelling. The prognosis in the adult horse is poor, although successful surgical treatment has been achieved. Better results are obtained in foals. Occasionally nondisplaced fractures in adult horses have healed spontaneously.

FRACTURES OF THE CARPUS (KNEE)

There are at least seven bones in the knee – the radial, intermediate, ulnar, accessory, second, third and fourth carpal bones – of which five commonly sustain fractures. Fractures occur most often in racehorses and are not usually associated with direct trauma but are the result of repeated stress on the front aspect of the bones, resulting in a small chip fracture of a corner of a bone or a larger slab fracture through the length of a bone. There is usually subtle swelling of the knee and resentment of flexion, with moderate lameness. Chip fractures commonly involve the radial, intermediate or third carpal bone and may be successfully treated by removal of the piece. Slab fractures occur most commonly in the third carpal bone. Thin slab fractures may be removed. Thick slab fractures are treated by inserting a screw through the fragment into the parent bone.

Fractures of the accessory carpal bone occur more often in older horses and are difficult to treat surgically, due to the odd shape of the bone. Prolonged rest renders some horses sound.

Occasionally fractures of several carpal bones occur concurrently; this results in instability of the carpus and merits a poor prognosis.

FRACTURES OF THE THIRD METACARPAL OR METATARSAL (CANNON) BONES

Fractures of these bones are usually the result of direct trauma and, because of the small amount of overlying soft tissue, bone is often exposed through the skin causing a high risk of infection (osteomyelitis - see p. 213). There are often several pieces. If there are not too many pieces, the fracture is not too contaminated and the soft tissues are in reasonable condition, then surgical treatment may be successful. Two bone plates are used, plus additional screws and a bone graft if necessary.

FRACTURES OF THE SECOND AND FOURTH METACARPAL OR METATARSAL (SPLINT) BONES

Fracture of a splint bone may occur spontaneously or associated with inflammation of the suspensory ligament (suspensory desmitis – see p. 274) or be due to trauma. Fractures occur most commonly at the junction between the top two thirds and the bottom one third of the bone, although they may be located anywhere, especially if they are the result of external trauma. In some instances it is possible to palpate a movable fracture fragment, but radiographs are usually necessary to confirm a diagnosis, especially if there is soft-tissue swelling associated with suspensory desmitis.

If the fracture is uncomplicated, that is, if there are only one or two fracture fragments, and the overlying skin is intact, conservative treatment is adequate. Most fractures heal spontaneously by bony union, even if there is some displacement of the fracture fragment. Initially a fairly large bony callus may develop to unite the pieces, but this will remodel and reduce in size. Persistent lameness is unusual, even if the bones do not become united (i.e. even if there is a non-union). Therefore in an uncomplicated fracture surgery is usually not warranted, except for cosmetic reasons, and rest is the treatment of choice. Subsequent radiographs will help to determine when the horse may resume work. If there is associated suspensory desmitis, the prognosis is more guarded.

Surgical treatment may be indicated if there are multiple fracture fragments, if the fracture occurs high up, thus separating the major part of the bone from the top, or if the bone becomes infected secondary to a concurrent skin wound. Infection may usually be managed by removal of infected bone and concomitant antibiotic treatment and a favourable prognosis may be offered. If the fracture has occurred high up, the prognosis must always be guarded. Removal of the fragment may mean that the remaining part of the bone is unstable, and repetitive, slight movement is likely to produce persistent lameness. Attempts have been made to stabilise this piece by inserting a screw through it into the cannon bone and, although this technique is successful in some horses, it is not uniformly so.

FRACTURES OF THE PROXIMAL SESAMOID BONES

Spontaneous fractures of both the sesamoid bones in one or both forelegs occur occasionally in foals and some recover without treatment. Otherwise sesamoid fractures are usually restricted to racehorses but do also occur in other types. There is moderate lameness and pain on pressure over the bone. Fractures of the top (apex) of the bone may be successfully treated by removal of the piece, provided that there is no associated severe suspensory desmitis. Fractures of the middle of the bone are more serious but screwing or the installation of a bone graft is sometimes successful. Fractures of the base warrant a guarded prognosis.

FRACTURES OF THE PROXIMAL (FIRST) PHALANX (LONG PASTERNBONE)

Fractures of the proximal phalanx are not uncommon in all types of horses. If the fracture is displaced and/or comminuted, it is identified readily, but nondisplaced fissure fractures may be difficult to diagnose and multiple radiographic views may be necessary. In young Thoroughbreds with a nondisplaced fissure fracture, box rest is sufficient. All other types of fracture require either casting or surgical fixation. The prognosis depends upon whether or not the fracture involves the fetlock and/or the pastern joint and how many pieces there are. Chip fractures of the top of the bone also occur and may be treated by removal of the piece with a good prognosis provided there is no arthritis of the fetlock joint.

FRACTURES OF THE MIDDLE (SECOND) PHALANX (SHORT PASTERN BONE)

Fractures of the second phalanx are rare in Britain but occur more frequently in racing Quarter horses in America.

FRACTURES OF THE DISTAL (THIRD) PHALANX (PEDAL BONE)

Fractures of the third phalanx which do not enter the distal interphalangeal (coffin) joint have a reasonable prognosis following box rest and the application of a bar shoe to immobilise the foot as much as is possible. These fractures often heal by fibrous rather than by bony union and can still be seen on radiographs. Fractures which enter the joint warrant a poor prognosis.

FRACTURES OF THE NAVICULAR BONE

Fractures of the navicular bone cause a sudden onset of moderate to severe lameness and may be the result of the horse kicking a solid object or a misstep. Without treatment the lameness may improve but usually mild lameness persists. Some horses with recent fractures may be treated successfully by screw fixation.

FRACTURES OF THE PELVIS see p. 323.

FRACTURES OF THE FEMUR AND TIBIA

Fractures of the femur and tibia in both adult horses and foals warrant a very poor prognosis, although successful surgical repair has been achieved in foals.

FRACTURES OF THE PATELLA (KNEE CAP)

Fractures of the patella usually occur as a result of a direct blow; surgical treatment offers the best prognosis.

FRACTURES OF THE FIBULA

Fractures of the fibula are extremely rare. The bone forms as several different pieces which look separate on radiographs and these separations must not be confused with a fracture.

FRACTURES OF THE HOCK

Fractures of the hock usually occur due to trauma and most have a poor prognosis.

Genetic Disorders

HEREDITARY MULTIPLE EXOSTOSIS

This is a rare hereditary condition characterised by numerous growths on the long bones, the ribs and the pelvis. The bony enlargements may rub on soft-tissue structures, causing enlargement of tendon sheaths and joint capsules and mild lameness. There is no known treatment. Affected horses should not be used for breeding.

POLYDACTYLY

Polydactyly is the presence, in the newborn foal, of an extra part of a limb. It can take a variety of forms, for example, an extra lower leg comprising a miniature third metacarpal bone and phalanges growing from the third metacarpal bone. The protuberance, which is hair-covered, can be amputated for cosmetic reasons and to avoid interference with the contralateral leg.

Examination Techniques

Radiography (X-rays) has traditionally been used to evaluate conditions of bone, and still plays an important role. However, it is relatively insensitive: a 40% change in bone density must occur before any change is seen on an X-ray. With very recent lameness, no abnormality may be detected. Nuclear scintigraphy, or bone scanning, provides a much more sensitive technique for the detection of abnormalities in bone, or where soft tissues attach to bone. A radioactive bone-seeking substance is injected intravenously, and is taken up first in the soft tissues and then into bones. If there is an increase in bone blood supply or bone activity, more of the radioactivity is taken up, resulting in a 'hot spot' (Figure 8). A hot spot may be present long before any X-ray change is apparent, and with some conditions X-ray changes are never detected. This may permit earlier diagnosis of some conditions, especially relatively recent onset lameness of moderate to severe degree. It is also useful in areas difficult to X-ray, such as the pelvis. However, with mild, chronic lameness a bone scan is often negative.

Ultrasonography is useful to evaluate bone contours in certain circumstances (See Chapter 18, Figure 6). Magnetic resonance imagery and computed tomography, by allowing three-dimensional assessment of bone, permits identification of abnormalities not detectable by other means.

Figure 8
A 'hot-spot' (arrow) in the knee

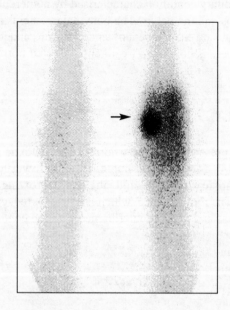

13
THE JOINTS

Joint structure and function

The basic structure and function of all limb joints (articulations) are similar. Articular (joint) cartilage covers the ends of the bones, protects the underlying bone and transmits forces to the underlying subchondral bone. Cartilage has no nerve supply, therefore damage to it does not itself cause pain. It has no blood supply and is dependent on the synovial (joint) fluid for nutrition. If movement of synovial fluid in and out of the articular cartilage is impaired, then the cartilage will receive inadequate nutrition resulting in cell death and a decrease in resistance to stress. Articular cartilage has limited powers of regeneration, therefore damage to it is incompletely repaired.

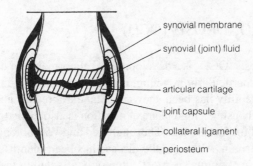

Figure 1   Structure of a typical joint

The synovial membrane controls the composition of the synovial fluid, which consists of some of the constituents of blood plus hyaluronic acid. Hyaluronic acid is produced and secreted by cells of the synovial membrane. Synovial fluid is vital for nutrition of the articular cartilage and has an important role in the lubrication of the synovial membrane and the joint capsule. The synovial membrane has a nerve and a blood supply. Pain is caused by inflammation of both the synovial membrane and the surrounding joint capsule. Distension of these structures due to the presence of excess synovial fluid also causes pain. Damage and inflammation of the synovial membrane and the joint capsule is usually associated with lameness; minor damage of the articular cartilage alone does not always cause lameness.

Both the joint capsule and the collateral ligaments provide stability to the joint and limit its range of motion. The joint capsule and the ligaments are attached to the periosteum, the thin membrane which covers the bone. Tearing of the attachments of the joint capsule or the collateral ligaments will lift the periosteum from the underlying bone, causing pain and subsequent new bone formation. These periosteal proliferative reactions are some distance from the joint surfaces and should not compromise the long-term function of the joint. Thus, when soft-tissue damage has repaired and the periosteal reaction has settled down, lameness should resolve, provided that the articular structures of the joint were not also damaged.

Conditions of Joints

Congenital joint abnormalities in the horse are extremely rare. Occasionally a foal is born with a joint which will not flex. Sometimes parts of a joint are underdeveloped (hypoplastic), predisposing to angular deformity at the joint or luxation (dislocation) of the joint.

OSTEOCHONDROSIS (OCD)

Osteochondrosis (OCD) is a developmental abnormality of cartilage and bone which occurs particularly in young, rapidly growing individuals.

Direct heritability has been shown in Standardbreds. Encouraging a horse to grow quickly using a high plane of nutrition is also likely to predispose foals with potential for fast growth, Thoroughbred and Warmbloods being the most common in Britain. Although the disease has been identified in most joints, the stifle and hock joints are most commonly affected in the hind leg and the shoulder joint in the front leg. The clinical signs of the disease are usually evident within the first two years of life.

During development of bone, cartilage is converted to bone. Impaired blood supply to the cartilage will delay conversion of cartilage to bone and result in abnormally thick cartilage on the joint surfaces, the lower layers of which may die. Therefore the cartilage on the joint surface is only loosely attached to the underlying bone and may become fragmented or detached. This causes inflammation within the joint and production of excess synovial fluid, with the result that the joint capsule becomes distended. Therefore the typical clinical signs of osteochondrosis are joint swelling and lameness. The diagnosis is confirmed by radiography. The disease often occurs at the same site bilaterally (in the opposite front or back leg) so it is important to take radiographs of both joints even if only one is obviously affected. Osteochondrosis seldom occurs at different sites in the same horse.

Although some joints may only have mild osteochondrosis without clinical signs the majority of lesions cause lameness and deteriorate if not treated, so the treatment of choice is surgical removal of the abnormal cartilage and bone fragments to leave healthy underlying bone. This reduces the inflammation within the joint.

SUBCHONDRAL BONE CYSTS

Subchondral bone cysts are holes in the bone close to the articular (joint) surface. They may or may not communicate with the joint surface via a narrow neck. The holes in the bone are filled with fibrous material and/or joint fluid. There is controversy about whether subchondral bone cysts and osteochondrosis are related conditions. The exact cause of subchondral bone cysts is unknown. Repetitive trauma resulting in tiny fractures in the bone may be important. Cysts occur in most bones, although they are found more commonly in some locations than in others, for example, in the bottom of the femur in the stifle joint. Most cysts which are close to a joint surface cause lameness, although with time this may resolve even though the cyst can still be seen on radiographs. Occasionally cysts fill in and are no longer visible on radiographs. If lameness persists, then surgical treatment may be successful.

DISTENSION AND ENLARGEMENT OF A JOINT CAPSULE

A joint may appear enlarged either due to thickening of the joint capsule or its distension by excessive amounts of synovial fluid. This may occur without lameness. Some horses seem particularly prone. Horses, especially the middle to heavyweight types with upright forelimb conformation, commonly have distension of the fetlock joint capsules, giving a rounded appearance to the joints. This becomes more obvious if the horse does a lot of work on hard ground. The swelling may be controlled by keeping the joints bandaged but this is not essential. These swellings are sometimes called articular windgalls.

BOG SPAVIN

Bog spavin is a distension of the joint capsule of the true hock (tarsocrural or tibiotarsal) joint (see Figure 7b). It does not normally cause lameness. One or both hocks may be affected. It is particularly common in young, fastgrowing youngsters, and both in these and in older horses usually resolves spontaneously. Distension of the joint capsule may reflect disease within the hock (e.g. osteochondrosis, secondary joint disease or bone spavin), but in the majority of cases is an innocuous swelling of no clinical significance and no treatment is required. If the swelling is associated with lameness, further investigation including radiography is indicated.

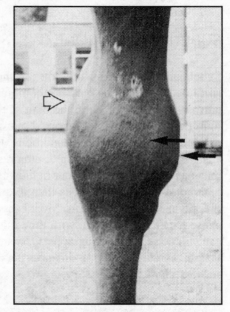

Figure 2
Soft, fluctuant swelling of the tarsocrural joint capsule: bog spavin. The swelling is most obvious on the front and inside of the hock (black arrows). There is also an out-pouching of the joint capsule on the outside of the hock (white arrow). Pressure applied to one swelling causes the other to enlarge

JOINT SPRAIN

Joint disease may be limited to the structures around the joint, that is, to the synovial membrane, the joint capsule and the collateral ligaments. Sprain of these structures is usually the result of the joint suddenly being positioned abnormally, for example, when it is twisted. Not all the structures need be affected simultaneously, or to the same degree. Inflammation of the synovial membrane (synovitis) and the joint capsule (capsulitis) alone is less serious than damage to the collateral ligaments, as the latter may impair the stability of the joint and predispose to damage of the joint itself (secondary or degenerative joint disease see below).

Clinical signs

There is heat around the joint and swelling due to distension of the joint capsule by excess synovial fluid. If the collateral ligaments are sprained, then there is more swelling around the joint. Passive flexion of the joint causes pain and lameness is accentuated by manipulation of the joint. With such obvious clinical signs additional diagnostic tests are frequently unnecessary, although it is prudent to examine the joint radiographically to exclude the possibility of a fracture. Radiographs will demonstrate the presence of concurrent bony damage but will often appear normal apart from showing soft-tissue swelling around the joint. Radiographs obtained ten to fourteen days after injury may show periosteal proliferative reactions (new bone formation) at the sites of attachment of the collateral ligaments and joint capsule. Unfortunately it is not always possible to appreciate fully the extent of the damage and to determine whether it is restricted to the soft-tissue structures of the joint or if it involves the articular cartilage, in which case the long-term prognosis is more guarded.

Treatment

Inflammation should be reduced by application of cold to the joint – cold hosing and cold-water bandages. Anti-inflammatory drugs, such as phenylbutazone, may help to relieve pain and minimize the inflammatory reaction. Immediate ultrasound treatment may help to reduce soft-tissue swelling. A firmly applied support bandage may maintain reduction of swelling. The horse is confined to box rest. The duration of rest required depends on the severity of the initial injury and ranges from two to three weeks to several months. Intra-articular medication with sodium hyaluronate alone or in combination with a low dose of corticosteroids may be used as a single treatment. This permits a more rapid return of normal joint function, or is used to alleviate persistent joint inflammation caused by synovitis and capsulitis.

SECONDARY (DEGENERATIVE) JOINT DISEASE (OSTEOARTHRITIS)

Despite extensive studies in man and in experimental animals, much controversy still surrounds the exact mechanism of development of secondary (degenerative) joint disease (osteoarthritis). The condition starts as a degradation (breakdown) of the articular cartilage, which may occur secondarily to inflammation of the soft-tissue structures of the joint (synovitis and capsulitis). Loss of substances called proteoglycans from the cartilage into the synovial fluid itself causes synovitis, creating a vicious circle. The structure of the cartilage is altered by loss of proteoglycans and collagens and its function is impaired. This contributes to the vicious circle.

Bony changes occur later in the disease and are a response to what is primarily a disease of cartilage. It may develop as a sequel to a traumatic incident such as a severe sprain, or it may have a more insidious onset. Conformational abnormalities may result in abnormal stresses on a joint and thereby predispose to development of degenerative joint disease. Back-at-the-knee conformation may result in abnormal stresses on the joints of the knee. This, together with the tendency of the joint to hyperextend when the horse is galloping, causing compression of the front faces of the bones of the knee, results in a high incidence of secondary joint disease of the knee in young racing Thoroughbreds. Although secondary joint disease is predominantly a problem of the mature horse, it is not exclusively so. The lower-limb joints - the knee, hock, fetlock, pastern and coffin joints – are more commonly affected than the upper-limb joints, bone spavin (see p. 250) and ringbone (see p. 233) being common examples.

Clinical signs
Lameness may be sudden or insidious in onset. There may be distension of the joint capsule by increased amounts of synovial fluid. Passive flexion of the affected joint may be resented and may accentuate lameness. The range of motion of the joint may be restricted due to fibrosis of the joint capsule. If there is extensive new bone around the joint, there is firm swelling around the joint.

Diagnosis
It is often necessary to use local anaethesia to determine the source of pain. Radiographs will not always provide enough information because there is often a poor correlation between radiographic abnormalities and clinical signs. The absence of radiographic changes does not preclude a joint as the source of the problem; in early degenerative joint disease no radiographic changes are detectable. Similarly the presence of radiographic abnormalities does not necessarily implicate that joint as the source of pain. There may be fairly extensive bony changes some distance from a joint which may reflect previous tearing of soft-tissue attachments which are currently of no clinical significance. Radiographs cannot demonstrate cartilage damage unless this is extreme with considerable loss of articular cartilage and narrowing of the joint space. Currently there is no reliable means of detection of cartilage damage, but this is commonly present in long-standing joint disorders and is how we define osteoarthritis; it is irreversible and potentially progressive. Radiographic changes diagnostic of secondary joint disease include periarticular bone spurs (osteophytes), narrowing of the joint space and sclerosis of subchondral bone. Their presence indicates a fairly advanced case.

Treatment

Treatment of chronic secondary joint disease is aimed at minimising soft-tissue inflammation and associated pain, facilitating joint lubrication and maintaining optimal nutrition of the articular cartilage.

Precise treatment involving medication, exercise and surgery, depends on the joint involved, the duration of lameness, the severity of the radiographic changes and the response to treatment. Oral, intra-muscular, intra-venous and intra-articular medications are available, and fall into three main categories. Non-steroidal anti-inflammatory drugs (e.g. phenylbutazone, meclofenamic acid, flunixin meglumine, carprofen) reduce soft tissue inflammation, thus reducing pain. They have no direct effect on the rate of cartilage degradation although pain relief may improve joint mobility and cartilage nutrition. Corticosteroids are potent anti-inflammatory drugs with the potential to cause further cartilage degradation if used incorrectly. They are given in small doses directly into the joint. 'Chondroprotective' drugs, including hyaluronic acid, polysulphated glycosaminoglycans (PSGAG's) and oral treatments such as glucosamine and chondroitin sulphate have gained in popularity more recently. There is no clear evidence to prove they have a 'cartilage sparing' effect but may help improve clinical signs in less severe cases. There is little scientific rationale behind the use of blistering or firing other than enforcing rest. Rest may permit soft tissue inflammation to subside, but some joint movement is essential and complete immobilization of the joint is contraindicated. Few surgical treatments can be performed. In some cases a joint may be fused (arthrodesis), or fragments of bone removed through keyhole surgery. Joint replacement, as in humans, is not possible at this moment in time.

Degenerative joint disease is a common problem which is, as yet, poorly understood. The different postures of man and the horse put different joints at stress; hence the relatively high incidence of hip osteoarthritis in man compared to the horse. In contrast to man, the incidence of rheumatoid arthritis in the horse is extremely rare. There is no firm evidence to suggest that there is a hereditary factor involved in the development of degenerative joint disease in the horse, although both the now obsolete Stallion Licensing Act and the recently introduced National Stallion Approval Scheme preclude recognition of stallions with ringbone. Ultimately the horse has to perform athletically as a sound animal, and at the moment management of degenerative joint disease is a major problem which remains unsatisfactorily answered.

LUXATION (DISLOCATION)

Luxation of a joint means that the bones forming a joint have been displaced relative to one another with resultant extensive damage to the surrounding soft tissues. It is a rare and serious injury in the horse and causes severe lameness.

Realignment of the bones may require anaesthetizing the horse in order to get adequate relaxation of the muscles to allow movement of the bones. Early treatment is essential for a successful outcome.

A more common occurrence is subluxation or partial displacement of two bones. Hind pastern joints in young Thoroughbreds are the most commonly involved. The cause is uncertain. It may be related to pain and analgesic medication can be beneficial. It resolves spontaneously in some horses.

JOINT INFECTION (SEPTIC ARTHRITIS, JOINT ILL)

Infection of a joint occurs most commonly in foals, but may be found in adult horses. In foals one or several joints may be infected and the condition is colloquially called 'joint ill'. Infection usually originates from the blood. A foal which is immunologically compromised because of failure to receive colostrum is most at risk. In the adult, infection is usually restricted to one joint and may originate from the blood or be a sequel to a penetration wound.

Clinical signs
There is a sudden onset of severe lameness associated with warm, painful enlargement of the joint capsule. The horse may be depressed and inappetent. Rectal temperature may be elevated.

Diagnosis
The results of infection of a joint are rapidly damaging, so an early diagnosis is essential. Naked-eye examination of the joint fluid may be highly suggestive. The normal yellow, translucent synovial fluid is orange-brown, discoloured and turbid and less viscous than normal. Estimation of the total number and type of white blood cells in the fluid confirms the diagnosis. Although the joint is infected, it is often not possible to isolate the causative organisms. If infection has been present for some time (several days), destructive bony changes may be seen on radiographs. This merits a poor prognosis.

Treatment
The aims of treatment are to kill the infectious microbes and to minimise further damage to the joint by enzymes produced by the bacteria and by the white blood cells which invade the joint cavity in response to infection. This is achieved by aggressive antibiotic treatment maintained for up to several weeks and by copious flushing of the joint to remove debris from within the joint. This may be possible with the horse standing, but sedation or general anaesthesia is often required. A large needle is inserted into the joint and sterile fluid is pumped into the joint and then allowed to escape either via a second needle or through the input needle. In some cases arthroscopy may be used to assess

the severity of the joint infection and help remove solidified debris from within the joint spaces. This procedure should be done as soon as possible after recognition of infection and sometimes must be repeated.

Prognosis
The prognosis depends on the duration of clinical signs prior to initiation of treatment, and the speed of response to treatment. The longer infection is present the greater likelihood there is of irreversible cartilage damage and development of secondary joint disease. A joint which is suspected of being infected should be treated as such until proven otherwise. Multiple joint infections in foals warrant a guarded prognosis.

Conditions of the Fetlock and Pastern

Functional anatomy
The metacarpophalangeal (fetlock) and proximal interphalangeal (pastern) joints are hinge joints. The joints flex and extend, but there is minimal movement from side to side. Side-to-side movement is controlled by the collateral ligaments. On the back of the fetlock joint are two smaller bones, the proximal sesamoid bones. The suspensory ligament attaches to the top of these bones. Three pairs of ligaments – the superficial, middle and deep distal sesamoidean ligaments – attach to the bottom of the sesamoid bones and to the top of the middle (second) phalanx (short pastern bone), to the back of the proximal (first) phalanx (long pastern bone) and to the top of the proximal phalanx respectively. The deep and superficial flexor tendons pass over the back of the sesamoid bones.

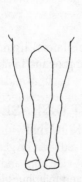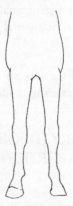

Figure 3   Toe-in and toe-out conformation

Horses with upright conformation of the pastern and fetlock are prone to enlargement of the fetlock joint capsule (articular windgalls) and the flexor tendon sheath (tendoinous windgalls). This is physiological and does not necessarily imply the presence of disease. Horses with a long sloping pastern are likely to stress the suspensory apparatus, i.e. the suspensory ligament, the sesamoid bones and the distal sesamoidean ligaments. Toe-in and toe-out conformation results in particular stress on the outside and inside of the fetlock and pastern joints respectively.

Fetlock injuries are not uncommon in all types of horses and ponies in both forelimbs and hind-limbs. Injuries and disease of the pastern joints occur less frequently.

SPRAIN OF THE FETLOCK JOINT

Clinical signs
The horse is lame. There is enlargement of the fetlock joint capsule and there may be more diffuse, warm, soft-tissue swelling around the joint. The horse resents flexion of the joint.

Diagnosis
Sudden onset of lameness associated with the development of such swelling is typical. If lameness is severe, or fails to improve rapidly with rest, radiographs should be obtained to preclude the possibility of bone damage.

Treatment
The aims of treatment are to reduce pain and soft-tissue inflammation. Cold hosing and cold-water bandages help to reduce swelling and inflammation. Phenylbutazone is beneficial. Ultrasound treatment is also useful in the early stage to reduce swelling but is not essential. Box rest should be continued until all swelling has dissipated.

Prognosis
Provided that there is no major damage of the collateral ligaments of the fetlock joint resulting in instability of the joint, the prognosis is favourable.

SECONDARY (DEGENERATIVE) JOINT DISEASE (OSTEOARTHRITIS) OF THE FETLOCK JOINT

Clinical signs
The horse is lame. Forelimbs are more often affected than hind limbs. There is usually, but not always, slight to moderate distension of the fetlock joint

capsule and resentment of passive flexion of the joint. The fetlock joint may also be abnormally stiff. Lameness is usually accentuated with the affected leg on the inside of a circle or by flexion of the joint.

Diagnosis
Lameness is alleviated by desensitization of the fetlock region by nerve blocks and by intra-articular anaesthesia of the joint. Early disease may be present in the absence of radiographic abnormalities. As the disease becomes more advanced, radiographic changes typical of secondary joint disease develop (see p. 227).

Treatment
In the early stages intra-articular treatment with sodium hyaluronate or a glycosaminoglycan polysulphate can resolve the lameness. When radiographic changes are advanced, the prognosis is poor.

SECONDARY (DEGENERATIVE) JOINT DISEASE (OSTEOARTHRITIS) OF THE PROXIMAL INTERPHALANGEAL (PASTERN) JOINT (RINGBONE)

Secondary (degenerative) joint disease of the pastern joint is known as high articular ringbone. It may arise spontaneously, or be secondary to an injury.

Clinical signs
Both fore- and hind-limbs can be affected. The horse shows a variable degree of lameness. If more than one leg is affected, the lameness may be difficult to pinpoint. There is firm swelling in the pastern region and there may be resentment of manipulation of the joint and/or limitation of its range of motion.

Diagnosis
In the early stages it is necessary to use local anaesthesia to confirm the site of pain. In more advanced cases radiographs confirm the clinical diagnosis. There is loss of joint space and production of new bone around the joint.

Treatment
The condition is incurable. The horse may be enabled to work sound by treatment with phenylbutazone or intra-articular medication. Some horses fuse the joint spontaneously and, provided that there is not an excessive production of new bone, may become sound. If there is excessive new bone production lameness may persist despite fusion of the joint. If only one joint is affected, surgical fusion can be performed. The prognosis is better for hind limbs than for forelimbs.

FLEXURAL DEFORMITY OF THE METACARPOPHA-LANGEAL (FETLOCK) JOINT (CONTRACTED TENDONS)
See p. 330.

ANGULAR DEFORMITY OF THE FETLOCK JOINT
See p. 331.

CHIP FRACTURES IN THE FETLOCK JOINT

It is not particularly unusual to see on radiographs a small bony piece on the top front aspect of the proximal phalanx (long pastern bone). If smooth, small and well rounded, this may be an insignificant radiographic abnormality and can be present in more than one leg. It may represent a separate centre of ossification or an old chip fracture. It can be present without causing lameness. If seen in a lame horse, its significance must be proven. It should not be assumed that it is the cause of lameness.

Figure 4
An oblique radiographic view of the metacarpophalangeal (fetlock) joint showing a small chip fracture or separate centre of ossification (arrow). Such abnormalities can be seen in both lame and sound horses and must be interpreted with care

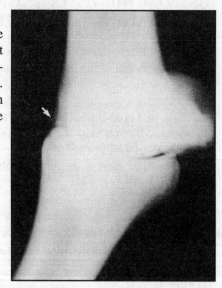

Diagnosis and treatment
The horse is sound after intra-articular anaesthesia of the joint. If the bony piece is slightly irregularly shaped or if some abnormality in the contour of the top edge of the proximal phalanx can be identified, the piece is likely to be significant.

Treatment is by surgical removal.

Prognosis
Provided that there are not major radiographic changes indicative of secondary joint disease, the prognosis is good.

CONDYLAR FRACTURES

Condylar fractures are fractures of the bottom end of the cannon bone which enter the fetlock joint and extend obliquely upwards. They occur almost exclusively in young racing Thoroughbreds and Standardbreds when working at speed. They can occur in both the forelegs and hindlegs.

Clinical signs and diagnosis
The horse is very lame and may be non-weightbearing on the limb. At the time of injury there may be little to see, but within twelve to twenty-four hours some swelling in the fetlock region usually occurs. There is pain on movement of the joint.
Diagnosis is confirmed by radiographs.

Treatment and prognosis
The fracture is stabilised surgically using screws and the lower leg is temporarily immobilized in a cast, which is then replaced by a heavy support bandage.
Provided that the fracture is non-displaced and is treated early, the prognosis is good.

FRACTURES OF THE PROXIMAL (FIRST) AND MIDDLE (SECOND) PHALANGES See p. 218.

FRACTURES OF THE PROXIMAL SESAMOID BONES See p. 219.

SESAMOIDITIS See p. 211.

WINDGALLS See pp. 225 and 261.

STRAIN OF THE DIGITAL FLEXOR TENDON SHEATH See p. 262.

CONSTRICTION OF A TENDON SHEATH BY AN ANNULAR LIGAMENT See p. 263.

Conditions of the Carpus (Knee)

Functional anatomy

The carpus consists of two rows of small bones. Three bones of the top row, the radial, intermediate and ulnar carpal bones articulate with the bottom of the radius. On the back of the knee is the accessory carpal bone. The top row of bones articulate with the lower row, the second, third and fourth carpal bones. The small first and fifth carpal bones may be present or absent. The lower row of bones articulate with the metacarpal (cannon and splint) bones. Most of the flexion in the carpus occurs in the top two joints, the antebrachiocarpal (radiocarpal) and middle (intercarpal) joints. The small bones in each row of carpal bones are connected to each other by short ligaments.

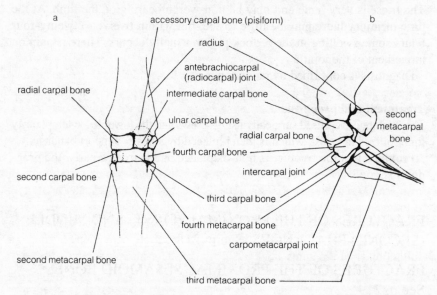

Figure 5   Anatomy of the carpus (knee) a) craniocaudal view b) flexed lateral view

When the carpus is hyperextended, as in the galloping horse, the front edges of the bones of the carpus move closer together. This effect is exaggerated in a horse with back-at-the-knee conformation. Bony carpal problems and degenerative joint disease are most common in racehorses, but are found in other types of horses as well.

Over the front aspect of the knee pass several tendons, the largest of which, the tendons of the extensor carpi radialis muscle and the common digital extensor muscle, are enclosed in tendon sheaths. On the back of the knee, on the inside of the accessory carpal bone, run the digital flexor tendons within a synovial structure, the carpal canal.

SECONDARY (DEGENERATIVE) JOINT DISEASE (OSTEOARTHRITIS) OF THE CARPUS

This is a common condition in racehorses, but occurs occasionally in other types of horses. Either or both the middle (intercarpal) and antebrachiocarpal (radiocarpal) joints are affected.

Clinical signs
The horse is lame. The leg may be swung outwards as the limb is advanced to minimise flexion of the carpal joints. There is slight palpable distension of the joint capsule of the affected joint. The horse may resent full flexion of the carpus and lameness may be exaggerated by flexion.

Diagnosis
In some cases the diagnosis can be based on the clinical signs and radiographs. The correlation between radiographic abnormalities and the degree of lameness is not very good. In particular, bony proliferation on the front face of the small carpal bones at the site of attachment of the intercarpal ligaments does not necessarily cause lameness. The diagnosis is confirmed by intra-articular anaesthesia. This is mandatory in early cases when there may be no radiographic abnormalities.

Treatment
In the early stages in young Thoroughbreds the condition may resolve with rest. A more rapid return to soundness is achieved by intra-articular treatment. If there are advanced changes seen on radiographs the long-term prognosis is poor. In older horses sodium hyaluronate or a glycosaminoglycan polysulphate is sometimes useful. Flexion of the carpus many times daily helps to maintain full mobility of the joints. This is especially important in a jumping horse.

BROKEN KNEES See p. 312.

FRACTURES OF THE CARPUS See p. 218.

PHYSITIS See p. 214.

HYPOPLASIA OF THE CARPAL BONES See p. 340.

HYGROMA (see also Acquired or False Bursae, p. 260)

A hygroma is an acquired bursa on the front of the knee as a result of repetitive trauma, such as banging the knee on the stable door. It results in a cosmetic blemish. If the swelling is very large, flexibility of the knee may be restricted. The swelling may be variable in size and a blow to the knee will cause temporary enlargement of the swelling and inflammation. Occasionally there is slight lameness.

If a horse with a 'big knee' is kept in work the swelling will usually persist, although it may fluctuate in size. If the horse is rested for several months the swelling usually diminishes and becomes firmer.

Treatment
If the swelling is small, no treatment is required. If the swelling is large, drainage and injection of a corticosteroid can be helpful if the limb is then bandaged and the horse confined to box rest for seven to fourteen days, but the results are not uniformly successful. Surgical removal of the false bursa gives the best cosmetic result.

Prevention
If possible, the cause should be removed. Lining the stable door with coconut matting is sometimes helpful.

DISTENSION OF THE TENDON SHEATHS OF THE EXTENSOR CARPI RADIALIS, THE COMMON DIGITAL EXTENSOR AND THE LATERAL DIGITAL EXTENSOR TENDONS

The tendons of the extensor carpi radialis, the common digital extensor and the lateral digital extensor muscles pass over the front of the knee. These tendons are each enclosed in a tendon sheath. Inflammation of the tendon sheath (tenosynovitis) causes production of excess synovial fluid and long tubular swellings around the tendon. Inflammation is usually the result of direct trauma. These swellings must be differentiated from the more diffuse swelling of a hygroma. Lameness can occur, but is rare, unless there is tendon damage or adhesions develop within the sheath. Treatment is usually unnecessary, but some swelling is likely to persist.

Conditions of the Elbow

With the exclusion of capped elbow (a cosmetic blemish which does not cause lameness), fractures of the olecranon and radial nerve paralysis, problems involving the elbow are extremely rare. Lameness associated with the elbow causes a similar type of lameness to shoulder lameness and the two are difficult to differentiate.

Functional anatomy

The elbow joint is a simple ginglymus or hinge joint. The main part of the joint is the articulation of the humerus with the radius. The ulna in the horse is not exactly similar to that in man. It lies on the back of the elbow joint and its upward projection, the olecranon, forms the point of elbow. The ulna fuses with the back of the radius and does not extend beyond the top half of the radius although a separate vestigial lower remnant is sometimes seen. The joint is supported on the inside and outside by the medial and lateral collateral ligaments.

CAPPED ELBOW   (see also p. 260)

Capped elbow is the name applied to an acquired bursa on the point of the elbow. It develops due to repetitive trauma, such as the heel of the front shoe pressing on the elbow when the horse is lying down. Although it may be unsightly, it is of no real clinical significance.

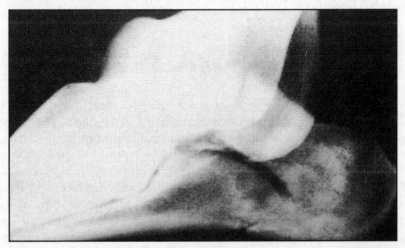

Figure 6   A simple displaced fracture of the olecranon of the ulna involving the elbow joint, sustained as the result of a kick. The fracture was treated successfully by reduction and internal fixation using a contoured bone plate

Application of a sausage boot around the pastern should prevent the heel of the shoe and the elbow coming into contact.

FRACTURE OF THE OLECRANON

Fractures of the olecranon of the ulna usually occur as the result of direct trauma, such as a kick or a fall, but sometimes occur spontaneously.

Clinical signs
One of the principal extensor muscles of the upper forelimb is the triceps muscle which attaches to the top of the olecranon. If the olecranon is fractured, the function of this muscle is compromised and the horse will tend to stand with the limb semiflexed and the elbow dropped. The limb is advanced with difficulty. There may be audible or palpable crepitus (grating of the bones), and manipulation of the elbow causes pain.

Diagnosis and treatment
Diagnosis is confirmed by radiographic examination.
    Although some simple, non-displaced fractures of the olecranon heal spontaneously with box rest, surgical stabilization of the fracture is the treatment of choice. Single fractures warrant an optimistic prognosis. If there are many bone fragments, the prognosis is poor.

RADIAL NERVE PARALYSIS See p. 281.

Conditions of the Shoulder

Although, in the absence of any obvious swellings or areas of heat or pain in the lower leg, the shoulder is often incriminated as the cause of lameness, genuine shoulder lameness in the horse is comparatively rare.

Functional anatomy
The scapula (shoulder blade) and the humerus form the shoulder joint, which is a ball and socket joint, which principally flexes and extends, but can also rotate. Unlike other joints, the shoulder joint has no collateral ligaments and support is provided by muscles which cross the inside and outside of the joint. In contrast to man, the horse does not have a collar bone. The foreleg is attached to the rest of the body by the serratus muscles, which attach to the lower neck and side of the chest and to the inside of the scapula.

SHOULDER LAMENESS

Most horses with a genuine shoulder lameness exhibit a gait with certain characteristics. The horse tries to limit the amount of movement of the joint by taking a much shorter stride. The flight of the foot is lower than normal to avoid flexion of the shoulder and the horse may drag the toe as the leg is advanced. There is a marked lift of the head as the lame leg is advanced, resulting in a very obvious head lift and nod. The horse is often lamer with the affected leg to the outside of a circle, especially in soft going. Because the horse is not using the leg normally, the muscles over the shoulder blade may become atrophied (wasted).

OSTEOCHONDROSIS (see also p. 224)

Osteochondrosis is a developmental abnormality of cartilage and bone and one of the more common sites is the shoulder joint. The condition affects either the scapula or the humerus or both.

Clinical signs
The disease is most often seen in young (six months to two years of age), rapidly growing horses, especially, in Great Britain, in Thoroughbreds. In the early stages the lameness is often intermittent and variable in severity. When the lameness is moderate to severe the gait abnormality is characteristic of shoulder lameness. The muscles over the affected shoulder tend to atrophy.

Diagnosis
In some instances it is necessary to use local anaesthesia to confirm the source of pain, but in most young horses the history and clinical signs are suggestive of the condition, which is confirmed by radiography. The condition may be bilateral and both shoulders should be radiographed routinely.

Treatment
Without treatment the disease usually deteriorates and secondary joint disease develops, resulting in permanent lameness. A small number of horses have been treated surgically with encouraging results.

FRACTURE OF THE SUPRAGLENOID TUBERCLE

The supraglenoid tubercle is a large bony projection on the front of the lower end of the scapula, to which is attached the biceps brachii muscle. This muscle is a powerful flexor muscle of the elbow and its downward pull tends to displace fractures of the supraglenoid tubercle. The fractures are usually the result of a fall on the shoulder, or a collision with either another horse or a solid object such as a gatepost.

Clinical signs

There is usually considerable soft-tissue swelling over the front of the shoulder and typical shoulder lameness. The swelling dissipates fairly rapidly and the lameness often improves significantly within seven to ten days so that a fracture is not suspected. Muscle atrophy over the shoulderblade may develop rapidly due to concurrent damage of the suprascapular nerve.

Diagnosis and treatment

Diagnosis is confirmed by radiographic examination.

Smaller avulsion fractures, which do not enter the articular surface of the glenoid cavity, may respond well to conservative management and occasionally the fragment may be removed. The prognosis for fractures involving the joint surface is much worse and the fracture fragment becomes displaced forwards and downwards due to the pull of the biceps tendon. Successful surgical repair has been performed in some small or young horses with improved results, but the repair can often fail due to the immense pull by the biceps tendon.

FRACTURE OF THE SCAPULA See p. 217.

FRACTURE OF THE HUMERUS See p. 217.

BRUISING OF THE SHOULDER REGION

Because of its prominent position the shoulder region is extremely prone to severe bruising due to a kick or a fall or a similar accident.

Clinical signs

The clinical signs can be extremely difficult to differentiate from those of a fracture of the supraglenoid tubercle (i.e. a severe shoulder-type lameness) and it is often necessary to obtain radiographs to exclude the possibility of the latter. The horse often remains very lame for weeks and then starts to make a rapid improvement.

Treatment
Ultrasound treatment is useful in the early stages, together with anti-inflammatory analgesic drugs to help to reduce the swelling and pain. Subsequent faradic treatment can help to prevent muscle atrophy due to disuse. Muscle atrophy may occur due to concurrent damage to the supras-capular nerve (sweeny).

The long-term prognosis is usually good.

INERTUBERCULAR (BICIPITAL) BURSITIS See p. 260.

MUSCLE STRAIN

Due to an abnormal step or exertion, a horse can strain muscles in the shoulder region, principally the triceps muscles, the brachiocephalicus muscle (a muscle at the base of the neck) and the pectoral muscles.

Clinical signs
Depending on the severity of the muscle strain, the horse will show a variable degree of lameness, which is often worse as the horse moves on uneven ground, on soft surfaces or up or down a gradient.

Diagnosis and treatment
Palpation and manipulation of the forelimb may enable a painful focus to be detected. Faradic stimulation is helpful.

Treatment consisting of rest and faradism, followed by a controlled exercise programme, usually results in a successful outcome.

SWEENY See p. 280.

INSTABILITY OF THE SHOULDER JOINT See p. 281.

NECK INJURIES (see also p. 317)

Occasionally injuries to the lower neck can cause forelimb lameness.

Conditions of the Hock

Functional anatomy

The tarsus or hock is not a simple joint, but consists of several joints. The largest joint, the tarsocrural (tibiotarsal) or true hock joint, is the top joint and is the articulation between the tibia and the talus (tibiotarsal bone). This is where most of the flexion of the hock occurs. Adjacent to the talus is the calcaneus (fibular tarsal bone).

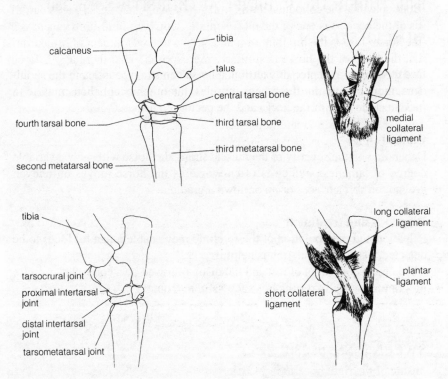

Figure 7a/b   The bones, joints and principal ligaments of the tarsus (hock)

It is this bone which forms the point of the hock. There are two layers of small hock bones. The joint between the talus and calcaneus and the first row of small hock bones is the proximal intertarsal joint. The next joint, between the two rows of small hock bones, is the centrodistal (distal intertarsal) joint. The bottom row of hock bones articulates with the cannon and splint (metatarsal) bones at the tarsometatarsal joint. Even in the normal horse little movement occurs in the three lower joints, the proximal and distal intertarsal and the tarsometatarsal joints. There are several strong collateral ligaments on the inside and outside of the hock which attach to the tibia and the next row of bones, the talus and calcaneus. There is a broad plantar ligament which attaches to the back of the fibular tarsal bone. There are several small ligaments which attach to the small hock bones.

SECONDARY (DEGENERATIVE) JOINT DISEASE (OSTEOARTHRITIS) OF THE HOCK (BONE SPAVIN)

Bone spavin is the colloquial term for degenerative joint disease or osteoarthritis of the hock. It is one of the most common causes of hind-limb lameness in the horse. Just as the hip joint of man is prone to development of osteoarthritis, the hock of the horse is similarly predisposed. That there are different predilection sites is probably attributable to the upright posture of man and the four-legged position of the horse. Bone spavin commonly affects the centrodistal (distal intertarsal) and tarsometatarsal joints and only occasionally involves the proximal intertarsal joint.

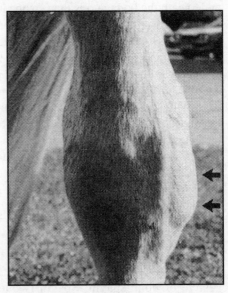

Figure 8
Firm swelling (arrows) on the inside of the right hock associated with bone spavin

Clinical signs
Because the disease is often bilateral, that is, affects both hind legs, one of the common presenting signs is a generalised hind-limb stiffness which is often worse when the horse first comes out of the stable and then improves with exercise. It is usually more obvious in horses that do some form of dressage or flat work, because lack of hind-limb impulsion is more readily apparent under these circumstances than when hacking. The horse may take a few unlevel steps, especially when moving in small circles. It may be difficult to

maintain a regular rhythm in lateral work, tending to hop. Frequently when working in medium and extended paces, the horse may lose rhythm or take obvious lame steps or break stride. There are many reasons for these symptoms – inadequate training, lack of suppleness, insufficient preparation for the movement – but if there is no good explanation, slight lameness may be the cause. If the horse is a jumper, he may start to stop uncharacteristically. Sometimes, because the horse is not pushing properly from behind, he appears rather restricted overall and the problem is wrongly attributed to back trouble. Many horses with a hind-limb lameness will develop back muscle soreness secondarily to an abnormal way of moving.

If the problem is unilateral or one leg is affected worse than the other, then the first sign may be obvious hind-limb lameness. This can be gradual or sudden in onset. If it develops gradually, the hindquarters may appear asymmetrical with the muscles on the affected side less well developed because the horse has been favouring the leg.

Although not characteristic of all horses with spavin, the limb flight may be altered so that, as the affected leg is brought forward in trot, it deviates in underneath the body and is then stabbed outwards as it comes to the ground. This results in excessive wear of the outside branch of the shoe. The stiff legged horse tends to drag the toes, which causes abnormal wear of the toes of the feet and shoes. Toe-dragging is a feature not only of spavin: lameness associated with the stifle or hip joints can cause a toe-drag; many young horses drag the hind toes, particularly if unfit; and toe-dragging may just reflect laziness. With spavin, restricted flexibility of the hind limb or resentment of flexion may be noticed first by the farrier. The horse may be reluctant to hold the leg hyperflexed for a long time.

Some horses develop a swelling on the inside of the hock at the so-called seat of spavin. This is at the level of the distal intertarsal and tarsometatarsal joints. Although the swelling feels very hard, it is not bony, but is a fibrous reaction around the joints.

Diagnosis
A history of hind-limb stiffness improving to an extent with exercise, or of hind-limb lameness characterized by stiffness and dragging of the toe is suggestive of bone spavin. Spavin is one of the most frequent cases of a hind-limb disability in the horse. Swelling on the inside of the hock and abnormal wear of the shoes are useful indicators. Careful observation of the horse moving may give additional clues. It is useful to watch the horse on a hard surface, such as a driveway or road. Then subtle abnormalities in the limb flight and unevenness in stride length may be detected. It is easiest to appreciate slight irregularities in rhythm by listening to the horse, as well as looking at him. A slight, intermittent toe-drag may be heard more easily than seen. In some instances lameness may be more apparent when the horse

moves in circles rather than in straight lines – either with the affected leg on the outside or on the inside. This is particularly so in deep going.

Lameness associated with spavin is accentuated by prolonged flexion of the leg in most horses, although failure to react to the spavin test does not preclude this diagnosis. The spavin test is performed by holding the leg in maximal flexion underneath the body for at least a minute, and then trotting the horse and reassessing the lameness. Although called the spavin test, it is nonspecific because it is impossible to flex the hock without also flexing the stifle and hip joints. Prolonged hyperflexion of the leg will stress all these joints and can accentuate the lameness associated with any of them. Whenever doing the spavin test, it is important to assess the reaction of both legs. It is best to test the sounder leg first because, if the lame leg is flexed first, lameness may be accentuated to such an extent and for so long a time that it is then difficult to interpret the reaction to flexion of the sounder leg.

Radiographic examination
Because the disease is often bilateral, although obvious lameness may only be seen in one leg, it is advisable to have a radiographic examination of both hocks.

Degenerative joint disease starts as a disease of the articular cartilage and only later progresses to involve the underlying bone. Cartilage cannot be seen on radiographs. It appears as a black line between adjacent bones – the joint space. In the early stages of bone spavin radiographs of the affected hock may look normal, but this does not necessarily mean that the joints are normal. In the normal horse the joint spaces are readily seen as black lines. The bones have a clear outline with no fuzziness. The corners of the bones are square or slightly rounded. The bones are of fairly uniform whiteness.

As the disease progresses the joint spaces may become narrower or even completely obliterated, due to destruction of the articular cartilage which normally fills the space between adjacent bones. Nature appears to try to stabilise the affected joints by producing new bone to bridge the joints. This can be seen either as bone spurs (osteophytes), which are smoothly outlined projections of bone, or as irregularly outlined, fuzzy periosteal new bone.

The destructive part of the disease may progress to involve the bones as well as the cartilage, and black areas become apparent in the normally white bone. All these changes are typical of degenerative joint disease (bone spavin). In some horses an end stage is reached. The joint spaces are completely obliterated and the bones look fused. At this stage the horse is usually sound again. Nature, by fusing the bones, has removed the source of pain.

The correlation between clinical signs and radiographic changes is often poor. The horse may be very lame but show minimal radiographic changes. Similarly radiographic changes may be very extensive but may not be associated with lameness.

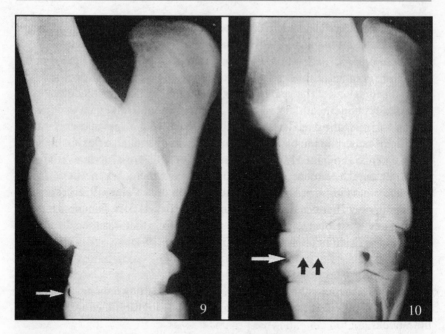

Figure 9   A side radiographic view of a hock with degenerative joint disease of the tarsometatarsal joint (bone spavin). There is a large bone spur (arrow) on the top of the third metatarsal (cannon) bone, bridging the joint. The radiograph has been deliberately underexposed to highlight the bone spur which is less dense than the normal bone. Therefore the joint spaces cannot be seen

Figure 10   An oblique radiographic view of a hock with degenerative joint disease of the distal intertarsal joint (bone spavin). The distal intertarsal joint is partly fused (black arrows). There is some bone destruction (white arrow)

Nerve blocks

In some horses the history and clinical signs do not clearly indicate a hock problem. In other horses with typical clinical signs the radiographs may not confirm the suspected diagnosis. In these situations it is necessary to use local anaesthesia to define the source of pain. This can be done in one of two ways. Either local anaesthetic may be infiltrated over the nerves which convey sensation from the hock region, effectively numbing the area, or local anaesthetic may be placed directly into the suspected joints. The latter is more specific but much more difficult.

In most cases the lameness is improved, but only rarely can it be eliminated totally by nerve blocks. It is therefore important that the horse is showing a sufficient degree of lameness, so that improvement can be appreciated. If the horse is only marginally lame, interpretation of the nerve block is extremely difficult. Therefore, although superficially it may seem contraindicated to work a lame horse, in some instances it is necessary to do so in order to accentuate or maintain the same level of lameness, so that a diagnosis may be reached. Nuclear scintigraphy also helps in the diagnosis of some cases.

Treatment
The end stage of the disease is functional fusion of the affected joints. In some horses this occurs spontaneously, but it is impossible to tell in which horses it will happen, or how long it might take. If an affected horse is rested, the clinical signs usually subside, but they tend to recur when work is resumed. The degenerative changes progress fairly slowly. Treatment aims to accelerate the degenerative changes in order to achieve effective stabilisation of the joints. Fortunately most of the flexion of the hock occurs in the tarsocrural joint, which is unaffected in this condition. Therefore, even if the affected joints do fuse, the ultimate flexibility of the leg should not be compromised unduly.

One method of accelerating the degenerative changes is to maintain the horse in work, while judiciously treating it with a pain-killing drug, such as phenylbutazone, to enable it to work sound. This is satisfactory provided that the horse is not too lame. It is not possible to predict for how long medication will be required – it may be for years. The toxic effects of phenylbutazone in the horse are much less than in man and many horses have been maintained on continuous treatment with phenylbutazone for months or even years without any untoward effects. A few horses do not tolerate the drug and develop soft faeces or diarrhoea quite quickly. Other horses will not eat the drug. It can be disguised by mixing it with milk of magnesia and injecting it into the mouth by syringe, but some horses become wise to this trick.

Many horses are helped additionally by appropriate shoeing. The foot should be trimmed as short as possible and the toe of the shoe rolled in order to help the foot break over. Shoeing the horse with a flat shoe, with an extension on the outside heel, an outside trailer, helps to widen the gait of affected horses and improve the lameness.

The type of work which the horse does can be important. Excessive hill work or deep going may aggravate the problem. Controlled exercise may be better than turning out. An over-exuberant horse which bucks and races round and stops suddenly in the field may twist the joints and accentuate the lameness. A careful, slow, progressive warm-up programme is probably important. Thus if treatment by work and pain-killing (analgesic) medication is adopted, then the work programme should be planned carefully and corrective shoeing performed concurrently.

An alternative treatment is to inject the affected joints with an anti-inflammatory corticosteroid drug. This provides local pain relief, although the use of corticosteroids in joints is controversial because at high doses these drugs will accelerate cartilage degradation, and thus in other locations may aggravate the disease long term, but in this instance destruction of the cartilage is beneficial. There are several problems associated with this treatment. The joint spaces are very small, and it is not at all easy to insert a needle accurately into the joints in order to administer the drug. The effects of the treatment are usually temporary and repeated injections may be necessary several times each year. Nevertheless this can be a useful method of treatment.

If the horse fails to respond to conservative treatment or is very lame, then surgical treatment may be contemplated. Drilling of the joint surfaces to destroy some of the articular cartilage may be used alone or in combination with screw and plate fixation. Several techniques have been described, with similar results, and like most orthopaedic operations in horses it is not uniformly successful. Approximately 60% respond favourably to bone drilling alone, becoming sound within six to twelve months of surgery. Some exercise post-operatively is beneficial, and again phenylbutazone is a useful painkiller to use in the interim period, before the horse becomes sound.

Other surgical techniques encountered are cutting of the cunean tendon to reduce forces on the hock and subchondral bone drilling to reduce pressure within the bone plates next to the degenerate joints. Chemical fusion by injecting a cartilage-dissolving drug can have serious complications if there is communication of the small hock joints to the tarso-crural joint and the treatment is very painful in the initial stages.

Occasionally the proximal intertarsal joint is involved. This warrants a very poor prognosis regardless of treatment because this joint communicates with the tarsocrural or true hock joint, where most flexion occurs. Inflammation in the proximal intertarsal joint induces inflammation in the tarsocrural joint, causing persistent lameness.

ENLARGEMENT OF THE TARSOCRURAL (TIBIO-TARSAL) JOINT CAPSULE (BOG SPAVIN)

Distension of the joint capsule of the tarsocrural (tibiotarsal, true hock) joint is colloquially called 'bog spavin'. It results in a soft, fluctuant swelling on the inside front aspect of the hock and another swelling, slightly higher, on the outside of the hock. If pressure is applied to one of these swellings, the other one is seen to enlarge because they represent outpouchings of a single joint capsule. The condition is often seen, either unilaterally or bilaterally, in big-jointed young horses. It does not cause lameness and usually resolves spontaneously. It is also seen in older horses and rarely causes lameness.

If the horse is lame in association with a bog spavin, then the hock should be radiographed. Horses with osteochondrosis usually develop distension of the tarsocrural joint capsule and there may or may not be associated lameness. Horses with degenerative joint disease (bone spavin) of the proximal intertarsal joint can have a bog spavin. The proximal intertarsal and tarsocrural joints communicate, and degenerative joint disease in the former can incite inflammation in the latter and therefore distension of the joint capsule.

If the hock is severely twisted and sprained there is usually not only distension of the tarsocrural joint capsule but also more extensive soft-issue swelling.

SPRAIN OF THE HOCK JOINT

Clinical signs
There is a sudden onset of lameness associated with soft-tissue swelling and usually some heat around the hock. Flexion of the hock may be resented and will accentuate the lameness. Lameness may be very severe.

Diagnosis
The clinical signs are fairly typical and, especially if there is a known history of trauma, further diagnostic tests are unnecessary unless the horse is very lame. Then the possibilities of a fracture or infection of the joint must be excluded by radiographs and by analysis of a sample of synovial (joint) fluid.

Treatment
Rest is mandatory. Initially anti-inflammatory analgesic drugs and ultrasound treatment can be beneficial. When the horse starts to improve, controlled exercise is useful. If marked lameness persists, then follow-up radiographs should be obtained at intervals to see whether any bony proliferations have developed at the site of ligamentous attachments. This would indicate severe ligamentous damage requiring a more prolonged recovery time. If the joint has been very severely sprained, secondary degenerative joint disease (bone spavin) may supervene.

Prognosis
The prognosis depends on the severity of the initial injury. Frequently a degree of swelling persists, due to some thickening and fibrosis of the joint capsule.

CURB See p. 276.

DISPLACEMENT (LUXATION) OF THE SUPERFICIAL DIGITAL FLEXOR TENDON See p. 272.

THOROUGHPIN See p. 263.

FRACTURES

Clinical signs

There is a sudden onset of severe hind-limb lameness. The horse is reluctant to bear weight on the leg and resents flexion of the hock. There is usually some soft-tissue swelling.

Diagnosis

Because of the complex structure of the normal hock joint, multiple, high-quality radiographs may be necessary to identify a fracture. In some cases a fracture line cannot be seen because the fragments cannot move apart due to the tight ligaments holding the small hock bones together. If there is a strong suspicion of a fracture then nuclear scintigraphy may help to diagnose the precise location.

Treatment

Most fractures warrant a guarded prognosis for future soundness. Small fractures originating from the bottom outside and inside parts (lateral malleolus and medial malleolus) of the tibia usually have a fair prognosis and, depending on the size of the fracture and its degree of displacement, can be treated either by rest alone or by surgical removal of the fragment. Slab fracture of the central or third tarsal bone can sometimes be treated successfully by internal fixation.

OSTEOCHONDROSIS (see also p. 224)

The tarsocrural (true hock) joint, is a common site for osteochondrosis in the horse.

Clinical signs

There is usually moderate to marked distension of the tarsocrural joint capsule (bog spavin). The horse may be lame or sound. If lame, the lameness can be accentuated by flexion of the joint. The condition may be unilateral or bilateral.

Diagnosis

Diagnosis is by radiographic examination. There are several sites at which osteochondrosis occurs in the hock – at the lower end of the tibia and on the trochlear ridges of the talus (tibiotarsal bone).

Treatment

Osteochondrosis of the lower end of the tibia can be an incidental radiographic abnormality, unassociated with lameness, in which case no treatment is indicated. Even if the separated bone fragment is removed, a bog spavin may persist, causing a cosmetic blemish. Osteochondrosis of the trochlear ridges of the talus often causes lameness. Early surgical treatment offers a good prognosis for future soundness, although mild distension of the tarsocrural joint may remain.

COLLAPSE OF THE THIRD AND/OR CENTRAL TARSAL BONES See p. 342.

See p. 342.

Conditions of the Stifle

Functional anatomy
Although the stifle joint is only a hinge joint it is one of the most advanced and complicated joints in the horse. Four bones form the stifle joint: the femur, the tibia, the fibula and the patella (knee cap). The joint is stabilised by ligaments and cartilage segments, the menisci, which are themselves held in position by meniscal ligaments. The cranial and caudal cruciate ligaments, in the middle of the joint between the femur and tibia, cross over to provide stability from front-to-back and rotational movement. The collateral ligaments provide side-to-side stability, and the wedge shaped menisci add to this support. The fibula is a small bone situated on the outside of the tibia and has little function. It is often formed from two or more separate ossification centres which sometimes never unite and this should not be confused with a fracture. The patella slides up and down the bottom end of the femur over the trochlear ridges. It is a sesamoid bone in the quadriceps muscle and its smooth movement depends upon normal function and strength of the muscle. Attached to the inside of the patella is a large cartilaginous extension. Three ligaments, the medial, middle and lateral patellar ligaments, run from the bottom of the patella to the tibia.

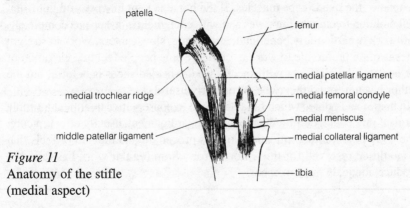

Figure 11
Anatomy of the stifle
(medial aspect)

This unique arrangement of the patellar cartilage and ligaments allows the horse to hook the patella over the top of the trochlear ridges of the femur and fix the stifle in extension. This means that the horse can stand with little muscular effort, so can sleep standing up. The stifle joint cannot flex independently of the hock because of another unique arrangement of muscles and tendons, the reciprocal apparatus, so stifle and hock lameness can appear similar.

INTERMITTENT UPWARD FIXATION OR DELAYED RELEASE OF THE PATELLA

Clinical signs

The clinical signs depend on the severity of the condition, which occurs most often in young horses and ponies, especially those which are unfit and poorly muscled. In the most severe cases the leg becomes stuck in extension and the patella is 'locked'. The horse may hop on three legs, dragging the affected leg behind it. The horse may release itself spontaneously. Some horses remain unable to flex the leg and it may be necessary to force the horse either to back or to jump forward in order to release the patella, which has become effectively stuck on the upper part of the trochlear ridges of the femur. This may happen intermittently several times a day, especially if the horse is kept in. One or both hind legs may be affected.

In less severe cases the patella moves jerkily and its release from the position when the leg is extended is slightly delayed. This may be most obvious as the horse walks up or down a slope, or when pushed sideways. If moved over in the box, the horse may move the leg very stiffly. It may find it difficult to make smooth downward transitions from trot to walk and the back legs may appear slightly uncoordinated and jerky.

It is usually not a painful condition and the horse is not as such lame.

Treatment

In many horses and ponies the condition appears to be related to poor muscular tone of the quadriceps muscles. If the horse is kept in work and got fitter, the condition frequently improves and with enough time disappears completely. Hill work is particularly beneficial, as are long, slow canters. Work in straight lines is often preferable to work in circles. Some people feel that elevation of the heels of the hind feet with special wedge-heeled shoes is helpful, but the author has not found this to be particularly useful.

In horses and ponies which fail to respond to conservative treatment a simple surgical procedure, cutting the medial patellar ligament, usually effects a cure. There are potential complications of this procedure and the author feels that it should be reserved for those horses for whom regular work has failed to produce adequate improvement.

CONGENITAL LUXATION OF THE PATELLA

This is a rare condition in which the patella slips sideways (usually outwards). In some cases the lateral trochlear ridge of the femur is unusually small and this predisposes to abnormal movement of the patella. The signs are usually present at birth. The foal finds extreme difficulty in standing because it is unable to straighten the hind-limb(s) and squats with all the joints of the hind-limb(s) flexed. The patella can be felt unusually positioned towards the outside of the joint.

If the lateral trochlear ridge is unusually small, the prognosis is poor. If there is no identifiable underlying bony abnormality surgery may be successful. A tuck is placed in the joint capsule of the femoropatellar joint to stabilize the patella.

OSTEOCHONDROSIS (see also p. 224)

The lateral trochlear ridge of the femur is one of the most common sites for osteochondrosis.

Clinical signs
The condition is usually seen in young horses (six months to three years old), but is occasionally identified in older horses. There is marked distension of the femoropatellar (stifle) joint capsule and slight to moderate lameness characterised by a stiff limb flight, lowered arc of flight of the foot with or without an intermittent toe-drag. Lameness may be accentuated by flexion of the limb. The condition may be unilateral or bilateral. Young horses with both stifles affected may become slightly roach-backed and have difficulties in getting up after lying down.

Diagnosis
Diagnosis is confirmed by radiographic examination.

Treatment
Without treatment lameness usually persists. Provided that the lesions are not too severe, surgery is generally successful.

SUBCHONDRAL BONE CYST (see also p. 225)

The stifle joint is a common location for subchondral bone cysts, which almost invariably occur at the point of maximum weightbearing in the lower end of the inside of the femur, the medial femoral condyle. They most commonly present when young horses begin training although the lesions may have been quiescent for some time. They are also seen in older horses.

Clinical signs
The horse shows a sudden onset of a variable degree of lameness. The lameness may be extremely subtle or very severe. The horse usually improves with box rest but the lameness recurs when work is resumed. There is only slight distension of the stifle joint capsule, if any.

Diagnosis
It is often necessary to exclude other potential sites of lameness first by nerve blocks. Diagnosis is confirmed by radiographs.

Treatment
Prolonged rest (six to nine months) results in soundness in approximately 60% of horses. In horses which fail to respond to rest surgery can be performed with a fair prognosis.

Soft tissue injuries of the stifle region

SPRAIN OF THE STIFLE JOINT

Clinical signs
There is a sudden onset of lameness associated with some swelling of the stifle joint capsule.

Diagnosis and treatment
Diagnosis is based on the clinical signs.

Treatment consisting of rest usually resolves the lameness. The duration of rest depends on the severity of the initial injury. If lameness persists, the stifle should be radiographed. If there has been severe ligamentous damage, there may be detached bony fragments at the site of ligamentous attachment or a bone spur. These warrant a poor prognosis.

BRUISING OF THE STIFLE REGION

Bruising of the stifle region is a common injury either as a result of a kick or hitting a fixed fence when jumping. The latter is a common injury of event horses.

Clinical signs
Trauma to this region may result in non-specific injury but severe or persistent lameness may indicate more serious injury to the bone or ligamentous structures supporting the stifle and may be investigated further with lameness examination by a veterinary surgeon including intra-articular anaesthesia, ultrasonography, radiography and nuclear scintigraphy.

Treatment
Anti-inflammatory analgesic drugs are extremely helpful in reducing swelling and removing pain. Plenty of slow exercise prevents the horse from becoming excessively stiff, so if it can be turned out in a small paddock or walked in-hand regularly, this is helpful.

Provided that there is no underlying bony damage the prognosis is good. If the horse does not improve rapidly the stifle should be examined radiographically. A fracture of the patella or other bony damage might otherwise be missed.

FRACTURE See p. 215.

INJURY TO THE CRANIAL CRUCIATE LIGAMENT

Clinical signs
There is usually chronic lameness, sometimes relatively severe, with a history of trauma or a fall whilst competing. Lameness is usually exacerbated by flexion tests and there is swelling of the medial femorotibial joint.

Diagnosis
Anaesthesia of the joint often improves lameness and nuclear scintigraphy may show uptake in the region of the ligament insertion on the tibia. In chronic cases X-ray changes are seen. Full assessment can only be performed with arthroscopy. In cases with severe injury the prognosis is poor, with many cases remaining lame, but partial injuries have a better prognosis.

INJURY TO THE MEDIAL COLLATERAL LIGAMENT

Clinical signs
Lameness is associated with swelling on the medial aspect of the joint, with pain on palpation of the medial collateral ligament. There may also be effusion of the medial femorotibial joint.

Diagnosis

Ultrasonography reveals changes within the ligament with enlargement and changes in longitudinal fibre pattern. X-ray changes at the ligament insertion (entheseophytes) may be seen in chronic cases. A careful examination should be made to check for other injuries. The prognosis is good for partial injuries and provided that there are no other injuries.

INJURY TO THE MENISCI

Meniscal injuries may occur alone, or together with damage of the cruciate or collateral ligaments. Ultrasonographic assessment of both the medial and the lateral menisci can be performed. Injuries to the front part of the meniscal cartilages can be more accurately assessed using arthroscopy, but other parts are not accessible for examination. Treatment by removal of torn portions will often improve the degree of lameness, but the prognosis for a return to athletic use is guarded.

14
BURSAE, TENDONS AND LIGAMENTS

BURSAE (TRUE BURSAE) AND TENDON SHEATHS

Bursae

Bursae are sacs lined by a synovial membrane. They contain synovial fluid. They are found over bony prominences and facilitate the movement of tendons or muscles over the bony protrusion. These are the so-called true bursae; they have standard anatomical locations and are present in all horses. They may become enlarged and/or inflamed, resulting in swelling with or without pain and lameness.

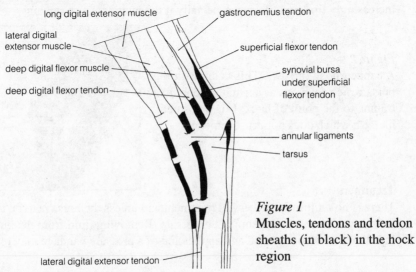

long digital extensor muscle

lateral digital extensor muscle

deep digital flexor muscle

deep digital flexor tendon

gastrocnemius tendon

superficial flexor tendon

synovial bursa under superficial flexor tendon

annular ligaments

tarsus

lateral digital extensor tendon

Figure 1
Muscles, tendons and tendon sheaths (in black) in the hock region

Conditions of Bursae

INTERTUBERCULAR (BICIPITAL) BURSITIS

There is a bursa over the front of the top of the humerus through which passes the tendon of origin of the biceps muscle. This bursa may become inflamed, resulting in severe lameness and a reluctance to advance the limb. Rest and administration of an anti-inflammatory drug is usually successful, but sometimes lameness persists despite treatment.

TROCHANTERIC BURSITIS

There is a bursa over the greater trochanter of the femur, a bony protuberance close to the hip joint. Inflammation of the bursa may cause hind-limb lameness. In the author's experience the condition is very difficult to diagnose and occurs rarely. There is said to be a high incidence in Standardbred trotters and pacers.

ACQUIRED OR FALSE BURSAE

Acquired or false bursae are synovia-filled sacs which develop as a result of repetitive low-grade trauma. They are not present in all horses and usually result in a cosmetic blemish but rarely cause lameness. Common examples are a capped hock, a capped elbow and a hygroma (an acquired bursa over the front of the knee). Once acquired, these swellings persist and may become increasingly firm and fibrous, especially if the inciting cause remains.

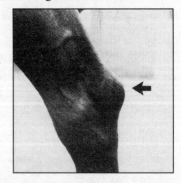

Figure 2
A capped hock (arrow). This is an acquired bursa which develops as a result of repetitive trauma to the point of hock. It is a cosmetic blemish which does not cause lameness

Treatment
There is no uniformly successful treatment and unless the horse is to be used for show purposes treatment is unnecessary. Removing fluid from the bursa, injection of a corticosteroid and application of a pressure bandage may result

in temporary resolution of the swelling. Most of the acquired bursae occur in places which are either difficult to bandage, or where repeated bandaging is likely to result in rub sores. Elasticated support bandages (Pressage bandages) are now available and are particularly good for the knee and hock. Some swellings remain permanently reduced, but others recur. There are potential complications with injection of a long-acting corticosteroid. The drug is a potent anti-inflammatory agent and can depress the body's response to infection, thus, to minimise risk of infection, it is of paramount importance that strict aseptic techniques are employed when injecting this drug into a synovial structure. Calcification within the soft tissues may occur as a result of injection of a corticosteroid.

Irritating solutions such as concentrated iodine have been injected into false bursae, the aim being to destroy the lining membrane which produces synovial fluid and to encourage fibrosis and fusion of the walls of the sac. The results are unreliable. Surgical removal gives the best long-term result for a large false bursa.

Tendon Sheaths

Tendon sheaths are long sacs which are lined by a synovial membrane which secretes synovial fluid. They enclose part or all of a tendon. The fluid provides lubrication for the movement of the tendon. Inflammation of the synovial membrane may result in excessive accumulation of synovial fluid and swelling of the sheath. Tendonous windgalls and thoroughpin are common examples. The sheath may become permanently stretched so that the swelling persists, although there is no longer inflammation. The sheath itself can become thickened.

Conditions of Tendon Sheaths

TENDONOUS WINDGALLS

Tendonous windgalls are enlargements of the digital flexor tendon sheath. Although the sheath extends above and below the fetlock joint, swelling is usually confined to above the fetlock and does not cause lameness. The swelling occurs between the suspensory ligament and the flexor tendons and should be distinguished from distension of the fetlock joint capsule (articular windgall – see p. 225) which occurs between the back of the cannon bone and the suspensory ligament. Windgalls occur in both front and hind legs and are often larger behind, especially in heavier types of horses. Although unsightly, these swellings rarely cause problems.

Figure 3
Normal fore-limbs demonstrating clear demarcation between the cannon bone, suspensory ligament and the deep and superficial digital flexor tendons. The site of distension of the metacarpophalangeal (fetlock) joint capsule (an articular windgall) (closed arrow) between the cannon bone and the suspensory ligament and the site of distension of the digital flexor tendon sheath (a tendonous windgall) (open arrow) between the suspensory ligament and the digital flexor tendons are in dicated

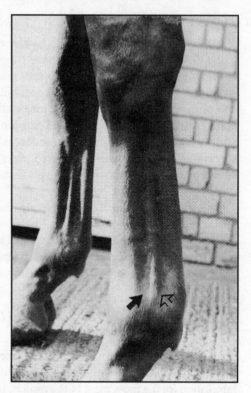

STRAIN OF THE DIGITAL FLEXOR TENDON SHEATH

Occasionally the digital flexor tendon sheath becomes suddenly very swollen and the horse is lame. The swelling occurs above the back of the fetlock, behind the suspensory ligament. This is due to an acute strain and inflammation of the tendon sheath, which can occur without damage to the flexor tendons contained within it. If the sheath is very swollen it may not be possible initially to detect whether or not one or both tendons have been damaged. This assessment can only be made when some of the swelling has subsided or by use of diagnostic ultrasound.

Treatment
Anti-inflammatory analgesic drugs, such as phenylbutazone, help to reduce the acute inflammation. Cold hosing for short periods is beneficial. The leg should be kept bandaged and the horse box-rested for a minimum of ten to fourteen days. Although slight swelling of the sheath may persist, the horse may slowly resume work. Some horses have recurring problems if excessive pressure is applied to the sheath by an over-tight bandage or boot. Occasionally fibrous adhesions develop within the sheath causing chronic lameness.

CONSTRICTION OF A TENDON SHEATH BY AN ANNULAR LIGAMENT

The annular ligament which passes around the back of the fetlock area can constrict the tendon sheath, resulting in a characteristic notching of the contour of the back of the fetlock. Fibrous adhesions may also form within the sheath, and both of these can cause lameness. In some cases medical therapy by direct injection into the tendon sheath can be used to manage the condition. Surgery is required for cases which respond poorly to treatment. The prognosis is more guarded when adhesions are present.

THOROUGHPIN

A thoroughpin is an enlargement of the deep digital flexor tendon sheath above the hock and must be distinguished from distension of the hock (tarsocrural) joint capsule (bog spavin – see p. 250). The swelling of a thoroughpin is higher up and farther back and may be pressed from inside to outside and vice versa.

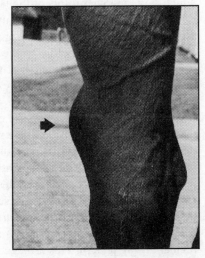

Figure 4 Soft, fluctuant swelling on the upper, outside aspect of the right hock (arrow). This is distension of the deep digital flexor tendon sheath: thoroughpin. The swelling is higher than a bog spavin

The swelling is usually innocuous and may resolve spontaneously. Topical application of a corticosteroid, dimethyl sulphoxide mixture, may speed its resolution. Drainage of excess synovial fluid and placement of corticosteroids within the sheath has proved successful for cosmetic results in more chronic cases. Occasionally lameness is associated with a thoroughpin. Radiograph views of the hock may show bony changes on the sustentaculum tali, over which the deep digital flexor tendon passes. This warrants a poor prognosis.

INFECTION OF A BURSA OR TENDON SHEATH

Infection of a bursa or tendon sheath is usually the result of a penetration wound, and, like an infection of a joint, is extremely difficult to treat unless recognized early. It can be helpful to clip in the region to identify the puncture wound. There is a hot, painful swelling and the synovial fluid is turbid. Treatment consists of the aggressive use of antibiotics combined with flushing the bursa or tendon sheath.

TENDONS AND LIGAMENTS

Tendons

Functional anatomy
Tendons attach muscles to bones and, in comparison to muscles, are relatively inelastic. The evolution of the horse has resulted in an animal which stands on its toes, with slender lower limbs. The bellies of the muscles which flex the lower joints of the legs are confined to the upper limbs, that is, above the knee and hock. The superficial and deep digital flexor tendons are long flattened cords of tissue, approximately oval in cross-section, which connect these muscle bellies to the middle (second) and distal (third) phalanges (short pastern bone and coffin bone). These tendons are covered only by skin and therefore are extremely susceptible to damage by a direct injury to the lower leg.

The structure of tendons is fairly complex (see Figure 7). Surrounding the tendon is a loose connective tissue sheath, the paratenon, and it is from this that blood vessels extend into the substance of the tendon itself. Contrary to popular belief, the tendon has a relatively good blood supply. It is subdivided into groups of fibres called fascicles, which are orientated in a longitudinal fashion, that is, in the direction of stress on the tendon. Within each fascicle the tendon fibres are arranged in parallel in a helical spiral.

The fibres also exhibit 'crimp': rather than being straight, they bend in a regular zigzag pattern. This arrangement confers a degree of elasticity to the tendon. When the tendon is stretched, the crimp straightens, but it can resume its original form provided that the maximum safe load is not exceeded. The fibres can further be subdivided into bundles of collagen fibrils. Collagen is a protein produced by special cells, tendon fibroblasts. These cells are arranged in long columns, parallel to the fibrils. There are several types of collagen which are found in different tissues in the body. Normal tendon is composed of type 1 collagen, which is relatively elastic. Unfortunately, if the tendon is damaged, repair tissue is formed from relatively less strong type 3 collagen,

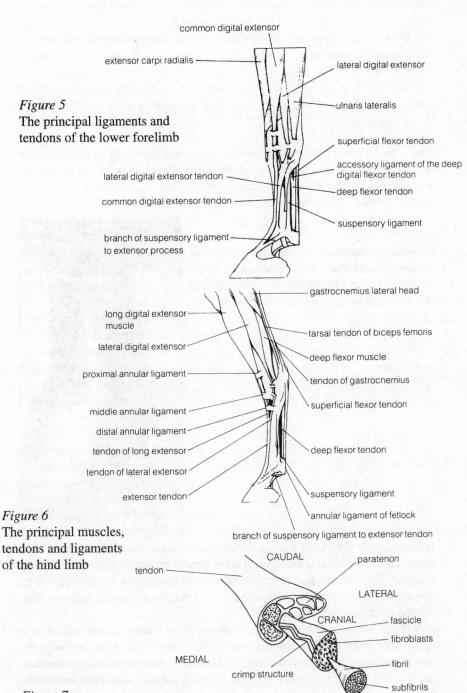

Figure 5
The principal ligaments and
tendons of the lower forelimb

common digital extensor

extensor carpi radialis

lateral digital extensor

ulnaris lateralis

superficial flexor tendon

accessory ligament of the deep
digital flexor tendon

lateral digital extensor tendon

deep flexor tendon

common digital extensor tendon

suspensory ligament

branch of suspensory ligament
to extensor process

gastrocnemius lateral head

long digital extensor
muscle

tarsal tendon of biceps femoris

lateral digital extensor

deep flexor muscle

proximal annular ligament

tendon of gastrocnemius

superficial flexor tendon

middle annular ligament

distal annular ligament

tendon of long extensor

deep flexor tendon

tendon of lateral extensor

extensor tendon

suspensory ligament

annular ligament of fetlock

branch of suspensory ligament to extensor tendon

Figure 6
The principal muscles,
tendons and ligaments
of the hind limb

CAUDAL

paratenon

tendon

LATERAL

CRANIAL

fascicle

fibroblasts

MEDIAL

fibril

crimp structure

subfibrils

Figure 7
Structure of a tendon

thus creating a mechanically inferior structure which is susceptible to re-injury. It is the complex arrangement of the fibres within the tendon which confers strength and elasticity, and disruption of this arrangement compromises the function of the tendon.

Conditions of Tendons

There are a number of types of tendon injury, and they vary in their severity and the long-term consequences for the horse. Constriction of the tendon by an overtight bandage causes the classical 'bandage bow' – localised inflammation around and within the superficial digital flexor tendon.

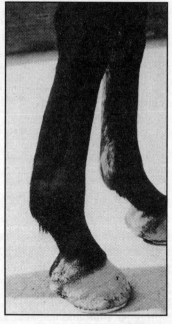

Figure 8
Typical appearance of an old, severely 'bowed', i.e. strained, superficial digital flexor tendon. The back of the leg above the fetlock has a convex contour instead of being straight

Inflammation results in the accumulation of fluid, causing swelling and distortion of the normal anatomical arrangement of fibrils within the tendon. Usually the fibrils are not themselves damaged, thus the long-term consequences for the horse are not serious, although a small, subtle swelling often persists at the site of injury.

A direct blow to the tendon is more serious because, although it is a relatively localized injury, there is usually rupture of some of the tendon fibrils and associated bleeding into the tendon. The fibrils will be repaired by mechanically inferior collagen, thus there is some potential for re-injury, although the prognosis is more favourable for this type of injury than for tendon strain.

In a strained tendon the normal pattern of fibrils and fibres is disturbed and some of the fibrils rupture. In more serious cases fibres or complete fascicles of fibres may be damaged. Occasionally the entire tendon is completely separated. There is bleeding into the tendon and accumulation of inflammatory fluid, which contains enzymes which may cause further damage to the collagen fibrils.

Incidence of tendon strain

The flexor tendons of the forelegs are strained much more often than those of the hind legs. In the forelegs the superficial digital flexor tendon is much more frequently injured than the deep digital flexor tendon. The most common site of injury is the middle of the superficial digital flexor tendon. The tendon has its smallest area of cross-section in this region, therefore the stress on the tendon per unit area is highest. Back-at-the-knee conformation and hyperextension of the fetlock joint associated with a long sloping pastern probably place additional stresses on the tendon, predisposing to injury.

Tendon strain is definitely an occupational hazard of moving at speed, especially if combined with jumping. Thus hunter-chasers, point-to-pointers and event horses are particularly prone. When a muscle becomes fatigued it contracts and relaxes less efficiently. Lack of complete muscular coordination means that the forces applied to the tendon may be more sudden in onset than usual and may not be transmitted evenly through the tendon, resulting in injury. Similarly a sudden change in the going or placing the foot on uneven ground can put abnormal stresses on the tendon.

Clinical signs

Haemorrhage into the tendon and accumulation of inflammatory fluid cause considerable swelling and pain. In the acute stage the degree and extent of swelling usually reflect accurately the severity of the injury. Careful palpation of the tendon with the leg weightbearing and non-weightbearing enables the experienced clinician to assess the degree of swelling and pain. When non-weightbearing, the normal tendon feels firm; damaged tendon feels slightly softer. Once the initial acute reaction has subsided, it is very much more difficult to assess the nature and extent of damage; therefore veterinary advice should be sought as soon as possible in order to obtain an accurate prognosis. It is important to differentiate between minor tendon strain and damage due to localised trauma. Sometimes the swelling associated with a tendon injury is very extensive and it is not possible to define precisely which structures are involved. It is necessary to initiate treatment in order to reduce the swelling before an accurate diagnosis can be made unless diagnostic ultrasound is available.

Significant tendon damage can be present without lameness. In the early stage of tendon injury the amount of swelling may be slight. Usually the vein on the inside of the leg is enlarged. A few days' rest and application of cold may resolve these clinical signs temporarily, but when work is resumed the problem is likely to recur and deteriorate. These early signs must not be ignored. It is important to know exactly what your horse's legs look and feel like, and subtle changes must be noticed and appropriate action taken if more serious damage is to be avoided. The most accurate method of assessing whether or not there is damage to a tendon is by an ultrasound scan. This produces images of the tendons and even very small areas of damage can be detected. The extent of the injury and its severity can be assessed and, by sequential scanning, healing can be monitored. If there is any doubt about the significance of slight swelling in the region of a tendon the author strongly recommends that an ultrasound scan should be performed. It must be remembered that tendon strains often do not cause lameness unless very severe, therefore small swellings should not be ignored just because the horse appears sound.

Treatment of an acute injury
Treatment of an acute tendon injury aims to relieve swelling as soon as possible in order to restore normal alignment of the tendon fibrils, to minimise the inflammatory reaction and to relieve pain. Movement should be limited to prevent further injury. Cold compresses, in the form of ice packs or purpose-built gel packs, should be bandaged to the affected limb for 20 minute periods at frequent intervals. Intravenous injection of anti-inflammatories such as non-steroidal anti-inflammatory drugs (NSAIDs) or corticosteriods will help both to minimise swelling and relieve pain. Corticosteriods are very potent, but should be used for a short-term only as they can result in side effects including delayed healing. The more rapidly the soft-tissue swelling is resolved the better the final functional and cosmetic results are likely to be. Careful use of therapeutic ultrasound can be very effective in dispersal of inflammatory fluid and is thus useful in the acute stage of the injury.

Tendon repair
Following the subsidence of the acute inflammatory reaction, fibroblasts, the cells that synthesize collagen, migrate into the damaged area in a fairly random fashion. It is important that the cells are arranged longitudinally if the repair fibrils are to be correctly aligned. Slight longitudinal tension applied to the tendon is important. Therefore, once the acute inflammatory reaction has subsided, short periods of controlled exercise by walking in-hand are beneficial. This also helps to prevent the development of adhesions between the tendon and surrounding structures. Obviously, an adequate blood supply to the area is necessary for repair tissue to be formed, but it is likely that this is not a limiting factor in tendon repair, therefore it is unnecessary to promote blood supply to the area artificially.

Complete repair of tendon tissue takes a long time. After significant damage to collagen fibrils, a minimum of fifteen months is necessary before the tendon has achieved its maximum healing. Rest, combined with controlled exercise, is probably the optimal treatment currently available. The author usually recommends total box rest until the acute inflammation reaction has subsided, with the leg being kept under bandage. Small periods of in-hand walking exercise are then commenced and gradually increased in duration until, after eight weeks, the horse is walking for up to an hour twice daily. At this stage ridden walking exercise is quite acceptable and short periods of trotting can start. The amount of trotting is progressively increased, up to a maximum of thirty minutes after three to four months. The horse is then turned out for a further convalescence until at least nine months after the initial injury. Slow ridden work is then recommended. Horses become sound long before repair of the damaged tissue is sufficient to withstand stresses of normal work, therefore the temptation to return the horse to work prematurely must be resisted strongly. Ideally, healing of the tendons should be monitored using diagnostic ultrasound because it seems that some horses heal more slowly than others. A premature resumption of work is likely to result in re-injury.

Firing
Much controversy surrounds the practice of either pin or line firing. There is no scientific evidence that either of these procedures is at all beneficial, although there is plenty of anecdotal support. A recent study by Professor Silver and his colleagues from the University of Bristol indicated that neither line nor pin firing accelerated tendon repair. Pin firing actually caused additional damage and prolonged the healing process. Scar collagen in pinfired tendons was not aligned along lines of stress and remained a cause of permanent weakness. Firing tended to be associated with development of peritendonous adhesions, thus compromising the normal function of the tendon. The study was performed on experimental animals, and the tendon injuries were artificially created and cannot be regarded as exact replicas of naturally occurring injuries. However, the basic results are irrefutable and, in the author's opinion, firing is contraindicated in the treatment of tendon injury.

Tendon splitting
Tendon splitting involves the insertion of a small knife into the tendon at several sites and the creation of multiple small cuts within the tendon. Various rationales for this treatment have been proposed, including drainage of inflammatory oedema from an acutely strained tendon and stimulation of an increased blood supply, especially in a chronically damaged tendon. It has also been suggested that tendon splitting can help to create better interdigitation of normal tendon and repair tissue, making re-injury less likely. Professor Silver concluded from his studies* that tendon splitting delayed repair and reachievement of a normal gait when compared to horses treated by rest alone.

*L A. Silver and P. D. Rossdale, 'A clinical and experimental study of tendon injury, healing and treatment in the horse', *Equine Veterinary Journal, Supplement* 1, 1983.

Used alone, or in conjunction with tendon splitting, or tendon injection, the accessory ligament of the superficial flexor tendon (superior check ligament) may be cut to relieve strain on the superficial flexor tendon. The results of this technique have been variable, with failure to prevent further injury in a significant number of cases. Some successfully treated horses go on to injure the suspensory ligament.

Tendon injections
A hole within the tendon or the surrounding region can be injected with the help of ultrasound guidance. There are several drugs now used with varying success rates between veterinarians. Further trial work needs to be completed but there are some promising results when combined with strict re-training programs.

Laser therapy
There are anecdotal reports of low-output lasers being used successfully for the treatment of tendon injuries. Although one cannot disprove the reports, there is no scientific evidence to indicate that such treatment is at all efficacious in accelerating tendon healing although unquestionably soft-tissue swelling is rapidly reduced and this may be beneficial in the long term.

Pulsating electromagnetic field (PEMF) therapy
A lot of interest has recently surrounded the use of pulsating electromagnetic field therapy (PEMF) and a number of products have been available, e.g. the Blue Boot, Magnetopulse. There is evidence that this treatment can accelerate the healing of delayed unions of bone fractures in people. Although there is anecdotal information concerning this treatment for various problems in the horse, one must be extremely sceptical about its interpretation. Unquestionably, if the current is applied at a specific frequency and strength, the behaviour of certain cells may be influenced, but the signal characteristics required to affect tendon cells is different from that for bone cells. The signal characteristics of the currently available devices are probably not ideal and much more experimental work is necessary before we can assess properly whether or not tendon repair can be accelerated or improved. At present we can say that probably there are no deleterious effects of PEMF on tendon healing, but with the present equipment one must be sceptical about any benefits.

Practical implications of tendon strain
From the preceding discussion it should be clear that optimal repair of a strained tendon requires time – at least nine months. The repaired tendon is functionally less efficient than a normal tendon, therefore there is a real danger of re-injury. The horse with poor conformation is particularly susceptible. The future work programme of the horse must be adapted accordingly. The horse

should be as fit as possible for the intended job. Many horses which are unable to withstand the rigours of racing are able to perform in other activities such as hunting.

Prevention of tendon injury

The use of boots and/or bandages can provide some protection to the flexor tendons from injury due to direct trauma. They cannot prevent tendon strain and can, incorrectly applied, actually cause damage to the tendon. Early detection of subtle abnormalities of the tendon is very important. Careful daily observation and palpation of the lower legs should enable an astute manager to detect early changes in the contour of the superficial digital flexor tendon or localised increases in temperature. Care must be taken not to confuse swelling of the tendon with the vein which runs down the inside of the leg just in front of the superficial digital flexor tendon; it is particularly obvious just below the knee. Compare like with like, one leg with another leg. If there is a suspect area, pick up the leg and gently squeeze each tendon between finger and thumb, starting at the top and working slowly down. Assess the consistency of the tendon and the reaction of the horse to gentle pressure. Is there any area of abnormal softness? Does the horse flinch? Is there a similar reaction in the same area of the normal leg? Recognition of the early warning signs is most important. A few days' rest and moderation of the training programme may prevent more serious damage. Initially there may be just localised inflammation without damage to the fibrils and, once the inflammation has subsided, the tendon is restored to normality. Assessment of this can only be done objectively using diagnostic ultrasound, therefore, if in any doubt, rest the horse and seek veterinary advice. It is helpful for the vet if the leg is not bandaged during the twelve hours prior to his examination. This helps him to assess the problem most accurately. If swelling increases without a bandage, this bodes ill.

Should one buy a horse with an old tendon injury?

Inevitably after any tendon injury there is always some slight conformational abnormality of the tendon, and careful palpation of the tendon with the leg non-weightbearing should confirm the presence of an old injury. The length of the tendon affected, the presence or absence of adhesions of the tendons to the surrounding tissues, and whether the deep or the superficial digital flexor tendon is involved must all be assessed. Generally speaking, injury to the deep digital flexor tendon is more serious than a similar degree of damage to the superficial digital flexor tendon, but deep digital flexor tendon injury is rare. The conformation of the horse and its intended use will also determine whether or not it is likely to stand up to work. If there is a known history of blunt trauma to the tendon, the prognosis is better than for a true tendon strain.

TENDON RUPTURE (BREAKDOWN)

Complete rupture of either or both of the superficial and deep digital flexor tendons occurs occasionally. Division of the superficial digital flexor tendon results in sinking of the fetlock. If the deep digital flexor tendon is disrupted, the toe of the foot tips up. The prognosis for either injury is poor.

TENDON LACERATIONS

Lacerations may partially or completely sever the superficial digital flexor tendon and the deep digital flexor tendon and are serious injuries. The wound must be very thoroughly cleaned and all badly damaged, dying tissue removed. This is best achieved under general anaesthesia. If the tendon has been severed completely, it may be possible to stitch it back together, provided that the ends are not too widely separated. Carbon fibre implants have been used in people and horses. However, the results have been poor, with no beneficial effects over suturing the tendon. Carbon fibre fragmentation in both horses and people can result in complications. Whichever of these techniques is used, the limb is then immobilised in a plaster cast. It is usually necessary to raise the heel of the foot so that the ends of the tendon are not pulled apart. The height of the heel is gradually reduced to avoid excessive contraction of the tendon during healing. The horse is box-rested. Although the horse may be pasture-sound, recovery cannot be completely guaranteed. A few horses are able to resume work twelve to eighteen months after the injury, especially if it involves a hind leg. If the laceration occurs within a tendon sheath, the prognosis is less favourable. Lacerations of extensor tendons are less important and surgical repair is often unnecessary.

DISPLACEMENT OF THE SUPERFICIAL DIGITAL FLEXOR TENDON OF THE HIND LIMB

The superficial digital flexor tendon is a flattened fibrous band as it passes over the tuber calcanei (point of hock). Here two fibrous bands detach on either side and insert on the calcancus and help to keep the tendon in position. If either or both of these bands is damaged, the tendon may be displaced either to the outside or, more rarely, to the inside. The injury usually occurs while the horse is cantering or galloping. The tendon may move on and off the tuber calcanei and the horse shows great distress and is unwilling to bear weight on the leg. Initially there is minimal soft-tissue swelling and careful palpation reveals the diagnosis. Within twenty-four hours considerable soft-tissue swelling may develop making accurate palpation more difficult.

Treatment
If the tendon has been displaced and remains displaced, a prolonged period of rest results in considerable improvement; some horses are able to resume work, although there may be some mechanical impairment of the gait. The prognosis is less favourable if the tendon is displaced medially or continues to move on and off the tuber calcanei. Anti-inflammatory medication may be contraindicated, as some inflammation and subsequent fibrosis may help to stabilise the tendon in a displaced position.

Numerous surgical techniques have been attempted to stabilise the tendon, with limited success.

Ligaments

Functional anatomy
Ligaments are fibrous bands which attach to bone. They are similar in structure to tendons, but are more fibrous and less elastic. Damage to collateral ligaments is discussed under joint injuries (see pp. 224 and 226).

The suspensory apparatus
The suspensory ligament attaches to the top of the back of the third metacarpal (cannon) bone. Two thirds of the way down the metacarpal region it divides into two branches, the medial and lateral branches, which attach to the proximal sesamoid bones.

There are also branches which cross onto the front of the pastern region. Attached to the bottom of the sesamoid bones are the distal sesamoidean ligaments, which insert on the proximal (first) and middle (second) phalanges (long and short pastern bones). These structures are important for support of the fetlock joint.

The normal suspensory ligament is uniform in width throughout its length

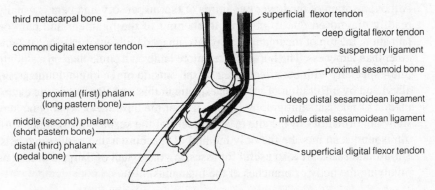

Figure 9 The ligaments and tendons of a lower limb

and has a firm consistency. Pressure applied to it does not cause pain, although some hypersensitive horses may show some reaction to its palpation, as may horses doing a lot of fast work.

Conditions of Ligaments

SPRAIN OF THE SUSPENSORY LIGAMENT (SUSPENSORY DESMITIS)

Clinical signs
The suspensory ligament may be sprained anywhere along its length. The top of the ligament is hidden beneath the digital flexor tendons and between the splint bones and cannot be seen or felt directly. Damage in this area may cause localised heat and/or enlargement of the medial palmar vein on the inside of the limb. Lameness may be extremely slight and only evident after fast work or very long periods of exercise. Injury may occur in the main body just above the site of the division into the two branches, and either, or both of the branches may be injured. An acutely damaged ligament is thicker and of softer consistency than a normal ligament. Pressure applied to the damaged area with the limb non-weightbearing causes pain. If one of the branches of the suspensory ligaments is damaged, there may be concurrent damage to the sesamoid bone to which it is attached.

Predisposing factors
Poor foot balance and pronounced toe-in and toe-out conformation may predispose to injury of the suspensory ligament. Horses which work at speed are most prone.

Diagnosis
Although sprain of the lower two thirds of the suspensory ligament is usually readily diagnosed due to obvious thickening of the ligament and pain on palpation, the top of the ligament may be damaged without overt clinical signs other than lameness. The horse is often more lame on a circle than on a straight line, especially with the affected leg on the outside of the circle. Lameness is alleviated by infiltration of local anaesthetic in this area. Radiographic examination or nuclear scintigraphy (see p. 222) of the third metacarpal bone may show abnormalities at the site of attachment of the suspensory ligament. An ultrasound scan may be the only method of reaching a definitive diagnosis. Ultrasound scans are also useful for assessing the extent of damage of lesions involving the body or branches of the ligaments.

Treatment

The principles of treatment are the same as those for tendon strain (see p. 269), although a recent development for the treatment of chronic cases is the use of shockwave therapy. Pulse waves of energy are used to stimulate healing. This needs further assessment before any final conclusions can be drawn regarding its effectiveness.

Prognosis

The prognosis depends upon the severity of the initial injury, the conformation of the leg and use of the horse. Re-injury occurs not infrequently.

Concurrent suspensory desmitis and fracture of a splint bone are a not uncommon injury in point-to-point horses and steeplechasers. Prognosis depends largely on the severity of the suspensory desmitis.

SPRAIN OF THE DISTAL SESAMOIDEAN LIGAMENTS

Clinical signs

The distal sesamoidean ligaments are not easy to feel. The middle pair of ligaments which attach to the back of the proximal (first) phalanx (the long pastern bone) are most frequently injured. This causes swelling on the back of the pastern region and lameness.

Diagnosis

This injury is most accurately diagnosed using diagnostic ultrasound. If the injury occurred some weeks previously, oblique radiographic views highlighting the areas of insertion of the middle distal sesamoidean ligaments may show periosteal proliferative reactions. In chronic cases there may be calcification in the ligaments.

Treatment

Rest is the best treatment. There is a relatively high rate of recurrence.

SPRAIN OF THE ACCESSORY LIGAMENT OF THE DEEP DIGITAL FLEXOR TENDON (THE INFERIOR CHECK LIGAMENT)

Functional anatomy

On the back of the knee are palmar carpal ligaments which connect the second and third carpal bones with the metacarpus. The accessory ligament of the deep digital flexor tendon is a direct continuation of these and lies between the suspensory ligament and the deep digital flexor tendon. It merges with the deep digital flexor tendon in the middle of the metacarpal region.

Clinical signs

Sprain of this ligament results in a variable degree of lameness. There is usually palpable enlargement of the accessory ligament of the deep digital flexor tendon, but it is vitally important to be sure that swelling is limited only to this structure and that the damage is not more extensive. Lesions are best identified using diagnostic ultrasound.

Treatment and prognosis

The principles of treatment are the same as those for tendon strain (see p. 269), although generally a shorter period of rest (three to six months) is adequate. Ideally, healing should be monitored using diagnostic ultrasound.

The incidence of recurrent injury of this ligament is less than for strain of the deep digital flexor tendon itself and for sprain of the suspensory ligament.

SPRAIN OF THE PLANTAR TARSAL LIGAMENT (CURB)

The plantar tarsal ligament is a long flat band which runs down the back of the hock and is attached to the back of the top of the tuber calcanei (point of hock) proximally and to the calcaneus, the fourth tarsal bone and the head of the fourth metatarsal (outside splint) bone.

Clinical signs

Sprain of this ligament results in a swelling, usually at its insertion on the lower part of the back of the hock. This swelling must be differentiated from the head of the fourth metatarsal bone, which can be very prominent. Strain of the ligament may cause mild lameness.

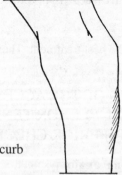

Figure 10 A hock showing the location of a curb

Treatment

Rest usually results in rapid resolution of lameness, although a mild swelling may persist. This swelling is difficult to eradicate. Swelling may occur without lameness. Although curbs can be a recurrent problem in Standardbred trotters and pacers, they are rarely a significant injury in other types of horses.

15
MUSCLE PROBLEMS

MUSCLE ATROPHY

Muscles control movement of the body. They are attached to bone via tendons. An adequate blood and nerve supply is essential for normal function. Muscles waste (atrophy) either due to lack of use or due to damage to the nerve supply. If a horse has a severe hind-limb lameness due to pain in the foot, the muscles of the hindquarters on that side may atrophy. The site of muscle atrophy does not necessarily imply that the problem is in that area.

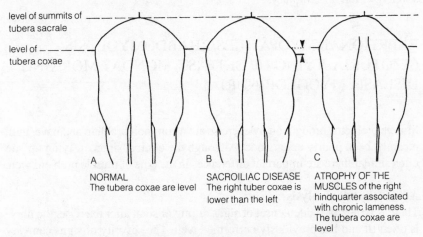

level of summits of
tubera sacrale

level of
tubera coxae

A
NORMAL
The tubera coxae are level

B
SACROILIAC DISEASE
The right tuber coxae is
lower than the left

C
ATROPHY OF THE
MUSCLES of the right
hindquarter associated
with chronic lameness.
The tubera coxae are
level

Figure 1   An assessment of muscle atrophy and pelvic symmetry

Although the lameness may resolve, it may only be when the horse is returned to regular work that the muscle mass is restored. If a nerve is damaged irreversibly, then associated muscle atrophy will not recover unless the muscle receives innervation from more than one source.

MUSCLE STRAIN AND MYOSITIS
(MUSCLE INFLAMMATION)

Muscle strain may be the result of a sudden incoordinate muscle contraction or overstretching of a fatigued muscle. The degree of lameness is variable. Muscle inflammation (myositis) is also present.

Diagnosis
Pressure applied to a strained muscle or manipulation of that muscle may cause pain. Faradic stimulation of a damaged muscle causes pain. A skilled operator can detect differences in the way a damaged muscle contracts in response to faradic stimulation compared with a normal muscle. A high resolution thermography camera is used by some veterinarians to detect changes in skin temperature associated with muscles close to the skin.

Treatment
Rest or a controlled exercise programme is required. Treatment with ultrasound or faradism aids resolution of inflammation and facilitates return to normal athletic function. Some muscles may go into spasm and this contributes to pain. Muscle spasm can be relieved by faradic treatment or, in some circumstances, by manipulation. The period of rest required depends on the severity of the initial injury.

EXERTIONAL MYOPATHIES/RHABDOMYOLYSIS
(AZOTURIA, TYING UP, SETFAST, MONDAY MORNING
DISEASE, MYOGLOBINURIA)

Muscle problems brought on by exercise are a common problem and have, until recently, been poorly understood. Although the clinical signs of 'tying up' are often similar there are important differences in the type of muscle problem seen.

Acute Rhabdomyolysis
There is typically sudden onset of signs during or soon after exercise, the horse is often fit and has previously performed well. The severity of signs can vary from mild muscle stiffness of the back and hindquarters to severe pain, muscle tremors and profuse sweating. Some cases are unable to stand or appear to have colic. Traditionally it has been seen following a period of rest whilst fed on full rations. The underlying cause is over-exertion of the muscles either at speed causing a build up of lactic acid or depletion of energy reserves over time, as in endurance horses. Alterations in cellular metabolism lead to membrane

disruption and breakdown with the release of muscle proteins such as myoglobulin, creatinine kinase (CK), asparate transferase (AST) and lactate dehydrogenase (LDH). Levels within the blood stream can be used to measure the severity of injury and monitor improvement. Some proteins are released into the blood stream and filtered by the kidney causing colour changes (dark brown) in severe cases and kidney damage in the most severe cases.

Treatment varies according to severity but in the initial stages further exercise will exacerbate the condition. Rest with anti-inflammatory medication may be all that is required, severe cases require tranquillisation, fluid therapy and supportive treatment if recumbent. A gradual and early return to exercise may be beneficial, but only if serum muscle enzymes have been closely monitored. Further attacks can be prevented by gradual changes in exercise regimes and encouraging endurance horses to drink electrolyte replacements.

Chronic Rhabdomyolysis (Recurrent Exertional Rhabdomyolysis RER)
Some horses seem to be predisposed to recurrent attacks, often following little exercise, it may be characterised by poor performance. The cause is not well understood with highly-strung individuals, particularly fillies or young mares, more commonly affected. Some, but by no means all horses have abnormal glycogen reserves stored within the muscle, as shown by a muscle biopsy used to diagnose the condition.

Dietary management and strict, regular exercise regimes are most important in the treatment of RER. A roughage only diet, such as good quality hay, can be fed to those horses in little work. Most commercially produced horse and pony cubes fed with hay provide a nutritionally balanced ration for hoses in light to moderate work, with carbohydrate replaced by soya oil or other fats as energy requirements increase further. Electrolyte and vitamin supplementation is also vital as exercise increases. It may be possible to protect excitable horses by altering their environment and some mares may benefit from hormonal control.

RUPTURE OF THE FIBULARIS TERTIUS MUSCLE

The fibularis tertius muscle, one of the muscles of the hind leg, is part of the reciprocal apparatus which prevents the horse from flexing the stifle without simultaneously flexing the hock. It is largely tendonous. Spontaneous rupture of the muscle can occur and is usually the result of the horse getting the leg stuck or left behind in, for example, a ditch. The horse is lame and has an odd hind-limb gait because the stifle may be flexed without flexing the hock. If the leg is picked up and extended behind the horse, there is a characteristic dimple in the contour of the back of the leg above the hock.

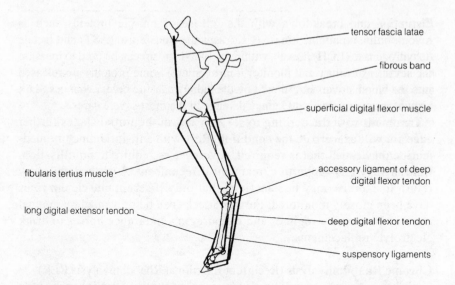

Figure 2 The 'stay apparatus' of the hind-limb. These structures allow the horse to sleep standing up

Treatment
Rest is the only treatment. Most horses become permanently sound.

Abnormal Muscle Function Secondary to Nerve Injury

SWEENY

Sweeny is atrophy of the supraspinatus and infraspinatus muscles, which cover the scapula (shoulderblade). It is a result of damage to the supra-scapular nerve, the nerve which innervates these muscles. This nerve passes over the front of the scapula and is liable to damage if the horse falls on the shoulder or runs into a solid object. If the nerve is damaged irreversibly, muscle atrophy will be permanent. Nerve damage takes a long time to recover and, after severe bruising of the nerve, it may take several months for normal muscle mass to return.

Some horses recover spontaneously. If there is no improvement, isolation of the nerve surgically and removal of a piece of bone over which the nerve passes can relieve pressure on the nerve and muscle mass may ultimately be restored.

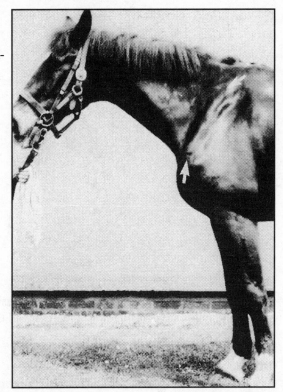

Figure 3
A horse with sweeny. Atrophy of the supraspinatus and infraspinatus muscles which cover the scapula results in abnormal prominence of the ridge on the shoulder blade, the scapular spine (arrow)

INSTABILITY OF THE SHOULDER JOINT

If the nerve supply to the muscles on the inside and outside of the scapula is damaged, then the shoulder joint can move much more than normal because these muscles normally provide stability to the shoulder joint. As the horse starts to take weight on the leg, the shoulder will appear to slip sideways. This injury is usually the result of the horse colliding with something and stretching or rupturing the nerves of the brachial plexus on the inside of the shoulder.

If the nerve damage is not too severe, the horse will slowly improve, but it may take many months. If the damage is severe, the horse will not recover.

RADIAL NERVE PARALYSIS

The radial nerve innervates the muscles which extend the elbow, carpus (knee) and digits. Damage to the radial nerve results in inability to use these muscles properly. Damage to the nerve usually occurs where it passes around the humerus and can be the result of a knock or a fall.

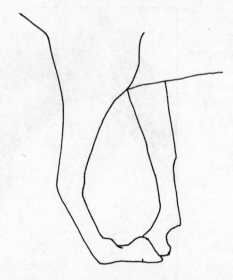

Figure 4   Radial nerve paralysis – the muscles which extend the elbow, carpus and digits are non-functional, therefore all these joints are held flexed, with the elbow 'dropped'

Clinical signs

The horse adopts a typical stance with the elbow dropped and sometimes with the fetlock knuckled forwards. It is unable to move the leg forward properly and may drag the toe, and is unable to walk over small obstacles. It may compensate to a degree by swinging the leg outwards as it is advanced. The muscles innervated by the nerve rapidly atrophy.

Treatment

The lower leg should be bandaged to prevent damage to the skin if the horse tends to knuckle over. Faradic stimulation of the affected muscles helps to retain muscle mass. Prolonged rest to allow time for nerve damage to recover is essential. This may take many months. If the damage is severe, the horse will remain permanently incapacitated.

16
THE FEET

Functional anatomy

There are three bones in the foot: the middle (second) and distal (third) phalanges (the short pastern bone and the pedal or coffin bone) and the navicular or distal sesamoid bone. The middle and distal phalanges articulate via the distal interphalangeal or coffin joint. The navicular bone lies on the back of this joint. The deep digital flexor tendon passes over the back of the navicular bone and inserts on the distal phalanx. Attached to the sides of the distal phalanx are the cartilages of the foot, which may become ossified from one or more ossification sites (sidebone). The distal phalanx is supported in the foot by the laminae. The sensitive laminae are attached to the distal phalanx and interdigitate with the insensitive laminae, which line the inside of the hoof wall. The wall of the foot is horny tissue secreted by the coronary band. The horn is produced at the rate of approximately one centimetre per month. The walls of the foot are infolded at the heels, to form the bars. The wall horn is covered by a thin membrane which helps control the movement of moisture into and out of the wall. The frog is a thick horny cushion on the sole of the foot. There is considerable controversy about its true function and whether it should make contact with the ground.

Most horses have symmetrically shaped and equally sized front and hind feet. The hind feet have more sloping walls than the front feet. The soles are usually slightly concave and only the wall makes contact with the ground. The soles are of variable thickness. A horse with relatively flat soles which are readily compressible by firm thumb pressure is more prone to bruising and sore feet than a horse with firmer, more domed soles. In the wild, constant roaming by the horse wears down the feet, so trimming is not required. With domestication it is necessary to trim the feet regularly every four to six weeks to maintain correct shape, size and balance.

Correct trimming is essential for normal function. Shoeing is not essential but helps to prevent excessive wear of the feet and provides some protection and grip. However, bad shoeing can create problems (see Chapter 20).

The foot is the most common site of lameness in the horse. The incidence of lameness of front feet far exceeds that of back feet.

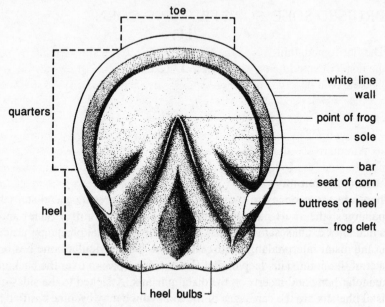

Figure 1a   The foot seen from below

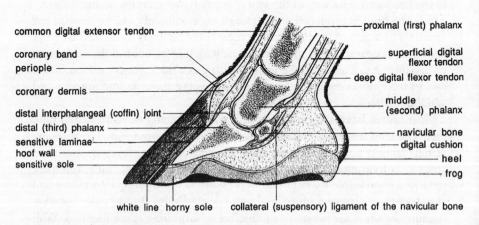

Figure 1b   Lateral view of a section through the foot

Conditions of the Foot

BRUISED SOLE, SORE FEET AND CORNS

The flat-footed, thin-soled horse is most prone to bruising. Bruising is usually the result of standing on a solid object, such as a stone, or repetitive trauma to the sole by a poorly fitting shoe, or excessive work on hard ground. A corn is a bruise which occurs between the wall and bar of the foot at the so-called seat of corn.

Having trodden on a stone, the horse may become suddenly lame and remain so. Alternatively after a few lame steps the horse may recover, only for lameness to recur the following day. Lameness associated with corns may only be obvious as the horse turns, especially with the affected foot to the inside. Generalised bruising or sore feet may be manifest merely as a slightly restricted, pottery, shuffling gait with shorter strides on corners, a reluctance to demonstrate medium and extended paces and a slight hesitation to jump. The horse usually shows more willingness and fluidity in the paces on soft ground.

Hard ground results in a greater concussive force being transmitted through the foot than does soft ground. If the foot is placed flat to the ground, the force is dissipated over the entire hoof wall. If the initial impact is concentrated on a smaller area, the force transmitted through that area will be greater. If the branches of the shoe are too small, the effective surface area making contact with the ground is reduced. If the foot starts to overgrow the shoe, especially at the heels, this predisposes to bruising at the heels. If one part of the foot is slightly higher than the other, that part will make contact with the ground fractionally earlier, concentrating stress on that area. This is a common trimming error. The same unbalancing effect is created by the use of studs, especially if a single stud is used on one branch of the shoe.

Diagnosis

The area of pain can usually be located by the careful use of hoof testers to apply pressure to discrete areas of the sole. Particularly in a white foot it may be easy to identify red areas which reflect subsolar haemorrhage. It may be necessary to remove several superficial layers of horn before an area of bruising can be found. The absence of visible subsolar haemorrhage does not preclude the existence of severe bruising. It is often necessary to remove the shoe before the bruised area can be found. If the horse is just footy or jarred, there may be neither visible bruising nor a discrete area of pain. The digital blood vessels may feel fuller and the pulse in the digital arteries may be more intense than in the normal horse. The diagnosis may be reached only by a careful evaluation of the way in which the horse moves and by exclusion of other potential causes of lameness.

Treatment

If there is a discrete area of bruising, some of the overlying horn is pared off to relieve pressure. Poulticing the foot for a couple of days is of benefit and is essential if a corn has become infected (a suppurating corn). Once the horse has significantly improved, the affected area of the sole must be rapidly hardened so that it can withstand pressure. Direct pressure to the affected area should be avoided. The shoe should be fitted accordingly. If the sole has been severely damaged, it may be helpful to place a rigid metal plate over the affected area, provided the sole is reasonably domed, so that the plate does not press directly onto it. The plate must be rigid to avoid any distortion. A horse with a narrow wall and flat sole should be shod with a wide-webbed shoe with a concave solar surface (a seated-out shoe). This provides some protection to the sole without the potential complications of pads. If possible, studs should be avoided on hard ground. A relatively new fullered shoe with rough-headed nails should provide adequate grip.

There is some controversy over the use of pads, particularly over the type of pad used and the way in which it is fitted. A simple leather pad may protect the site from direct bruising on stony ground and may be of definite temporary value on flinty terrain, or for a horse with a recently bruised foot. These pads do little to alter the concussive force transmitted through the foot and at the same time encourage the foot to sweat. It is much more difficult to fit the shoe so that force is transmitted evenly over the wall. Thus, a leather pad may protect against direct trauma, but will do little to moderate concussion. There are a number of commercially available pads which are claimed to absorb concussion, although there is little scientific evidence to support this; indeed, there is some evidence that pads may actually increase the forces accepted by the sole of the foot, a structure not designed to bear weight. It is important that, if a pad is used, it should not alter the balance and angle of the foot.

PEDAL OSTEITIS

The term pedal osteitis implies that there is active inflammation of the pedal bone or distal phalanx. Traditionally the diagnosis has been based on clinical signs (lameness associated with pain in the foot) and radiographic abnormalities of the distal phalanx. However, there is tremendous variation in the radiographic appearance of the distal phalanx in normal horses. Many horses have distal phalanges with fuzzy outlines, especially at the heels, prominent vascular channels, which appear as broad black lines radiating through the bones or a large notched area at the toe. Therefore it is extremely difficult, in the authors' opinion, to assess which radiographic abnormalities are clinically significant. The authors reserve the term pedal osteitis for those horses with severe radiographic abnormalities in which other potential causes of lameness have been eliminated. It is often possible to localise pain to the foot and not be able to reach a definitive diagnosis, despite good-quality radiographic views. Many of these horses are diagnosed as having pedal osteitis, thus implying a specific condition. The authors believe that this is incorrect and that veterinary surgeons and owners should acknowledge that it is not possible, with the current diagnostic techniques available, to give a name to every lameness. Often we just do not know.

If there are major radiographic abnormalities of the distal phalanx, e.g. periosteal proliferative changes (new bone) on the front of the bone and a marked reduction in the overall density of the bone, this is pedal osteitis and warrants a poor prognosis for future soundness. The bony abnormalities are permanent. A horse with this condition will always be inclined to be footy, especially on hard ground.

LAMINITIS

Laminitis is inflammation of the sensitive laminae of the foot. In Great Britain it occurs most commonly in overweight ponies and horses kept at grass, especially when the grass is growing rapidly. Small ponies are particularly susceptible. It occurs commonly in overweight show ponies and horses. It is also associated with excessive consumption of carbohydrates (grain overload) or with generalised toxaemia (e.g. severe diarrhoea). Excessive weightbearing on one leg may induce laminitis, as can excessive work on hard ground.

Clinical signs
Usually only the forefeet are involved, although sometimes the hind feet are as well. Initially the pony shows extreme reluctance to move and stands with the hind legs well underneath the body, rocking back on the heels of the forefeet to take some weight off the toes. The feet feel hot and the pulses in the blood vessels which supply the foot are pounding. The pulse in the digital arteries is most readily felt at the level of the fetlock joint. Here the arteries supplying the foot are relatively close to the skin surface on the inside and outside of the fetlock.

What causes the pain?
The normal blood flow to the foot is disturbed so that some areas, notably the sensitive laminae, receive an inadequate blood supply, especially in the toe region. The blood supply brings oxygen and nutrients to the tissues, without which the cells become damaged and ultimately die. Damage to the cells induces inflammation (laminitis) and chemical mediators are released, which cause pain. The inflammation also causes swelling which, within the close confines of the rigid hoof wall, contributes to pain.

Treatment

The aims of treatment are to eliminate the cause and to alleviate pain. The cause - overconsumption of lush grass – is removed by confining the pony to a box or a 'starvation square' where there is no grass. The diet should be severely restricted and limited solely to hay and water. It is vitally important not to overfeed and constant access to hay is not necessary. Pain is alleviated by the use of veterinary drugs. These may initially be administered by injection in order to achieve rapid onset of action; subsequently they may be mixed with fluid and squirted into the mouth by syringe, or given as a paste.

Figure 2a
Forces acting on the normal foot

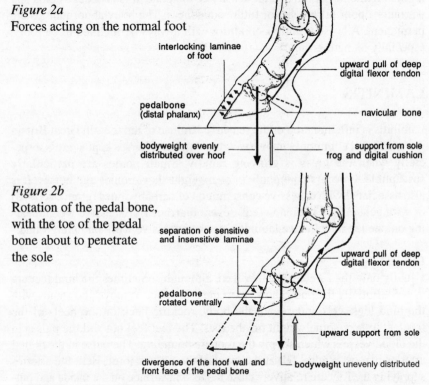

Figure 2b
Rotation of the pedal bone, with the toe of the pedal bone about to penetrate the sole

Walking is important for blood flow within the foot, but excessive exercise carries with it a risk. The sensitive laminae, which clothe the distal phalanx (pedal bone), interlock with the insensitive laminae and thus suspend the pedal bone in the foot. If the laminae are damaged, the interlocking is liable to break down. The deep digital flexor tendon attaches to the back of the pedal bone, and if it pulls upwards and the interlocking mechanism is no longer holding the pedal bone firmly, the pedal bone is likely to rotate so that its toe drops. This can ultimately result in the tip of the bone penetrating through the sole. Overexercise may have dire consequences. Rotation may occur very rapidly and is difficult to control. It may be beneficial to bed the pony on a bedding, which will pack up into the foot and provide some support to the sole.

Within the first twenty-four to thirty-six hours of treatment most affected ponies show improvement, but treatment usually has to be continued for considerably longer to avoid recurrence of clinical signs. Any pony which has once had an attack of laminitis must be regarded as a prime candidate for future attacks and therefore must be managed accordingly: access to pasture, control of bodyweight and farriery must be carefully managed.

Chronic laminitis

Regardless of the initial treatment, some cases of laminitis become chronic, so that there is persistent lameness of variable severity. It is usually associated with some rotation of the pedal bone. Often the toe of the foot is excessively long and the sole appears remarkably flat or even convex. Successful treatment can sometimes be achieved by appropriate trimming of the foot and dietary management. Trimming necessitates cooperation between the vet and the farrier. Radiographs of the foot can reveal the amount of rotation of the pedal bone and its position relative to the hoof wall. Based upon these observations the vet can advise how much of the toe of the foot can be safely removed. Careful, regular trimming is the key to success and a normal shape of the foot and alignment of the pedal bone can slowly be re-achieved.

In severe cases of laminitis which do not respond to more conventional treatment, removal of the entire hoof wall from the coronary band to the ground around the front half of the foot can provide some relief. The hoof must be kept scrupulously clean and under a bandage until firm protective tissues redevelop. Provided that the coronary band is not damaged then the wall will slowly regrow.

In selected cases application of a heart-bar shoe can produce considerable relief. The shoe provides some support over the frog; it is essential that it is fitted correctly or the problem may be compounded.

In any horse with laminitis as a result of poor blood supply to the hoof wall, development of new wall may be impaired, especially in the toe region. Rings on the hoof wall reflect circumferential hoof growth. In a horse with chronic laminitis these rings may be very prominent and may diverge at the heel because the heel has grown faster relative to the toe. Biotin and methionine are amino acids required for the manufacture of keratin, one of the essential components of the hoof wall. Supplementation of the diet with these amino acids may be beneficial to the laminitic pony, but there is little scientific evidence to support this.

In a minority of cases these measures do not achieve complete resolution of the problem and blood tests are performed to determine if other medical conditions may be present as underlying predisposing problems.

Treatment of chronic laminitis is a long-term project. It may be a year or more after the initial onset of clinical signs before the pony is able to resume work and its successful management requires a concerted effort from the triad of owner, farrier and veterinary surgeon.

PROBLEMS ASSOCIATED WITH TRIMMING AND SHOEING

The importance of correct shoeing and trimming cannot be overemphasised. Each foot should be symmetrically shaped with equal-height heels, so that the foot lands on the ground squarely. However well a shoe fits, unless the foot is prepared properly first, the end result may cause uneven distribution of forces through the foot and predispose to lameness either in the foot or in the lower joints of the limb.

The foot should be trimmed so that there is a straight pastern-foot axis to which the heels of the foot are parallel. The medial and lateral halves of the foot should be symmetrical, with the heels of equal height, so that when the horse is standing the foot is in the same plane as the rest of the limb. If one heel is higher than the other, this may predispose to bruising of the foot, damage to the sensitive laminae, disease of the lower limb joints and sprain of the suspensory ligament. Collapse and contraction of the heel may predispose to the navicular syndrome. Poor trimming and its relationship to bruising are discussed above (see p. 285).

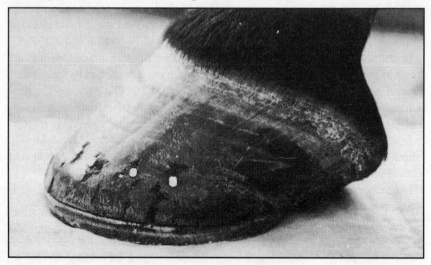

Figure 3   Poor foot conformation typical of many horses with the navicular syndrome. The toe is over long and the heels are low and collapsed and are no longer parallel with the front of the foot. The shoe is too small and gives no support to the heels

The concept that the shoe must be made to fit the foot and not vice versa is not strictly correct. The shape of a foot can be improved by fitting the shoe to an ideal shape (for example, wide or long at the heels) to encourage the foot to grow to that shape. If the shoe conforms exactly to the shape of the foot when the horse is shod, then the foot will soon overgrow the shoe and the shoe

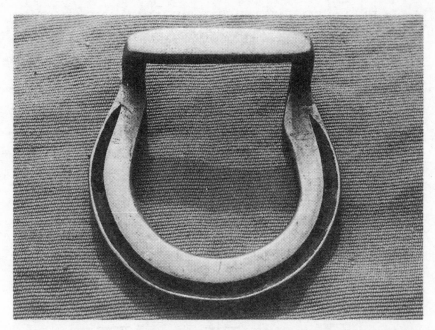

Figure 4
A raised-heel shoe
used for horses with
traumatic disruption
of the superficial
and/or deep digital
flexor tendons

Figure 5
A bar shoe used to
provide stability to
the foot. It is useful
for the treatment of
fractures of the distal
(third) phalanx (pedal
bone), for sheared
heels, and for cases of
severe imbalance of
the heights of the
heels

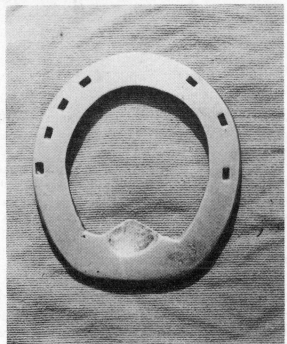

will tend to migrate inwards, predisposing to bruising at the seat of corn. Fitting the shoe wide at the heels does not cause problems with brushing or losing the shoe, provided the horse does not move excessively closely and the shoe is properly finished with the inside edge bevelled.

If the horse is shod with shoes that are too small, this will encourage the heels to become more contracted and to collapse, especially if the toes are left too long. The area through which forces are transmitted is also artificially reduced. This may be compounded by the use of pads. All these factors can cause the horse to move less freely.

NAIL BIND

The shape of a horseshoe nail is designed so that, as the nail is driven into the hoof wall, it is directed upwards and outwards, rather than inwards towards the sensitive laminae. If the nail is placed too close to the white line, it will put pressure on the sensitive laminae causing pain. This is more likely to occur if the wall is very thin. Lameness is evident soon after the horse has been shod.

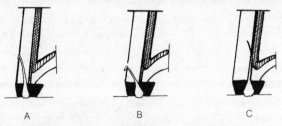

Figure 6   Nail problems: a) correct position of a nail; b) nail angle too great so that nail emerges too low; c) pricked foot – nail penetrates sensitive laminae

If the wall is struck with a hammer over the offending nail, then the horse will flinch. Removal of the nail usually provides adequate relief, but it is sometimes necessary to remove the shoe and obtain veterinary advice about subsequent care and management of the foot.

NAIL PRICK

If a nail is driven into the sensitive tissues of the foot, the horse is said to have been pricked. This is more serious than a nail bind and usually causes more severe lameness. There may be a trace of blood when the nail is removed. Provided that the nail prick is recognized immediately and the nail withdrawn and the hole flushed with a suitable antiseptic solution, then complications should not ensue. If the nail is left, infection is likely to develop.

INFECTION IN THE FOOT, PUS IN THE FOOT, UNDERRUN SOLE

This is the most common cause of lameness in the horse.

Infection in the foot may develop following a puncture wound (e.g. nail prick) or as a sequel to a crack in the white line. In some cases, particularly in the early stages of the infection, when lameness is only slight, it is not always possible to identify the site of infection. Infection in the foot causes inflammation and the production of pus within an enclosed space (abscessation). Because the hoof wall is rigid, pressure increases within the foot, causing extreme pain.

Clinical signs

Although only slight lameness may be evident initially, this may develop so that the horse is reluctant to bear any weight on the limb, sweats profusely, blows and refuses to eat. The foot feels warm and the digital blood vessels have a bounding pulse. The site of infection can usually be identified by applying light pressure with hoof testers to the sole. A discrete area of pain can be located, surrounded by less sensitive areas. Even finger pressure may cause pain and pus may be heard squeaking beneath the sole. The sole may be thinner at this area and a small amount of pus (usually black) may exude through it. The pus will tend to track along paths of least resistance and will migrate beneath the sole (underrun sole) and up between the laminae, eventually to burst out at the coronary band. Before this happens an area of sensitivity and swelling at the coronary band may be identified. There may be diffuse soft-tissue swelling above the foot extending as far as the knee which may make the horse reluctant to flex the fetlock joint.

Treatment

The aims of treatment are to relieve pressure within the foot by draining the abscess and to eliminate infection. If a discrete area of pain is identified by pressing on the sole, then removal of the overlying sole will allow drainage of pus and reduction of pressure and this will produce considerable pain relief. Although a large hole may facilitate drainage, it is likely to result in exposure of sensitive tissues, which can itself cause pain. Therefore it is best to create a medium-sized hole and then encourage further drainage by daily poulticing of the foot for several days. Provided that drainage is established, the horse usually resolves the infection spontaneously. Tubbing the foot, that is, standing the horse in a tub or bucket of warm water and Epsom salts, also helps to draw infection. The bacteria which cause infection in the foot usually thrive in an environment with small or negligible amounts of oxygen (anaerobic bacteria). Flushing the hole with an oxidising agent such as hydrogen peroxide creates an unfavourable environment for the bacteria, which helps reduce the infection. In very severe cases the use of special antibiotics effective against anaerobic bacteria, are extremely helpful. The drug is injected directly into the drainage hole daily for two to four days. The use of other antibiotics injected intravenously or intramuscularly is usually unnecessary and, unless adequate drainage is established, may prolong infection in the foot.

Once the infection is resolved, any sensitive tissues that have been exposed must harden and some new protective horn must develop before the horse is likely to be completely sound. If infection bursts out at the coronary band, horn production in the area will be temporarily impaired. This will result in a horizontal defect in the hoof wall which will gradually grow out.

Puncture wounds create ideal conditions for the multiplication of the bacteria which cause tetanus, so it is essential that if the horse has not been vaccinated against tetanus it should receive tetanus antitoxin.

Any soft-tissue swelling above the foot will resolve spontaneously if the foot is treated appropriately.

Complications
Occasionally a deep puncture wound in the region of the frog can result in infection of the pedal bone and/or the navicular bursa. This is a very serious condition and early surgical treatment is essential. All infected and dead tissues must be removed. This inevitably causes damage to vital structures of the foot such as the deep digital flexor tendon, but without such radical treatment the horse will remain permanently lame. In such cases aggressive antibiotic therapy is necessary.

Prevention
Horses which are turned out unshod and develop hoof wall cracks are particularly prone to pus in the foot. The hoof walls should be regularly trimmed, and if they are inclined to break up excessively the feet should be kept shod.

THRUSH

Thrush is a degenerative condition of the frog which results in the accumulation of black, foul-smelling, moist material in the frog clefts. In the early stages the horse is sound. If the condition is allowed to progress and extends into the sensitive tissues, the horse may become lame. The condition usually develops due to poor hygiene, failure to clean the feet regularly and leaving the horse standing in dirty, moist conditions. A horse with deep clefts is particularly susceptible. Horses with long toes and contracted heels will tend to develop deep frog clefts.

Treatment
Treatment aims to eliminate the cause, to clean the foot thoroughly and to control any infection. The frog and frog clefts must be aggressively trimmed to remove all loose dead tissue. The foot should be thoroughly scrubbed with antisceptic solution. An antibiotic spray may be applied to the affected tissues. This will help to dry and harden them. Alternatively the clefts may be packed with a drying powder. The feet must be cleaned and treated daily until the condition is resolved. The horse should stand on a clean dry bed.

Prevention
The condition is easily prevented by good hygiene – daily, thorough cleaning of the feet and a clean dry bed. Foot shape is important: the toes should be kept short.

SEEDY TOE OR SEPARATION OF THE WALL

Separation may occur at the white line. The separation is usually greatest at the sole and becomes progressively less higher up the wall. If the separation occurs at the toe, it is called seedy toe. The zone of separation is filled with dry, dead, cheesy-type material. It is often seen in horses whose toes have been allowed to become too long. It does not cause lameness unless infection occurs, or there is severe instability of the attachment of the wall to the foot, resulting in inflammation of the sensitive laminae.

The cause of seedy toe is not properly understood.

Provided that the horse is not lame, then the condition can be managed by the farrier by careful trimming of the foot. Gradually the defect should grow out. The toes should be kept short because the tip of the toe tends to act as a lever and may increase separation between the laminae.

HOOF-WALL CRACKS (SANDCRACKS)

Vertical cracks in the hoof wall either develop from the lower, bearing surface of the wall and extend upwards (grass crack) or develop at the coronary band and extend downwards (sand crack). The latter develop as a result of injury to the coronary band so that the function of the horn-producing cells is impaired either temporarily or permanently. The length of crack which develops reflects the severity of the injury. If the cells permanently lose function, there will be a permanent crack down the length of the wall. If the cells recover function, then the crack will grow out slowly, at a rate of approximately one centimetre per month. Cracks which develop at the bearing surface of the wall are usually the result of the foot being overgrown and splitting. Some feet seem particularly prone.

Clinical signs

The clinical signs depend on the depth of the crack. If the crack is only superficial, then the horse is usually sound, but if the crack extends deeper into the sensitive tissues, the horse may be lame, either due to the edges of the crack moving, which causes inflammation of the sensitive laminae, or due to infection.

Treatment

Cracks which are only superficial usually require no treatment other than regular careful trimming of the foot. Applying a shoe helps to stabilise the crack. If a deep crack becomes infected, then the infection must be controlled before an attempt is made to stabilise the crack. Immobilisation of the edges of a deep crack is not easy and the method used depends on the location and depth of the crack and the proposed use of the horse. Cooperation between the vet and farrier is essential. A well-fitting shoe with a clip on either side of the crack is sometimes satisfactory. In some horses the edges of the crack can be laced together or bonded using an acrylic resin. When the resin is applied, it can incite inflammation and temporarily accentuate the lameness.

BRITTLE FEET

Some normal horses develop multiple splits around the bottom of the hoof wall, especially during the summer months. In the unshod horse this predisposes to infection. The shod horse becomes prone to losing shoes. The cause of brittle feet has not been properly established.

The moisture content of the hoof wall is probably partly controlled by the membrane which overlies the wall, the periople. This permits moisture both to enter and to leave the wall. It has been suggested that damage to the periople can lead to excessive desiccation of the wall, making it prone to cracking. If the horse's feet are allowed to become too long and overgrow the shoes, this also encourages the walls to crack. If the shoe becomes slightly loose, there will be more movement of the nails within the wall, predisposing to cracking.

Treatment

Regular trimming and shoeing are extremely important. Some horses seem to benefit from hot shoeing rather than cold shoeing. If the horse is turned out on hard ground, a shoe will help to protect the wall. Horn growth requires certain amino acids, including methionine and other keratogenic agents such as biotin. Although there is little scientific evidence proving their efficacy as dietary supplements in the horse, their use is recommended. The application of a mild blister to the coronary band seems to improve the hoof growth in some horses. Hoof oil is of doubtful benefit and may impair normal movement of moisture through the wall.

NAVICULAR SYNDROME

Navicular disease is most accurately described as a syndrome rather than a single disease, as the term 'disease' implies that there is one specific condition with a single cause. There are probably multiple causes of pain in the navicular bone giving rise to a variety of pathological changes which result in similar clinical signs.

Functional anatomy

The navicular bone lies on the back of the distal interphalangeal (coffin) joint. It is supported by suspensory ligaments which attach to its top border. The deep digital flexor tendon passes over the back surface of the navicular bone and, interposed between it and the bone, is the navicular bursa, a small fluid-filled sac which communicates with the coffin joint. Infoldings of the synovial membrane project upwards into the lower margin of the navicular bone, forming synovial outpouchings.

Many theories have been postulated as to why navicular disease occurs. These include impaired blood flow in the back part of the foot due to poor venous return from the foot, perhaps related to the conformation of the foot. As a result the pressure within the bone may be elevated, causing pain. Thickening of the walls of the blood vessels within the navicular bone have been reported, as have bloodclots (thrombi) in the blood vessels. An alteration in blood flow through the bone may alter bone cell metabolism.

In some horses with the navicular syndrome there is evidence of increased bone turnover within the bone. This may represent a regenerative process. In some cases the primary problem may involve the navicular bursa or the distal interphalangeal joint. At present the cause or causes of pain associated with the navicular syndrome are poorly understood.

Clinical signs

Navicular disease occurs almost exclusively in the front feet of horses. Ponies are rarely affected. It occurs in all breeds of horse, although there is a higher incidence in some breeds, for example, the Quarter horse. Usually both front feet are affected, resulting initially in an insidious shortening of the stride and slight unlevelness on turns rather than obvious lameness. The condition appears worse on hard ground. In the early stages the horse may appear reluctant to go forward properly or to lengthen the stride. The horse is described as 'footy'. The horse may show slight, intermittent lameness on one or both legs, especially when working in circles. In some horses more obvious lameness develops in one or both legs. The horse may point one or both feet when standing at rest. Horses with all types of foot conformation develop the disease. Many affected horses have poor foot balance, long toes and low, collapsed heels. The disease is also seen in horses with upright, narrow feet. In some horses with navicular disease the feet appear to become more contracted at the heels.

Diagnosis

The horse with navicular syndrome tends to place the foot to the ground slightly toe first. This is most readily appreciated when the horse is on a hard, flat surface. The stride length is shortened. Lameness may be accentuated by flexion of the fetlock and lower joints. Obvious lameness may become apparent when the horse is lunged on a hard surface, left forelimb lameness on the left rein and right forelimb lameness on the right rein.

The pulses in the digital arteries may be stronger than usual although the feet are of normal temperature. Hoof testers rarely cause pain.

Desensitisation ('nerve-blocking') of the back part of the foot should make the horse sound on that leg. If the horse is affected in both legs and previously demonstrated a shortness of stride without obvious lameness, lameness may become obvious in the leg which has not been nerve-blocked. This lameness should be eliminated by desensitisation of the back of the foot and the horse should then move more freely.

Diagnosis is confirmed by radiography but cannot be based on radiographic examination alone. There is a large variation in appearance of navicular bones in normal horses. Along the lower border of the navicular bone are a variable number of black triangular areas which represent the synovial outpouchings and vascular channels (nutrient foramina). In some horses with navicular disease these areas are increased in number and size and are more variable in shape. It can be difficult to delineate strictly between what is normal and what is abnormal and the radiographs must be interpreted in the light of clinical observations. In some horses black radiolucent areas develop in the middle of the navicular bone and these are considered diagnostic of navicular syndrome. Erosion of the back (flexor) aspect of the navicular bone is also diagnostic. There is controversy regarding the significance of bone spurs on the upper edge of the navicular bone, especially those which occur on the top corners. Occasionally horses with typical clinical signs of navicular syndrome have small chip fractures along the lower border of the bone. Some horses with clinical signs typical of the navicular syndrome have no radiographic abnormalities.

Treatment

No single treatment alone is uniformly successful. A number of the treatments outlined below can together produce marked improvement provided that there are no erosions on the flexor surface of the bone as these merit a poor prognosis.

Trimming and shoeing Although some horses show significant improvement if the heels of the feet are artificially raised, either by a wedge-heeled shoe or by the use of a wedge pad, this tends to perpetuate or accentuate abnormalities of the shape of the foot. Pads are also difficult to fit properly.

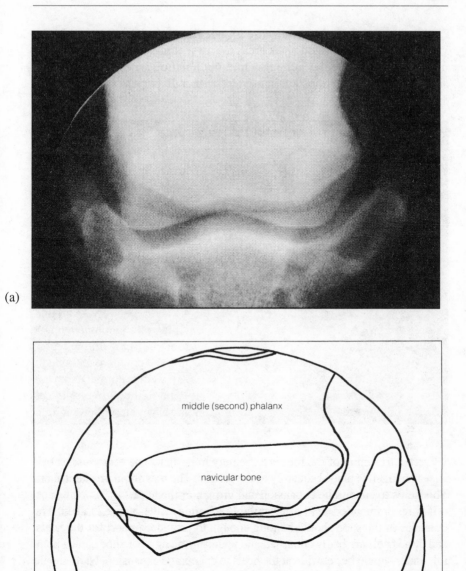

(a)

(b)

middle (second) phalanx

navicular bone

distal (third) phalanx

Figures 7a and b   Radiograph and diagram of a normal navicular bone

Figure 8   Radiograph of a diseased navicular bone. There are multiple, variously shaped and sized black areas (arrows) along the sloping and lower borders of the navicular bone. Seen in conjunction with typical clinical signs, these abnormalities are consistent with a diagnosis of the navicular syndrome

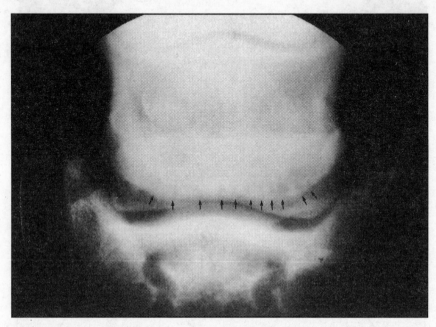

Correct trimming of the foot is extremely important. The foot must be balanced so that it is placed squarely to the ground. The toes should be kept short. This helps to encourage expansion and growth of the heel.

It is recommended that, after suitable trimming, a flat shoe is used. The branches of the shoe should be long enough to provide support for the heels, and if the heels are badly collapsed and underrun, an egg-bar shoe can be helpful. Shoes should be set wide at the heels to encourage expansion. Nails should not be placed farther back than the quarter of the foot, so that hoof-wall expansion is not restricted.

Exercise   Although rest may produce temporary improvement, lameness usually recurs when work is resumed. Regular exercise is important for normal blood flow through the foot, so any treatment should be combined with exercise to try to maintain normal blood flow. Provided that the horse is not very lame, then work may be done on hard or soft surfaces. The horse should also be turned out daily if possible, so that it is standing in its stable for the minimum possible time.

Drugs

Analgesics   Phenylbutazone and meclofenamic acid are drugs which have both anti-inflammatory and analgesic properties and will relieve lameness in most horses with navicular disease while they are being treated. These drugs merely alleviate the pain and do not treat the disease itself.

Warfarin   Warfarin is a drug which prolongs blood clotting time. Some horses with navicular syndrome are improved by the use of this drug, which is administered in the feed. It is a potentially dangerous drug and the horse's blood clotting time must be monitored carefully. Permanent medication is usually necessary, but in some horses which have been treated for two years or more treatment can be withdrawn. Why the drug works is not understood.

Isoxsuprine   Isoxsuprine is a drug used to dilate peripheral blood vessels in man. Some horses with the navicular syndrome improve while being treated with this drug, which is given in a feed or as a paste into the mouth. The drug is most helpful in the early stages of the disease and some horses may remain sound after a course of treatment. Results of treatment have been poor in horses in which the disease is more advanced.

Surgery

Neurectomy   The back of the foot can be desensitised by removing a small piece of each of the two nerves which innervate this area (palmar digital neurectomy). This relieves the pain associated with navicular disease. The procedure is successful in some horses but lameness may recur because the nerves regenerate. There are a number of potential complications of a neurectomy, including the development of painful neuromas (fibrous swellings at the cut end of the nerve) and necrosis (death) and rupture of the deep digital flexor tendon. Because the horse cannot feel the back part of the foot, daily foot care is essential so that puncture wounds, etc., are recognised early.

Desmotomy   The navicular bone is suspended by the collateral (suspensory) ligaments. Cutting of these ligaments (desmotomy) results in improvement in lameness in some horses, at least in the short term (months). Longer-term results (years) are less good. It is likely that the ligaments rejoin and there do not appear to be any long-term adverse effects.

Radiographs and the pre-purchase examination
There is considerable controversy about the interpretation of radiographs of the navicular bone in clinically sound horses. There is an area of overlap

between radiographic abnormalities seen in sound horses, which do not necessarily go on to develop the navicular syndrome, and changes seen in horses with this condition. Vets naturally tend to be cautious and may advise against the purchase of a horse with radiographic abnormalities in this category. However, these horses may never have a problem, whereas a horse with apparently normal navicular bones may subsequently develop the navicular syndrome. The authors recommend that the feet should be radiographed if they are of unequal size or of abnormal shape; if there is any suspicion of a subtle gait abnormality; if the horse has not been in regular work prior to the examination; or if the horse is being purchased with a view to resale. The horse's shoes should be removed and its feet thoroughly trimmed and cleaned before radiography, and the resulting views must be of excellent quality.

FRACTURE OF THE NAVICULAR BONE

Clinical signs
There is a sudden onset of moderate to severe lameness. The horse may have trodden on a stone or kicked a solid object. Old, non-healed fractures of the navicular bone cause a similar lameness to the navicular syndrome. Fractures of the navicular bone occur both in forefeet and in hind feet.

Diagnosis
The horse is sound after desensitisation of the back part of the foot. The fracture is visible on radiographs but must not be confused with a shadow from the frog, which can also appears as a black line crossing the bone.

Treatment
Without treatment a variable degree of lameness persists. A neurectomy can be performed to desensitise the back part of the foot. Similar complications occur as for a neurectomy to treat navicular syndrome (see above). Degenerative joint disease of the proximal interphalangeal joint often develops subsequently. A few horses have been successfully treated surgically by having a screw placed through the bone. If the fracture is displaced or has been present for some time, the prognosis is poor.

ARTHROSIS OF THE DISTAL INTERPHALANGEAL (COFFIN) JOINT

Usually one forefoot is affected and the condition causes a unilateral forelimb lameness, which is worse when the horse is turned towards the affected leg. The lameness is improved by injecting local anaesthetic into the distal interphalangeal joint. No abnormalities of the joint can be identified on radiographs.

The foot must be correctly trimmed and shod. The condition may improve with rest, but often recurs when work is resumed. Some horses are made sound by injecting sodium hyaluronate or a glycosaminoglycan polysulphate into the joint.

SECONDARY (DEGENERATIVE) JOINT DISEASE (OSTEOARTHRITIS) OF THE DISTAL INTERPHALANGEAL (COFFIN) JOINT (LOW ARTICULAR RINGBONE)

The horse is lame. The forefeet are most often affected and the condition may be unilateral or bilateral. Sometimes there is swelling just above the coronary band on the front of the pastern. Lameness is alleviated by desensitisation of the foot by nerve blocks. Changes typical of degenerative joint disease are seen on radiographs.

There is no effective treatment, although the use of analgesics and/or anti-inflammatories may relieve the pain sufficiently to allow the horse to be worked.

FRACTURE OF THE EXTENSOR PROCESS OF THE DISTAL (THIRD) PHALANX (PEDAL BONE)

The horse is lame, with the forefeet most commonly affected. Lameness is alleviated by desensitisation of the foot by nerve blocks. The fracture can be seen on a lateral radiographic view of the foot.

Small fractures may be successfully treated by surgical removal. Larger fractures which involve part of the joint surface warrant a poor prognosis.

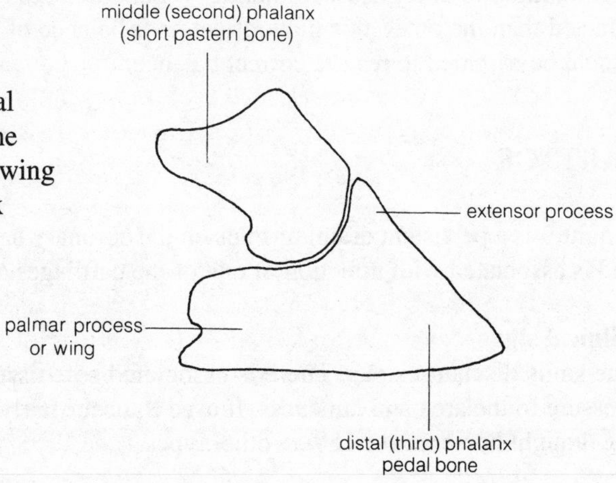

Figure 9
Lateral view of distal phalanges to slow the extensor process or wing of the distal phalanx (pedal bone)

middle (second) phalanx
(short pastern bone)

extensor process

palmar process
or wing

distal (third) phalanx
pedal bone

WING FRACTURE OF THE DISTAL (THIRD) PHALANX (PEDAL BONE)

There is a sudden onset of severe lameness. Pressure applied with hoof testers across the affected heel may cause pain. Lameness is alleviated by desensitisation of the foot. The fracture is visible on radiographs, although oblique views may be necessary.

If the fracture does not involve the distal interphalangeal (coffin) joint, box rest and application of a bar shoe for three to six months usually produces satisfactory results. If the fracture enters the joint, the prognosis is poor.

SIDEBONE

Sidebone is ossification of the cartilages of the foot. The whole cartilage may ossify from a single centre or from more than one centre. The latter results in two apparently separate bony masses, which should not be confused with a fracture.

Clinical signs
Sidebone occurs most commonly in the front feet of heavier types of horses (hunters, cobs, etc.) The cartilages above the coronary band feel firmer than usual. Many normal horses have sidebone. Both the inside and outside cartilages can be affected equally. In horses which place one heel to the ground momentarily before the other the sidebone may be more obvious on the side hitting the ground first. Only rarely does sidebone cause lameness.

Diagnosis and treatment
The diagnosis is confirmed by radiographic examination.

The condition rarely causes lameness. If one side of the foot is more severely affected than the other, this may reflect poor balance of the foot and the foot should be trimmed to restore correct balance.

QUITTOR

A quittor is a persistent draining sinus on the coronary band towards the heels and is associated with infection of one of the cartilages of the foot.

Clinical signs
The sinus discharges pus. There is associated soft-tissue swelling, pain on pressure to the area and lameness. It used to occur fairly frequently in working draught horses, but rarely in other types.

Treatment
The chronically infected tissue must be removed surgically.

KERATOMA

A keratoma is a tumour of the horn-producing cells of the foot. It is a rare
condition. Forefeet and hind feet are affected equally.

Clinical signs
The shape of the foot becomes distorted. There is a variable degree of lameness.

Diagnosis and treatment
The diagnosis is confirmed by radiographs and/or histology. Although the
tumour is usually not radiopaque, and therefore cannot itself be seen, it often
presses on adjacent structures, such as the distal phalanx (pedal bone), and creates a defect in its outline. This must be differentiated from the radiolucent
defect which results from infection.
   Surgical removal of tumours is possible, and recurrence is unlikely.

Developments in Imaging the Horse's Foot

Additional imaging techniques are sometime needed when a diagnosis cannot
be reached by clinical examination and radiography. Thermography, detection
of surface heat, may be useful for identification of relatively superficial acute
inflammatory reactions e.g. abscess, corn. Scintigraphy can be used for the
identification of abnormal bone activity unassociated with X-ray abnormalities. Ultrasonography allows limited evaluation of some soft tissue structures.
Computed thermography and magnetic resonance imaging permit evaluation
of all the bony and soft tissue structures of the foot in three dimensions.
Knowledge of other causes of foot pain is advancing rapidly, particularly with
the use of MRI.

OVERREACH

An overreach is caused by a horse striking the coronary band or heels of a forelimb by the toe of a hind limb.

Clinical signs

An overreach results in a laceration of variable depth and severity and associated soft-tissue bruising. Depending upon the site and severity of the injury, the horse may be sound or extremely lame – much more lame than would be anticipated from the appearance of the wound itself. This is the result of bruising rather than the wound itself. Although most commonly the back of the foot is injured, the inside or outside coronary band may be damaged. In these lateral locations the horizontal split at the coronary band must be differentiated from that caused by pus, which comes up the white line from a subsolar abscess, bursting out at the coronary band. In both instances pressure applied around the lesion causes pain. If there is bruising due to trauma the surrounding tissues may also be sore. If there is a subsolar abscess, pressure applied to the sole with hoof testers should identify a focus of pain.

Treatment

The wound should be thoroughly cleaned with a suitable antiseptic. If there is a large skin flap, it may be beneficial to cut this off. An antibiotic spray should be applied and this is most easily done by dabbing on the solution using cotton wool. Greasy ointments should be avoided as these tend to attract dirt. Wound powders have poor adherent qualities. The wound should be kept clean and dry and the horse is best kept in until satisfactory healing has occurred. If the horse is lame due to severe bruising, treatment with an anti-inflammatory and/or analgesic drug may be beneficial. Local laser treatment may accelerate healing of a severe wound.

Complications

Wounds involving the heels may take a long time to heal as repetitive movement in this area pulls the skin edges apart. Sometimes secondary infection may occur, which should be treated by poulticing and, if necessary, the administration of antibiotics. Damage of the horn-producing cells of the coronary band may cause either exuberant horn production or temporary failure of horn production, resulting in a horizontal crack in the hoof wall which will gradually grow out. Occasionally horn production is permanently arrested at the site of injury.

Overreach boots provide some protection.

CRACKED HEELS, MUD FEVER

Mud fever and cracked heels are synonymous terms for an identical condition, which is also referred to as scratches in America.

Clinical signs

The clinical signs are variable in severity, but essentially the underlying disease is the same. The disease is characterised by inflammation of the skin and subcutaneous tissues on the back of the pastern resulting in soft-tissue swelling, stretching of the skin, exudation of serum through the skin and ultimately cracks in the skin. The skin cracks are usually horizontal and may extend deeply. Constant motion of the skin on the back of the pastern encourages the skin cracks to gape. All these factors cause pain, resulting in a stiffness of gait or lameness. Secondarily, there may be diffuse inflammatory oedema of the affected leg(s), resulting in a filled appearance. The fissures in the skin may permit entry of pathogenic bacteria which cause infection and increased severity of the clinical signs. More than one limb may be affected.

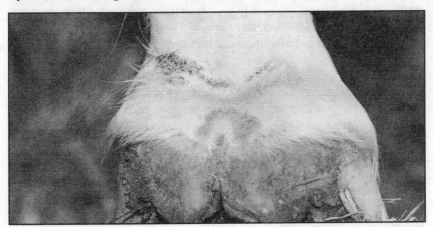

Figure 10   A cracked heel

Cause

The condition may occur in stabled horses or horses turned out and is usually associated with wet conditions. Even heavy dew in the autumn may be a predisposing factor. The condition is seen in both heavily feathered horses and those with clipped legs. In grass-kept horses the incidence is higher in horses with a lot of feather, which presumably traps an excessive amount of moisture. Prolonged wetness of the skin may damage it, making it more susceptible to irritation by mud. There is potential for secondary infection. Some horses seem prone to recurrent attacks and in some years there appears to be a higher incidence. Horses may be more severely affected on some soil types. Poor hygiene, combined with a failure to recognise early clinical signs, contributes to development of overt disease.

Treatment

Treatment is aimed at removing the offending cause, reducing inflammation and eliminating infection if present. If at all possible, a grass-kept horse should be brought into drier conditions. Excessive feather should be removed and the area cleaned thoroughly and kept dry. A dilute iodine solution is a most effective cleansing agent. This treatment may be adequate for a mild case, but if there is considerable inflammation, then a soothing ointment containing corticosteroids, with or without antibiotics, should be applied. An oil-based cream will provide a barrier to water and corticosteroids will reduce inflammation. Ointments containing corticosteroid oil, and antibiotics are commercially available. In a very severe case it may be necessary to administer antibiotics by intra-muscular injection.

Usually clinical signs resolve fairly rapidly, although careful management must be practised to avoid a re-exacerbation. The skin must not dry out excessively, as this in itself will predispose to further cracking. Once the acute inflammation has resolved, a lanoline-based ointment may help to keep the skin supple, as well as providing a barrier to water.

Prevention
Careful management of the stable-kept horse, including thorough cleaning and drying of the legs after exercise, usually prevents occurrence of the disease. Excessive feather should be removed, but clipping the legs is not recommended. Much controversy surrounds whether or not horses' legs should be washed clean and then dried, or whether they should be allowed to dry and then brushed clean. It has been suggested that washing legs while the skin pores are open permits the entry of dirt through the pores. The authors have had no problems associated with washing, provided that the legs are dried properly afterwards. Many horses tolerate this better than having dried mud brushed off their legs. Leaving the legs wet will not necessarily create a problem in a normal horse, but in a susceptible horse drying is important. Bandaging the legs is the best way to dry them effectively. Prevention in the grass-kept animal is more difficult, due to the ubiquitous mud. Excessive feather should be removed and the horse examined daily.

DISTAL INTERPHALANGEAL JOINT FLEXURAL DEFORMITY (CONTRACTED TENDONS, CLUB FOOT)
See p. 330.

17
MISCELLANEOUS CONDITIONS OF LAMENESS

STRINGHALT

Traditional stringhalt is a poorly understood condition in which the horse hyperflexes one or both hocks. It usually occurs in adult horses, is gradual in onset, and may be slowly progressive. In Australia a different type of stringhalt has been recognized, occurring mostly in pasture-kept horses in certain geographic locations, especially after periods of drought, often affecting several of a group of horses. Australian stringhalt is rapid in onset and invariably affects both hind limbs and sometimes the forelimbs as well. The majority of horses recover completely, but a few deteriorate progressively. The condition may be caused by ingestion of a plant toxin. The following discussion refers to traditional stringhalt.

Clinical signs
The horse exaggeratedly flexes one or both hind limbs when in motion. The abnormality is sometimes evident at all paces, but it is usually most apparent at walk, especially if the horse is turned or backed, and may disappear at trot. The condition may be intermittent and remain static or deteriorate.

Treatment
The cause of the condition is unknown. Some horses are successfully treated by the removal of a piece of the lateral digital extensor tendon at the level of the hock.

Prognosis
Unless the gait abnormality is extremely severe, affected horses are usually able to perform adequately, including jumping, but are unsuitable for dressage. A guarded to fair prognosis is warranted after surgery. Some horses improve initially but subsequently relapse.

SHIVERING

Shivering rarely results in a horse being unridable unless it cannot be shod. Therefore very few horses with this condition are humanely destroyed, so opportunities for post-mortem examination of affected horses are rare. As a result very little is known about the cause or causes of shivering.

Clinical signs
The horse involuntarily picks up a hind leg and holds it partly flexed, slightly away from the body. The leg shakes. Usually both hind legs are affected. The tail may be raised and quiver simultaneously. It is a rare condition seen most often in big horses, especially draught type. The symptoms are intermittent and are most reliably provoked by making the horse move backwards.

Treatment and prognosis
The cause of the condition is unknown, and there is no known treatment. Mildly affected horses are still able to work, but the condition is usually progressive, and may result in the farrier being unable to hold the affected limb in the shoeing position in order to shoe the horse.

LYMPHANGITIS

Widespread swelling of a limb below the knee or hock occurs for many reasons, including lymphangitis. A careful clinical examination of both the foot and the swollen region of the leg is necessary to establish the cause of the swelling.

Clinical signs
One or more legs are diffusely swollen. Hind legs are more commonly affected than forelegs, and usually the entire leg is swollen up to the level of the stifle, resulting in moderate to severe lameness. Surface lymph vessels are prominent and local lymph nodes are enlarged. Serum may exude through the skin. The rectal temperature may be raised. Heavy-hunter types seem especially prone.

Diagnosis
The clinical signs are fairly typical. The inflammation is often secondary to a chronic low-grade infection of the leg and careful inspection usually reveals an old wound or wounds. The condition must be differentiated from other causes of filled legs (see below).

Treatment

Treatment aims to eliminate the primary infection and reduce the soft-tissue swelling. Relatively long-term treatment with appropriate antibiotics is combined with cold hosing of the leg, bandaging and exercise.

Prognosis

Vigorous treatment can produce rewarding results, although the leg may remain permanently thickened. The problem may be recurrent, especially in hind limbs, and careful vigilance is necessary to detect and treat small wounds as early as possible.

FILLED LEGS

Filled legs are usually a managemental and cosmetic problem rather than one causing lameness.

Clinical signs

The condition is usually confined to the stabled horse. Heavy-hunter types are especially prone. There is diffuse swelling of the lower legs if the horse is kept in for more than twenty-four hours without exercise. The swelling is usually restricted to the areas below the knees and hocks and results in loss of definition of the tendons and suspensory ligaments. The hind legs are more commonly affected than the forelimbs, although all four may be affected simultaneously. Usually both hind legs are involved, and although the presence of soft-tissue swelling may impede mobility and cause stiffness, this resolves with exercise.

Diagnosis

The clinical signs are fairly typical but the condition must be differentiated from other problems which cause diffuse swelling of the legs. These include purpura haemorrhagica, congestive heart failure, recurrent lymphangitis (see above) and excessively low blood protein levels due to malnutrition or chronic liver disease.

If there is only one hind limb or forelimb affected, it is more likely that there is a more serious underlying reason for the filling, such as cracked heels, pus in the foot, a puncture wound or a chronic low-grade infection.

Treatment

The condition usually resolves with exercise. Keeping the legs bandaged helps to prevent recurrence. If the horse has a day off it should be turned out for a few hours if possible.

BROKEN KNEES

Broken knees is the colloquial term used to describe lacerations on the front of the carpi (knees), caused by a fall onto the knees. It does not imply that any of the bones of the knee have been fractured. Because the horse is usually moving when the accident occurs, the knees tend to scrape along the ground for a short distance, resulting in tearing of the skin and underlying structures and bruising.

Clinical signs

There is usually an area of complete skin loss and moderate haemorrhage (bleeding). The severity of damage is extremely variable. Sometimes only the skin is torn, but in more serious cases the underlying soft tissues may be stripped off to reveal the bones. The sheath of one of the tendons which passes over the front of the knee (extensor carpi radialis, common digital extensor, lateral digital extensor) may be torn so that there is leakage of synovial fluid. Very occasionally the joint capsule of one of the knee joints may be disrupted.

Treatment

The extent of the damage must be assessed carefully and this is only possible after thorough cleaning of the wounds. The hair in the area immediately around the wound should be trimmed and each knee hosed for at least five minutes to remove any debris which may have accumulated in the wound. Any pieces of tissue which have been severely damaged and are likely to die due to disruption of their blood supply should be trimmed off. This is called débridement of the wound. The wound should be further cleaned using an antiseptic such as a dilute iodine solution. At this stage it should be possible to evaluate which structures have been damaged. Thorough cleaning is essential to minimise the risks of secondary infection. Administration of a short course of antibiotics may also help to reduce the likelihood of infection occurring.

Unlike a cut, where the two skin edges remain close together and heal by so-called first intention, with minimal scar formation, broken knees must heal by second intention. This is the ingrowth of skin epithelial cells from the edges of the wound. The skin defect is first filled by granulation tissue. Constant movement of the edges of the wound and the granulation bed will delay healing, therefore comparative immobility is important. For this reason it is necessary to restrict the horse to a box and ideally he should be tied up for twenty-four hours a day to prevent him from lying down until healing is well established.

Bruising usually causes swelling and this will tend to draw the skin edges farther apart. To minimise swelling it can be beneficial to administer an anti-inflammatory drug such as phenylbutazone as soon as possible after the injury. Application of a light bandage over the knees is also helpful. A non-adherent dressing (e.g. Melolin) is placed over the open wounds, followed by Gamgee and a crepe bandage, held in place by either Elastoplast or a Pressage bandage.

Bandaging the knees until healing is progressing satisfactorily helps to keep the wounds clean. Granulation tissue tends to dry and crack if left exposed; keeping the wounds covered helps to keep them moist, which probably aids healing. Bandaging may also reduce the likelihood of production of exuberant granulation tissue (proud flesh). Horses are particularly prone to development of excessive granulation tissue, especially in wounds on the limbs. This must either be cut off, a pain-free procedure since granulation tissue has no nerve supply, or controlled using a suitable substance applied directly onto the tissue. There are many such preparations, including corticosteroid creams, copper sulphate solution and lead lotion.

Normal wound healing may be accelerated by laser therapy and this treatment can be extremely helpful, although it needs to be repeated. Under normal conditions the wounds may take four to six weeks to heal completely. The horse may need to be kept tied up for at least two weeks but may be given small amounts of walking exercise in-hand. Wound healing may be delayed if the horse is permitted to move about or, especially, if it is allowed to lie down.

Tetanus prophylaxis is mandatory. The horse should be fed maintenance rations only.

Complications
If a tendon sheath has been damaged, it is occasionally possible to repair it surgically. However, often it is too badly torn and must be left to heal spontaneously. Sometimes a synovial sinus develops: there is a small hole in the skin through which synovial fluid drains. This will close eventually, although it may take considerably longer to heal than the original skin wounds.

Prognosis
The wounds will ultimately heal satisfactorily but some residual fibrous swelling may persist. The amount of scar tissue which develops is related to the size and severity of the initial injury and the speed of healing. White hairs may grow at the sites of injury and there may be small areas of permanent hair loss.

Prevention
If a horse is prone to stumbling, then knee boots should be worn when it is worked on roads or hard tracks. The toes of the feet should be kept short. Rolling the toes of the shoes may facilitate breakover, thus reducing the chances of stumbling.

GENERAL TRAUMA WITH SECONDARY INFECTION

One of the most common causes of lameness is trauma causing bruising and laceration, with secondary infection, or a puncture wound. Infection may develop due to failure to recognise and treat the wound or due to inappropriate treatment. The horse is generally found with a so-called big leg.

Clinical signs
There is diffuse, warm, painful swelling. A wound which exudes pus may be readily identifiable. Alternatively it may be necessary to clip the hair to identify the nature and extent of the wounds. Lameness is moderate to severe and the horse may be depressed and inappetent and have an elevated rectal temperature.

Treatment
The hair around the wound should be clipped and thoroughly cleaned with a suitable antiseptic. If the wound is severely contaminated, preliminary hosing may be helpful. If the wound is of puncture type, a hot poultice may help to draw the infection. The poultice should be replaced twice daily. Depending on the nature and extent of the wound, a dry, non-adherent dressing may be applied if the area is accessible to bandaging.

If infection is severe, then appropriate antibiotic therapy is required for at least five days. Tetanus prophylaxis is essential. If the horse has received regular tetanus vaccinations, no further preventive treatment is required. However, if the vaccination history of the horse is uncertain, tetanus antitoxin should be administered and a course of tetanus vaccination started. If possible the horse should be confined to a box or covered yard. If infection is not resolved completely within five days or if no improvement is observed after three days of treatment, then swabs should be collected from the wound for bacterial culture and antibiotic-sensitivity testing to check which antibiotics are effective against the bacteria causing the infection.

If appropriate antibiotic treatment fails to resolve the infection, then radiography should be performed to identify bony changes, if any, typical of infectious osteitis or osteomylitis and to preclude the presence of a radiopaque foreign body. Diagnostic ultrasonography can be used to identify a non-radiopaque foreign body. Surgical exploration is indicated if neither is identified.

HEREDITARY MULTIPLE EXOSTOSIS See p. 321.

18
THE NECK, BACK AND PELVIS; INCOORDINATION

Functional anatomy

The horse's neck consists of seven cervical vertebrae. The back comprises eighteen thoracic vertebrae, five or six lumbar vertebrae, the sacrum and the coccygeal vertebrae. The vertebrae are complex in their structure and lock firmly together. The bones are held together by ligaments and muscles which attach to them. The back is a relatively rigid structure capable of only limited movement and it is the author's opinion that vertebrae cannot become displaced relative to each other. Each vertebra has a large hole in it, the vertebral canal, through which passes the spinal cord. On the top surface of each vertebrae is a bony projection of variable size, the dorsal spinous process. These are longest in the withers region. The tops of the dorsal spinous processes can be felt in poorly muscled horses. Particularly in the cranial lumbar region (the area behind the saddle, in front of the 'jumper's bump') prominence of the dorsal spinous processes due to muscle wastage may make the back appear 'roached' (i.e. an upward, convex curvature). Attached to the top of the dorsal spinous processes is the supraspinous ligament (Figure 4). On either side of the dorsal spinous processes are the paired longissimus dorsi muscles.

The pelvis, consisting on each side of the fused ilium, ischium and pubis, is attached to the sacrum via the sacroiliac joints. The pelvis is bound tightly to the sacrum and lumbar vertebrae by the sacroiliac ligaments. The so-called jumper's bump is the tubera sacrale (part of the ilium). These are more or less prominent depending on the horse's conformation and degree of muscling. The tubera sacrale are normally level when viewed from behind (see Figure 1, p. 277). The tubera coxae are also normally level.

There is considerable variation in the normal conformation of the horse's back. Long-backed horses seem more prone to muscular injuries. Short-backed horses are more likely to have impingement (rubbing together) of the dorsal spinous processes.

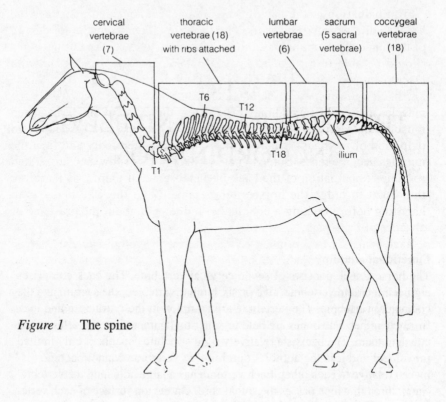

Figure 1	The spine

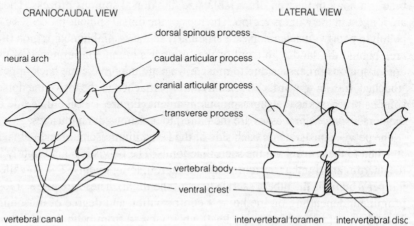

Figure 2	A typical equine vertebra

Firm palpation of the back in the area behind the saddle induces the horse to dip its back. This is a normal reaction. Firm palpation of the top of the hindquarters stimulates the horse to arch its back. The normal horse should be able to dip and arch the back repeatedly without showing resentment and without the back muscles going into spasm. If the horse has back pain, it may be reluctant to dip and arch the back; the back muscles may feel firm and may fasiculate – that is, show small, localised muscle contractions – and the horse may demonstrate resistance to palpation of the back. It may initially sink exaggeratedly and then the muscles become tense. Some hypersensitive horses show an exaggerated response to palpation of the back in the absence of pain. It is therefore important to judge the horse's temperament and the way it reacts to handling before making a conclusive judgement about the presence or absence of back pain.

Back pain may be a primary problem or may develop secondarily to an altered way of moving due to lameness. A careful assessment of the whole animal is essential when examining a horse with suspected back pain.

It is the author's opinion that certain methods of palpating the back can relieve muscle spasm and associated pain, thus producing clinical improvement. The author does not believe that any method of manipulation can move vertebrae or move the pelvis relative to the back.

Conditions of the Neck

Many normal horses are slightly less well muscled on one side of the neck compared with the other and are stiffer to the right than to the left or vice versa. A horse with neck pain usually shows stiffness of the neck – it is unable to flex the neck from side to side and may find it difficult to raise and lower its head. The neck may be held abnormally low at rest. In order to graze, the horse may need to straddle the forelimbs or even go down on one knee. With the exception of the wobbler syndrome (see p. 326) and congenital malformations of the cervical vertebrae, most neck problems are the result of a fall or other traumatic incident.

MUSCLE DAMAGE

Clinical signs
There is neck stiffness and pain on manipulation of the neck. Faradism may help to identify the affected muscles.

Treatment

Treatment is aimed at relieving pain and facilitating muscle repair. Non-steroidal anti-inflammatory drugs such as phenylbutazone alleviate pain. Treatment with faradism or ultrasound facilitates muscle repair. The horse should be rested until the clinical signs have resolved. The prognosis is usually good.

FRACTURES OF THE CERVICAL VERTEBRAE

Clinical signs

Fractures of the cervical vertebrae cause neck stiffness and pain. There may be an area of localized sweating and some of the neck muscles may atrophy. The horse may also show signs of incoordination (see pp. 326-8). The diagnosis is confirmed by radiography.

Treatment

Most fractures are not amenable to surgical treatment and must be allowed to heal spontaneously. The horse should be confined to a restricted area. It should be fed at chest height if unable to raise or lower its head. If there are signs of incoordination, treatment with corticosteroids or dimethyl sulphoxide may be beneficial during the first forty-eight hours after the accident. If signs of incoordination persist the prognosis is guarded. Some fractures heal spontaneously with excellent results; sometimes there is a degree of permanent neck stiffness.

NECK ABSCESS

An abscess in the neck can be the result of an intramuscular injection, a penetrating foreign body or, rarely, a blood-borne infection.

Clinical signs
There is localised heat, swelling and pain, and neck stiffness.

Treatment
Hot compresses applied to the area may resolve the problem if it is the result of a reaction to an intramuscular injection. Oral administration of phenylbutazone will resolve pain. In more serious cases antibiotic therapy, preferably administered orally, may be necessary. If the abscess does not resolve then an ultrasound scan may be used to define better its extent, before surgical drainage is performed.

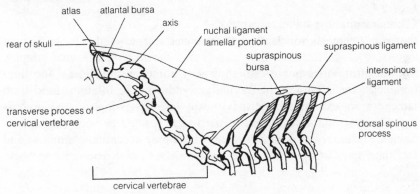

Figure 3   Anatomy of the neck and withers region

TORTICOLLIS (WRYNECK) See p. 742.

Conditions of the Thoracolumbar Spine

BACK PAIN

The clinical signs of back pain are often subtle and result in a reduced standard of performance. The horse may move in a restricted fashion with limited hind-limb impulsion with or without intermittent dragging of the toes. Obvious uni-lateral hind-limb lameness is rarely associated with a primary problem involving the thoracolumbar spine. The horse may be stiff and reluctant to work on a circle. It may also be difficult to keep on the bit. A horse which formerly made a well-shaped bascule over fences may start to hollow the back, find combination fences difficult and rush on the approach or refuse. The horse may be difficult to turn. The clinical signs can be more obvious when the horse is ridden rather than moving freely on the lunge. The horse is often poorly muscled over the back.

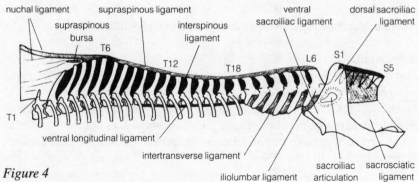

Figure 4
The thoracolumbar spine, showing
the major ligaments which attach to the bones

Similar clinical signs are also shown by horses with bilateral forelimb lameness, for example, the navicular syndrome, or bilateral hind-limb lameness, for example, bone spavin. Any horse showing these symptoms must be assessed as a whole. In particular it must be seen working in circles, preferably on a hard surface, which may accentuate lameness and facilitate diagnosis.

IMPINGEMENT AND OVERRIDING OF THE DORSAL SPINOUS PROCESSES (KISSING SPINES)

The dorsal spinous processes of normal horses tend to be closest together in the mid-back region (the caudal thoracic area) and may touch (impinge). This is most common in short-backed horses, especially Thoroughbred types. A moderate degree of impingement is often unassociated with clinical signs. However, severe crowding of the dorsal spinous processes can cause back pain.

Clinical signs
The horse is reluctant to dip the back and will tend to hold it rigidly with the muscles in partial spasm. If the horse is rested, these clinical signs disappear temporarily. Because many of the horses show a degree of impingement, the diagnosis of a clinically significant problem is made using a combination of clinical examination, radiographic examination, nuclear scintigraphy and possibly local anaesthesia.

Treatment
In young horses the dorsal spinous processes may remodel and form false joints and the clinical signs improve after approximately six months' rest. If the

clinical signs do not resolve completely, then phenylbutazone is often helpful. Some clinicians advocate local treatment of the impinging spines with injection of various cocktails of anti-inflammatory drugs. Accurate injection of the region requires ultrasonographic or radiographic guidance. In selected horses surgical removal of the summits of one or two dorsal spinous processes is successful.

MUSCLE STRAIN

Muscle strain is usually the result of a fall, an awkward jump or a mis-step.

Clinical signs
Palpation of the back may reveal an area or areas of sensitivity and/or muscle spasm. Both sides may be similarly affected or one side may be worse. This can be confirmed using faradism. Damaged muscle cells leak, releasing creatine kinase and aspartoaminotransferase into the blood; therefore, if muscle damage is severe, concentrations of these enzymes in the blood may rise.

Treatment
The aims of treatment are to relieve muscle spasm and to facilitate repair of damaged muscle. Local treatment with faradism or ultrasound, combined with rest and controlled exercise, is beneficial. Muscle spasm can also be relieved by manipulation. The period of rest necessary is extremely variable: sometimes up to three months is required, but in many cases ten to fourteen days is sufficient, followed by a slow resumption of normal work. Premature resumption of work may result in chronic muscle pain, which can be much more difficult to diagnose and treat.

SPRAIN OF THE SUPRASPINOUS LIGAMENT

This usually is the result of a fall when jumping at speed.

Clinical signs
Muscle atrophy over the back develops rapidly. The horse's movement is severely restricted. The history and clinical signs are fairly typical. Sometimes the diagnosis can be confirmed by radiographic examination. Associated with strain of the supraspinous ligament, small flakes of bone are detached from the summits of the dorsal spinous processes in the midthoracic region.

Treatment
A prolonged period of rest (six months) usually results in total remission of clinical signs with a favourable prognosis.

Figure 5
Thoracic spines –
normal and impinged

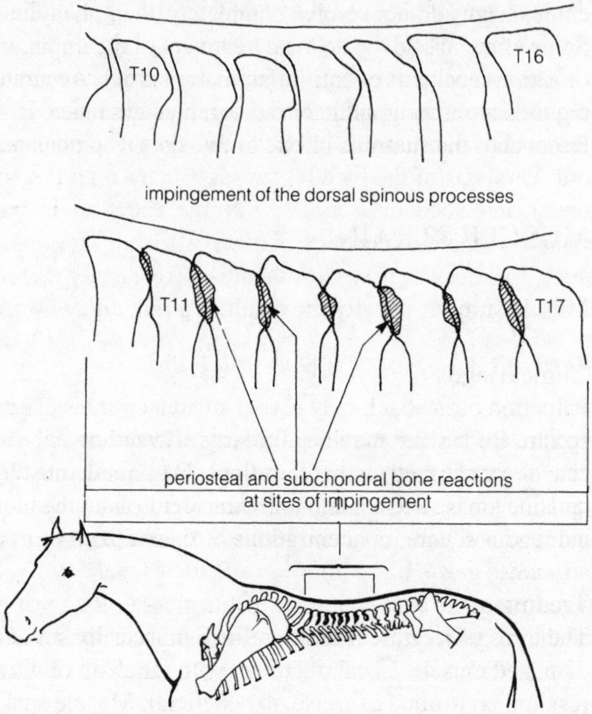

impingement of the dorsal spinous processes

periosteal and subchondral bone reactions
at sites of impingement

OTHER CAUSES OF BACK PAIN

As in man, the causes of back pain in the horse are poorly understood.
Nevertheless the clinical signs of other problems are frequently wrongly
attributed to back pain. The horse which is moving poorly should be assessed
as a whole; bilateral fore-limb lameness or bilateral hind-limb lameness is
often confused with a primary back problem.

FRACTURES OF THE BACK

FRACTURES OF THE THORACOLUMBAR SPINE

Fractures of the thoracolumbar spine or the sacrum are uncommon and are
usually the result of an accident such as a fall. The horse exhibits pain and
patchy sweating and may show complete or partial paralysis of the hind-limbs
due to damage to the spinal cord. Paralysis may not be immediate in onset, but
usually develops within twelve to twenty-four hours. There is no treatment
and the prognosis is hopeless.

FRACTURES OF THE SACRUM

A horse with a fracture of the sacrum may show less severe clinical signs initially, because nerve function of the hind-legs remains intact. However, paralysis of the bladder and tail usually result due to damage to the cauda equina, part of the spinal cord. Paralysis of the bladder causes urinary retention and overflow (incontinence) and secondary cystitis. Nerve function is rarely restored, so the prognosis is poor if bladder function is affected. The rare fractures of the sacrum which do not cause nerve dysfunction have a better outlook for recovery.

FRACTURES OF THE WITHERS

Fractures of the dorsal spinous processes in the cranial thoracic (withers) region occur as a result of trauma: for example, a horse rearing up and falling over backwards. There is swelling in the withers region and crepitus may be felt. The horse tends to stand with its forelimbs close together and is reluctant to lower its head and neck to graze. It may move in a restricted manner. The diagnosis is confirmed by radiographic examination. Treatment other than rest is usually unnecessary and the prognosis is favourable, although a specially fitted saddle may be required.

Conditions of the Pelvis

FRACTURES OF THE PELVIS

Fractures of the three bones of the pelvis – the ilium, the ischium and the pubis occur spontaneously in two- and three-year-old Thoroughbred horses, especially fillies, when galloping. Fractures in foals and yearlings are usually a sequel to rearing up and falling over. Fractures in older horses are less common and are usually the result of a fall or collision with a solid object.

Clinical signs
There is a sudden onset of severe hind-limb lameness. Fractures of the tuber coxae (knocked-down hip) may demonstrate only mild lameness. Careful palpation of the hindquarters and/or an internal examination via the rectum may reveal crepitus. There may be localised patchy sweating over the hindquarters. If the ilium has been fractured, the pelvis may appear asymmetrical when viewed from behind.

Diagnosis
A fracture may be suspected from the presentation and clinical signs. Ultrasonography and nuclear scintigraphy can be used to localise the site of

the fracture although it takes two or three days for the fracture to become 'hot' on a bone scan. Ultrasonography can detect a defect in the bone and overlying haemorrhage soon after injury. In some horses further investigation with radiography may be performed, but usually requires general anaesthesia.

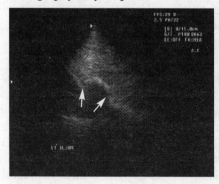 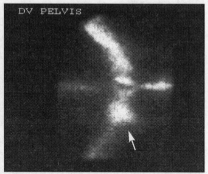

Figure 6   Ultrasonographic image (left) and nuclear scintigraphic image (right) of a fractured pelvis. In the ultrasonographic image the normal regular contour of the bone surface is disrupted by a fracture (arrows). The scintigraphic image is looking down on the pelvis (tail end to the right); there is a focal 'hot spot' (arrow) at the fracture site

Treatment and Prognosis

The horse is box rested for a lengthy period. Occasionally fragments of bone will become loose and form a foreign body, bursting out of the skin below the point of the tuber coxae. The prognosis depends on the location and configuration of the fracture. Horses with fractures of the tuber coxae or ischium often become sound. Stress fractures of the ilium have a good prognosis. Some fractures result in permanent lameness, but mares can be used for breeding. A fracture involving the hip joint carries a very poor prognosis because of secondary osteoarthritis.

SECONDARY (DEGENERATIVE) JOINT DISEASE (OSTEOARTHRITIS) OF THE COXOFEMORAL (HIP) JOINT

Unlike in man, this is a rare condition in the horse and is usually the result of getting a hind leg trapped and severely wrenching the joint, or an awkward fall, or it may develop secondary to a fracture. There is severe wastage of the muscles of the hindquarter and moderate to severe lameness. The horse may swing the leg outwards as it is advanced to avoid flexion of the joint, or may move on three tracks with the hindquarters deviating from the lame limb, so that the lame leg is placed between the imprints of the two forelimbs. The lameness may be accentuated by hyperflexion of the hind leg or by pulling the hind leg outwards or forwards. Diagnosis is confirmed by radiographic examination, but this is only possible with the horse lying on its back under general anaesthesia. There is no treatment and the prognosis is hopeless.

SACROILIAC DISEASE

Clinical signs
Slight unilateral or bilateral hirid-limb lameness or poor hind-limb impulsion is associated with asymmetry of the bony prominences of the pelvis, the tubera sacrale and the tubera coxae (see Figure 1, p. 277). Symmetry or levelness can only be assessed with the horse standing perfectly squarely on level ground. Muscle wastage may give a false impression of asymmetry (unlevelness) of the tubera sacrale and tubera coxae. There may be muscle wastage in association with the unlevelness. A marked disparity in height of the tubera sacrale is suggestive of disease of the sacroiliac joints, although many clinically normal horses show slight asymmetry.

Diagnosis
Clinical signs can be misleading and all other possible causes of hind-limb lameness must be excluded. Ultrasonography may show changes in the dorsal sacroiliac ligaments and nuclear scintigraphy may demonstrate a 'hot-spot', but there are false positives and negatives. Occasionally changes involving the sacroiliac joints can be seen on radiographs. This merits a poor prognosis.

Treatment
Some horses respond to rest. Slight hind-limb unlevelness may persist, though this is thought to be related to mechanical instability of the sacroiliac joints, rather than to pain.

Prognosis
Many horses are able to perform adequately despite slight unlevelness especially if they are kept fit. A few horses have recurrent problems. Big horses seem especially prone. The condition is rarely seen in ponies.

SPRAIN OF THE SACROILIAC LIGAMENTS

There is a sudden onset of hind-limb lameness which may be associated with a fall or a mis-step. Palpation of the hindquarters in the region of the tubera sacrale and tubera coxae causes pain. Manipulation of the leg may be resented.

Rest is the most important treatment. Faradism and ultrasound may be helpful. The prognosis is usually fair, although some horses may develop signs of chronic sacroiliac disease.

INCOORDINATION

Incoordination is a general term used to describe abnormal placement of a limb or limbs due to lack of awareness of the precise position of the limb. In some cases there may also be motor dysfunction due to an inability to use certain muscles. There are many potential causes of incoordination, the most common of which is the wobbler syndrome.

WOBBLER SYNDROME

The wobbler syndrome describes a number of conditions which result in compression of the spinal cord in the neck and cause a typical incoordinate gait. Hind-limbs are more severely affected than forelimbs and, because the horse lacks awareness of where it is placing its limbs and often has some hind-limb weakness, it has a loose, wobbly gait – hence the name wobbler syndrome.

Clinical signs
The syndrome occurs most commonly in young, rapidly growing Thoroughbreds. The incidence in colts is higher than in fillies. The syndrome can also occur in older horses of all types. Ponies are rarely affected.

The clinical signs may be sudden and severe, or subtle and insidious in onset, and may remain static or progress. If the syndrome develops gradually, at first the horse may show slight, intermittent, shifting hind-limb lameness. The toes may be dragged. When turned in small circles, the horse may place the hind-legs abnormally and may swing one leg outwards (circumduction). As the condition progresses the horse will tend to stand with the hind legs in odd positions. When the horse walks and trots the legs may be placed very deliberately to the ground. The hindquarters may look bouncy. The forelimbs are usually much less severely affected, but may show a stiff, stilted, spastic gait. If the clinical signs are sudden and severe in onset, the horse may appear normal one day and have little control over limb placement the next. If it has to stop or turn suddenly, it may fall over.

Diagnosis
The clinical signs are typical. The reason for compression of the spinal cord can sometimes be determined by radiographs of the neck. It is important to try to establish the cause of the problem if breeding is being considered.

Treatment
The condition is incurable, and may or may not be progressive. Some horses learn to accommodate to an extent but are not safe to ride, although they are suitable for breeding. However, in some forms of the syndrome there is

probably a hereditary predisposition for development of the disease, so these horses should not be used for breeding. Surgery has been performed on selected cases, resulting in some improvement in the clinical signs, but rarely are treated horses completely normal.

Prevention
One form of the syndrome is related to osteochondrosis (see p. 224), for which there is a hereditary predisposition. High planes of nutrition which encourage rapid growth may encourage manifestation of the condition; therefore young animals should be restricted in their plane of nutrition and growth rate.

CONGENITAL MALFORMATION OF THE CERVICAL (NECK)VERTEBRAE

Congenital malformations of the cervical vertebrae may cause abnormal pressure on the spinal cord resulting in incoordination. Although the bony abnormality is present at birth, the clinical signs of incoordination are sometimes not apparent until the foal is several months old. The most common condition is called occipito-atlanto-axial malformation, which occurs most frequently in Arabs and in this breed is an inheritable disease (see p. 742). There is no evidence that other congenital malformations are inherited.

NEUROAXONAL DYSTROPHY OR EQUINE DEGENERATIVE MYELOENCEPHALOPATHY

Equine degenerative myeloencephalopathy is a primary degenerative condition of the spinal cord, the cause of which is uncertain. It occurs most commonly in Arabs and Morgans suggesting a familial incidence, but is not directly heritable. Clinical signs usually develop within the first year of life and may be slowly progressive. As in the wobbler syndrome, the hind-limbs are usually more severely affected than the forelimbs. The disease cannot be diagnosed definitively except at post-mortem examination. There is no treatment.

FRACTURES

A fracture of a cervical vertebrae is usually the result of a fall and may cause compression of the spinal cord resulting in incoordination. There is usually associated neck stiffness and pain. The diagnosis is confirmed by radiography.

In some horses, depending on the site and configuration of the fracture, incoordination persists. In a few horses the signs of incoordination resolve rapidly, suggesting that there is not permanent pressure on the spinal cord. Some fractures heal spontaneously, and although the horse may have some permanent neck stiffness, it may otherwise be normal. However, if a large amount of callus is produced during fracture healing, the callus itself may press on the spinal cord and cause incoordination. It may be impossible at the time of the accident to predict the eventual outcome for the horse; it may be necessary to monitor its progress for several weeks or months.

BRUISING OF THE SPINAL CORD

The spinal cord may be severely bruised following a fall. Inflammation around the cord results in the formation of oedema, causing pressure on the spinal cord. Either of these conditions will result in incoordination. Treatment with anti-inflammatory agents such as corticosterolds or with the drug dimethyl sulphoxide may facilitate recovery. Signs of improvement are usually apparent within twenty-four hours, although it may take considerably longer before the horse appears completely normal. Persistence of severe incoordination for more than forty-eight hours warrants a guarded prognosis and usually indicates that there is additional, irreversible, damage.

MIGRATING PARASITES

Parasites which migrate through the spinal cord causing damage are a rare cause of incoordination. In contrast to the wobbler syndrome, the clinical signs are usually asymmetrical – one hind limb may be much more severely affected than the other. There is often muscle wastage. The diagnosis is usually based upon the clinical signs, lack of significant radiographic abnormalities and the progression of the disease. Most cases are not amenable to treatment but some early presumed cases of equine protozoal myelitis have been treated successfully.

CEREBELLAR HYPOPLASIA See pp. 160, 741

OTHER BRAIN LESIONS

Conditions of the brain are rare in the horse but can cause incoordination together with other clinical signs involving the head: for example, a head tilt, drooping of an ear or one side of the lips, blindness, abnormal position of the eyes or patchy sweating. Treatment is usually unsuccessful.

19
FLEXURAL AND ANGULAR LIMB DEFORMITIES IN FOALS

Limb deformities in foals are quite common and can be divided into flexural deformities and angular limb deformities. Some foals may have both types of deformity.

FLEXURAL DEFORMITIES

Flexural deformities of the limbs (so-called contracted tendons) may be congenital, i.e. present at birth, or acquired, i.e. develop after birth.

Congenital Flexural Deformities

A number of foals are born unable to straighten one or more limbs. If the limbs are manipulated passively they can usually be straightened. This condition is thought to be in part related to the position of the foetus in the uterus. The majority of these foals show progressive improvement over the first few days of life and no treatment is required. Occasionally it is not possible to straighten the affected limbs passively, and this warrants a more guarded prognosis. Such cases require the careful application of splints by a veterinarian in order to encourage the foal to walk on its toes and correct the flexure with limited exercise. Some veterinarians have had success injecting contracted foals intravenously with high doses of oxytetracycline (an antibiotic) which slackens the muscles and tendons at the back of the limb.

Similarly many foals are born with apparently lax flexor tendons, so that the fetlocks are overextended and drop towards the ground. This condition usually improves spontaneously and exercise is beneficial (see p. 341).

Acquired Flexural Deformities

DISTAL INTERPHALANGEAL (COFFIN) JOINT FLEXURAL DEFORMITY

Although this has been called contracture of the deep digital flexor tendon, there is no evidence to support the hypothesis that the tendon is contracted.

Clinical signs
Rapidly growing foals between six weeks and six months old are most commonly affected, the condition appearing in one or both forelimbs. The position of the limb becomes more upright and affected foals have been called toe dancers, as the foot becomes upright and boxy. The condition may occur apparently spontaneously or secondarily to a painful condition such as pus in the foot.

Diagnosis
The clinical signs are typical. Any underlying primary condition must be identified and treated accordingly. If the condition has been present for longer than two to three weeks the foot should be radiographed to establish whether any secondary problems have developed.

Treatment
Any primary problem must be treated and appropriate analgesics administered. If the condition has occurred spontaneously, the diet must be reduced and the foal should have exercise restricted or it should be confined to the stable. The feet should be carefully trimmed to lower the heels as much as possible. The toes should be kept well rounded to facilitate breakover. Some longer standing cases benefit from the farrier fitting a toe extension using equilox. If the disease is recognised early and treated quickly, the condition may resolve. As with congenital flexural deformities, some veterinarians have had success treating these cases with high doses of intravenous oxytetracycline. If no improvement is observed or if the condition deteriorates, surgical treatment (cutting the accessory ligament of the deep digital flexor tendon – the inferior check ligament) is indicated.

Prognosis
The prognosis is usually favourable unless secondary changes (for example, degenerative joint disease of the distal interphalangeal joint) have supervened. Pedal osteitis may be a sequel.

METACARPOPHALANGEAL (FETLOCK) JOINT FLEXURAL DEFORMITY

This condition has also been incorrectly called contracted tendon.

Clinical signs
The condition occurs in the forelimbs and hindlimbs, usually left and right limbs are affected simultaneously. It is seen in older foals and well-grown yearlings. The fetlock and pastern joints become more upright and the fetlock starts to knuckle over and may be held permanently so. It often occurs secondary to painful conditions such as osteochondrosis.

Diagnosis
The clinical signs are typical. In contrast to distal interphalangeal joint flexural deformity (see above), the foot shape is not usually deformed.

Treatment
In mild cases conservative treatment may be successful. The diet must be restricted and analgesics administered. Corrective shoeing is sometimes helpful. A toe extension can be placed on the shoe to delay breakover. Slight elevation of the heels may also help. Treatment of any osteochondrosis present improves this conformation.

If conservative treatment falls, surgical treatment is indicated. Some cases are improved by cutting the accessory ligament of the deep digital flexor tendon (the inferior check ligament). If this fails desmotomy of the accessory ligament of the superficial digital flexor tendon (superior check desmotomy) may help.

Prognosis
The prognosis is more guarded than for distal interphalangeal joint flexural deformities, especially if surgical treatment is required.

ANGULAR LIMB DEFORMITIES

Many foals are born with legs that are not completely straight: for example, the knees may deviate inwards (knock knees) or the fetlocks deviate outwards. Such foals usually show progressive and fairly rapid improvement. The condition usually affects both front legs and less frequently the hind legs. One leg may be more severely affected than the other. There is cause for concern if the deformity is severe, or if no improvement occurs.

There are many causes. If a foal is born prematurely or is one of a twin, the small bones of the knee or hock may not be properly formed and may be unable to withstand the stresses of weightbearing, which tends to compress and distort the bones. In other foals the bones are completely formed but, for various reasons, growth may occur more rapidly on one side of the leg compared with the other (imbalance of metaphyseal or epiphyseal growth – see below), so that the leg is crooked. If one of the physes (growth plates) of a bone is injured, the growth in that area will be decreased.

IMBALANCE OF METAPHYSEAL OR EPIPHYSEAL GROWTH

In this condition one side of the growth plate is growing faster than the other due to the imbalance of growth in the metaphysis or the epiphysis (Figure 1). This imbalance causes the limb to deviate away from the side of fastest growth.

Precise nomenclature is necessary to describe accurately the direction of angulation of the affected leg. This is accomplished by using a line bisecting the leg (Figure 2). The term 'carpus valgus' is used when the leg below the carpus (knee) falls outside this line (Figure 2a).

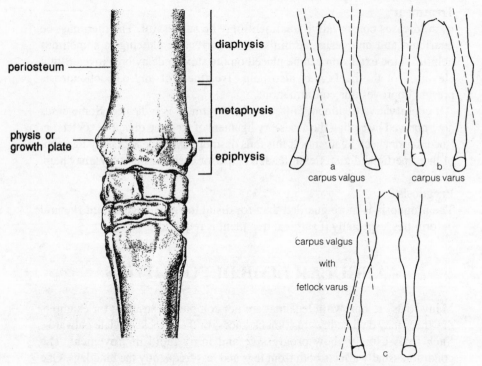

Figure 1   Anatomy of the carpus (knee) of a foal
Figure 2   Angular limb deformities

The term 'carpus varus' is used when the leg falls inside this line (Figure 2b). In these cases the direction of the fetlock follows the line of the third metacarpal (cannon) bone. However, there may be a combined situation in which the third metacarpal deviates to the outside of the line bisecting the carpus but the fetlock deviates towards the midline (Figure 2c). This is described as 'carpus valgus with fetlock varus'. In addition, some degree of rotation of the third metacarpal bone usually occurs with a valgus deformity.

Location

These deformities are seen in a variety of locations:

   (a) the carpus (valgus more commonly than varus);

   (b) the fetlock (varus more commonly than valgus);

   (c) the distal tibia (valgus more commonly than varus);

   (d) other locations (very rare).

Cause

The cause of angular limb deformities in foals due to asynchronous longitudinal growth is complex. Certain factors that contribute to this condition also contribute to the syndrome of physitis (see p. 214).

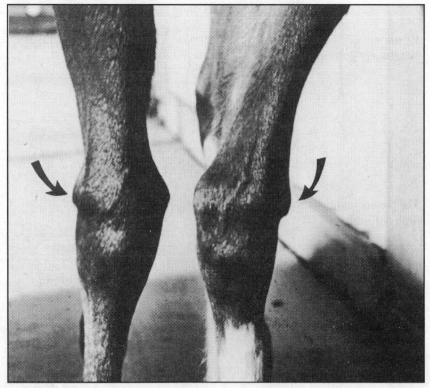

Figure 3   A case of angular limb deformity (carpus valgus) with physitis (arrows)

Both physitis and angular limb deformities can be seen in the same individual, although physitis is generally seen in older animals (Figure 3).

Trauma   Trauma in the form of abnormal pressure on the growth plate is believed to be one of the main underlying causes of angular deformities in foals. This pressure can cause cartilage cells within the growth plate to die and bone growth at this site to cease. If the pressure is asymmetrical, the growth plate damage is uneven and this leads to retarded longitudinal growth on the side of excessive pressure (the concave side of the joint). If the asymmetric loading is not severe, nature responds by increasing growth on the concave side to achieve normality. If the loading is excessive and nature cannot respond adequately, a vicious circle ensues with the resulting angulation leading to an even greater asymmetry of load. Virtually all forms of treatment (surgery, hoof trimming and extensions, etc.) are directed at interrupting this cycle (Figure 5). Factors which can cause asymmetrical loading on the growth plate include joint laxity, malpositioning in the uterus (windswept deformity), poor foot trimming, heavy muscling, overactivity or lameness in the opposite limb.

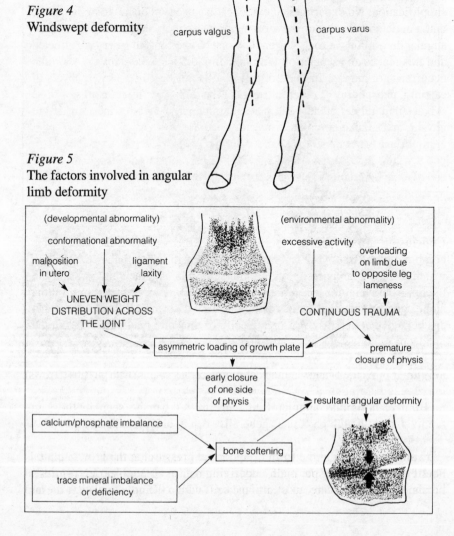

Figure 4
Windswept deformity

carpus valgus   carpus varus

Figure 5
The factors involved in angular limb deformity

(developmental abnormality)   (environmental abnormality)

conformational abnormality   excessive activity

malposition   ligament   overloading
in utero   laxity   on limb due
                                                                to opposite leg
                                                                lameness

UNEVEN WEIGHT
DISTRIBUTION ACROSS   CONTINUOUS TRAUMA
THE JOINT

asymmetric loading of growth plate   premature
                                               closure of physis

early closure
of one side
of physis   resultant angular deformity

calcium/phosphate imbalance

                           bone softening

trace mineral imbalance
or deficiency

Developmental abnormalities Hypoplasia (underdevelopment) of the carpal bones can also produce asymmetric loading. The end result in these foals is angular limb deformity due to the collapse of the hypoplastic bones as well as a growth imbalance at the level of the growth plate. Incomplete development of the second and fourth metacarpal (splint bones) can lead to a similar end. These syndromes are discussed in detail below.

Nutrition The role of nutrition is more complex and poorly understood. Previously deficiencies in calcium, phosphorus, vitamin A, carotene and vitamin D have been suggested and the condition has been erroneously called rickets by horse owners and veterinarians alike.

Rickets is a vitamin D deficiency and, although some features of the disease are seen in angular limb deformities, likening the two conditions is an over-simplification. No experimental evidence has been produced to demonstrate that a deficiency in one of the aforementioned vitamins or minerals leads to angular deformities in foals. Often only one or two foals in a herd are affected and this makes an association with nutrition difficult. Perhaps the sporadic occurrence of angular limb deformity can be attributed to varying levels of calcium, phosphorus or other nutrients in the milk of different mares.

Trace mineral deficiencies, in particular copper, have been incriminated in physitis and angular deformities in cattle and may play a role in horses. Copper is important for bone strength and a deficiency may result in so-called soft bones which angulate easily. Radiographically, the metaphysis appears to flare and overlap the epiphysis. The role of zinc, manganese, molybdenum and other minerals appears unclear, but excessive zinc from industrial pollution may cause a copper deficiency to develop.

Conclusion Most cases of angular limb deformities are the result of a combination of trauma plus a non-specific nutritional imbalance. Cases in which there is a lameness in one limb resulting in angular limb deformity in the opposite weightbearing limb are obviously trauma-induced, but trauma alone cannot explain all cases of angular limb deformities. Some veterinarians believe that heredity, through the sire or the dam, may play a part in the incidence of congenital angular limb deformities in foals.

The history of foals with angular limb deformities is variable. Some are normal at birth then begin to deviate, while others are crooked at birth and improve to varying degrees. An attending veterinarian needs to ascertain the rate, if any, of improvement in order to decide if surgery is necessary.

Treatment
With an understanding of the effects of trauma on the growth plate, the rationale behind certain aspects of management of angular limb deformities becomes apparent. The most important factor behind correction of an

angular deformity is restriction of exercise.

Foals, by their nature, will do everything possible to stay near their dams early in life, and overactivity in this regard produces increased trauma to the growth plate. Trauma should be minimised by restricting the foal's exercise by confining it to a loosebox. This must be done until the limb has straightened.

Foot trimming (or balancing) also helps correct conformation and subsequent asymmetrical loading. In addition, the application of appropriate extensions using Equilox or similar materials can encourage angled or flexed limbs to achieve correct conformation. Frequent evaluation, including radiographic examination by a veterinarian, is necessary to monitor the progress of conservative therapy.

These two factors can correct a large proportion of angular limb deformities and should always be used as a first step in correction, provided there is no evidence of hypoplasia or immaturity of the carpal bones. With careful management most angular limb deformities make significant improvement when the foal is between one and three months of age.

Because of the relatively early closure of the growth plates at the end of the cannon bones, surgery should be attempted as soon as the deformity is noted in these areas. Surgical treatment for such angulations after sixty to eighty days of age is unsuccessful.

Casting and braces have often been regarded as conservative methods, but these have no scientific basis and are fraught with pressure-sore problems because of the thinness of young foals' skin.

In cases in which there is another orthopaedic problem that causes excessive loading on the 'good' limb the solution is not as clear-cut. Sometimes the resultant lameness is so severe or protracted (for example, a healing fracture) that the animal has no option but to take excessive weight on the good limb during convalescence. Clearly the solution is to minimise the convalescent time on the injured limb so that normal weightbearing can resume as soon as possible.

Surgery is indicated in the case of the carpus (knee) and tarsus (hock) if the angular limb deformity is unchanged at age sixty days or is getting progressively worse. If the limb is nearly straight at this time the veterinarian may wait an additional thirty days before a final decision is made. Occasionally a severe deformity at the carpus will be considered a surgical candidate at forty-five days. Fetlock deformities must be operated on between thirty and sixty days or, preferably, as soon as the deformity is noticed.

Surgical treatment for angular limb deformities has two main objectives: first, to stimulate growth on the retarded side (concave) and, second, to slow down growth on the opposite side (convex).

Stimulation of growth on the concave side
Stimulation of growth on the concave side is achieved by lifting the periosteum away from the bone at the affected site.

There are two explanations as to why this technique is successful: first, the procedure is thought to disrupt the blood supply on the operated side and thus stimulate growth there; second, the periosteum is supposed to have a tethering effect on the growth rate. Thus by surgically incising it, this effect is lost and growth rate increases. This latter explanation is the more likely.

Because periosteal stripping is a stimulation procedure (i.e. it increases bone growth), it is performed on the side of the metaphysis with retarded growth (the concave side). Experimentally it has been shown that making an incision on the inner periosteum *causes* a valgus deformity. Thus, clinically, an incision on the outside (lateral) periosteum is to *correct* a valgus deformity. Therefore, for a valgus deformity of the carpus, the periosteum is transected and lifted on the outside of the lower radius.

Periosteal stripping is the primary surgical technique for angular deformities of the lower (distal) radius and tibia. This technique, in combination with transphyseal bridging (discussed below), is used for angular deformities of the fetlock.

Technique   The surgery for periosteal stripping is performed under a general anaesthetic. The veterinarian makes an inverted T-shaped incision just above the growth plates on the concave side of the deformity and the periosteum is peeled away from the bone at this site. It is then left apart and the subcutaneous tissues and skin are closed. The surgery itself is quite simple.

Post-operative management   The skin incision is covered with a non-adhesive dressing and the entire joint wrapped with adhesive bandaging. Antibiotics are not given prior to surgery unless screws and wires are also to be used (see below).

The wound is kept wrapped for at least ten days with the bandage changed every three or five days. Skin sutures are removed at ten to fourteen days.

During the convalescence (while the limb straightens) the foal must remain relatively confined to minimise concussion to the growth plate. Although complete confinement of the mare and her foal to a loosebox is desirable and recommended, this often meets with resistance from owners. They frequently prefer the mare to be out in sunlight to help induce regular ovulation. As a compromise mare and foal should be placed in a stall that has a small run attached to it. Under no circumstances, however, should the foal be running free with the mare in a large pasture.

The advantages of periosteal stripping over other techniques are that it is relatively straightforward to perform, it does not require expensive implants nor a mandatory second operation to remove screws and wires. The hospitalisation period is also slightly shorter and therefore the overall operation is less expensive. It is cosmetically appealing but may not result in complete correction of the deformity. However, the surgery can be repeated if necessary. Of interest is the fact that the technique, if used as the sole procedure, has not resulted in overcorrection of an angular limb deformity.

Deceleration of growth on the convex side

The second surgical technique used for asymmetrical growth is a retardation by various transphyseal bridging methods. These usually involve the insertion of staples or screws and wires spanning the growth plate on the convex side of the limb. The metal implants create a compressive force causing a change in the blood supply to that side of the growth plate and thus a gradual decline in growth. Continued growth on the opposite side causes the sides of the metaphysis to equalise; thus the leg returns to its normal axis. At this point the implants are removed and normal leg growth continues.

Technique   Metal staples can be used to bridge growth plates in both foals and children. The technique was modified in 1972 and bone screws can be placed on either side of the growth plate with wire tied in a figure of eight connecting the heads (Figure 6). For severe angulations this is the preferred method as immediate compression is applied across the growth plate, thereby hastening correction. Although a larger surgical incision is required for insertion of the screws and wire, they can be removed through two small stab incisions when the limb has straightened (Figure 7).

The procedure can be used alone or in combination with hemicircumferential transection of the periosteum and periosteal stripping for certain deformities, particularly in the fetlock joint.

Post-operative management   A sterile non-adhesive dressing is placed over the incision and then the affected joints bandaged. A full-limb bandage using cotton may be needed, but a light gauze and elastic adhesive bandage covering only the affected joint may be all that is required if it is carefully applied. Antibiotics are given before and following surgery because implants increase the likelihood of infection.

The foal should be confined during convalescence to reduce concussion on the growth plates. The hooves should receive appropriate trimming. Frequently foals are fed mineral supplements or given injections of various vitamins. These are unnecessary in most cases unless a true deficiency can be identified. Certainly older animals presented for this surgery (e.g. weanlings) should be fed a ration containing the appropriate calcium-phosphorus ratio. Analysis of the diet of these older foals frequently reveals a mineral imbalance. The role of other trace minerals as an adjunct to the treatment of angular limb deformities in foals is less well understood. A zinc excess and/ or a copper deficiency may exist in isolated instances.

Removal of implants   When the axis of the limb is straight, removal of the implants must be performed to prevent overcorrection of the deformity. Thus

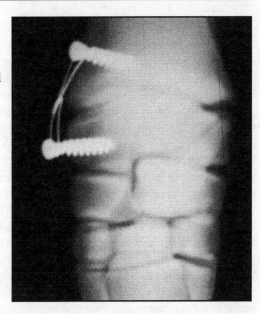

Figure 6
A radiograph of a foal's carpal joint showing two screws bridged by a piece of wire (transphyseal bridging) to retard growth on that side of the limb to correct a carpus valgus deformity

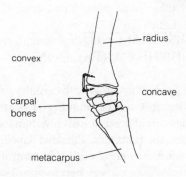
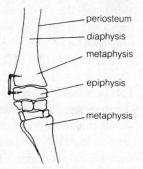

periosteum
diaphysis
metaphysis
epiphysis
metaphysis

radius
convex
concave
carpal bones
metacarpus

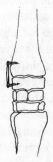

Figure 7
Screws and wire to correct an angular limb deformity of the lower radius

owners must observe the leg closely and return the foal to the veterinarian when the limb is straight. Removal of screws and wires can be done with the foal standing under local anaesthesia if it can be adequately restrained.

Wedge osteotomy
If the limb is severely deviated and the growth plate has closed (typically a foal six to nine months old with a severe varus deformity of the fetlock), the only hope of straightening the limb is a wedge osteotomy. Here a wedge of bone is removed with a motorised saw and the limb straightened and held in position with one or two bone plates. It is a radical procedure but has a place with a valuable animal that requires saving for breeding purposes. Wedge osteotomy is performed far more commonly in dogs than in horses but the principles are the same. It is not the type of surgery done routinely in all equine practices and is best referred to a specialised orthopaedic practice.

Occasionally a wedge osteotomy is performed in a foal that has diaphyseal angular limb deformity. Here the bone is bent in the middle of the shaft. Usually the cannon bones are affected. Diaphyseal angular deformities occur in areas of the tubular long bones unrelated to a growth plate. They can be congenital (in-*utero* positioning). The only treatment for this is a wedge osteotomy, in which the bone is cut into two. Bone plates are then used to immobilize the bone while it heals. Again, such cases are best left to specialists experienced in orthopaedics.

HYPOPLASIA, NECROSIS OR INCOMPLETE OSSIFICATION (COLLAPSE) OF THE CARPAL BONES

This condition is rare but should be suspected when a foal with carpus valgus or carpus varus has not responded to confinement or is becoming progressively worse. It is usually present at birth. Various carpal bones are involved, in most cases at least two, and commonly the ulnar, the fourth and the outer aspect of the third carpal bones. There is usually some distention of the joint capsules due to excess synovial fluid.

The diagnosis is made using radiographs. The affected carpal bones are smaller and more rounded than usual and may be deformed (collapsed) in shape. This is because in this condition the carpal bones are still partly cartilaginous and not completely bony, so they are less well able to withstand the normal forces transmitted through the limb during weightbearing and therefore are susceptible to being squashed.

The bones in the hock joints of these foals should also be checked for signs of collapse. Advanced cases of collapsed carpal bones will show radiographic signs of arthritis. It mostly occurs in premature foals or those which for unknown reasons have some degree of softness of the cartilage base of the carpal bones during immaturity.

Treatment
Mild cases will respond to conservative therapy as described for growth

imbalance (see p. 335 above). Rest and restriction of exercise are particularly important. Some will be candidates for surgery if there is a concurrent imbalance of metaphyseal growth. Severe cases will not respond simply to temporary transphyseal bridging (screws and wires). In severe cases of hypoplasia or collapse of the carpal bones the only hope is casting to remove pressure from the bones to allow normal bone formation (ossification) to proceed.

This is done by the use of tube or cylinder casts. These extend from the top of the radius to the top of the sesamoid bones and prevent the tendon laxity and osteoporosis (breakdown of bone cells) seen with casts that encase the entire foot. Foals with casts should be hospitalised and the casts changed every two to fourteen days under general anaesthesia.

Cast application in foals and adults is difficult and must be performed by a veterinarian. After three to four weeks' casting, ossification and the natural formation of the carpal bones should have been completed and usually the bones can then withstand the strength of normal loading without collapsing. Even after ten to fourteen days some improvement will be found. The key to success is early recognition of the problem before complete collapse and arthritis has occurred.

INCOMPLETE DEVELOPMENT OF THE SMALL METACARPAL (SPLINT) BONES

This is a relatively uncommon cause of any limb deformity and is manifest by a less than normal degree of attachment of the splint bones to the carpus.

LIGAMENT LAXITY

This is present to some degree in *all* foals at birth and can be manifested as laxity of the flexor tendons.

Laxity will appear as an angular limb deformity of one kind or another (usually a valgus deformity of the carpus). Some foals with ligament laxity show carpus valgus in one front leg and carpus varus in the other (windswept deformity – see Figure 4). Windswept deformities more commonly occur in the rear limbs.

Treatment
Nature will usually correct these and exercise is beneficial for cases involving the hindlimbs. Box rest may be more appropriate (perhaps with access to a small run) for those affecting forelimbs in order to reduce the trauma of asymmetric loading on the growth plates. Very few of these cases are appropriate for splinting.

Casting is contraindicated and will usually exacerbate the condition by preventing exercise, which has a physiotherapeutic effect. Everything loses strength and mass in a cast, not only muscles but tendons, joint cartilage and ligaments. Thus casts are not recommended.

TRAUMATIC LUXATION AND FRACTURE OF THE CARPAL BONES

This dislocation is a rare cause of carpal deviations. These foals usually have a history of severe trauma, such as being caught under a fence or stepped on or kicked by the mare. The prognosis for future soundness is grave because of irreversible damage (structural change) in the affected bones.

COLLAPSE OF THE THIRD AND/OR CENTRAL TARSAL BONES OF THE HOCK

This has also been called necrosis (cellular death) of the third and/or central tarsal bones.

It is a condition in which, early in postnatal life, the third and sometimes the central tarsal bones of the foal's hock begins to collapse. The end result is a severe and crippling arthritis of the distal rows of tarsal joints. The condition generally occurs in both hocks but is worse in one. It is found most commonly in foals born prematurely or as one of a twin. As in hypoplasia of the carpal bones (see above), the tarsal bones are not completely bony (incompletely ossified) at birth and are therefore susceptible to being squashed. An affected foal shows sickle and slightly curby hock conformation (see Figure 14 , p. 722). If examined early (within the first fourteen days of life) the tarsal bones are found to be smaller and more rounded than usual and treatment at this stage can prevent the more debilitating secondary changes. If left untreated the condition progresses and an affected foal usually develops signs of a stiff, stilted gait in the first two months of life. It lies down a lot and is less active than other foals. It will have a cow-hocked and/or sicklehocked conformation. Such foals eventually develop a severe degenerative tarsitis (arthritis) of the hock resembling bone spavin. Usually an enlargement can be felt in the inner fore aspect of the lower hock because, as the bone collapses, a piece of bone becomes pushed forward. Treatment of collapsed tarsal bones is usually unsuccessful.

Casting in very early cases can be successful but foals are usually presented to the veterinarian when collapse has already occurred, in which case there is no effective treatment. Eventually severe bone spavin (arthritis) and chronic lameness result and the prognosis for future athletic soundness is poor. Obviously more work is needed to establish the exact cause of this condition.

20
SHOEING

Shoeing is a necessary evil, carried out for two basic reasons: first, to prevent undue wear to the hoof, which can result in damage to the foot, leading to pain and lameness; and, second, to spread the load around the hoof wall so that small segments of the horn do not come under high pressure, which can result in damage to that segment.

In the wild, the wear of the hoof wall against the ground is counteracted by the continual growth of the wall down from the coronary band. Nature will adjust the growth rate so that it is roughly equal to the rate of wear. This means that unshod horses can do light work without causing excessive wear and damage to their feet, particularly in countries with a dry climate, or when worked on light or sandy soils. Where the soil is heavy, or on hard surfaces such as metalled roads, work for any length of time will cause excessive wear and damage to the hooves. Wet or moist conditions result in softening of the horn, and the foot will wear down more quickly than in dry conditions.

Horses' hooves, like the nails in a human's hand and feet, grow continually and need constant wear or trimming if they are to remain properly 'balanced' and shaped. Thus shoeing, which reduces foot wear, inevitably leads to the need for regular trimming of the feet. The feet of young horses, even if unshod, should be inspected and if necessary, trimmed at least once a month. This practice pays dividends in the long run by ensuring the growth of well-shaped feet; it also enables corrective trimming to be carried out at an early age to encourage formation of straight limbs.

Horses working on the road almost invariably need shoeing. However, depending on the degree of work, shoeing of the hind feet may sometimes not be necessary. Horses working predominantly on a soft surface or in indoor schools may not require shoeing at all, although regular trimming is essential in order to maintain correct foot shape.

The period between shoeing varies with the type of shoe and the work carried out by the horse. Re-shoeing may be required for two reasons. First, the shoe may be so worn that it is liable to break, causing damage to the horse, or the position of the shoe on the foot may have altered so that the branches are putting pressure on the sole. Secondly, the foot is continuously growing and, although some wear occurs at the heels as they rub against the shoe, no wear occurs at the toe. This means that the foot gets gradually longer, and the toe becomes disproportionately long compared with the heels. The foot therefore needs trimming in order to maintain its shape, and the shoes should be removed or replaced at least once every four to six weeks. In exceptional cases re-shoeing may be needed as frequently as every two to three weeks.

Traditionally, shoes are made of iron, and this has the advantage that the farrier can shape them with a high degree of precision to fit the vagaries of individual feet. It has one disadvantage, however: on hard road surfaces shoes become polished and horses are apt to slip. Various devices have been introduced to combat this, ranging from the use of Carborundum on the ground surface of the shoe to small studs or hardened heads on the horseshoe nails. Recently, experiments have been carried out with different materials, including rubber and plastic as alternatives to the traditional iron shoe, but to date none of these has proved very satisfactory. A degree of slip is required as part of the mechanism to reduce concussion as the foot is placed on the ground. If this slip is totally eliminated, then excessive strain is placed on the fetlock and pastern joints.

Growth and function of the hoof
In the natural state the hoof wall grows at a rate that compensates for the normal wear. In the average horse it takes between eight and twelve months for new horn formed at the coronary band to grow down to the lower border of the foot. The rate of growth varies in different animals depending on the work carried out, the wear on the foot, and the season of the year.

The quality of the horn is a reflection of the bodily condition of the animal, and a sick horse or one in poor condition will produce poor horn at the coronary band. This may not be noticed until this region of horn has grown to the bearing surface of the foot some eight to twelve months later, and wears excessively or breaks away when loaded.

There is a suggestion that black horn is stronger than white. However, it has now been proved that the mechanical properties of horn of both colours are identical, the colour being due purely to pigment granules in the horn which do not affect its strength although they may reduce the rate of wear.

The horn of the hoof wall is formed entirely at the coronary band and grows downwards to the bearing surface of the foot. The horn is composed of a large number of tubules of horn growing down from the coronary band, and these are bound together by intertubular horn. The pedal bone is attached to the hoof wall by the sensitive laminae; under normal circumstances the laminae do not form horn themselves, although they may do so if the hoof wall is damaged. The sole and the frog are formed from a layer of young cells (the solar corium), which form a sheet across the sole of the foot. In the normal foot the sole is not a prime weight bearing area, only coming into contact with the ground on soft surfaces. The bulk of the horse's weight is carried by the hoof wall, with some weight being taken by the frog.

There are many theories about the function and movement of the foot, many of which are unproven. It is well recognised that the heels of the foot normally expand during weight bearing and that the hoof wall itself distorts as it takes weight. The expansion of the heels results from the loading of the sloping hoof walls, resulting in the ground surface sliding outwards. It is not related to frog pressure as was once thought. Indeed it has been shown that excess frog pressure can in fact result in contraction of the heels.

The process of weight bearing is also responsible for pumping blood from the foot back towards the heart, and this may play a dual role, the vascular pressure acting as a hydraulic cushion to absorb concussion as the foot takes weight. As the foot comes in contact with the ground, the arteries and veins within the foot (across the sole and in the hoof wall) come under pressure. The pressure forces the blood along the vessels and through the digital veins up the limb. At the same time the resistance to the blood being forced through the veins may help to absorb concussion as the foot is placed on the ground. There are also veins in the bulb of the heel, which are squeezed when the fetlock and pastern are flexed. These may also help pump blood back up the limbs.

The movement of the limbs and feet are affected and controlled by the action of muscles. These muscles and their tendons are attached to appropriate sites on the skeletal framework, so that when a muscle contracts (works) precise movements take place and the joints are flexed or extended. There are no muscles present below the knee or hock of the horse, all the actions in the lower limb being transmitted by the long tendons.

The principle movements in the limb are those of flexion and extension. The flexor muscles and tendons lie behind the skeletal column of bones and the extensors in the front. When the horse is standing at rest, the flexor tendon to the foot is under tension, pulling on the pedal bone and around the back of the fetlock in order to maintain the horse in a standing position. When the horse moves, the muscle attached to the flexor tendon shortens, increasing the pull on the tendon and thus flexing the pastern and fetlock joints as the heel is raised from the ground.

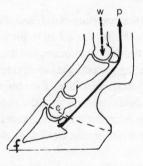

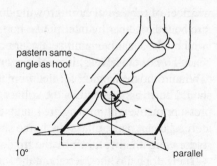

Figure 1
The mechanics of the foot

Figure 2
Normal hoof conformation

This can be considered in mechanical terms (Figure 1). In effect the pull of the tendon P supports the weight of the horse bearing down on the fetlock W. At the end of the stride the pull P lifts the heels, the toe of the foot F acting as a fulcrum. Hence it is evident that the longer the toe grows the greater the leverage it exerts and the greater the strain put on the tendons. Lowering the heels of the foot excessively also increases strain on the tendons. The ideal angle for the front of the hoof varies from one horse to another, depending on the individual's conformation. The angle of the hoof, however, should be the same as that of the pastern (and this in turn is the same as the angle described by the shoulder). Thus a line drawn from the front of the fetlock to the coronary band and then on down the front of the hoof should be straight, with no deflection forwards or backwards at the coronary band (Figure 2).

In the natural state the length of the hoof is determined by the rate of wear and the rate of growth of horn. In the shod horse length is determined by the farrier trimming the feet when the horse is shod. There is no simple guideline as to how long a foot should be; one has to rely on the experience of an expert farrier for the foot to be trimmed correctly.

Weight bearing surfaces of the foot

The horn of the foot is not sensitive, being formed in a similar manner to the human fingernail. The hoof wall is formed exclusively from the coronary band, but the sole and frog are derived from the solar corium, a sheet of cells that covers the bottom of the pedal bone. This corium is very sensitive, and the foot is designed with an arch to the sole in such a manner that weight is not normally carried on the sole itself. The arch of the sole is greater in hind feet than in front feet, and if it is flattened (as in dropped soles), the foot and deeper structures become more liable to bruising, which may result in lameness.

When standing normally on a hard surface the weight of the horse is supported on the ground surface of the wall and on the immediately adjacent rim of the sole, the bulk of the sole remaining clear of the ground. The bars, which are a continuation of the wall turned forward at the heel of the foot, may also be weight bearing in unshod horses. The frog is normally just clear of the ground in the standing animal, but may be responsible for a degree of weight bearing when the horse is in motion, particularly on soft ground, and in flat feet.

When a horse is shod all the weight bearing structures described above should be utilised as fully as possible. The shoe should normally not only put pressure on the wall of the foot but also cover the white line and the immediately adjacent part of the sole. In the shod horse, however, the bars of the feet seldom play their full role in weight bearing.

The wall of the hoof is an equal thickness and strength all round the foot. Because it grows to the ground at an angle however, it appears thicker at the toe, becoming relatively narrower at the quarters of the foot. It is normal practice however to make the shoe of an equal width around the entire foot. The portion of sole, which lies in the angle, formed by the wall and the bar at the heel of the foot (the so-called seat of corn) should not bear any weight in a well-shod horse, as this area is very prone to bruising. If the shoe is properly fitted, it may cover much of the seat of corn and protect it from bruising.

Because it is generally not weight bearing, the sole is not subject to much wear. In the normal horse there is continual flexing of the sole during weight bearing, and this causes exfoliation of the superficial layers of the horn of the sole preventing a build-up in thickness of horn. In some circumstances, for example, in dry conditions, exfoliation may not take place and it may be necessary for the farrier to trim excessive horn away from the sole.

Similarly the size of the frog is normally regulated by wear, and a well balanced, well-shaped foot shows a healthy frog. When trimming the foot, any excessive growth of the frog should be trimmed away in order to prevent moisture and infection collecting around the loose leaves of horn that can sometimes form in the frog and frog clefts.

Preparing the foot for shoeing
The shoe is applied to the foot in order to protect the hoof from excessive wear. When the foot is prepared for re-shoeing it is trimmed (to replace the normal wear that would have taken place in an unprotected foot) taking great care to maintain the normal slope and contour of the hoof. The heels, quarters and toes grow at approximately the same rate. When the animal is shod the shoe protects the toe from wear, but the branches of the shoe are not fixed to the heels and therefore there is a degree of movement and attrition of horn as the heels expand and contract with the horse's movement. When the shoe has been on for some time the toe will need shortening rather more than the heels in order to maintain the balance of the foot. For this reason it is common practice amongst farriers to shorten the toe with hoof cutters, but to trim the heels only with a hoof rasp.

Some confusion exists with regard to the meaning of the terms 'lowering the toe' and 'shortening the toe'. In lowering the toe the horn is removed from the ground surface of the foot. In shortening the toe, the long anteroposterior (front to rear) axis of the hoof is reduced by vertical removal of the horn of the hoof wall at the toe.

Although it is generally accepted that the shoe should be fitted to the hoof and not the hoof to the shoe, the advantage to be gained by judicious manicuring of the toe of the foot should not be overlooked. Long toes affect the balance of the foot and increase the stress on the flexor tendons. There is also evidence that a long-toed, low-heeled foot increases the loading on the heels and may interfere with blood flow through the foot as a whole. This conformation certainly predisposes to the development of navicular disease. Shortening the toe in these cases is an essential practice. In some circumstances the shoe may be set back under the toe of the foot and the projecting superfluous portion of horn rasped off. This is common practice in the shoeing of the hind feet in order to avoid the dangers of overreaching.

When the hoof is being prepared for shoeing, the bearing surface (the portion of the foot against the ground) should be perfectly level. When the limb is viewed from in front, the bearing surface from medial to lateral sides should be at right angles to the long axis of the limb. When viewed from the side, the angle the wall at the toe makes with the ground should be the same as the angle of the pastern. Some trimming of the sole and frog may be necessary to remove flakes of horn from the sole and remove any ragged portions of the frog, and the bars may be trimmed to prevent them from growing across the sole of the foot. Undue thinning of the sole or paring of the frog or the bars should be avoided; thinning should be just sufficient to maintain the shape of the foot.

Trimming and balancing the foot

Although trimmimg and balancing the foot are probably the most important and skilled aspects of shoeing a horse, unfortunately the significance of trimming is not immediately obvious to the casual observer; it is far less impressive than the working of red-hot iron. For this reason, in recent years, probably insufficient attention has been paid to trimming, balancing and, in particular, maintaining the shape of the heel.

The horn at the heels of the foot should grow down in a line parallel to the horn at the toe, and the quarters of the foot should not be allowed to spread. If the heels are over lowered or the shoe is placed rather short under the heels, there is a tendency for the heels to collapse forwards and inwards, and this has been incriminated as one contributory cause of foot disease.

Evidence of hoof function currently suggests that the continual expansion and contraction of the heels as the horse moves are necessary for healthy normal horn growth and also for normal blood flow through the foot as a whole. Contraction of the heels may result in the horn losing much of its elasticity and the frog tending to become wasted. There is no doubt that regular exercise and careful trimming to maintain correct balance of the foot play an important part in maintaining the health and function of the hoof itself.

The current fashions for 'natural balance' and 'four point' shoeing should be treated with caution until scientific evaluation of the techniques is available. At present these theories are unproven, based on observation of the wear of the feet of feral horses. The interpretation of the significance of these wear patterns is still at best equivocal.

The shoe

Steel or aluminium alloys are still the commonest materials used in shoes. Much has been written about the 'unbiological' nature of these materials, but they have stood the test of time, and it seems unlikely that they will be replaced for routine shoeing with any other materials in the foreseeable future.

Modern economic constraints have resulted in the majority of farriers now using machine-made shoes. There is little doubt, however, that the farrier who makes his own shoes from straight iron has an expertise and ability to fit shoes with an accuracy unlikely to be equalled by the farrier using ready-made shoes. There is nothing inherently wrong with a machine-made shoe, providing the shoe is the correct size and shape for the animal to which it is fitted. This, however, entails keeping a large selection of ready-made shoes available, considerably more than if each shoe is purpose made from straight iron stock.

Figure 3
Application of the
shoe to the foot.
A: a concave fullered
shoe, B: a flat seated
out shoe

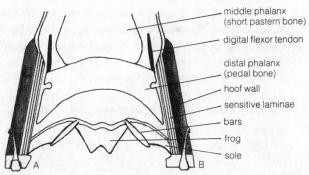

middle phalanx
(short pastern bone)

digital flexor tendon

distal phalanx
(pedal bone)

hoof wall

sensitive laminae

bars

frog

sole

In Britain the majority of horses are shod with concave fullered shoes (Figure 3). The iron has a ground surface with a deep groove (the fuller) around its entire length, which gives additional grip. Many shoes used in continental Europe are flat and do not have this groove.

The foot surface of the shoe, whatever type it may be, should be flat and level. The weight should be distributed evenly around the foot, and no pressure points should be caused by twisted or unlevel shoes.

The width of iron should be adequate to cover the entire wall and a small portion of sole inside the white line. In some horses a slightly wider shoe may be used in order to give a degree of protection to the sole. In such cases the inner portion of the solar surface should be bevelled so that it does not come in contact with the sole of the foot; this process is called 'seating out' (Figure 3). In theory the use of seated- out shoes may increase the likelihood of stones getting caught between the sole and the shoe, which is almost impossible with a concave fullered shoe. Many competition horses have a large bodyweight and comparatively weak feet, making the use of a flat, seated- out shoe essential, in order to give additional support to the foot by taking a small amount of pressure on the periphery of the sole.

In order for the frog to bear weight in a relatively normal fashion, and to prevent the shoe from being too heavy (which may interfere with the horse's gait) the shoe should be as thin as practicable. However, this reduces the life of the shoe and may result in it becoming distorted if it wears too thin. For this reason the farrier must compromise by choosing a shoe which has adequate width to give the support needed and adequate thickness to give good wear, but which at the same time is not too heavy for the horse's foot. The fullered shoe serves this purpose well in that it is relatively light for its thickness; however, the very act of fullering reduces the area of shoe in contact with the ground and thus increases the rate of wear. A flat shoe will show better wear for its thickness, although it is relatively heavier.

A normal shoe is of uniform thickness from the toe through the quarters to the heels. Thus, when fitted, it does not disturb the trim and balance of a foot that has been correctly prepared. Some shoes are made with varying thickness from toe to heel, but these are only used in special cases to correct abnormalities of the hoof. The width of the shoe should also be uniform from the toe to the heels; the practice of narrowing the inner branch of the shoe (which is supposed to minimise damage caused by brushing) should be discouraged as this tends to allow the shoe to press on the seat of corn.

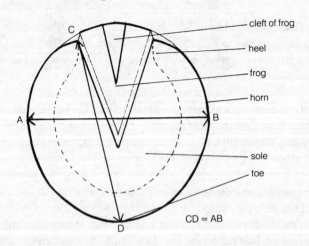

Figure 4   The correct shape of a shoe

In shape the shoe should follow the general form of the weight-bearing surface of the wall of the foot. It should be the same dimension at the widest point of the quarters as it is from the middle of the toe to the ends of the branches at the heel (Figure 4); if two shoes are superimposed they should form a smooth elliptical shape. (A horse's hind feet are slightly narrower and longer than the front feet.) The outline of the shoes should follow a smooth curve and should not turn in at the heels. The heels of the foot are not restrained by nails, and are able to expand and contract as the horse moves. For this reason the heels are fitted wide, allowing sufficient margin for the heels not to slip over the edge of the shoe as they expand.

Front shoes frequently have a clip at the toe, and hind shoes a clip either side of the toe. Side clips help prevent lateral rotation of the shoe, and side slips and toe clips tend to stop the shoe moving backwards on the foot as the shoe comes into contact with the ground, taking some of the stress off the nails. Some people consider that clips on shoes are unnecessary, and many horses are shod without clips and show no resulting problems. Many horses are shod with a rolled toe, in which instance no clip is provided.

The shoes should be fitted so that they project slightly beyond the ends of the horn at the heel (any risk of a fore shoe getting caught by a hind foot is obviated if the toe of the hind foot is dressed well back). As the foot grows, the horn growing down at an angle tends to pull the shoe forwards, and it is important that the heels should remain on the shoe. If the heels of the shoe are fitted slightly in front of the heels of the foot, then they will soon become embedded in the hoof wall and the heels will not be maintained at the correct angle, gradually collapsing forwards and inwards.

With wear, the toe of the shoe (or an unshod foot) is generally worn more than the rest of the foot. This can be imitated by thinning the toe of the shoe from the ground surface (rolled-toe shoe) or even turning up the entire shoe at the toe (Blenkinsop shoe). Whereas the rolled-toe shoe is quite commonly used nowadays, particularly for animals that tend to stumble, Blenkinsop shoes are seldom used because of the difficulty and time involved in making and fitting them.

Heavy shoes change a horse's action slightly and they are sometimes deliberately used to encourage a hackney action. One disadvantage of heavy shoes is that they require larger nails to fix them, increasing the amount of damage to the hoof wall.

Calkins, studs, cogs, etc., which are supposed to increase the grip of the shoe, should only be used after careful consideration. If used they should be kept as small as possible, and be fitted on both branches of the shoe, rather than on one alone, because they interfere with the normal balance of the foot. The use of a single calkin or road stud in just one heel can seriously affect the growth of the horn and the action of the foot, and in some cases will result in lameness. A single stud will cause increased pressure on the horn above it, slowing horn growth. It will also unbalance the foot, increasing joint strain, and reduces the slip on one side of the foot, tending to cause a rotatory distortion of the hoof wall. The use of studs on soft ground, where the protuberance can dig into the surface, is less damaging, but protuberances from the ground surface of the shoe should always be kept to an absolute minimum.

Traditionally many hunters and driving horses are shod behind with a calk and wedge shoe, and this is a satisfactory practice for increasing the grip. The calk and wedge are relatively small, and balance each other, one on each branch of the shoe, so there is a minimum of interference with the balance of the hoof. Many heavy draught horses were traditionally shod with high calkins on the inner and outer heels, coupled with a toe piece. This practice should no longer be continued. It was developed to give a good grip on the traditional cobbled road, the calks and toe grab lodging over the edges of the cobbles. With modern roads there is nothing for them to grip, and they simply unbalance the feet, cause pressure points on the hoof wall, and in fact reduce the horse's grip. If the calkins are removed, and the foot is balanced and trimmed in the normal way, after an initial period of sliding, the horses will regain their previous degree of grip, but will develop better quality horn and feet.

Nail holes

With thin fullered shoes it is normal practice to leave the nail, once driven home, slightly proud of the ground surface of the shoe. The taper of the head of the nail is shaped to fit tightly into the fuller of the shoe, and the taper of the shank of the nail is similarly shaped to fit tightly into the hole in the shoe. In this way, as the nail head and shoe wear, the shank of the nail still remains tight in the hole and a loose shoe does not result. If the tapers on nail and shoe do not match, the shoe will rapidly work loose. If the nail head becomes wedged in the fuller, then as the shoe wears the head of the nail will be worn away, and so rapidly work loose. If the shank of the nail binds but the head is left loose, then there is a tendency for the nails to break as they pass through the shoe.

With a flat unfullered shoe the nail hole is stamped to coincide with the shape of the head of the nail. The hole narrows downwards (looking at the shoe from the ground surface). In this manner the nail head lodges securely and solidly in the hole without weakening the shoe.

One advantage with the flat unfullered shoe is that the nail hole can be more readily placed towards the inner or outer margin of the shoe and the angle of the hole altered to suit different shapes of foot. With the fullered shoe the fullering is at an equal distance from the outside edge all around the shoe and the nail holes tend to be punched inside the fullering without reference to the thickness of the horn. Thus, although this method of fullering is labour saving, it may not always result in the ideal positioning of the nail hole or the angle of the nail.

Ideally the nail holes should not be punched through the shoe until the foot is dressed and ready for the shoe to be applied. In this way the farrier can position the nails to avoid driving them through the weak parts of the hoof wall, or through areas which may have been chipped, split or pierced by previous nails.

Normally three nails are used on the inner branch of the foot and either three or four on the outer branch. The posterior nail hole should not be more than half to two thirds down the branch from the toe of the shoe. If the last nail is placed too far back in the branch of the shoe, it will either restrict the movement of the heel of the foot or, more commonly, work loose or be torn from the horn as the heel spreads.

Fitting the shoe
The outside margin of the shoe should coincide exactly with that of the hoof, unless the hoof wall is being shortened in order to correct the balance of an abnormally shaped foot. The portion of shoe behind the last nail hole should be set a little wide of the outer edge of the hoof wall as otherwise, with constant use from being hammered on the ground, the hoof wall will spread over the shoe which will become embedded in the horn near the heel.

Traditionally the shoe is fitted at a dull red heat and held briefly in contact with the horn of the foot. Where the horn and shoe are in contact the horn will be discoloured, so that it is possible to see which areas of foot have not been in contact with the shoe. The shoe can then be adjusted or the foot levelled as necessary. With 'hot shoeing' in this way the shoe can rapidly be altered if its shape does not conform exactly to the foot. Exact juxtaposition of iron and hoof is obtained, with consequent increased security of the shoe.

It has been suggested that burning the hoof wall also renders the bearing surface of the wall and sole impervious to water and the hoof less liable to split when the nails are driven. There is no scientific evidence to confirm or refute this at the present time.

The practice of 'burning on the shoe' is to be deprecated. This is when a shoe, which is not quite even, is held in contact with the horn for a longer period of time than normal in order that the unlevel areas of hot iron will burn themselves into the horn. This practice, which is an abuse of hot shoeing, can result in severe charring of the hoof wall with subsequent weakening. It allows the poor farrier to bed an inadequate shoe onto a foot, which could not be done with a cold shoe.

The practice of applying shoes cold is spreading, particularly with the increasing tendency for the farrier to visit the horse rather than the horse to visit the forge. The horse can be shod perfectly adequately in this manner, provided the shoe is made flat and the foot is dressed level so that the two surfaces meet. Minor alterations to the shoe, such as spreading or closing the heels to fit the curve on the foot, can be made cold. Although cold shoeing can be carried out perfectly satisfactorily, it is probably more difficult to shoe well cold than to shoe well hot. However, in shoeing a horse with poor or weak heels, hot shoeing may create a problem if the heels are inadvertently burned when the shoe is applied.

Nailing on the shoe

The nails should normally take a short hold on the wall of the foot, coming up not more than 1 inch from its ground surface. The ends of the nails are then twisted off approximately an eighth of an inch from the hoof wall and the end turned down to form the clench. After the nails have been driven the rasp should not normally touch the hoof wall, except to file a little horn away from under the end of the nails so that the clenches seat down tight and, if necessary, to shorten the toes slightly. The clenches should all be level at an equal distance from the ground surface of the foot. Nails should be positioned so they do not pass through areas of weak or broken horn and should avoid previous nail holes if possible.

The shoeing nail is made with a bevel on one side of the point only, so that as it is driven into the hoof wall it gradually turns outwards, taking a curved course through the horn prior to breaking out through the wall.

Hoof dressings

There is considerable controversy over the value of hoof oils and dressings. There is little or no evidence that oiling hooves is of value in the normal animal and it is probably far more important that the feet should be kept cleaned out (particularly the sole of the foot) and the horse not left to stand in damp conditions. Dressings applied to the surface of the hoof can have little effect on horn quality.

There is evidence that massage to the coronary band may improve the quality of horn. Horn quality also reflects the bodily condition of the horse and its nutritional state. An improved diet may therefore help hoof quality and there is some evidence that in some animals the amino acids methionene and biotin may be beneficial. When assessing dietary supplementation it is important to remember that the hoof wall is formed at the coronary band and so any improvement in the horn is seen first in that area, the new horn gradually growing downwards; improvement in hoof quality throughout the wall will not be seen until some nine to twelve months after supplementation of the diet.

The Reproductive System

Reproduction is based on the female and male genital organs and glands. These have special functions which determine sexual behaviour leading to mating and fertilisation of the egg. The foetus is housed in the genital tract of the mare, specifically in her uterus. Here it is nurtured for eleven months until expelled at the time of foaling. The newborn foal must adjust to the new environment and then start the two-year or so development before puberty is reached and the reproductive cycle starts again in the new generation.

The process of reproduction is described in the chapters of this section against the background of anatomical features on the one hand and the function of sexual organs on the other:

* Reproduction from the stallion's viewpoint is dealt with first, followed by a chapter on artificial insemination;

* Next are chapters covering reproduction from the mare's viewpoint;

* The section ends with chapters on foaling and the development of the newborn foal.

An understanding of the reproductive process is essential to good stud management and as a basis for the management and care of the stallion, barren mare, pregnant mare, and newborn foal. It should be possible for the reader to use these chapters for reference or for reading about the subject as a whole, starting with the male and passing to the female, through pregnancy, foaling and the development of the foal.

21
THE MALE GENITAL ORGANS AND THEIR ENDOCRINE GLANDS

Functional anatomy of the testis and adnexa

The reproductive organs of the male consist of the testes, situated within the scrotum, the epididymis, the spermatic cord, the accessory glands and the penis within its sheath. The functioning of these organs depends on both nervous and hormonal stimuli. The hormones control the way the organs develop and the substances or cells they produce and the nervous stimuli control the response of the stallion to the presence of a mare in oestrus.

Hormonal control

Stimuli from the outside affect that part of the brain known as the hypothalamus through nervous pathways leading from the sense organs. In particular, lengthening periods of daylight stimulate the hypothalamus to produce increasing amounts of a hormone called gonadotrophin releasing hormone (GnRH).

GnRH is carried in the bloodstream to the anterior pituitary causing this gland to release follicle-stimulating hormone (FSH) and lutemizing hormone (LH). These hormones are identical to those secreted in the female but in the male FSH stimulates the tubules in the testes to form sperm, whereas LH stimulates the Leydig cells (specialized interstitial cells which lie between the tubules which produce the sperm) to produce testosterone.

Testosterone is responsible for the development of the male genitalia in the foetus, the growth of the male genitalia at puberty, the final stages of sperm maturation, and the growth, maintenance and function of the accessory glands. It stimulates the central nervous system in producing libido (sexual drive) and male sexual responses, and is responsible for the secondary sexual characteristics such as muscular development and the crest of the neck.

Thus significant increases in semen volume, sperm density, total sperm per ejaculate (and a reduction in reaction time of the stallion to mating) occur during spring and summer compared with autumn and winter.

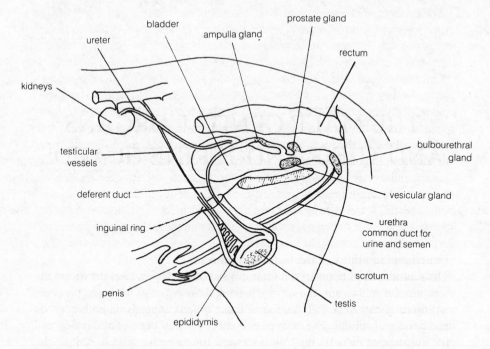

Figure 1   The male reproductive organs

TESTES

Normal descent and growth

In the foetal foal the testis develops near the kidney, but it moves into the scrotum during the last month of gestation. Newborn foals, therefore, usually have both testes in their scrotum. The testes are quite small at this stage and grow very little during the ensuing twelve months. The gubernacular structures, which help to move the testes out of the abdomen, are quite large at birth, shrinking afterwards as their function is completed. The contents of the scrotum can therefore actually become smaller during the first few weeks of life.

In rapidly maturing breeds the testes begin to grow significantly in the second summer and autumn while the animal is a yearling; most growth, however, occurs over the next winter. By the spring of the year in which the horse is a two-year-old, the testes are almost fully grown. This growth is controlled by hormones from the brain (see above), and these hormones are also responsible for sperm production; most testes weighing over 70g are capable of producing fertile sperm. In particular, the male hormone testosterone appears at this time.

The testes continue to grow after two years of age, but the rate of growth is much slower. By three years of age the horse is also producing large quantities of the female hormone oestrone sulphate, which can be used as the basis of a blood test for cryptorchidism (retained testicle – see p. 361*)*.

The mature testes hang horizontally in the scrotum at the front of the pelvis. Normally they measure 6-12 cm long, 4-7 cm high and 5 cm wide. The testis consists of very small tubules lined by cells which divide and change into spermatozoa – the sperm cells are nursed during their development by specialised cells called Sertoli cells. When the spermatozoa are formed, they are shed into the tubules and pass into the epididymis.

Each epididymis lies just above its testis, to which it is attached by a sheet of tissue. The epididymis (Figure 2*)* can be divided into three parts – head, body and tall – but it is in fact one very long, much-coiled tube, and the spermatozoa enter the epididymis at one end and pass along it, maturing as they go. The mature sperm are stored in the tail of the epididymis prior to ejaculation and this tail can be seen as a discrete swelling at the back of the testis. (Some horses have the tail of the epididymis at the front of the testis but this is unusual.)

At ejaculation (see p. 367) the sperm leave the epididymal tail and enter the deferent duct, which is part of the spermatic cord. This cord (which is actually a triangular sheet of tissue with its base at the testicle and its apex high up in the groin) contains not only the vas deferens but also the blood vessels and nerves which supply the testis and epididymis. The cord is severed when a horse is castrated (see p. 629).

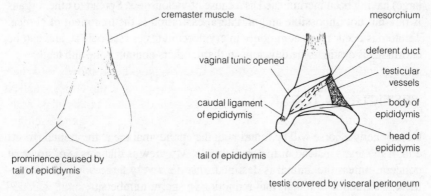

Figure 2 A detail of the testis

Each testis lies enveloped in a sac called the vaginal tunic, and attached to this tunic is a powerful muscle, the cremaster muscle. This is quite capable of pulling the vaginal tunic and its enclosed testis up into the groin and will do so in response to fear, sometimes to excitement and invariably to the touch of cold hands.

Conditions of the Testis

For castration and related conditions see p. 629. Disorders of the testis are relatively rare in horses but they include the following:

ORCHITIS

This disease is characterised in the acute phase by pain and swelling of one or both testes and can be caused by a kick, by migrating strongyle larvae or by infectious agents. The horse will be infertile. Treatment is aimed at keeping the testis cool with a spray of cold water, and includes systemic antibiotics and painkillers. As the condition resolves the pain abates and the testis often shrinks and degenerates, no longer producing sperm.

TESTICULAR TUMOURS

Various types of tumour can be found in the testis but differentiation depends ultimately on histological examination. The commonest and most striking are seminomas, which produce gross distortion of the testes and eventually degeneration, often preceded by a high proportion of abnormal sperm. Other types are Sertoli cell tumours and interstitial cell tumours, the latter (which are not always large) having been incriminated as a cause of viciousness. Spread to other organs is rare but not impossible and unilateral castration is the treatment of choice. Teratomas occur more commonly in cryptorchid testes (see below) and can be enormous if cystic tissue develops in them; others contain bone and teeth.

TESTICULAR TORSION

Occasionally a horse will be found with the epididymal tail at the cranial (front) end of the testis instead of the caudal pole. My view is that this is of no great concern, unless the animal is destined to serve a very large book of mares – there is evidence of a marginal reduction in sperm numbers.

More serious, however, is when a testis and its vaginal tunic twist through 360°, producing symptoms of acute colic and a markedly swollen, oedematous scrotum. As the testis gets cut off from its blood supply, it dies (undergoes necrosis) and the pain may ease, though the swelling remains for longer, resolving only to reveal a shrunken testis. In the early acute phase testicular torsion needs to be differentiated from strangulated inguinal hernia (see pp. 626), though both are serious and require surgical intervention.

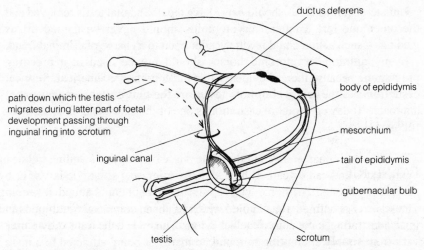

Figure 3 The descent of the testis. It has passed through the inguinal canal but is not fully in the scrotum

CRYPTORCHIDISM (RIG, RIDGELING)

Most testes reach the scrotum in the last months of gestation but some fail to pass out of the abdomen, resulting in abdominal cryptorchidism; or fail to descend from the abdominal opening to the scrotum, resulting in inguinal cryptorchidism. Cryptorchidism may be unilateral, the other testis reaching the scrotum normally and sometimes being much larger than expected, or (in about 10-20% of cases only) bilateral, both testes then usually being retained in the same place.

Any testis which does not reach the scrotum will not produce sperm and will be infertile; a unilateral cryptorchid, however, will be fertile from his scrotal testis. All testes, however, whatever their location, produce hormones in the usual way and any mature animal, even those with only one testis, will behave like a stallion.

A testis which is retained in the abdomen will never descend to the scrotum after the first few weeks of life – the opening through which it passes becomes too small.

Most of these testes are quite small and flabby, weighing about 20g. Others may be teratomas (i.e. tumorous, see above).

Some testes retained in the inguinal region are simply late developers which grow in size and descend into the scrotum during the transition from two-year-old to three-year-old. Removal of the contralateral testis will *not* make it descend. Some inguinally retained testes, however, never descend. These are often high up in the groin and are difficult to feel, even with the animal anaesthetised and on its back.

Unilateral cryptorchids should *never* have the one scrotal testis removed and the other one left. Bilateral cryptorchids should never be passed off as geldings – such action could lay the vendor open to a charge of criminal fraud.

In my opinion, cryptorchid horses should not be used in a breeding programme because there is evidence that the condition is inherited. Surgical castration and the removal of both testes are the only suitable management approach. Today cryptorchid castration is one of the safest and most successful operations.

FALSE RIG

The false rig is defined as an animal which has been completely castrated but is demonstrating some masculine behaviour. The male behaviour shown may vary from simply attempting to round up mares or being attracted to a mare on heat, to a full erection and intromission (see below) and, occasionally, ejaculation.

A male horse whose castration history is uncertain and which has no visible or palpable testes, but which is exhibiting stallion-like behaviour should first be subjected to a blood test. This will determine whether it is in fact a cryptorchid horse, with one or both testes retained (see above), or whether it is a false rig. If the animal is less than three years of age or is a donkey, it is necessary to take two blood samples, one before and a second sample thirty to 120 minutes after the intravenous injection of human chorionic gonadotrophin (hCG) (see p. 167). A reputable laboratory, used to analysing samples from horses, should be asked to measure testosterone in both samples. If the horse in question is aged three years or older, then a single sample will suffice, but the concentration of oestrone sulphate must be determined. Most laboratories have a range of values for this hormone which helps the vet to make a diagnosis of whether a particular individual is a false rig.

Masculine behaviour in castrated horses is not due to the animals having been improperly castrated – recent scientific investigation has totally discredited the idea of false rigs being 'cut proud'. Rather, most horses behave the way described because such behaviour patterns are part of normal social interaction between horses meeting and living together for the first time; the unpleasant and unwelcome aspects of that behaviour usually wane with time.

Geldings which are simply difficult to handle or ride and show no sexual behaviour usually behave so because of a failure of discipline. Sometimes the rider and horse may just be incompatible.

No treatment is likely to be effective for a false rig, but if a blood test has been performed and a diagnosis has been made, you will know exactly where you are and will have to decide whether the individual's behaviour is acceptable or not.

ACCESSORY SEX GLANDS

The spermatozoa which are ready to achieve fertilisation leave the tail of epididymis and pass along the vas deferens (deferent duct). This tube passes through the inguinal canal, the opening in the body wall through which the testes descend, and opens into the urethra at the neck of the bladder (see Figure 3). The watery products (secretions) of four sets of glands are added to the spermatozoa to make up the semen, which is eventually ejaculated into the mare.

These four glands (Figure 1) are:

1 The ampulla of the deferent duct (paired)
2 The vesicular gland, often wrongly called the seminal vesicles as it was believed they stored semen (paired)
3 The prostate gland (bilobed)
4 The bulbourethral gland (paired)

The first three lie around the neck of the bladder where it opens into the urethra. Complex mechanisms come into play to prevent urine becoming mixed into the semen. The bulbourethral glands lie farther back, just underneath the anus.

It is very uncommon for these glands to be affected by disease. Occasionally, however, the vesicular gland becomes infected (vesiculitis) and pus cells are added to semen, rendering the stallion infertile. Some horses with vesiculitis have their vesicular glands removed but fertility does not always return.

In castrated horses these glands become very small and insignificant.

PENIS

The horse's penis normally lives inside its sheath, out of sight. It is held in position by muscles within the body of the penis and is extruded initially by relaxation of those muscles, producing a flaccid penis. The horse can then fill the spaces between the muscles with blood and he may do this at two different pressures, a low one producing a turgid penis, and the second a very high pressure producing the erect penis necessary for entering the mare (intromission). On erection the penis doubles its length and thickness. After ejaculation the rose at the end of the penis enlarges to three times its resting size.

Besides the muscles and blood spaces, the penis also has passing along all its length the tube that carries urine at urination and semen at ejaculation. This tube is called the urethra and is housed on the lower aspect of the penis.

The penis begins just below the anus, but the only part which is seen is that which lies within the sheath, covered by a special fold of skin called the preputial fold. When the penis drops out of the sheath, the fold of skin unrolls over it. The very end of the penis has an opening for the urethra, which protrudes slightly beyond the end, forming the urethral process and surrounded by a cavity called the urethral sinus. Occasionally debris may accumulate in the cavity causing obstruction to the passage of urine, but its major significance today is that this fossa may harbour potential venereal-disease-producing bacteria, e.g. the contagious equine metritis organism or *Klebsiella* or *Pseudomonas* (see p. 481).

The sheath is quite voluminous and movement of the penis within it may cause a sucking noise when the horse is trotting. Deep inside the cavity of the sheath, debris from the glands and skin lining the cavity accumulates. This accumulation is called smegma. Occasionally so much smegma can accumulate, or it can turn so hard, that it causes the horse discomfort.

A number of bacteria normally live on the skin covering a horse's penis and it is not a good idea to wash them away with strong antiseptics or antibiotics because this may actually encourage the development of serious infections. In order to clean a horse's penis the penis should be caught at staling and washed gently with soap and water.

Conditions of the Penis

PROLAPSE

Most horses will drop at least part of their penis out to stale (urinate), but usually withdraw it quite readily. Occasionally, however, the penis hangs out of the sheath and the horse seems unable to retract it. Thus, prolapse can occur in an exhausted horse, but usually recovery takes places readily. Similarly, the horse prolapses his penis under the influence of many sedatives but the effect usually wears off.

Overdosage, however, or certain types of tranquillisers in stallions may result in prolonged relaxation, and persisting prolapse may occur in certain systemic diseases such as rabies and in some debilitating diseases like parasitism, malabsorption or enteritis. In such cases the paralysis can be reversed if the disease causing the prolapse is also reversible. Paralysis, accompanied by swelling, is also seen as a sequel to a painful kick or to a sadistically inflicted whip wound.

A prolapsed penis is in greater danger from kicks and bruising, either of which may produce such swelling as will make it impossible for the horse to pull his penis back in. In addition the free end of the penis is susceptible to drying and cracking, and if this is prolonged it will lead to further swelling and a worsening of the prolapse.

In the early stages cold-water hosing may help to reduce the swelling, but the most important things about treating a prolapsed penis are support and the prevention of drying and cracking. The former may be done in a variety of ways – that most commonly used today is a previously-unused pair of pantihose, held in place by appropriately placed bandages attached to a surcingle and crupper. Every day, the penis must be washed and dried and then smeared with a bland ointment such as petroleum jelly to prevent it drying out and cracking and becoming scalded with urine.

Your veterinarian should be involved in giving advice on this, as well as in providing supportive therapy *and* a diagnosis of the cause.

TUMOURS

Two sorts of tumour may be associated with the horse's penis.

Skin tumours generally occur only on the outside of the sheath and the outer layer of the preputial fold. These tumours can be any of the various types of skin tumours, including sarcoids (see Chapters 7 and 42).

Cancerous growths usually occur on the free end of the penis of aged horses. They look like angry cauliflowers. Although cancerous, these tumours usually grow slowly and do not spread throughout the body. They can be dealt with by amputation of the free end.

EQUINE COITAL EXANTHEMA (HORSE POX)

This is a contagious disease transmitted naturally at coitus and characterised by vesicular or pustular lesions of the external genitalia. It is caused by an equid herpesvirus (see p. 488), but not the same type as is responsible for rhinopneumonitis or abortion. Mechanical transfer may occur, for example, by nuzzling, by direct contact with mares or teasers, or by handling the part.

The incubation period varies from three to six days, but in many instances it may be from twelve to twenty-four hours. The disease is most commonly observed during the spring months, this being the time at which mares are sent to the stallion. It is widespread throughout the world, but is often not noticed unless there is routine veterinary inspection of the stallion prior to mating.

In the mare the eruption occurs on the inner surface of the lips (labia) of the vulva, on the vaginal mucosa (especially in the vicinity of the clitoris), and to a lesser extent on the external surface of the vulva and undersurface of the tail. Dark red spots the size of a pin head first appear; these become papules which develop into vesicles (sacs containing fluid) or pustules (collection of pus within or beneath the epidermis).

The vesicles are transparent in the early stages, then change to various tints of yellow, then darken to a brown colour; in some cases the contents are of a red colour, due to the presence of blood. The pustules develop into flat ulcers with a deep red base and discharge a yellowish glutinous fluid.

Frequently two or more ulcers become confluent and are covered by a brown scab. When healing takes place, smooth white scars or depigmented areas remain. As a rule, fever and constitutional disturbances are absent, but discomfort may be displayed by apparent sexual excitement, frequent attempts at staling and rubbing of the tail.

In the stallion the penis is rarely affected, but vesicles and pustules develop, which later form ulcers. When healing occurs, depigmented scars are left. Occasionally the outer surface of the sheath and scrotum may be affected, also the inside of the thighs and undersurface of the abdomen, extending to the inside of the fore-limbs, probably due to contact with infected secretions. A urethral discharge may be present in some cases and frequent attempts at staling may be observed. The affected stallion may be unwilling to mate mares because of the discomfort.

The eruptions in both sexes generally heal spontaneously in from three to four weeks, and sometimes in fifteen days if mating is prevented.

Severe secondary infection with bacteria can occur occasionally and the animal may then be systemically ill, discharges may be gross, and swelling due to oedema extensive. Fertility, however, is not usually affected, although the stallion may be unwilling to serve due to discomfort. It has been suggested that the virus can cause short cycles (i.e. oestrus cycles that are less than the usual twenty-one day cycle) in mares.

Preventive measures
These consist of strict isolation of the affected animals; they should not be used for breeding until perfectly cured. It is important not to overlook such simple measures as wearing disposable gloves when handling infected animals. A careful examination should be made of all mares before mating. It is probably best not to attempt to treat infected animals, as handling can spread the disease; isolation is more important. If secondary infection with bacteria has occurred, then spraying the affected parts with an antibiotic or weak antiseptic, perhaps incorporating a bland oil, can be beneficial in accelerating healing. Animals may be bred again when the lesions are no longer infective; that usually means when a scab has formed.

DOURINE

This venereal infection of the horse's penis is discussed on p. 506. It does not occur in the UK, Australia, South Africa or Argentina.

SEMEN

At ejaculation spermatozoa leave the epididymal tail and pass along the deferent duct, entering the pelvic urethra near the neck of the bladder. The secretions of the accessory glands are added to the spermatozoa, so producing the semen. This passes along the pelvic urethra by muscle action and then along the penile part of the urethra by a hydraulic system involving muscle pumping and bloodflow.

The stallion is believed to engage his urethral process in the cervix of the mare on heat and so deposit the semen within the uterus. The semen is deposited in four to seven spurts and this process is often accompanied by flagging of the tail by the stallion.

Examination of semen
The penis can be diverted into an artificial vagina into which the stallion can then be persuaded to ejaculate and so allow the semen to be collected and examined.

Semen has a white, opaque appearance and usually consists of three fractions. The first fraction is watery and contains little or no sperm; the second is also thin and watery and contains the sperm; the third is viscous, contains gel and comes mainly from the vesicular gland.

Semen is usually examined as soon as possible after ejaculation for volume (often divided into gel volume and gel-free volume), for sperm numbers and for motility and for the proportion of dead or abnormal cells.

Stallions vary enormously in all these characteristics and different collections from the same stallion also vary considerably. Therefore stallions with poor fertility may need to have several semen collections made before a positive diagnosis can be reached, though some with specific sperm abnormalities can be identified on a single examination.

There is general agreement now that for a stallion to approach normal fertility he should have the following minimum values:

total volume	35 ml
gel-free volume	25 ml
sperm concentration	20 x 10,000,000ml
total number of sperm	1.5 x 10,000,000,000,000
total number of live sperm	1 x 10,000,000,000,000

However, fertility also depends on the number of mares to be mated and the frequency with which they are mated. Examination of semen, therefore, *is not* a fertility examination.

Problems arise with young horses in their first season and this may be because they have been discouraged in training from displaying interest in mares; or it may be due to overuse early in the year before the advent of spring and summer when sperm output is at its highest.

22
ARTIFICIAL INSEMINATION

Introduction

Artificial Insemination (AI) involves collecting semen from a stallion and transferring it artificially into the mare's uterus with the intention of obtaining a pregnancy. Today, the technique is approved for use by most horse and pony breed authorities with the notable exception of the General Stud Book, regulator of the Thoroughbred breed. Internationally, artificial insemination gained widespread use during the final two decades of the twentieth century. Either fresh, chilled or frozen semen can be used.

Artificial insemination in the equine species has a long history. Arabian texts from the thirteenth century describe how mares were successfully inseminated with fresh transported semen. In the late eighteenth century an Italian biologist, L. Spallanzani, performed successful inseminations in the canine species and concluded that spermatozoa carry 'fertilizing power'. In 1803 he published the observation that '... freezing stallion semen in snow or winter cold did not necessarily kill the *spermatic vermiculi* , but kept them in a motionless state until exposed to heat, after which they continued to move for seven and a half hours.'

The use of artificial insemination in European horse breeding dates back to the beginning of the twentieth century. The first AI programmes were introduced on Imperial Russian Stud Farms by the pioneer of the method, E.I. Ivanoff. In Western Europe the technique was used on a large scale in the breeding region of Hanover, Germany, immediately after the Second World War. The objective was to combat the spread of the venereal disease Dourine (caused by *Trypanosomas equiperdum*). By 1955 with the advancing mechanization of agriculture and a significant reduction in mares being bred the Hanoverian AI station closed. The first use of frozen semen in horses was reported in 1957.

The use of AI regained popularity in Europe in the 1970s. Its use has become the standard reproductive method in several of the largest breeding regions of Germany, France, and The Netherlands etc. It is reported that very large numbers of mares are inseminated annually in China with fresh and chilled semen.

The regulation of artificial insemination varies from country to country and from one breed registry to another. Semen collection, processing and insemination are generally performed either by veterinary surgeons or trained technicians. In the United Kingdom the British Equine Veterinary Association has established a Code of Practice, manages a list of veterinary practices approved for the use of frozen or chilled semen and runs courses for veterinary surgeons and technicians working with artificial insemination techniques.

The success rate of artificial insemination using a healthy fertile stallion depends on the gynaecological health of the mare, quality of mare management and type of semen being used. In well managed fresh and chilled semen programmes the fertility rates do not differ greatly from natural covering using comparable mare management techniques. Frozen semen schemes require very intensive veterinary mare management and are likely to result in lower pregnancy per oestrus cycle rates than the other forms.

Types of Artificial Insemination
The choice of the type to be used depends on the availability of semen and the location and fertility of the mare. Stallion semen can be used in three different forms:

Fresh or raw
Raw semen is used within six hours of collection. The gel fraction of the ejaculate is removed prior to insemination. Semen extender can be added to the sperm rich fraction.

Chilled or cooled
This is suitable for use in most breeding situations and mares. Semen longevity varies from stallion to stallion. There is also variability from one ejaculate to another. Most semen is viable for up to 48 hours. Semen extender is always used.

Frozen
It has been found that only 50-60% of stallions produce semen that is suitable for freezing. The thawing procedure and the sperm cells resistance to changes in temperature are critical. Once successfully thawed the semen doses have a short lifespan necessitating immediate insemination. Mares have to be inseminated within a few hours of ovulation. The per cycle conception rate is lower than with the other types of preserved semen and natural cover. Therefore, only optimally fertile mares should be subjected to frozen semen insemination. Good breeding prospects are young maiden mares or those that have foaled without complications during the current breeding season. Older barren or maiden mares over 14 years of age require careful assessment before being bred with frozen semen.

Factors affecting a successful AI programme

Good communications between the mare, stallion owners and the inseminator are essential. The semen delivery must be coordinated with the anticipated time of ovulation. Therefore, the logistics of semen delivery must be arranged prior to the mare being in oestrus. The instructions from the stallion owner to the inseminator concerning the handling of the semen dose must be clear. For frozen semen the exact thawing instructions must be obtained. The mare owner should have access to facilities at which the mare can be examined and inseminated safely. Storage facilities for frozen semen must be available, i.e. a storage container filled with liquid nitrogen. The semen characteristics and information concerning fertility rates should be considered when a breeder selects a stallion.

Working with semen for AI

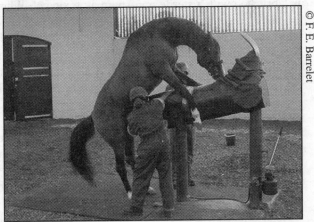

© F. E. Barrelet

Figure 1   Semen collecting using a phantom mare

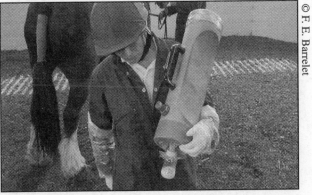

© F. E. Barrelet

Figure 2   Semen sample collected using Cambridge Model Artificial Vagina

The procedure consists of four steps:

Semen collection

Semen is collected using an artificial vagina (AV) while the stallion mounts either an in oestrus mare or a phantom (dummy). Occasionally, a stallion condom is used for semen collection. Different types of artificial vaginas are commercially available. Their use depends on the collector's preferences and the individual stallion's requirements. The most popular models are: Missouri AV, Hanover model, Colorado model, Nishikawa (Japanese) AV and the Cambridge Model.

In principle, they consist of a hard or firm outer shell surrounding a soft inner mantel. This is filled with warm water (38°-50° C). The pressure inside the AV is adjusted to suit the stallion. A disposable inner liner is inserted through the AV. This empties into a semen collection receptacle. Prior to use, the liner is lubricated with a sterile non-spermatotoxic gel. When the stallion mounts the mare his erect penis is deviated into the AV for collection of the ejaculate. Most stallions can be trained to ejaculate into an AV. Naturally shy coverers require the most patience. For continuous safe semen collection it is essential that the stallion and mare handlers as well as the collector are experienced with the procedure. All those involved with semen collection should wear protective headgear.

Semen processing

Initially, the gel is separated from the sperm rich fraction of the ejaculate. The gel originates from the accessory sex glands and is detrimental for sperm longevity. The gel free volume is measured. A sample is used to determine the sperm cell concentration and estimate their progressive motility with a microscope. Based on these results, the number of semen doses that can be obtained from the ejaculate is calculated. Semen extender is then immediately added to the sperm rich fraction. The extended semen can be subjected to centrifugation prior to resuspension to a predetermined concentration. The resuspended semen can be used for immediate insemination, cooled to 4°C or frozen in liquid nitrogen.

Semen extenders are used to provide a protective environment for the fragile sperm cells. They consist of nutrients, cryoprotective agents and contain low concentrations of antibiotics to suppress bacterial contamination in the ejaculate. The nutrients are sugars that are an energy source for the sperm cells. In the case of frozen semen the cryoprotective substances are of particular importance to protect the sperm cell from the effects of freezing and thawing. The extenders are made either from milk constituents or egg yolk.

The Kenney extender is the most popular milk based diluent:

Nonfat dried milk	2.4g
Glucose	4.9g
[Antibiotics]	
Distilled water to	100ml

The addition of antibiotics is recommended if the semen is not for immediate use. The choice of antibiotics should be discussed with a veterinary surgeon. The Kenney extender is suitable for immediate use or for chilling semen.

It is reported that a minimum of 150 million progressively motile and morphologically normal sperm cells are required to achieve fertilization. However, a semen dose intended for commercial use should contain at least 250 - 300 million progressively motile and morphologically normal sperm cells at the time of insemination. There are no internationally recognized standards for commercially used semen.

Semen storage

Semen should be protected from light, oxygen and temperature fluctuations.

Fresh extended semen can be kept for up to six hours at constant room temperature (20°C).

Semen chilled to 4°C is generally viable for 24-48 hours. In extreme cases a minimum of 12 and a maximum of 96 hours have been reported. By trying different types of extender, the maximal storage time can be determined for each stallion. Also, on a day-to-day basis the semen quality can vary considerably. Chilled semen can either be stored in a refrigerator or purpose made shipping containers. The ideal cooling rate appears to be –0.3° C. The Equitainer[R] (Hamilton-Thorne) is designed to cool semen at this defined rate and maintain the temperature for 72 hours whilst in transport.

Frozen semen is packaged in 0.25 or 0.5ml straws (Paillettes) or 4ml straws (MacrotubR). These are stored in special containers filled with liquid Nitrogen at -196°C.

Semen Transport

Raw extended semen is not usually shipped off the stallion farm. Chilled and frozen semen can be shipped by road, sea or air in a suitable container. The international shipping of semen requires import and export certification. Import and export certificates are issued by the pertinent government agencies in each country. They are issued subject to the stallion and semen fulfilling stringent health requirements. These requirements vary according to the demands made by the importing country. In the United Kingdom DEFRA is responsible for issuing these documents.

Insemination

Only healthy mares should be inseminated. A teaser stallion or gelding should be used to determine whether a mare is showing signs of oestrus behaviour. By measuring serum progesterone levels associated with a gynaecological examination the stage of the mare's sexual cycle can also be established. When the mare is in oestrus a gynaecological examination is recommended to ascertain whether she is suitable to be bred. A swab and smear should be obtained from the cervix or uterus. The cytological and bacteriological analyses will determine the presence of endometrial inflammation and infection. Mares suffering from endometritis should not be bred until the condition has been successfully treated.

The manual rectal and ultrasonographic examinations of the mare's uterus and ovaries will help determine the optimal time for insemination. Insemination should be as close to ovulation as possible. Ovulation occurs at the end of the oestrus cycle. The use of human Chorionic Gonadotropin (hCG) helps to steer ovulation and synchronize it with the time of insemination. This hormone is effective 24-48 hours after injection.

A successful protocol used in managing mares that are to be inseminated with chilled semen is:

1 Examine the mare every other day during oestrus until her cervix is relaxed and a follicle with a diameter of 30mm is detected.
2 Administer hCG.
3 Arrange for semen delivery the following day.
4 Re-examine one day after insemination to determine whether ovulation has occurred. If not, a further delivery is arranged for the following day.

A similar protocol is recommended when frozen semen is used. However, on the day following the hCG application the mare should be examined every six to eight hours until she has ovulated. Ovulation is diagnosed using an ultrasound scanner. Upon ovulation the mare is immediately inseminated. A follow up examination should be performed one day later to ensure that she has not accumulated any inflammatory fluid in her uterus. This reaction may require treatment to assist the establishment of a pregnancy. The correct thawing procedure for frozen semen is critical. The instructions for thawing must be obtained from the semen provider prior to attempting insemination.

Following insemination a residual sample of semen should be examined microscopically for quality control purposes. This is done by placing a drop of semen on a pre-heated microscope slide and allowing five minutes at 37° C for equilibration prior to examination. The vitality of the semen is judged by estimating the progressive motility of the sperm cells. At least 30% of the sperm cells should be progressively motile. However, progressive motility is only a rough indicator for fertility. There are no simple laboratory tests available to predict the fertilizing power of an individual ejaculate.

An ultrasonographic pregnancy examination is recommended from 14 days after ovulation onwards to diagnose pregnancy and exclude the presence of twins.

23
THE FEMALE GENITAL ORGANS AND THEIR ENDOCRINE GLANDS

The female genital tract consists of the ovaries, the Fallopian tubes, the uterus, the cervix and the vagina. It extends from the vulva to the ovaries, receives the male organ, forms a pathway up which the sperm cells travel to meet the ovum, houses the developing embryo and provides a passage for birth of the foal.

FUNCTIONAL ANATOMY

Ovaries

The two ovaries contain the female ova (or eggs). Many thousands of eggs are present in the two ovaries at birth and no more develop during the animal's lifetime. After puberty ova are extruded from the ovaries at intervals determined by reproductive hormones.

The ovaries are typically bean-shaped and vary in size, depending on age and season of the year. Individual variations also occur. The ovaries of maiden mares in winter are usually about 2-4cm long and 2-3cm wide. The ovaries increase in spring to 5-8cm x 2-4cm in size. In winter they may feel hard, and in spring or during sexual activity they usually feel soft.

The size of older mares' ovaries varies considerably, irrespective of the season of the year. During sexual quiescence (anoestrus) their size is minimal, i.e. 3-6cm long. During seasons of sexual activity they grow, but do not normally become larger than about 10 x 5cm. In many cases the ovaries lose their typical bean shape and become rounded or irregular in contour and one ovary may be much larger than the other. Typically the ovary has a convex border (hilus) to which the broad ligament containing blood vessels and nerves is attached. The opposite or free border has a narrow depression (the ovulation fossa) through which the ova are shed.

The ovarian tissue is composed of spindle-shaped cells and connective substance. Bundles of cells and fibres run in various directions giving a swirly appearance. There is a tough fibrous capsule which encloses the ovary except at the ovulation fossa.

The ovaries are situated high in the abdomen beneath the fourth or fifth lumbar vertebrae. The average distance from the ovaries to the vulva is 50-55cm in a mare of medium size. A veterinary surgeon can easily pick up the ovaries on rectal examination and identify by palpation the rounded extremities.

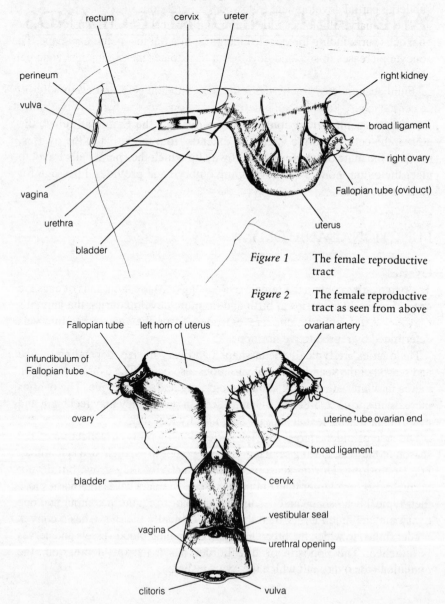

Figure 1   The female reproductive tract

Figure 2   The female reproductive tract as seen from above

Follicles

There are several hundred thousand ova in the two ovaries at birth. In the immature ovary the germ cell is surrounded by a layer of follicular epithelial cells. At puberty some of the oogonia develop into larger cells (primary oocytes) which undergo the first stage of meiosis (division). They do not complete meiosis until after puberty when the follicle is mature.

Of the many primary follicles present in the two ovaries at birth only a fraction reach maturity and liberate ova. Most of the follicles degenerate or undergo partial development followed by regression.

The primary follicle is about 45mm in diameter. As it develops the epithelial cells surrounding the oocyte change from a flat to a columnar shape. The oocyte increases in size and develops a thick outer membrane, the zona pellucida.

Fluid accumulates among the follicular epithelial cells and eventually fills a central cavity lined by follicular cells. The oocyte is attached to one side of the cavity on a mound of follicular cells known as the cumulus oophorus.

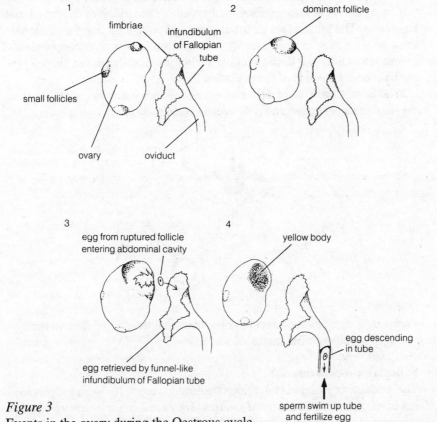

Figure 3
Events in the ovary during the Oestrous cycle

Yellow body

Follicular development continues until the follicle reaches about 3-5cm in diameter. It then bursts at the ovulation fossa and discharges its contents towards the open end of the Fallopian tube. After the ovum and part of the follicular wall have been extruded, the follicle collapses and the lining and remaining epithelial cells are thrown into folds. Bleeding occurs into the centre of the follicle and a clot forms.

The follicular or granulosa cells grow into the clot and, together with thecal cells, constitute the yellow body (YB) or corpus luteum. The yellow body produces progesterone. It has a variable life span and at the end of its life becomes non-functional and ceases to produce this hormone. The diagnosis of the presence of the functional yellow body can be made by measuring progesterone in the mare's bloodstream (see p. 162). Blood vessels and fibroblasts (connective-tissue cells) enter the yellow body, which changes from a soft consistency and a reddish-purple colour to a firm consistency and reddish-brown. As the yellow body becomes non-functional it turns yellow and eventually brown or white as the active cells are replaced by scar tissue.

If an ovary is cut into sections some or all of the structures described may be present. The follicles are distributed throughout the stroma; they may have thick non-vascular or thin vascular walls. Yellow bodies of varying ages and colour may be found. Recent yellow bodies are usually wedge-shaped with the base on the far side of the ovulation fossa.

In addition to its role of ovum producer, the ovary acts as a gland forming the hormones oestrogen and progesterone (see p. 383).

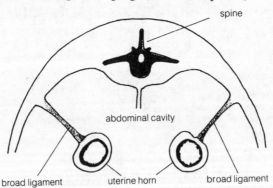

Figure 4   Location of the broad ligament and the uterine horn in the abdominal cavity

Fallopian tubes (oviducts)

The oviducts or Fallopian tubes are two tortuous tubes 20-30cm long, extending from the uterine horns to the ovaries. They are 2-3mm in diameter at their uterine end and 4-8mm in diameter at their ovarian end. Each tube is enclosed in a peritoneal fold (mesosalpinx); the ovarian extremity is funnel-shaped and its edge irregular with projections (fimbriae) attached to the ovulation fossa. The tube communicates with the peritoneal cavity via a small opening through which the ovum can pass at ovulation.

Cysts and embryological remnants are sometimes present in the fimbriae and mesoalpinx.

Uterus and cervix
The uterus is a hollow muscular organ continuous with the Fallopian tubes anteriorly and opening posteriorly through the cervix into the vagina. It is attached to the sublumbar region by two folds of peritoneum (the broad ligament) and consists of two horns, a body and neck (cervix). The horns are about 25cm long, and the body 18-20cm in length and 10cm in diameter.

The wall of the uterus consists of three coats: an outer serous layer continuous with the broad ligaments; a muscular layer (myometrium) containing an external layer of longitudinal fibres and an internal layer of circular fibres; and a mucous membrane (endometrium) comprising luminal epithelium (lining cells), stroma of connective tissue, glands and their ducts.

The uterus is supplied by the uterine artery and the uterine branch of the utero-ovarian artery, and its nerves are derived from the uterine and pelvic sympathetic plexuses.

The cervix is the constricted posterior part of the uterus. It is about 7cm long and 4cm in diameter in the sexually inactive phase and projects into the anterior vagina.

Vagina
The vagina extends horizontally through the pelvic cavity from the cervix to the vulva. It is about 20cm long and up to 12cm in diameter but its walls are normally in apposition. Most of the vagina is surrounded by loose connective tissue, veins and fat. Its wall is composed of muscular and mucous coats. The mucous coat is very elastic and covered with stratified epithelium.

The vagina is divided into anterior and posterior parts by a transverse fold (hymen) which is usually patent (open). The arterial supply comes from the pubic arteries and the nerves are derived from the sympathetic pelvic plexus.

The vulva is covered by mucous membrane. It is continuous in front with the vagina and opens externally about 7cm below the anus. It consists of two lips connected by a dorsal (upper) and ventral (lower) commissure. Immediately inside the ventral commissure is the clitoris. The vulval lips are covered by thin pigmented skin which is supplied with sebaceous and sweat glands. Beneath the skin are muscles that fuse above with the anal sphincter.

Perineum

The perineum (Greek *perineas* = space between anus and scrotum) is a loosely defined region in the mare, including the anus, vulva and adjacent skin. Its conformation is of clinical importance because of the part it plays in protecting the genital tract from the entrance of air (pneumovagina – see p. 625) and bacteria through the vulva. It is also subject to lacerations, wounds and bruising during birth or from kicks by other horses.

The entrance to the anterior vagina is protected by the arrangement of the vulva, posterior vagina and hymen, which form a valve preventing air from entering the vagina. The valve may be defective because of poor conformation or breached by introduction a speculum into the anterior vagina.

The optimal conformation is one in which the vulval labiae are vertical and 80% below the pelvic floor. If the pelvic floor is low relative to the labiae, there is a tendency for the anus to retract anteriorly and the upper part of the vulva to fall into the horizontal plane.

24
THE OESTROUS CYCLE

The oestrous cycle is a pattern of physiological and behavioural events under hormonal control, forming the basis of sexual activity and conception. The cycle has two components: oestrus (heat), in which the mare is receptive to the stallion and the ovum is shed, and dioestrus, which is a period of sexual inactivity.

The cycle typically lasts twenty-one days (five days of oestrus and sixteen of dioestrus) and may recur throughout the year, although in the horse sexual activity is characteristically confined to a restricted breeding season (spring and summer) and outside this period the cycles cease (anoestrus).

There is considerable individual variation in cycle length and character. Oestrous periods are longer and less intense in behavioural terms at the start and end of the season than in the middle. The cycle starts at puberty (about one and a half years) and continues throughout the mare's lifetime.

It is convenient to discuss the cycle under the separate headings of its physiological and behavioural components.

Pituitary gland
The pituitary gland lies immediately below the base of the brain, to which it is attached. From a functional viewpoint the pituitary is divided into the posterior lobe, which is innervated by nerve tracts originating in the hypothalamus, and the anterior lobe, which has no direct nerve supply.

The posterior lobe secretes the hormones oxytocin and vasopressin, and the anterior lobe secretes the gonad-stimulating (gonadotrophic) hormones, follicle-stimulating hormone (FSH), luteinizing hormone (LH) and prolactin. The character and actions of these hormones are discussed below.

The anterior pituitary also secretes adrenocorticotrophic hormones (ACTH) and thyroid-stimulating hormone (TSH), which influence the reproductive system indirectly but are not usually considered true reproductive hormones.

The hormones vasopressin and oxytocin are made in the hypothalamus and stored in the posterior pituitary lobe until released by the appropriate stimuli. For example, oxytocin is released by reflexes initiated during parturition by the stretching of the vaginal wall and, later when the foal approaches the mammary region.

The anterior pituitary is connected to the hypothalamus by a system of blood vessels which conveys releasing and inhibiting factors from the hypothalamic cells.There are about ten of these factors. The FSH and LH releasing factors and prolactin-inhibiting factor are of particular interest because of their effects on the oestrous cycle and mammary secretions respectively. Although work on the practical application of these substances is in its infancy, future development could have far-reaching significance in equine medicine and the management of the reproductive process.

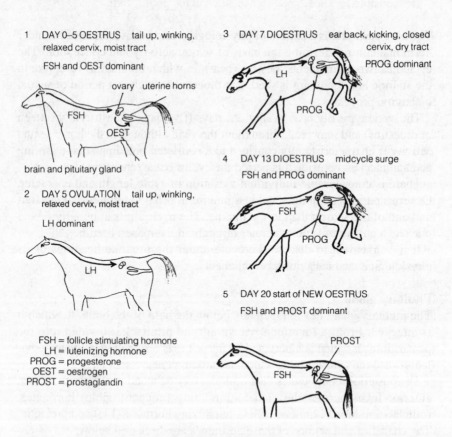

1   DAY 0–5 OESTRUS   tail up, winking, relaxed cervix, moist tract

    FSH and OEST dominant

    ovary   uterine horns
    FSH
    OEST
    brain and pituitary gland

2   DAY 5 OVULATION   tail up, winking, relaxed cervix, moist tract

    LH dominant

    LH

    FSH = follicle stimulating hormone
    LH = luteinizing hormone
    PROG = progesterone
    OEST = oestrogen
    PROST = prostaglandin

3   DAY 7 DIOESTRUS   ear back, kicking, closed cervix, dry tract

    PROG dominant

    LH
    PROG

4   DAY 13 DIOESTRUS   midcycle surge

    FSH and PROG dominant

    FSH
    PROG

5   DAY 20 start of NEW OESTRUS

    FSH and PROST dominant

    PROST
    FSH

Figure 1   Hormone changes in the oestrous cycle

Physiology

The classic view of the endocrinology of the oestrus cycle is as follows:

1   Follicle-stimulating hormone (FSH) stimulates the development of ovarian follicles which secrete oestrogen. These hormones are responsible for oestrous signs and changes in the genital tract.

2   Rising blood levels of oestrogen stimulate the anterior pituitary to produce luteinzing hormone (LH) and reduce the secretion of FSH. Ovulation occurs and a yellow body forms which produces progesterone.

3   Falling oestrogen and rising progesterone levels in the blood are responsible for dioestrous signs and changes in the genital tract.

4   The secretion of a hormone (now identified as prostaglandin) from the uterus ends dioestrus by arresting the functional life of the yellow body and causing blood progesterone levels to fall to zero.

5   Falling progesterone levels stimulate the anterior pituitary to secrete FSH and restart the cycle.

This account is a simplified one for ease of understanding and, as with all simplifications, it represents but part of the truth. There are many facets to the interaction of hormones on their target organs (see Chapter 8) and it is usually the net effect or balance which determines the outcome in any given instance. For example, oestrus represents a dominance, rather than an absolute status, of FSH and oestrogen relative to LH and progesterone. The activation of endocrine glands may also be based on their sensitivity to changing levels of hormones and the rapidity with which these occur. Many hormones leave their endocrine gland in an inert form and become potentiated by the target cells. In the mare, oestrus cycles are promoted by outside factors such as daylight and nutrition.

Controlling the oestrous cycle

Before discussing how we may control the oestrous cycle of mares we must be clear as to the states which require treatment.

Oestrus is the period of heat in which ovulation occurs. This normally takes place twenty-four hours before the mare goes out of heat, that is, enters dioestrus. Typically oestrus lasts five days. However, it may last for much longer, especially in spring. In February, March and maybe the beginning of April, heats may last for one, two or even four weeks. In some of these prolonged oestrous periods ovulation may occur at the end in the normal fashion. However, in other instances no ovulation occurs at all.

Prolonged dioestrus is a condition in which the normal dioestrus period of fourteen to sixteen days is prolonged by the abnormally continuing function of the yellow body (producing progesterone). This may last several weeks or even months in some cases.

Anoestrus is the condition of inactivity of the ovaries and sexual organs during winter.

Controlling the oestrous cycle therefore implies that treatment is used to bring mares from anoestrus into full fertile oestrous cycles combining five days oestrus and fifteen days dioestrus. Let us now consider how this may be done in our present state of knowledge.

Our aims at controlling the oestrous cycle are, essentially, to manipulate events so that one ovum is shed at a particular time, convenient to the interests of owner and manager in arranging a mating for the mare on a given day in a given month during an arbitrarily selected breeding season. Various therapies involving the administration of follicle-stimulating hormone (FSH), luteinizing hormone (LH), pregnant mare's serum gonadotrophin (PMSG), prostaglandin, gonadotrophin releasing hormone (GnRH), progesterone and/or oestrogen have all been tried with varying degrees of success at different points of the oestrous cycle. The most successful of these appears to be prostaglandin for inducing oestrus and luteinizing hormone for inducing ovulation. The effect of artificial light in promoting oestrous cycles during the early part of the breeding season is well know, as is the efficacy of intra-uterine irrigation of mares in dioestrus.

However, many therapies fail for reasons which are unclear or because they are based on insufficient knowledge of the physiological state of the individual at the time of application, or, indeed, because they are fundamentally incapable of action for reasons at present unclear. An example of the last category is the failure of PMSG (see p. 167) to stimulate follicular development or to cause ovulation, a fact which is peculiar considering that it is composed of FSH and LH. The refractory state of the mare's ovaries to administration of this hormone remains a mystery.

Advancing the onset of the cycle

The onset of the breeding season can be advanced artificially by exposing mares to artificial light. Temperature, nutrition and other environmental factors appear to play a secondary part, and prolonged periods of oestrus without ovulation occur commonly in mares during transition from deep anoestrus to complete sexual function.

There are a number of differing regimens. In all, exposure to artificial light is meant to 'trick' the mare into thinking that spring is approaching by artificially lengthening the daylight hours. The programme must begin at least one month prior to the required breeding time. One researcher found that 200 and 400-watt lamps caused mares to come into oestrus sixty-five to eighty days earlier than anticipated. Another used 15-watt bulbs three and four months prior to the beginning of the breeding season and 200-400 watt bulbs one and two months before the season, gradually increasing the length of artificial daylight until the mares were in light for sixteen out of twenty-four hours. There was a time lag of forty to a hundred days before the onset of oestrous behaviour in light-exposed anoestrous mares.

A practical disadvantage to light stimulation is the need to continue the programme until spring conditions occur. It is useful, therefore, only for mares that are resident on one stud during the whole period in which they are being treated. Should the mare be moved from one stud to another, the programme on the second stud should be phased to meet the protocol under which the mare has started her treatment.

If a mare is in anoestrus or prolonged spring oestrus, progesterone may be given for about ten consecutive days. This may be injected, but nowadays potent pregesterone-like substances are available (e.g. allyl trenolone) and may be given by mouth for about ten days. Progesterone therapy used in this manner causes accumulations of FSH and LH in the pituitary gland. When the treatment is stopped there is a rebound effect and the hormones are released from the pituitary in more substantial quantities than would otherwise have been the case. This causes the mare to come into heat and for a follicle to mature. This occurs at about seven to ten days following ceasing the treatment.

The incidence of ovulation

The oestrous cycle of the mare represents a coordinated sequence of events in which ovulation occurs towards the end of a limited period of behavioural receptivity. In this way the ovum and spermatozoa are able to meet under optimal conditions for fertilization to take place. From a practical point of view this shedding of the egg from the mare's ovary provides an opportunity for conception. Once the egg has been shed and remains unfertilised, a further opportunity for conception does not appear until the next oestrus, some twenty days later. Under ideal conditions, in which dioestrus lasts for two weeks and oestrus for one week, there are four opportunities during three calendar months. Within the Thoroughbred breeding season there is a maximum of six opportunities.

There are unfortunately a number of reasons why this number is reduced in many cases. The breeding season is arbitrarily arranged so that two thirds of it occur during the winter or early spring, when the oestrus cycle in many individuals is naturally absent or contains prolonged oestrus often without ovulation. Then there are mares which undergo prolonged periods of dioestrus which, if mating has taken place, resemble pregnancy, and by prolonging the cycle they cause a corresponding decrease in the number of ovulations that can occur during the breeding season. There are also foaling mares that cannot start their post-foaling oestrous cycle for some weeks or even months after the start of the breeding season.

We have to accept, therefore, that under average conditions of stud management there may be only three or four ovulations, i.e. eggs or opportunities for conception, per individual mare per breeding season. In most circumstances this is a more than sufficient number for the purpose of obtaining annual conception in a herd of broodmares. Indeed, the 60-70% conception rates obtained on average bear witness to this claim. However, when we, as veterinarians, are considering our contribution to the problem, we must, of necessity, concentrate on the substantial incidence of non-conceptions, i.e. barrenness and foetal loss. In this context, the more ovulations that occur the greater the chance that a satisfactory outcome can be achieved.

For example, in an individual suffering from endometritis (inflamed lining of the uterus) and therefore presenting a particularly hostile environment to the spermatozoa, repeated attempts to achieve fertilisation may be required. Nor can we dismiss the importance of semen quality and the libido of the stallion from the equation in establishing the balance for or against individual success.

Inducing oestrus

The need to induce oestrus occurs in the following circumstances:

1   When a mare has either been found to be not in foal at a pregnancy examination or is in a state of prolonged dioestrus without having visited the stallion.

2   When mating has to be arranged to suit managerial requirements as, for example, in synchronising oestrus in a herd, reducing the length of the cycle in cases that have, inadvertantly or deliberately, been missed in a previous oestrus (e.g. when ovulation has occurred before mating or when foaling or other heats have been avoided for reasons of infection, etc.), and, out of the breeding season, to promote oestrus for bacteriological tests of the genital tract.

Essentially there are two methods of inducing oestrus: uterine infusion with saline and the injection of a natural or a synthetic prostaglandin. However, it must be stressed that in both cases treatment can only be successful if the failure to show oestrus is due to the presence of an active yellow body. Prostaglandin acts directly to dissolve the yellow body and this causes the mare to come into heat within two to five days. Uterine infusion acts indirectly, probably by stimulating the release of prostaglandin from the uterus. Mares do not respond in either instance if treated within about five days of a new yellow body forming. The judgement of when to inject the mare is, of course, a veterinary decision.

Inducing follicle development

Gonadotrophin releasing hormone may be used to promote the development of mature follicles in the ovary. The use of gonadotrophin releasing hormone has exciting possibilities. However, this hormone acts by causing the pituitary gland to release FSH and LH. It does so only if administered in a pulsatile (rhythmic) manner and not if given in a single bolus dose. Implants releasing small doses over a period of days or a programme of injecting doses two or three times a day has been found to be most effective.

If a mature follicle is present in the ovary it may be assisted to ovulate by administering the luteinizing hormone hCG (human chorionic gonadotrophin). This treatment brings oestrus to an end and enables mating to be arranged just before ovulation occurs.

Use of treatments

As with abnormal mares, the treatment of normal mares is very much a matter for veterinary judgement in the context of the particular individual that requires treatment. It is not therefore in the scope of this book to argue the various methods that may be used and how these should be applied. However, there are some fundamental points which should be made in order for mare owners to appreciate the advantages and disadvantages of therapy aimed at altering a mare's sexual activity.

The reality of the changing hormonal concentrations in the body of a mare relative to changes in her sexual behaviour during the oestrous cycle is a complex interaction, not just a simple relationship of cause and effect. For example, although we know that follicles mature under the influence of FSH, they do so in relation to other hormones such as LH, progesterone and oestrogen.

Changing the level of hormones in the body by artificial means can never, therefore, be simplistic. Administering one hormone at any given time may be likened to increasing one ingredient of a cake without reference to the other ingredients. The outcome may, in effect, be the same type of cake as the one we started to make but its balance depends on the quantity of each ingredient. There may, therefore, be too much fruit or too little flour depending on the ingredients with which we started. And when we give hormones to a mare much of the effect depends on the makeup or state of the mare at the start of the treatment.

Unfortunately we do not have very precise means of diagnosing the exact state of a mare at any given time. We may say that she is aneostrus but we cannot determine the finer details which lie behind this state. We cannot measure directly the activity or inactivity of the pituitary gland and identify the control of this gland being exerted by cells in the brain producing GnRH. This inability to make a precise detailed diagnosis is one reason why our treatment works in only a proportion of cases, even if this proportion is sometimes as high as 70%. The failure of the 30% may be ascribed to a lack of current methods of distinguishing differences between individuals.

It is no coincidence that the most successful means of changing the mare's sexual state from one of inactivity (anoestrus) to one of activity (oestrous cycling) is by increasing the length of daylight artificially over a period of six to eight weeks. This mimics the natural stimulus more effectively than any combination of drugs can achieve in a shorter period of time.

25
PREGNANCY

PLACENTATION

The foal, unlike the young of smaller nesting mammals such as the rat, mouse, rabbit, cat or dog, is born at an extremely advanced state of development. It can stand within minutes after birth and is capable of highly coordinated movement within a matter of hours. The preparations for this dramatic entry into the world take place unseen in the mother's uterus, which is part of the female reproductive tract (see Chapter 23).

Attachment of the blastocyst and the development of the foetal membrane
After mating, sperm meets the egg (ovum) within the Fallopian tube, and the single cell of the egg begins to divide. The fertilised ovum enters the uterus as a hollow ball of cells, the blastocyst.

The blastocyst of the horse, like those of the other large domestic mammals, does not erode the endometrial lining of the uterus but remains within its central cavity. It comes to lie at the base of one or other uterine horn, where, on or about the thirtieth day of gestation, certain specialised cells on its outer surface begin to invade the endometrium. The cells form the structures known as endometrial cups which secrete the hormone eCG into the maternal bloodstream. The hormone is also excreted in the mother's urine and detection of its presence is the basis for one of the methods of the early diagnosis of pregnancy. The concentrations of eCG in the serum rise until about the seventieth day and then begin to decline. This pattern is reflected in the development and regression of the endometrial cups, which seldom persist longer than the 120th day of gestation. The endometrial cups have nothing whatever to do with the development of the placenta, which does not become fully established before the 100th day.

From its original position at the base of the uterine horn, the spherical conceptus expands to fill the whole of the cavity of the uterus, extending through the body and into the non-gravid horn. Nevertheless the foetus itself remains in its original position at the base of the gravid horn. By forty days it has become enclosed by three membranes, which together form two concentric fluid-filled sacs (Figure 1). The inner sac, the amnion, contains a slimy fluid. The outer sac, the allantois, not only wraps itself completely round the amnion, but also forms an inner lining to the outer limiting membrane, the chorion. The space between the two double membranes, the allanto-amnion and the chorio-allantois, is filled with watery allantoic fluid. The chorion, the outermost component of the chorioallantois, forms the foetal side of the placenta.

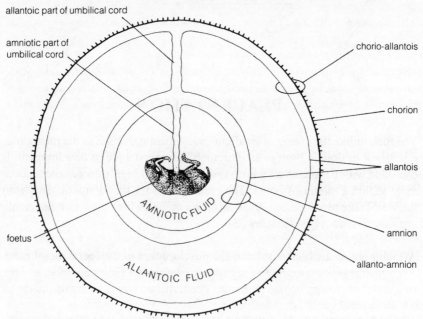

Figure 1   The placental membranes in the uterus

Flattened, oval, leathery bodies known as hippomanes float free in the allantoic fluid. They are aggregations of cell debris which have no known function, though they feature prominently in horse-related folklore. Tales may still be told of hippomanes lodging in the mouth of the foal and shaping its tongue, or of dried and powdered hippomanes having aphrodisiac properties. Unfortunately for the romance of folklore, neither of these tales is true.

The embryo is connected to the placenta by the umbilical cord, which passes first through the amnion and then crosses the space between amnion and chorion. Thus, unlike the situation in many other mammals, the umbilical cord has two distinct divisions: these are known as the amniotic part and allantoic part respectively. The umbilical cord carries blood from the foetus to the placenta in paired umbilical arteries, and oxygenated blood is returned to the foetus in a single umbilical vein. Foetal and maternal circulations are entirely separate, but they come into very close apposition within the placenta. It is within the placenta that oxygen and nutrients are transferred to the foetus, while carbon dioxide and the majority of waste products are passed in the opposite direction.

The development and structure of the placenta

The chorion is at first avascular, but blood vessels from the embryo spread across its inner surface shortly after the primitive circulation of the foetus becomes established. Along the course of these blood vessels tiny finger-like outpocketings of the chorion push into corresponding depressions which form in the lining of the uterus. The outpocketings of the chorion are known as foetal villi, and the depressions in the endometrial lining of the uterus as maternal crypts. The original villous outpocketings branch repeatedly to form very small tufts which, together with the correspondingly more complex maternal crypts, form minute globular structures known as microcotyledons. These are the functional units of the equine placenta: they number many thousands and are found in all parts of the uterus except the cervix and the points of entry of the Fallopian tubes.

The tiny tufts of foetal villi can be seen on the red side of the afterbirth after delivery. If a small piece of afterbirth is immersed in water, the villi float out like miniature sea anemones closely packed together on the surface of the membrane.

Placentae in twin pregnancy

The birth of live twin foals is a newsworthy event, but the conception of twin embryos is hardly a cause for celebration. The reason is that twin foals are usually aborted; survival seems to depend on the placenta of each foal occupying exactly half of the surface area of the uterus (Figure 2).

If the placentae are asymmetrically distributed, the foal attached to the smaller placenta will die (Figure 3). If this happens early in pregnancy, the embryo may mummify and the placenta of the living twin may expand its territory and enclose the mummified embryo (Figure 4). The result is the birth of a single living foal, and the evidence of twinning may never be suspected or discovered. More tragically, and usually not later than the ninth month of pregnancy, the death of one foal results in the abortion of both.

PREGNANCY

Length of pregnancy

Pregnancy lasts, on average, 340 days in the Thoroughbred and larger breeds. In ponies and other small breeds pregnancy is shorter by up to twenty days. However, individuals within all breeds vary quite considerably. The range for a Thoroughbred is some 320-65 days or even longer.

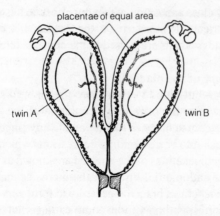

placentae of equal area

twin A

twin B

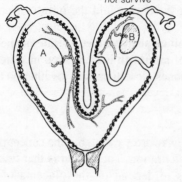

Placenta of B occupies less
than half the uterus, it will
not survive

A

B

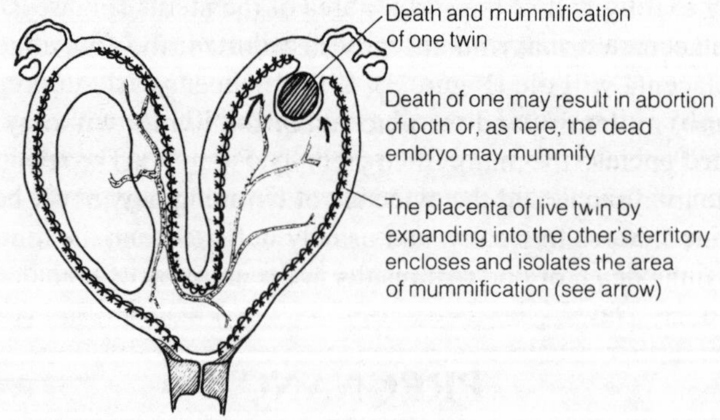

Death and mummification
of one twin

Death of one may result in abortion
of both or, as here, the dead
embryo may mummify

The placenta of live twin by
expanding into the other's territory
encloses and isolates the area
of mummification (see arrow)

Figure 2   Arrangement of the placentae of twin foals which are born alive.
Each placenta occupies half the uterus

Figure 3   Asymmetrical distribution of the placentae in twin foals

Figure 4   Twinning mummification

Pregnancy lasts about 365 days in donkeys and about 350 days in a horse mare carrying a foal by a donkey stallion. These differences illustrate that the genetic makeup of the foetus determines in part, at least, the length of pregnancy and that this may be influenced by the genetic contribution of individual stallions and mares.

The length of pregnancy is also influenced by nutrition, for well-fed mares tend to have shorter pregnancies than poorly fed ones. The time of year is also important: mares delivering in winter have longer pregnancies than those delivering in summer.

Pregnancy diagnosis

Pregnancy diagnosis is important to those who manage broodmares for a number of reasons. First, during the breeding season an early (seventeen to twenty days) diagnosis enables management to make a decision as to whether or not a mare requires further mating or whether measures should be employed to bring her into oestrus so that she is given a further chance of conceiving. Second, mares that are pregnant may be identified for purposes of sale, insurance or in continuing plans for the subsequent mating season. Third, it is important to determine whether or not twins are present and, if so, the measures to be taken to eliminate one or both members. Finally, it is helpful to be able to confirm barrenness in cases where diagnosis of conditions or treatment of the uterus is being considered at some stage following mating.

Rectal examination   The traditional method of pregnancy diagnosis in the mare is rectal examination. The operator places a gloved and lubricated arm in the rectum and feels the uterus. This method is accurate from about forty days after mating, depending on the individual. Experienced operators can achieve an accurate diagnosis earlier than this, even at twenty days.

Echography (ultrasound scanning) More recently the advent of ultrasound has enabled operators to make accurate diagnosis as early as fifteen days after conception. In practice the seventeen-to twenty-one-day period is usually the first routine examination made with scanning (Figure 5a).

At this time the fluid sac representing the foetus and its membranes may be visualised. By Day 24 the foetus itself may be identified and progressively, with time, further structures may be seen (see Figure 5b).

After about Day 80 the foetus may be visualised by an external examination placing the probe in the region of the udder.

Scanning has the advantage of very much improved accuracy in early pregnancy, while at the same time providing the means of diagnosing twins. Twins may be contained one in each horn of the uterus (see Figure 2) or together in one horn. In the first instance a diagnosis can lead to squeezing of one of the two members of the twins and its elimination with the probable normal

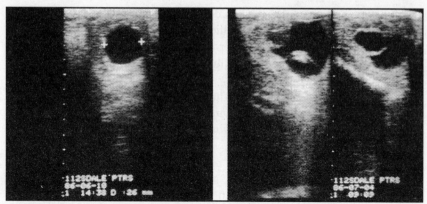

Figure 5a/b Ultrasound scans at (left) 21 days and (right) 29 days (two views)

continuation of the other one. This procedure is best performed before about Day 25. After this time the chances of successfully eliminating one without the other member are markedly reduced.

If twins are in the same horn, i.e. adjacent to one another, the usual approach is to abort them with prostaglandin. The importance of eliminating twins by one means or another (i.e. by removing one or both) are discussed on p. 396.

Detection of eCG   As discussed on p. 168, eCG is a hormone present in the bloodstream of pregnant mares between about Day 45 and Day 100. A blood sample taken during this period and tested for the presence of eCG is used as a pregnancy test.

More recently, an immunological test has been developed. This is based on the fact that the hormone acts as an antigen and, when mixed with an antibody, a reaction occurs. This reaction can be identified when red blood cells are incorporated into the test system . This is usually referred to as the MIP test (mare immunological pregnancy test).

The MIP test has certain limitations. For example, once the endometrial cups (see p. 389) from which the hormone eCG is secreted are established in the uterus, the hormone is produced until about Day 100 irrespective of whether or not the foetus lives. In other words, we may have a situation in which the foetus has died at, say, Day 45 and, when the test is performed at perhaps Day 80, the test is positive despite the mare having lost her pregnancy. The accuracy of the test is high, probably over 95%, apart from this one proviso. It is possible to rely on the test almost to a 100% if the result is negative but only to about 90% if it is positive.

The test is favoured by those who believe that the rectal examination may in itself cause abortion. It cannot be denied that such an examination may cause abortion, but in mares used to being handled for examination the chances of abortion are very small.

Cuboni test   The Cuboni test is based on a chemical test-tube reaction in the laboratory. Urine from the mare is mixed with hydrochloric acid and heated for ten minutes. After cooling, the hydrolysed urine is removed with benzene and transferred to a test tube. Concentrated sulphuric acid is poured down the side of the tube to lie under the benzene. The tube is stoppered, inverted once and heated. Under an ultra-violet lamp in reflected daylight a positive result shows as a green fluorescence.

Conditions of Pregnancy

ABORTION

Abortion means the expulsion of the foetus before it has any chance of living, that is, while it is non-viable. Thus abortion may occur at any time before Day 300 of pregnancy. After this time it is more usual to describe an abnormal termination of pregnancy as prematurity, dysmaturity or stillbirth (see p. 450).

It should, however, be appreciated that these terms are arbitrary definitions and do not represent different disease conditions. It is necessary to use the terms so that we have some convenient headings under which to discuss these conditions.

When abortion occurs early (before about Day 100) it may be described as foetal loss, embryonic death or resorption. Again, these descriptions are largely technical and need not concern the reader except, in so far as they may be used by vets, some understanding is necessary. For the purpose of description here the term 'abortion' is used to describe abnormal loss of pregnancy at any stage of pregnancy up to about Day 300.

Abortion concerns two beings, the mare and her foetus. It is the mare that expels the foetus but the cause of this may be the foetus itself dying. On the other hand, the foetus may be expelled in a relatively healthy state and it is the mare that is responsible for the event. An obvious example of this type of abortion is if a drug such as oxytocin is given to the mare.

The distinction as to whether the abortion is of maternal or foetal origin is a technical matter and outside the scope of this book. However, the expression of this difference is of interest practically because, when the foetus and placenta are failing, the mare springs an udder and may run milk. When no such development is present, this implies that the foetus has died suddenly or that the mare herself has been responsible for initiating the expulsion of her foetus.

The causes of abortion
Infection   Any microbe which is found in the genital tract of the barren mare may be responsible for abortion at any stage of pregnancy. The most

common bacterial infections are streptococci, staphylococcl, *Escherichia coli* and *Klebsiella* (see Chapters 29 and 30).

Fungus (mycosis – see Chapter 29) is responsible for abortions occurring in the second half of pregnancy. These microbes usually infect the placenta and cause substantial thickening of and damage to this membrane. Eventually the microbes may enter the foetus itself where they cause lesions in the liver and lungs.

Viruses, especially equid herpesvirus 1 (EHV-1, rhinopneumonitis), cause abortion typically from about the seventh month onwards. However, cases can occur as early as five months and frequently in mares that are near to or at full term. The condition may be epidemic and it has an especial place in veterinary and stud management practice (see p. 398).

Arteritis virus may cause abortion, particularly in the first half of pregnancy. The abortion is, however, usually a secondary event associated with general infection of a pregnant mare. For a description of this condition, see pp. 494-6.

Non-infectious causes   **Twin conception** leads to abortion. The reason for this is the nature of the horse's placenta (see p. 391). In all other species twins can be carried successfully because there is space on the uterine wall for the attachment of more than one placenta. In the horse, however, the area of placental attachment in single pregnancy normally involves the whole of the uterine wall. Thus, in twin pregnancy there is an inevitable reduction of the placental area available to each foetus, usually to the detriment of both. In most cases one twin dies and both are aborted. If twins are born alive, they are often smaller than usual, are especially susceptible to infectious disease, and may be subject to deficiencies in normal skeletal development.

Twisting of the Umbilical Cord around the hind limb sometimes results in abortion because of strangulation of the blood supply to the foetus. This may also occur, less commonly, because of abnormal twisting, which has the same effect. Many of these cases are probably due to abnormally long cords. The average length of the umbilical cord is in the order of 80 cm with about half of that being contained within the amniotic and the other half in the allantoic cavity, as the cord passes through these. Cord lengths of 100 cm length are thought to make the cord vulnerable to compression and interference with blood supply leading to abortion.

In other species it has been established that early abortions are due to chromosomal abnormality in the foetus. This is nature's way of ensuring that defective individuals do not survive pregnancy. This type of abortion has not been proved to occur in the horse but probably accounts for a number of the early abortions, i.e. those occurring before Day 100.

It is often difficult if not impossible to diagnose the cause of every abortion. This is because it may be the result of failure in the relationship between the uterus and the placenta, e.g. bloodflow or immunological and hormonal failure. States of incompatibility may develop between the uterus and the placenta. In making a diagnosis of the cause of any particular case of abortion the pathologist is presented with material that provides evidence only of death, that is, the pathology of shortage or absence of oxygen.

If a mare aborts up to about Day 150 it is probable that the foetus itself will not be found. The reasons for this are either that it is too small or it has been resorbed. The abortion is only established by the fact that the mare comes into heat or suffers a vaginal discharge. However, in other cases the event will be recognised only because the mare is found, at a subsequent examination, not to be pregnant. These abortions require veterinary interpretation of the cause and treatment of the mare if required.

EQUID HERPESVIRUS 1 (EHV-1, RHINOPNEUMONITIS, VIRUS ABORTION)

After Day 150 of pregnancy the abortion will probably be evident in the form of the expelled foetus and its membranes. The same approach as to earlier abortions should be made, namely, a veterinarian should be called to decide whether the mare requires treatment. However, whereas early abortions are almost certainly the result of causes which are not a threat to other mares, later abortions may, if they are caused by a virus, be a threat to other mares. For this reason all abortions after Day 150 should be regarded as being potentially cases of equid herpesvirus 1 (EHV-1) infection unless demonstrated otherwise by post-mortem examination of the foetus.

Herpesvirus causing abortion in mares is essentially a respiratory virus, causing the snotty-nose condition of foals and yearlings. The virus can be transmitted from one individual to another by two means and in both cases the mare inhales the virus. The virus may either be exhaled from the lungs of another infected mare in the vicinity, or it may be spread from an aborted foetus. At the time of an abortion a large amount of virus is spread into the atmosphere; any pregnant mare in contact with the abortion can inhale the virus and herself become infected.

The herpesvirus may be present in many individuals, especially foals and yearlings. There are two strains: subtype 1, which is usually associated with abortion, although it may cause the respiratory (snotty-nose) type of infection; and subtype 2, which is almost entirely respiratory and rarely causes abortion (see p. 490).

Following infection, immunity to either strain is short-lived and lasts only about two or three months. Further, infection with one strain does not necessarily confer immunity to the other. This presents a problem when we use vaccines. Most vaccines against herpesviruses are relatively ineffective and have to be administered frequently, say, every two months.

When any mare aborts, it is prudent to place the foetus and all its membranes in a leak-proof plastic container or bin. These should then be taken for post mortem at an appropriate veterinary establishment. Here the possibility of the case being one of herpes infection will be established. The diagnosis depends on histological examination of the liver and lungs for typical lesions and by growing the virus in tissue culture. It may take only twenty-four to forty-eight hours for a positive diagnosis to be made, but up to a week for a negative diagnosis to be confirmed.

The precautions that should be taken on a stud where other pregnant mares are stabled should be applied until a definite diagnosis has been achieved. These precautions are as follows:

1. A mare that has aborted should be confined to the loosebox in which she aborted. If she aborted in a paddock she should be brought in and placed in her own loosebox or in one which is isolated from any other pregnant mare. All areas which have been contaminated by the fluids of the foetus and placenta should be thoroughly disinfected.
2. All pregnant mares that have been in contact with the aborting mare for at least the previous three weeks should be regarded as being potentially infected. These mares should therefore be isolated as a group and not brought into contact with any other pregnant mare.
3. All other mares on the premises should be isolated as a potentially non-infected group. And all traffic of horses into or out of the studfarm concerned should be stopped.

If the abortion is subsequently diagnosed as being not due to herpesvirus, these restrictions can then be lifted. However, it cannot be overemphasised that the measures taken immediately after an abortion may mean the difference between a simple case, the condition spreading to only a very few other mares, and a widespread epidemic affecting more than one studfarm.

The immediate measures described above should be followed in every case of abortion. However, some cases of virus infection may occur at full term, and foals which are born sick should also be considered as possible cases of virus infection. In these circumstances they too may be a threat to other mares that have not yet foaled.

If a case of abortion or a foal dying in the first week of life is confirmed as being the result of virus infection, the long-term precautions have been stated by the Thoroughbred Breeders Association in their codes of practice. The following is abstracted from the HBLB 2000 Codes of Practice used by kind permission of the Horserace Betting Levy Board. The Code is reviewed and re-published by the Board annually.

Code of Practice for EQUID HERPESVIRUS-1

1. What is EHV-1

EHV-1 is a common and contagious virus which causes abortion, respiratory disease and paralysis.

It should be noted that EHV-4 can also cause abortion but more usually causes respiratory disease only.

2. How does infection occur?

All classes of horses and ponies can be a source of EHV-1. Pregnant mares should therefore be kept separate from all other stock to avoid infection which may lead to abortion and to disease in live foals.

The virus usually spreads via the respiratory tract, but aborted foetuses, foetal membranes and fluids are a particularly dangerous source of infection. All aborted foetuses and carcases from newborn foal deaths must therefore be handled hygienically and sent to a competent laboratory for examination.

Infected foals can pass on infection, via the respiratory route, to healthy mares, other foals and other in-contacts.

Mares which have aborted or whose foal has died are a source of infection to other foals and horses, also via the respiratory route. Disease can be transmitted to healthy foals from any infected horse as well as from infected mares and foals.

Mares and other horses can be 'carriers' of the virus, meaning that they may transmit infection without showing signs of illness themselves. Illness may become apparent in carriers from time to time, especially after stress or after suffering another disease. The virus is always contagious at this time.

The virus can survive in the environment for several weeks; indirect infection is therefore possible.

3. When does abortion Occur?

Abortion usually occurs in late pregnancy (8-11 months) but can be as early as 4 months.

Following infection, abortion can happen from 2 weeks to several months later.

Prolonged transport and other types of stress during late pregnancy may increase the risk of infection of the foetus.

4. What about live infected foals?

Infected foals are usually abnormal from birth, showing weakness, jaundice, difficulty in breathing and occasionally nervous symptoms. They usually die within 3 days.

These foals are highly contagious through direct contact via the respiratory route and through shedding virus into the environment. All horses can become infected but mares which have recently foaled are probably at greatest risk.

5. What about respiratory disease?

EHV-1 usually causes respiratory disease in weaned foals and yearlings, most often in autumn and winter. However, older animals can succumb. These are more likely than the younger animals to transmit the virus without showing signs of infection.

The signs that are seen are mild fever, coughing, discharge from the nose and other signs of respiratory disease.

6. How is EHV-1 diagnosed?

The presence of EHV-1 can only be diagnosed in a laboratory.

For abortion and newborn foal death, the laboratory requires the foetus or foal carcase. Blood testing the mare is not appropriate for diagnosing an EHV-1 abortion.

Members of the Thoroughbred Breeders' Association in Great Britain are reminded that a contribution may be available towards laboratory costs for aborted foetuses or foals which die within 14 days of birth. Further details are available from the TBA.

For confirmation of EHV-1 as the cause of respiratory disease or paralysis, blood samples and swabs from the throat are required.

7. Is EHV-1 notifiable?

There are no legal notification requirements for EHV-1 in the UK.

However, because the disease is spread easily between horses and can have severe consequences, it is very important to alert owners of horses which might be at risk of infection or might spread infection away from your premises following an outbreak at your premises. These owners can then arrange to take their own precautions against the spread of infection at their premises. Recommendations for reporting are given in Section 9 below.

On no account should any horse known or suspected to have disease caused by EHV-1 be sent, during the breeding season, to a stallion stud or to other premises where there are pregnant mares or brood mares.

8. Preventing EHV-1 – recommendations

A. Management

Where possible, mares should foal at home and go to the stallion with a healthy foal at foot.

Where this is not possible, pregnant mares should arrive at the stallion stud ideally one month before foaling is due. They should be put in isolated groups with other healthy pregnant mares; these groups should be as small as possible. Mares in late pregnancy and those from sales yards and abroad are a particular risk and should be isolated alone.

The isolated groups and individuals should be separated as far as possible from weaned foals, yearlings, horses out of training and competition horses. Fillies out of training are a particular risk to pregnant mares.

Mares in late pregnancy should not travel with other stock, particularly mares which have aborted recently.

If a foster mare is brought to the stud, she should be isolated – particularly from pregnant mares – until it has been proved that her own foal's death was not caused by EHV-1.

Stallions should ideally be housed in premises separate to the mare operations.

B. Hygiene

EHV-1 is destroyed readily by heat and disinfectants. Stables and vehicles for horse transport should therefore be cleaned and disinfected regularly as a matter of routine, using approved disinfectants and steam cleaning. If cleaning and disinfection are inadequate, the virus may survive in the environment for several weeks.

Ideally, separate staff should deal with separate groups of mares. If this is not possible, pregnant mares should be handled first each day.

C. Vaccination
The vaccine Duvaxyn EHV 1.4 (Fort Dodge) is licensed in the UK for use as an aid in prevention of EHV-1 abortion. Vaccination of mares is recommended.

This vaccine is also licensed for use against the respiratory form of EHV-1 and 4 in the UK.

Vaccination of all horses/ponies on any stud using these vaccines under veterinary direction may be advantageous to raise the level of protection against EHV-1. However, this may not necessarily provide total protection.

9. Controlling EHV-1 – recomendations
If: **-abortion occurs**
     -a foal is born dead
     -a foal is born ill
     -a foal becomes ill within 14 days of birth:

a. Seek veterinary advice IMMEDIATELY.
b. For abortions and foals born dead:
-place the mare in strict isolation
-send the foetus and its membranes or the foal carcase to a competent laboratory for examination as instructed by the veterinary surgeon; use leakproof containers
c. For sick live foals:
-place the mare and foal in strict isolation
-send samples (usually nasopharyngeal swabs and heparinised blood) to a competent laboratory for examination as instructed by the veterinary surgeon; use leakproof containers.
-the attendant should have no contact with pregnant mares
d. Stop movement off the stud. Do not allow any pregnant mare onto the stud until EHV-1 has been excluded as the cause of the abortion or foal death or illness.
e. Notify owners due to send mares to the stud.
f. Disinfect and destroy bedding; clean and disinfect premises and vehicles used for horse transport under veterinary supervision.
g. If preliminary laboratory results indicate EHV-1, divide pregnant mares in the contact group into even smaller groups to minimise the spread of any infection (NB: some may still abort).

B. If EHV-1 is confirmed:
a. Maintain isolation and movement restrictions and hygiene measures for at least one month.
b. Notify:
    • Your breeders association
    - by telephone
    - in writing
    • Owners (or their agents) of:
    - mares at the stud
    - mares due to be sent to the stud
    • Others:
    - Those responsible for the management of premises to which any horses from the stud are to be sent.

- Those responsible for the management of premises to which any horses have been sent in the previous 30 days, with the condition that owners must be notified immediately.
- Those responsible for the management of premises to which any pregnant mares (that have been in contact after the first 3 months of pregnancy) have been sent, with the condition that owners must be notified immediately.

Notification is extremely important. Failure to notify the disease can contribute to the spread of infection to the detriment of all owners and their horses, particularly mare owners.

C. After EHV-1 abortion at a stallion stud:
a. The stud can accept barren mares, maiden mares and mares which have produced healthy foals at home, providing there is no sign of infection at the home premises.
b. Non-pregnant mares which have been on the stud can visit other premises after one month from the date of the last abortion, providing they can be isolated from all pregnant mares for at least 2 months at the premises they are visiting.*
c. Pregnant mares due to foal in the current season must stay at the stud until they foal.
d. Walking-in mares can visit the stud, but cannot return to their boarding studs until one month after the last clinical case has occurred.*
e. Mares which have aborted must be kept in isolation from mares in late pregnancy for 8 weeks after abortion. Present evidence indicates low risk of spread of infection if mares are mated on the second heat cycle after abortion.
f. Mares that returned home pregnant from studs where abortion occurred the previous season should foal in isolation at home. Where this is not possible, the stud to which the mare is to be sent in the current season must be informed so that precautions can be taken.

* The managers and veterinary surgeons of the stallion stud and other premises must agree these arrangements before the mares are moved.

D. If paralytic EHV-1 is suspected in any horse:
a. Seek veterinary advice IMMEDIATELY.
b. Stop mating and teasing.
c. Stop all movement on and off the stud.
d. Send samples as directed by the veterinary surgeon to a competent laboratory for examination; use leakproof containers.
e. Divide horses into small groups, keeping pregnant mares separate from all others.
f. Implement Ae, Af and B above.

E. If paralytic EHV-1 is confirmed, policy should be decided with the veterinary surgeon. This should include screening and clearance of each group before individuals in the group return home. Individuals should then be isolated at home, especially pregnant mares until after foaling.

26
PARTURITION

Birth marks the end of pregnancy and the beginning of life as we know it outside the security of the womb. It is, as the name 'parturition' implies, a bringing forth of the offspring or foaling, the delivery of a foal. Birth is, in fact, a partnership between mare and foetal foal, as we will discuss shortly. Because birth is a dramatic event and sometimes hazardous, man plays some part in the partnership and foaling is often supervised. However, we must not forget that the event is natural and that problems arise only in a small percentage of cases.

Maternal preparation for birth
The first external sign that the mare is preparing for the event is the development of the udder or mammary glands. These start to enlarge about three weeks before foaling. However, there is quite a marked variation, and movement in mammary size occurs earlier in some mares and later than average in others. Younger mares tend to have a longer preparation time and this often occurs in two distinct stages: an earlier period, perhaps four to five weeks prior to foaling, followed by a pause of about two weeks, then a final preparatory enlargement terminating as a full udder a week or ten days prior to the event.

Secretions within the gland also change, becoming thicker in consistency and changing colour from gold to white. The calcium content rises sharply within four or five days of foaling, sodium levels fall and potassium levels rise.

We can estimate the date of foaling from changes in mammary size and from an analysis of the content of the pre-foaling milk. Traditionally, mammary size and the appearance of wax on the teats has been used for this purpose. Wax is the beads of milk that ooze from and dry at the end of the teats about twenty-four hours prior to foaling (see Figure 9, p. 411). However, some mares do not form wax, while others run milk, i.e. squirt milk from the teats, hours, days or even weeks prior to foaling.

Most mares foal during the hours of darkness, but the prediction as to which night the event will take place has always been a problem to those responsible for supervising foaling. More recently, studies in the changes in the milk composition have enabled us to make predictions more scientific and accurate. By measuring the calcium, sodium and potassium levels in pre-foaling secretions we can determine that foaling is not likely to occur on a particular night.

Measurements are less reliable for predicting the actual night of foaling, although they can be used to indicate foaling within two or three days once calcium content has increased (above 10 mmol/litre) and sodium levels are higher than potassium levels.

A strip test has been devised by Robert Cash and Jenny Ousey, based on a test for water hardness. There are four squares on the strip and these change colour according to the ionic level in the secretions with which the strip is brought into contact. This test is most appropriate for people who have a limited number of mares and therefore find it inconvenient or uneconomical to have someone present each night in case a mare foals. The test can predict that a mare will not foal (less than two squares changing colour) or that she is likely to foal (three or four squares changing colour). However, as with all tests of this nature, exceptions can occur. The test strips are available from Beaufort Cottage Laboratories, High Street, Newmarket.

Colostrum   The milk in the udder at birth is called colostrum, sometimes referred to as first milk because it is the first milk of the foal once it is born. It contains antibodies or protective substances which provide the foal with protection against infection (see p. 431). These protective substances do not appear suddenly in the mammary secretions before birth, but increase slowly to a peak during the preceding two to three weeks.

Foetal preparation for birth
People do not always realise that the foetus plays its own substantial part in preparing for and initiating the birth process. The foetal foal and its placenta produce hormones such as oestrogen, progesterone, prostaglandin, cortisol, etc. It is these hormones which start and control the birth process.

Readiness for birth   The foetal foal develops during the pregnancy to a state of maturity. Maturity means that its organs and the cells and tissues of which they are composed are ready to function normally after birth and thereby sustain the foal in the world outside the uterus – a very different environment from that it has experienced previously. Maturity has, therefore, two components.

First, there is a structural development in which organs become shaped and formed so that we recognise them as the kidneys, the lungs, the liver, etc. For example, the lungs are at first solid, but by two thirds of the way through pregnancy potential air sacs (spaces)and a branching system of air tubes have formed, albeit, at that stage, they are filled with fluid. At the end of pregnancy these potential airways are fully formed and ready for the first breath, in which the fluid they contain will be replaced by air.

The other component to maturity is a functional one. The organ cells and tissues are able to function because of a complex system of enzymes, hormones and other substances which control and regulate their activity. These systems do not appear suddenly but are evolved during pregnancy, and it is only when the foal is ready for birth (functionally mature) that their potential is fully realised.

For example, the lungs may have the structure (airways and alveoli) of maturity but lack that vital function which enables them to stay inflated when breathing air. This depends on the system known as surfactant.

Surfactant is a chemical substance secreted by cells lining the air sacs (alveoli) and small air tubes. It forms the lining of the air sac and reduces the surface tension. If surfactant is not present in sufficient quantities, the surface tension causes the air sacs to collapse, just as a bubble of water collapses unless lined by soap which is itself a surface-tension-lowering substance.

Unreadiness for birth or prematurity may involve a surfactant deficiency which makes the lungs unable to stay expanded although structurally they appear normal. This is discussed further on pp. 448-50.

Initiation of birth

In the previous chapter the average length of pregnancy was said to be 340 days with variation of about 15 days. Each individual has, therefore, a selected date for foaling varying between 325 and 355 days. Some individuals may foal outside this range and the foals still be normal.

From this we may assume that each individual has a selected length of pregnancy which is normal for that individual in that particular year. The actual date is determined more by the foetal foal rather than by the mare herself. It is probable, if we assume the mare is similar to other mammals which have been studied more closely by scientists, that the foetus triggers the process of hormonal events leading to birth.

However, because most foalings occur at night it would seem that mares have some control over the timing of birth and they may be able to hold up the event until darkness arrives. They may also be able to delay the event because of threats in their own environment. This control was probably evolved in order to allow mares to foal at times when predators were less active; and it may be one reason why today some mares appear to be able to foal only when people are not present.

In summary, it seems probable that the foetus determines the overall length of pregnancy and that the mare has some fine-tuning capacity which determines the actual hour, or even night, of delivery.

The exact hierarchy of changes that precipitate birth is unknown in the horse. The mechanism on which all mammalian birth depends is the contraction of the uterine muscle. This is largely under hormonal control, and any hormone which stimulates contraction or which increases the contractability of the muscles contributes to the initiation of the birth process.

The hormones most associated with this are oxytocin and prostaglandin, which cause contractions to occur, and oestrogens and cortisol, which make the muscle more susceptible to their action. However, progesterone prevents contractions and can override the action of the others, depending on the amount available. A decrease in progesterone levels is therefore a prerequisite for normal birth.

The way in which these hormones play their part need not concern us here; it is a process not as yet fully understood and quite complex. What is important for the reader is to recognise that these hormones play a part in contractions of the uterus and that they are produced from the foetus and the placenta as well as by the mare's pituitary gland.

Once contractions start the mare goes into first-stage labour. When the contractions are strong enough, the cervix dilates and the foal is pushed through the birth canal during second-stage labour.

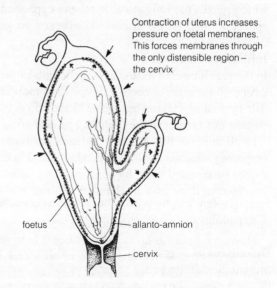

Contraction of uterus increases pressure on foetal membranes. This forces membranes through the only distensible region – the cervix

foetus

allanto-amnion

cervix

Figure 1
The first stages of labour

Forces of birth

The foal is pushed through the birth canal by the forces brought to bear on it from contractions of the uterus and the abdominal muscles. During the first stage of labour increasingly powerful contractions of the uterus cause pressure to rise in the fluids surrounding the foetus and these press against the placenta. So long as the cervix remains closed these pressures are contained, but as the cervix dilates it leaves a weak spot through which the placental membrane (the chorio-allantois) bulges, forced by the pressure of the foetal fluids into the birth canal. This action has often been likened to that of a hydraulic wedge.

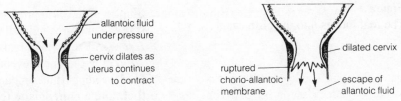

Figure 2   The rupture of the chorio-allantoic membrane

The end of the first stage of labour is normally marked by the rupture of the chorio-allantois and the escape of allantoic fluid. The cervix, now fully dilated, is prepared for the second stage of labour, and delivery of the foal. The pressure of the contracting uterine muscle, supplemented by the powerful straining action of the abdominal muscles and the diaphragm, propels the foetus through the opening in the cervix and the ruptured part of the placenta, and through the birth canal. Because the contours of the foal are relatively smooth, birth is usually a fairly rapid process.

Positioning of the foal for delivery
At the start of birth the foetal foal is typically lying on its back with its legs, head and neck flexed (Figure 4). As uterine contractions begin, so the foetus extends its forelimbs and head, turning into the upright position (Figure 5). Its forelegs and muzzle press against the cervix and may play some part in causing this to open. By the time the second stage is under way the foal lies in the most advantageous manner, namely with its head resting above its outstretched front legs and the body lying slightly to one side of the midline of the mare's pelvis (Figure 6).

If we examine the pelvis of the mare (Figures 10-11), we can see the optimal alignment by which the foal negotiates the birth canal with least risk of impediment.

Definitions of alignment   It is usual for vets to refer to the manner of presentation at the pelvis in terms of the parts that appear or present first in the birth canal. The only normal presentation is anterior, i.e. head and feet first. Posterior presentation (hind legs), breach (tail) and transverse (body) are comparatively rare and all abnormal.

The term 'posture' refers to the way the limbs, head and neck are arranged. They should be extended for normal delivery. Flexed posture is abnormal and obstructs the foal's delivery (dystocia).

'Position' describes the relative proximity of the foal's backbone to that of the mare. For example, the normal position is with the foal's backbone to the uppermost, i.e. in the dorsal position. During pregnancy and in the first stage of labour the foal's backbone is lowermost, i.e. in the ventral position.

Figure 3
The foal moves into the birth canal

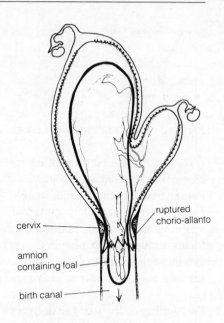

cervix

ruptured
chorio-allanto

amnion
containing foal

birth canal

Delivery of the afterbirth

The afterbirth consists of the outer membrane, the chorio-allantois, the long allantoic part of the umbilical cord, the amnion and the shorter amniotic part of the cord. After the foal has been born, the weight of the amnion hanging from the vagina pulls on the allantoic part of the cord and thus on its attachment to the inner surface of the chorio-allantois. As a result the chorio-allantois is usually delivered inside (or white side) out, with the placental (or red side) hidden within the inverted sac. Sometimes the afterbirth is delivered red side out, but this is less usual.

The afterbirth, covered in straw on the stable floor, is not a prepossessing sight. Nevertheless it should not be thrown away without examination, for if any of it has been left behind in the uterus, professional help is required to remove it and avert the danger of infection.

When spread out on a clean concrete floor, the chorio-allantoic part of the afterbirth looks like a baggy pair of trousers. The legs are the parts which lie within uterine horns, and the hole at the waist is the tear at the cervix through which the foal was born (Figure 7). The umbilical cord is attached near the top of one of the legs; the amnion is the separate membrane which surrounds the severed end. Apart from the tear at the cervix, the chorio-allantois should be undamaged and complete. Fortunately missing parts of the membrane are relatively rare (see p. 415).

Mares, unlike cattle, sheep and goats, do not usually eat the afterbirth. The one reported case which came to my notice could not be substantiated.

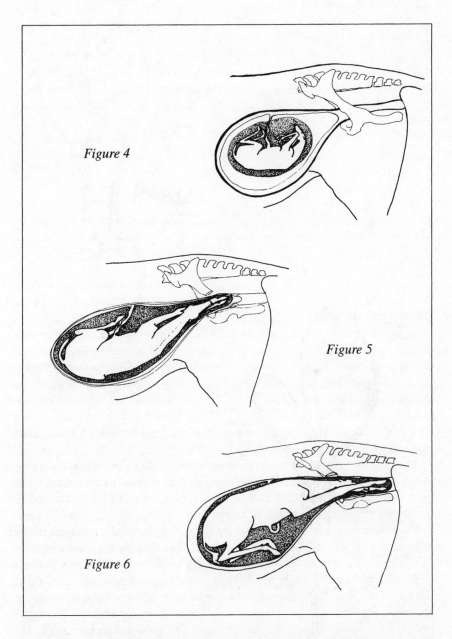

Figure 4

Figure 5

Figure 6

Figure 4   The position of the foal during the first stage of labour – ventral
Figure 5   The foal swivels to a dorsal position during the first stage
Figure 6   Normal presentation during the early second stage

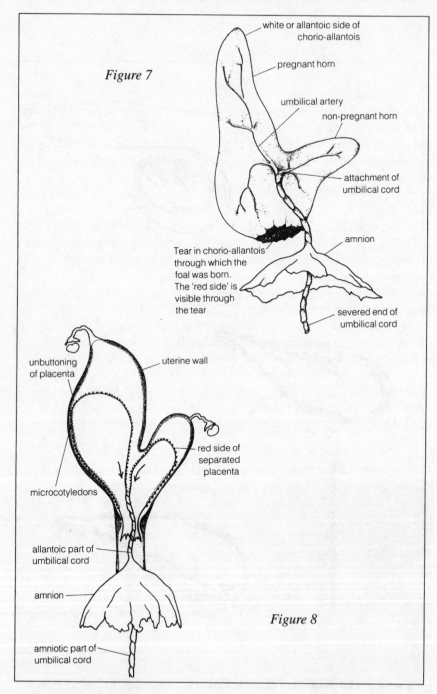

Figure 7

white or allantoic side of chorio-allantois

pregnant horn

umbilical artery

non-pregnant horn

attachment of umbilical cord

amnion

Tear in chorio-allantois through which the foal was born. The 'red side' is visible through the tear

severed end of umbilical cord

unbuttoning of placenta

uterine wall

red side of separated placenta

microcotyledons

allantoic part of umbilical cord

amnion

Figure 8

amniotic part of umbilical cord

Figure 7   The structure of the afterbirth
Figure 8   The placenta is usually delivered white side out

Description of Foaling

When we attend a foaling we must appreciate those matters described above, many of which we cannot see. We must appreciate them because this helps us to understand the normal birth process and, more particularly, to diagnose and correct matters when they are abnormal. This description is therefore an explanation of those points considered to be important in this process of understanding.

First stage

Mares become uneasy, pace the box, paw the ground, look round at their flanks and sweat. These are all signs of first-stage labour arising for the simple reason that contractions of the uterus are painful. The signs may vary according to the degree of pain caused and the appreciation of the individual. There is, therefore, considerable variation as to the length of the period and severity of first stage according to each individual.

The contractions of the uterus are caused largely because of the release of oxytocin from the pituitary and its effect on the uterine muscle. However, it also has an effect on the muscle of the mammary gland and may cause milk to spurt from the gland (milk-ejection reflex). This is another sign of first stage. Other signs include lengthening of the vulva and slight puffiness of the vulva labiae (lips).

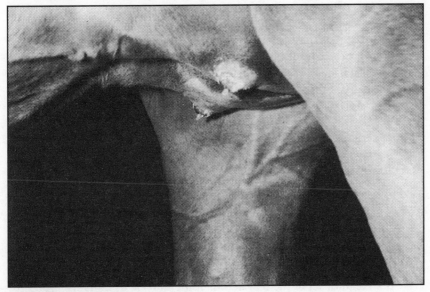

Figure 9   Waxed teats

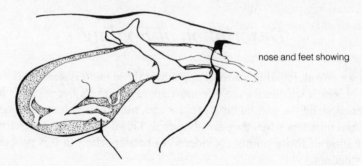

nose and feet showing

Figure 10   The second stage of labour – normal presentation and posture

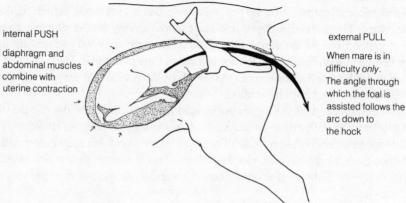

internal PUSH

diaphragm and
abdominal muscles
combine with
uterine contraction

external PULL

When mare is in
difficulty *only*.
The angle through
which the foal is
assisted follows the
arc down to
the hock

Figure 11   The forces at work during parturition

First-stage signs may be apparent long before a mare actually foals. The reason for this is that the contractions may not be strong enough to open the cervix. This remains closed and first-stage signs diminish as contractions cease. This is usually referred to as cooling off. It is not unusual for a mare to show first-stage signs one night or for several nights prior to actually foaling.

Second stage
Second-stage labour follows the first stage when the cervix relaxes and the placenta ruptures. This allows escape of allantoic (placental) fluid. This marks the start of the second stage; from this point there is, for the mare, no turning back from the act of foaling.

The escaping fluid is the first evidence that foaling is to take place and the foal will necessarily be delivered within the next hour at most. If the foal is in normal presentation and posture, the next landmark is for the shiny white membrane, the amnion, to appear between the vulval lips.

Next we can observe the feet and then the muzzle as delivery proceeds. These should be evident within five to ten minutes following rupture of the placental membrane (breaking water). Failure of the amnion to appear suggests that the foal may be in the wrong posture and not able to enter properly into the birth canal.

The mare may lie down during first stage but it is more usual for her to go through this in the standing position. However, the opposite is the case in second stage. The mare lies down, perhaps first on one side and then on the other. Occasionally she may roll.

It is tempting to suppose that this behaviour is an attempt to help the foal lie in the correct position. There is, of course, no way of proving that the mare has this intention, but those who have attended many births agree that the action of a mare appears to be purposeful. In many instances it is certainly helpful.

One aspect is obvious; lying down helps the propulsive force as the foal does not have to be pushed upwards over the brim of the pelvis against the force of gravity (see Figure 10). If the mare is lying on her side, the arc through which the foal is pushed through the pelvic canal lies in the same plane as the mare's forces are directing it. The drag of gravity is thereby avoided.

The foal is presented and its posture and position are such that it forms the minimum cross-sectional area. This is why one foreleg is usually delivered in advance of the other. The bulk of the elbows thereby pass through the pelvic outlet of the mare with the least risk of impediment. Sometimes one of the elbows may become lodged against the pelvic brim, and it is helpful in these cases to case it forward so that the forelegs come together rather than have a marked discrepancy between the two.

Pulling on the forelimbs during second stage introduces a different force to that applied by nature, which, as we have seen, is from behind the foal – a push not a pull. We must bear this in mind when we apply traction to assist the foal and recognise that it is an unnatural force. This is not to suggest that such a pull may not be helpful or even necessary in certain instances.

When the foal's chest is delivered, the hind legs become, probably passively, extended. At this stage the umbilical cord is being dragged across the pelvic floor and may suffer pressure. Once the foal's chest has been delivered it is important that delivery is completed as quickly as possible, within a few minutes. The chest is then freed for respiratory movements and the foal can breathe air instead of relying on the blood circulation in the cord, which may at this time be compromised.

The final stages of delivery are illustrated in Figures 12. It will be noted that the direction of delivery completes the arc towards the hocks of the mare. The important matter to emphasise here is that any pull applied to the foal should follow the line of this arc if it is to be helpful and successful.

In 96% of cases final delivery is completed with the mare lying on her side. Few individuals foal completely in the standing position and those that do are usually nervous and become disturbed by the presence of people. Second stage lasts sometimes as little as five or ten minutes and seldom as long as an hour.

Figure 12
The final stages of labour

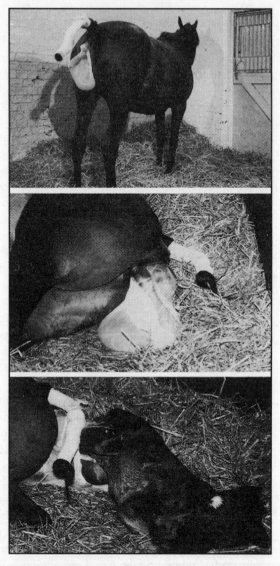

Mares foaling for the first time generally take longer than those that have had a number of foals. However, old mares may appear to be lazy and lie in the recumbent position without straining for long periods unless someone activates them by pulling on the forelegs of the foal.

Third stage
Third stage is the expulsion of the placenta or afterbirth. Although, so far as the foal is concerned, it is not strictly speaking part of delivery, it is an essential element of maternal function.

The placenta, as explained in Chapter 24, is held to the uterine surface by the interlocking of the small button-like structures known as microcotyledons. Successful expulsion of the membrane depends, therefore, on the unbuttoning of this arrangement. This seems to occur as the placental circulation ceases and blood is transferred from the placental circulation to the foal.

The circulation within the placenta, through the cord into the foal gradually diminishes in the minutes during which the foal, completely delivered, lies close to the mare, who usually remains lying down for up to twenty minutes after delivery. If this process is allowed to occur and the mare does not get up, thus breaking the cord, the microcotyledonary buttons on the placenta shrink and become detached, thus releasing the whole of the uterus from the placental membrane.

Other factors may play a part: for example, the contractions of the uterine muscle and the weight of the membranes hanging behind the mare help to pull the placenta through the cervix.

Expulsion of the placenta normally occurs within half to one hour of foaling. It may take considerably longer and, in this case, may only be shed as the placental tissue (the microcotyledonary buttons) shears and is left in situ. This may have a somewhat harmful effect on the resolution of the uterus back to the barren state after foaling and thus make a mare more difficult to get in foal at the foaling heat.

Duties of Personnel Present at Foaling

Those present should be quiet and discreet, especially if the mare is of a nervous disposition. They should observe rather than interfere.

They should know whether the mare has had a previous Caslick (sutured vulva) operation (see p. 625) and whether she has run milk and thereby lost colostrum (see p. 404). They should know whether the mare has suffered any problems in the past (such as a fractured pelvis or a difficult foaling) which might complicate the present birth.

Someone should note the exact time of the breaking of water. This is obvious in most cases but sometimes only a trickle of water appears. If there is any doubt the vulval lips should be parted to observe whether or not the amnion is in the vagina.

Soon after second stage has started any part of the vulva which has been previously stitched should be cut. This can be performed with the mare in the standing position or when she is lying down. The cut should be made with a pair of straight scissors with the blade about 12 cm long. The cut should be in the midline and carried out in one or two strokes.

It is usual for the vulva to lose feeling at this stage but some individuals retain sensation, so care should be taken when making the cut with the mare standing. It may be best to leave attempts to cut the vulva until the mare is lying down. However, this may not be possible in all cases because some individuals get to their feet on any approach to the hindquarters.

The safety of the operator is, of course, paramount and, if necessary, the mare's foreleg should be raised or the procedure carried out by a vet. Although it is preferable to make the cut at the time of foaling, those who are not experienced yet have responsibility for foaling may prefer the cutting to be carried out professionally some days prior to the event. In these circumstances a local anaesthetic is administered.

Early in the second stage an examination should be made to ascertain that the foetal foal is normally presented and in the extended posture. This examination may be conducted with the mare either standing or lying down. A washed or gloved hand should be inserted into the vagina and the presence of two feet and a muzzle confirmed. If the mare is standing, it will be necessary to reach farther into the birth canal than if she is lying down.

If one or more of the three appendages are not felt to be present in the birth canal, the person concerned should consider whether or not his/her experience is sufficient to correct any abnormality. If not, someone of experience should be called immediately.

If attempts at correction are to be made, these should be performed with the mare standing because its weight pulls the foetal foal back into the uterus and away from the pelvic inlet. This action allows more room for the operator to correct an abnormal posture. Sufficient room for manoeuvre is essential if corrections are to be made.

Straining and contractions of the uterus force the foal into the birth canal, and these may have to be reduced or suppressed in some cases before posture can be changed. The vet may inject drugs (beta adrenergic) to reduce uterine contractions and/or spinal anaesthesia to abolish them completely.

The responsibility of those attending birth is to decide whether they have the experience to correct the malposture or whether to call for professional assistance. It is better to err on the side of caution in this respect because the earlier a vet is called to the case the more chance of success.

Vets do not mind being called to a case only to find that the foal has been successfully delivered between the call and their arrival. But, conversely, it is disappointing for them to arrive too late and leave feeling that they might have achieved a happy outcome had they been called earlier.

Although there is considerable variation in the manner in which mares deliver, for example, the time they take, the effort they make and their individual behaviour, such as rolling or getting up and down frequently – there are certain signs that the onlooker may discern which indicate that all is not normal.

In the early stages of the delivery a mare that falls to strain and does not get on with the job may be reflecting a difficulty in passing her foal – a leg back or wrong positioning. On the other hand, a mare may show the opposite behaviour, getting up and down repeatedly or lying first on one side and then the other, especially when the foal's position is incorrect.

Positive, firm yet gentle assistance may be all that is required to help delivery in these instances. A forelimb may be pulled level with the other or traction on both limbs may be applied, provided the attendant bears in mind the fact that the forces of pulling are unnatural, as explained above. Inexperienced people may feel a compulsion to speed delivery, and this should be resisted.

These decisions and the approach to foaling are largely matters of experience, and instruction cannot be given in a text. The best advice is that those who have to be responsible for foaling should attend as many births as possible in the company of those that already have experience.

A moment of risk of which those present should be aware comes when the front feet have entered the vagina but not yet cleared the vulva. At this point the front legs and body of the foetal foal are pointing upwards, arrow-like, when the mare is standing. As she becomes recumbent she may, inadvertently, drive the outstretched forelimbs of the foal into the roof of the vagina. In most cases the feet, with their soft covering of horn, slide along the roof and out of the vagina so that no harm befalls the mare. But if the feet become caught in the roof of the vagina, as will occur if they are trapped by the suturing of the vulva, they may be driven through the roof of the vagina, into the rectum and appear from the anus. Thus creates a serious fistula (opening) between the rectum and the vagina.

If those present are aware of the risk, they can take quick action to guide the feet out of the vulva at this stage. However, the damage may already have been done by the time that they get to the mare and the feet may already be coming through the anus. In these circumstances it is essential to push them back into the vagina and redirect them through the vulva. In this event professional assistance should, of course, be called immediately.

There comes a moment in delivery (Figure 12b) when the foetal chest has been delivered through the vagina and only the back and hindquarters remain. This is the moment of no return, when delivery needs to be completed as quickly as possible so as to avoid pressure on the umbilical cord, which is being dragged across the floor of the mare's pelvis.

Although this is usually achieved through a combination of uterine contractions pushing from behind and the weight of the foal's body dragging it down and out of the vagina, there are some instances in which the hips of the foal lock against the pelvic inlet surrounding the birth canal.

This leaves the foal in a situation in which its umbilical cord is being squeezed and its source of oxygen from the placenta being compromised, while it cannot start respiratory movements in an unrestricted way because the chest is still in part surrounded by the vagina. It is therefore in danger of being asphyxiated.

The contraction at this stage may not be sufficient to unlock the engagement of the foal's hips and it is necessary to release them by pushing the hindquarters of the foal first one way and then the other until they slip easily from the mare. Here, it should be emphasized, the problem may be due to the direction in which we are pulling the foal. If, at this stage, we pull on the foal's forelimbs and body in a line which is a direct continuation of the axis of the vagina, we may be compounding the problem. If we change the line of direction of pull so that it is towards the hocks of the mare, this simulates the natural arc of delivery referred to above. This change of direction may in itself release the hindquarters of the foal for delivery.

A word of warning is required: any twisting of the forelegs of the foal in order to rotate the hind parts of the body may inadvertently fracture ribs or cause undue pressure on the heart. Twisting movements should be carried out only when essential. If possible, the body should be grasped behind the thorax and this should be supported gently as the rotational movements are conducted.

Again, it is prudent to remember that these manoeuvres are best learned by practice with others more experienced than oneself and are not really within the province of instruction in a text or classroom.

When dealing with the afterbirth it is good practice to tie the amnion to the cord as it hangs from the mare to prevent her from trampling on or kicking it. The weight of the amnion (about 2 kg, 5 lb) may help to pull on the placenta, thus aiding its expulsion from the uterus. The amnion may be knotted and then tied by string to the cord.

Some mares, especially those of heavy breeds, are susceptible to infection of the uterus and to laminitis if the placenta is not expelled soon after foaling. How soon, depends on the mare's susceptibility to the breakdown products of the foreign protein contained in the placenta.

In Thoroughbred practice the usual veterinary advice is that assistance should be called after about ten hours from foaling if the placenta has not come away. This gives ample time for the placenta to come away naturally while, at the same time, allows a reasonable time for it to remain in situ. As already described, most afterbirths are evacuated within about an hour of foaling.

In larger breeds it may be advisable to seek veterinary assistance before ten hours, while in ponies it may not be necessary for considerably longer. However, because it is abnormal for the membranes to remain in situ for longer than about two hours, some understanding with the veterinarian in advance of the event should be established. This gives an opportunity for the vet to give guidelines according to the circumstances of the client and the interest of the patient. For example, if the mare is prone to laminitis, special arrangements may have to be made for earlier removal of the placenta.

It is general practice to administer small doses of the hormone oxytocin and, if this does not achieve the desired evacuation, to remove the majority of the offending membrane manually. The remainder may then be removed hours, even days, later. Again, the manner of approach is a veterinary matter and may differ somewhat from one clinician to another.

The afterbirth, once it has been voided, should be checked to ensure that all of it has been discharged. In particular the horns should be examined to make sure they are intact (Figure 7) and no fragments have been left in the uterus. If there is any reason to suspect that some have been left behind, veterinary advice should be sought.

The surface of the placenta should be examined for any abnormal thickening or discolouration. The normal appearance depends to some extent on the length of time the membrane has been held in the uterus. It may go brown and have a parchment-like appearance the longer it remains attached.

The fresh appearance is of a velvet-like nature, dark to light red in colour. Blotching may be apparent, but areas of brown discoloration with a sticky surface may indicate that the placenta was diseased. These observations are important should the newborn foal suffer any illness. The placenta, cord and amnion, together with the fluids they contain, are valuable evidence in these cases (see p. 439).

Having checked the membrane and, if necessary, reported abnormalities to the vet, they should be placed immediately in a leakproof plastic sack and tied securely. They may then be placed in an isolated area until such time as the foal is diagnosed as being quite normal, for example, after twelve hours.

They should then be disposed of by burying, burning or in some other manner which avoids any possibility that, should they be contaminated with infection, this will not come in contact with other pregnant mares. This is a particularly important part of good management in the event of an outbreak of viral infection (for example viral arteritis, p. 494; equid herpesvirus 1, p. 488).

Abnormal Birth (Dystocia, Bad Birth)

Birth is a partnership between the mare and her foetus. Abnormal birth encompasses any untoward happening to either or both participants.

Foetal contribution

We have already discussed the problems arising from the malpositioning, malpresentation or malposture of the foetal foal and how this may result in an impeded passage through the bony ring formed by the mare's pelvis around the birth canal (see Figures 13, 14 and 15). Foetal abnormalities are, broadly speaking, either the result of a normally formed foetal foal lying incorrectly or consist of abnormal conformation of the limbs or body. The most common cause of malposture is a depressed reflex state of the foetus, often the result of infection or malfunction of the placenta; in other words, some disease process of pregnancy has diminished the normal activity of the foetal foal. The foetal body and/or limbs with abnormal conformation, may result from the way in which the foal has been lying in the uterus or because the development has been affected by infection and other forms of stress.

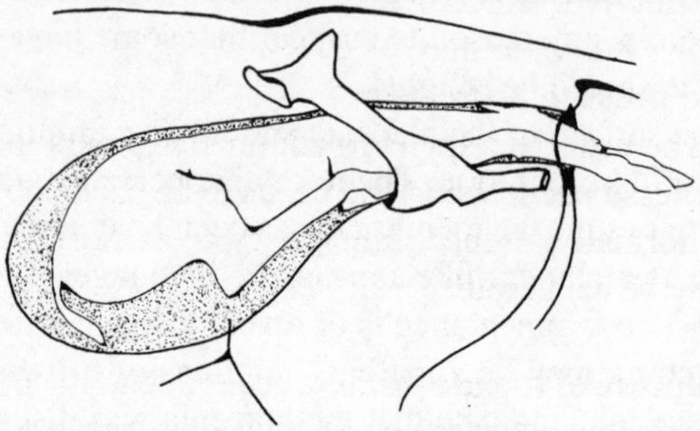

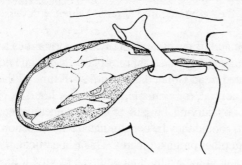

Figure 13
Postural abnormality- hind
legs too far forward

Figure14
Head bent back

Figure 15
Head and forelimbs bent down

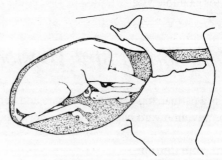

Compression on the umbilical cord restricts oxygen supply to the foetus and may result in death or in cerebral damage causing the newborn foal to be seriously ill (see pp. 448-50). This compression may be caused by the cord becoming entangled around the foal's hind leg or prolapsed in front of the chest as it passes through the birth canal, or it may be the result of the weight of the foal's belly in the final stages of delivery but prior to the foal being able to establish a normal respiratory rhythm.

Maternal contribution

Difficult birth may be the result of imperfect straining or uterine contractions. This condition is often described as uterine inertia. We have already considered this condition in relation to the age of the mare and the apparently instinctive reluctance of mares to strain if the foal is lying incorrectly. However, there may be cases in which uterine inertia has hormonal origins and needs to be treated.

The usual therapy is to administer oxytocin. However, this is obviously a professional decision and needs to be backed by an assessment that the foetus is normally aligned, otherwise the extra stimulus provided by the oxytocin may be dangerous.

Rupture of the uterus may occur due to the powerful contractions against an obstructed passage, as a result of a weakness in the uterine wall or from vigorous movement of the foetal limbs. Rupture may be associated with lack of straining efforts or the tear may only be found after the foal has been delivered normally.

Rupture of the large intestine may sometimes occur and is associated with signs of pain (sweating and rolling, getting up and down) that may be indistinguishable from the normal signs of foaling, except they are more severe and prolonged. Rupture of the intestines is rare but when it occurs it is usually fatal and may prevent the mare from delivering her foal normally.

Uterine torsion is a condition well recognized in breeds heavier than the Thoroughbred, but is probably less common in smaller breeds. In this condition the uterus twists on its long axis, thus preventing any chance of the foal being delivered through the cervix and birth canal.

The condition is very painful and the mare shows signs of severe colic before any chance of going into first- and second-stage labour. In practice, delivery cannot start and it is essential to have veterinary assistance if this condition is suspected. The uterus can then be returned to the normal position under general anaesthesia followed by a laparotomy (an incision through the abdominal wall).

Uterine haemorrhage is of two types. Haemorrhage from the lining of the uterus is less common and certainly less severe in the horse than that experienced by women. The essential difference is that, in the mare, the placenta does not erode the tissue of the uterus as it does in its human counterpart (see p. 391).

At the end of foaling the uterus may contain fluid tinged with blood and this may give the erroneous impression of bleeding on a large scale. This may occur in cases of delayed uterine involution (see below).

The dangerous type of bleeding associated with birth is haemorrhage into the broad ligament, which suspends the uterus (see p. 379). An artery may rupture during second stage or following delivery.

The initial symptom is acute pain: the mare may roll violently, sweat and tremble. Pain is caused by stretching of the peritoneum as the membrane of the broad ligament is dissected by the haemorrhage. Eventually the pressure of the ligament restrains the bleeding or, if the haemorrhage bursts through into the peritoneal cavity, the mare literally bleeds to death, her membranes becoming white, as she collapses gasping in her final death throes.

If the haemorrhage is contained within the membrane it causes symptoms of shock. The mare, besides showing signs of pain, develops a rapid heart beat, a cold clammy sweat, pale membranes turning to jaundice colour and, as the haemorrhage tracks back towards the vagina, a swelling may appear to one side of the vulva and anus.

The outlook for these cases is usually good, although it may take several weeks for the mare to recover fully. Symptoms of pain usually subside within a few days but the mare remains anaemic and slightly jaundiced for much longer.

The haemorrhage into the ligament may be felt per rectum as a large firm swelling in the wall of the uterus. The vet may advise against having the mare mated in the following breeding season. The swelling usually subsides and disappears completely within about nine months.

The bleeding may occur into the wall of the vagina. **Haematomas**, as these sacs of blood are called, bulge into the vagina and may burst, releasing considerable quantities of blood. If the bleeding comes from one of the major branches of the uterine artery, the haemorrhage can be fatal.

Mares foaling for the first time or those that deliver oversized foals or experience difficult delivery for other reasons may suffer **bruising of the vagina** and perineum (the area of the vulva and anus). A complication of haematomas and bruising is infection; in these cases it may be advisable to administer antibiotics for several days following foaling. Those responsible are advised to consult their vets if any signs of these untoward happenings develop following foaling.

A further complication, especially if infection is present, is the development of laminitis (see p. 287). This results from the combination of the products of dead tissue and bacterial infection. The products are toxic and, together with the proteins released into the circulation, cause severe vascular changes with constriction of the blood supply to the foot and consequent laminitic disease. Mares which suffer lameness after foaling, especially if reluctant to move, and stand with their feet bunched under the body and show excessive heat in one or more hooves should be suspected as suffering the acute stage of laminitis. In such cases professional advice should be sought.

Delayed uterine involution is the term used to describe a failure in the normal process of contraction of the uterus following foaling. It is not a specific condition but reflects differences in the degree and rate of elimination of the residual products of pregnancy.

These include foetal fluids which may have escaped through tears in the placenta, debris from the placenta itself and blood, fluid and cells which may have come from the uterine lining. Usually the accumulation (lochia) is expelled or absorbed following birth.

The lochia is normally a brown, somewhat sticky material. The fluid passes from the uterus through the cervix into the vagina and thence is voided to the outside, partly as a result of the uterus contracting and partly as a result of movement by the mare, e.g. walking, trotting, coughing, etc. This is the reason why it is important to turn mares out in a paddock or exercise them in hand in the first few days after foaling.

Normal involution also entails the uterine wall becoming less oedematous (waterlogged) and regaining the tone which is consistent with the barren state, i.e. ready for receiving the stallion's sperm and, after the egg is fertilized, the new conceptus at the start of another pregnancy.

The uterine lining must also be restored to a healthy and receptive state. Thus normal involution is a process involving the voiding of extraneous material and the resolution of the uterine lining into the condition required for 0successful reconception.

This situation may be achieved by the first heat (foal heat) at seven to fourteen days following birth. However, satisfactory resolution at this early stage is probably the exception rather than the rule and in many individuals it takes much longer for the uterus to be ready for reconception to take place.

Uterine prolapse sometimes occurs following delivery. The ligaments of the uterus are stretched by the weight of the foetus and the enormously enlarged uterus during pregnancy. However, they normally retain the organ, but in some instances the restraining mechanism fails and the organ turns inside out, being inverted through the cervix, vagina and vulva.

If this should occur, those present should call immediately for veterinary assistance and, if possible, keep the mare standing until help arrives. This position keeps the organ off the ground but increases the problem of gravitational effects. It is therefore helpful if the organ is supported, employing a moistened pillowcase or sheet.

If the mare is allowed to lie down this removes the gravitational effects but increases the risk of damage from straw bedding. When the mare is lying down it is therefore helpful gently to introduce a sheet under the organ to protect it from the straw.

Prior to the vet's arrival the protruding uterus should be kept wet by washing with normal saline. This may be prepared by adding a level teaspoonful of common salt to every 600 ml (1 pint) of warm water. Sluicing the saline frequently over the surface will keep the surface moist and remove debris.

The vet will replace the organ, probably employing spinal anaesthesia. This technique involves placing a needle between the vertebrae at the base of the tail and injecting an appropriate amount of local anaesthetic. Further measures may include injection of oxytocin to reduce the size of the uterus, anti-inflammatory drugs and antibiotics. Laminitis is always a risk following prolapse.

THE NEWBORN FOAL IN HEALTH

This chapter is intended to provide the reader with an understanding of the healthy foal in terms that lead to an appreciation of ill health. It is only by a knowledge of the normal that we can interpret the abnormal state. For example, the manner in which foals get to their feet is dictated by a nervous reflex action inherent in the species.

Horses raise their foreparts before their hind parts, in contrast to cattle, which use the reverse sequence. Foals instinctively adopt the adult pattern almost from their first efforts to stand and certainly when an hour or two old. Both the manner and the ease with which they achieve the standing position provide a general impression of the health of the foal. If it displays lethargy or difficulty in accomplishing the standing position, we may suspect illness.

Adaptive period

Behaviour of a newborn foal is dictated largely by the urge to seek and suck from the udder. The learning period is remarkably short, considering that the foal has spent all its previous life without either the need for feeding in this manner or the means of coordinating the reflexes of standing and the movement involved in sucking from the mare. Thus, within the space of about two hours, the foal has stood and sucked for the first time, a remarkable achievement of nervous coordination.

This change from a way of life in the uterus to one of independent existence outside requires a period of adaptation in respect of all the organs and functions of the body. This change has to be appreciated if we are to understand the difference between normal and abnormal changes. In the older animal changes occur as a result of outside stimuli rather than as an internal need for adjustment.

For example, the independent individual takes food into its alimentary canal and digests it. The changes which occur in this process do not alter fundamentally; the only variations are related to the type and quality of the food and the demand for energy and growth dictated by age and status.

However, the change from feeding *in utero* to that outside is profound. *In utero* the foal's supply of nourishment comes indirectly from the mare through the placenta. The mare digests food and the products of digestion (amino acids, carbohydrate, fatty acids) cross passively by diffusion or actively by selection through the placenta into the umbilical vein.

Thus the foetal foal has a continuous supply of nourishment in an already digested form. The substances it requires enter its body and are received directly by the liver through the umbilical vein.

After birth, food is imbibed and swallowed; it is digested in the stomach, small and large intestines, absorbed through their walls into the bloodstream, and transported through the portal vein to the liver. Unlike the continuous supply present in the umbilical vein, food is taken at intervals, so that peak levels of nutritive material (amino acids, etc.) may occur. Although these are dealt with adequately by the organs and systems of the body when in health, there may be problems in a premature or otherwise impaired newborn foal.

We may contrast the needs of the newborn with the foetal situation by reference to Table 1.

Dealing with the newborn foal

The essential basis of dealing with a newborn foal is, as with a foaling mare, patience and observation rather than interference, unless there are definite reasons for taking action. Those responsible for foals should therefore make themselves familiar with the normal patterns of behaviour so that they can judge when action is required or when veterinary assistance should be called.

Once the foal has been delivered completely there are a number of duties which those present should perform. The first is to avoid any sudden movement or disturbance within the loosebox which might cause the mare to rise to her feet prematurely.

Most mares, even with several people present in the foaling box, remain lying down for up to twenty minutes after the end of their exertions. During this time the foal turns onto its brisket and withdraws its hind legs from the vagina. The cord remains intact and the circulation of blood between the placenta and the foal gradually diminishes. This means that a substantial quantity of blood is drained from the placenta and received by the foal over the period of two or three minutes.

Premature rupture of the cord may deprive the foal of as much as a third of its circulating blood volume. It is for this reason that mares should be left, as far as possible, undisturbed and encouraged to remain lying down after they have delivered their foal.

Although every effort should be made not to disturb this relationship, it is

Table 1 Essential Differences between Intrauterine (Inside) and Extrauterine (Outside) Life of the Foal

System	Foetal	Newly born
Respiration	Oxygen and carbon dioxide exchange in mare's lungs and transported in maternal bloodstream; exchange at the level of the utero-placental junction	Gases exchanged in foal's lungs, used for first time
Digestive	Mare eats and digests food; products circulate in bloodstream; pass between uterus and placenta into foetal bloodstream. Metabolism controlled by mare	Food taken into alimentary tract and digested; products absorbed into bloodstream. Independent metabolism
Alimentary excretion	Faecal matter stored in caecum, colon and rectum as meconium. Foetus swallows amniotic fluid into stomach but does not defaecate	Meconium (first dung) evacuated within the first 48-72 hours after birth. Subsequently waste material eliminated as dung in the usual independent manner
Urinary	Waste products filtered by kidneys and passed by urine through urachus into placenta (i.e. mixes with allantoic fluid). Kidney function minimal; most waste products pass across placenta into mare's bloodstream to be eliminated in urine of mare	Enormously increased output of kidneys to match increased metabolism and waste products of digestion; volume of urine output correspondingly increased; bladder filled under tension for the first time as urachus closes after birth
Senses (hearing, sight, feeling)	The foetus may hear and certainly has feeling but acuity and response are much reduced	Sight, hearing and feeling are present almost immediately after birth
Temperature control	Body temperature controlled by mare	Balance of heat established by metabolic rate, activity and, in the first six hours, by shivering matched by heat loss through conduction, evaporation and radiation
Neurological function	Nervous system becomes increasingly mature throughout pregnancy. By full term reflex activity is established in preparation for post-natal adaptation but activity while in *utero* is reduced	Neurological basis of reflex activity for getting up, sucking, following the mare and galloping are activated and well established by 12 hours
Coat	In the uterus saturated with fluid; fine hair becoming coarser towards full term	Dry coat and sweating may form part of heat balance

usual, and probably good practice, for someone to be present during the final stages of the delivery in order to assist the foal should this be necessary.

Peeling the amniotic membrane from the foal's head and raising this above any pool of amniotic fluid in which it might take its first breath is unnecessary in a healthy foal but may be life-saving in one that is experiencing breathing difficulties. Because the diagnosis of a sick foal is often only possible in retrospect, assistance for all foals may be justified.

Foals should start regular breathing movements almost as soon as they are delivered. Gasping or delayed onset of a breathing rhythm is indicative that the foal has suffered some problem before or during birth that makes it less healthy than normal. We discuss in the next chapter what measures should be taken in these circumstances.

A further check on the foal's normality is to record the heart rate immediately after the foal is born. This may be accomplished by placing the hand gently on the left (or right) side of the chest over the heart just behind the elbows and counting the number of beats in 15 seconds. If we then multiply that number by four we obtain the number of beats per minute; this should be in the range of 50-100 beats per minute.

If the number of beats is outside this range, especially if the heart rate is slowed, some form of stress is indicated and the foal may not be entirely healthy. An arrhythmic (irregular) heart beat may also denote a problem, although this may be of a temporary nature only.

In performing these duties, as the delivery is completed, anyone present should crouch behind the mare and make slow movements, keeping his/her voice down and trying to be as quiet and unobtrusive as possible. Literally keeping a low profile is recommended for anyone moving round the box, and crouching behind the mare is preferable to standing, particularly if the mare is nervous or inclined to get to her feet. People should avoid walking past the front end of the mare because this may cause her to jump to her feet.

The next duty is to wait discreetly, observing both mare and foal to make sure their behaviour is normal. It is good practice to record on a sheet of paper the time at which the water broke and the time of complete delivery.

The next landmark is the time at which the cord breaks. This may be the result of the mare getting to her feet or the foal struggling in its attempts to stand. In both instances the cord breaks because of a tug.

It should be appreciated that cord thickness varies from relatively thin to quite thick and strong. Very thin ones may rupture as the mare makes her final expulsive effort and shoots the hips of the foal clear of her vagina. This will depend to some extent on the length of the cord itself.

Whatever the method or time of rupture, the cord breaks at a point about 3 cm (1 inch) from the abdominal wall. It will be remembered from Chapter 24 that the cord contains two arteries and a vein. These rupture in such a way that the arteries are immediately sealed and retract into the stump left at the umbilicus (navel).

This describes the usual happenings. However, a number of exceptions may occur. Some cords are quite thick, but they become brittle at the point of rupture providing the cord is left intact and the circulation of blood diminishes with time as already described. However, if the mare gets to her feet prematurely, separation in these cases may be abnormal and the arteries may not contract but may continue to spurt blood.

Pinching the stump between the finger and thumb for a minute or so will usually be sufficient to stop the bleeding completely. If this is not the case a ligature of tape should be applied; it is prudent to have such an item in one's foaling kit (see below).

It is usual to dress the stump of the navel with iodine or antibiotic powder. Before deciding on the approach, those responsible should consider the following points of view. Iodine dries the stump but also damages tissue and causes a hard scab to form. This may seem, therefore, to be an over-harsh approach to the delicate tissues.

Antibiotic powder does no such harm, but it is probable that the mare will lick the foal's coat and the navel, thus removing most of the powder. In any case, the stump seals naturally and the powder will not penetrate into the stump where infection, if it is to occur, will develop.

Because the stump seals on its own, the risk of infection is slight and probably depends more on the condition of the foaling box and on the particular circumstances of the stables. A clean foaling box and allowing the navel stump to form naturally (i.e. without cutting the cord, as used to be common practice) should be sufficient to avoid infection.

If there is a particular problem in the stables, as might result from contamination with a specific virulent microbe, some extra precautions may be necessary. But in these circumstances it is best to obtain veterinary advice. Changing management (for example, using different boxes) and/or the administration of antibiotics by injection in the first few days of life, together with checking on the immune status of the foal (see p. 438), will probably be recommended.

This last precaution may also apply to foals born with abnormally large cords which bleed from the navel or whose navel stump looks abnormal in any way. In addition, if the mare has run milk and the foal has been deprived of its protective antibodies, extra veterinary precautions will be required (see p. 443).

Once the cord has broken, the foal can be left to get to its feet, which it will do after numerous unsuccessful attempts. The duty of those present is to ensure that there is sufficient bedding on which the foal can rest. It will tend to push straw to one side in its struggles and thus allow its hocks to rub on the bare floor below. This may cause sores on the outside of the hocks. Someone should, from time to time, enter the box and rearrange the straw bedding to avoid this happening.

There is little point in trying to help the foal because it has to learn how to coordinate its actions in getting to its feet unaided. However, once on its feet it may be steadied for a minute or two by gently holding the tail. But it should be appreciated that any manipulation of foals at this stage may be resented and be counterproductive in attempts to help rather than hinder its actions.

Helping the foal find the mammary gland and suck requires considerable patience. The adage that you can lead a horse to water but you can't make it drink certainly applies to foals. The temptation to hurry completion of foaling by seeing that the foal sucks from the mare and thus confirms its wellbeing naturally influences those present, especially as foaling takes place mostly at night and the prospect of returning to bed depends on the mare's and foal's cooperation to this end.

The bonding of mare to foal and foal to mare takes place through a combination of sight and smell. Whatever help we give the foal towards obtaining its objective of finding and sucking from the udder, we must be careful not to break or delay this bonding process. The mare smells and tastes her amniotic fluid in which the foal's coat is saturated at birth. This fixes its identity in the mare's memory, eliciting maternal instincts towards the foal and evoking antagonism towards other, foreign, foals.

The foal is much less sophisticated in its instinctive powers of recognition. For the first week or two after birth the bonding of the foal to the mare depends almost entirely on recognition of the udder as a source of food, and it is not particular about whose gland the milk is coming from. It is, however, aware of the shape and movement of its dam and will follow and keep close to her instinctively.

If it strays away and tries to suck from another mare, it is the mare that shows antagonism and rejects the approach. This rejection is the negative aspect of the bonding process and is complemented, in the positive sense, by the foal's own instincts of being attracted to its own dam.

If mares foal outside with other mares present crossing over of one foal for another can occur. This is most likely to happen if foaling takes place on the same night and the mares have not bonded each to her own progeny.

The pedigrees of two Thoroughbreds were shown to be incorrect by blood typing. On tracing back their history it was found that they had been foaled on the same night on a studfarm in Newmarket and had been turned out together in a paddock soon after foaling.

It appears that the foals had switched dams without anyone realising it. This is a rare happening in Thoroughbreds because it is more usual for foaling mares to be segregated for sufficient time to prevent switching because bonding occurs soon after birth. Where mares foal in herds in the open this type of switching may be more common.

The foal should stand on its own for the first time within about an hour of birth. There is considerable variation in this period, depending on the size and strength of the individual. Some foals may get to their feet within 15 minutes of being delivered and others take 90 to 120 minutes. However, at the longer end we are entering a period that may indicate that the foal is abnormal and that professional assistance is required.

Once the foal is on its feet the next objective is to have it sucking from the mare as soon as possible. The average time from birth to sucking for the first time is about two and a half hours. However, foals vary quite considerably in the time taken to find and suck from the udder. It is important that they imbibe a substantial quantity of colostrum at their first suck and that this should occur within the first five or six hours after foaling.

The protective substances (antibodies) in the colostrum are absorbed from the small intestines of the foal, providing it is under about twelve hours of age, but probably the younger it is at the first suck, the more efficient the transfer into the bloodstream. But even more important is the fact that, once protein has been swallowed, the pathway is blocked to further transfer. Thus, if the foal sucks only small amounts over several hours, less antibody is transferred than if a large amount is sucked at first and then the foal does not feed for several hours.

This principle is particularly important if a foal has to be fed by bottle or through a stomach tube for its first feed. However, it should be appreciated that giving ordinary milk before the foal receives colostrum will block the pathway and this must if possible be avoided.

A foal is attracted towards its dam's udder by inborn instincts that depend on certain visual and olfactory (smell) senses. In the first place it is attracted towards dark undersurfaces. Thus it may be seen seeking the brisket, belly and finally the region of the udder. Here it is undoubtedly attracted by the odours emanating from the mammary glands of the mare and also from the milk.

The suck reflex is stimulated by contact with warm soft surfaces, as can be appreciated when the foal's muzzle comes in contact with the mare's skin or tongue in the period after birth before the foal has even got to its feet. It may then be seen with its lips and tongue curled in the manner characteristic of sucking from a teat.

Anyone who has been present at birth and watched a foal getting to its feet and sucking from the mare cannot but help to be impressed with this miracle of nature. We should now turn to how we may help or hinder the foal in this natural process of bonding.

We may use the information of natural behaviour and the instinctive basis on which it is built to avoid some of the pitfalls that may present in helping a foal to establish the sucking relationship with its dam.

Perhaps the simplest basis of help is to mimic the assistance given by the mare. A good dam will stand still while the foal is attempting to reach the mammary glands. However, she will stand in such a way that the udder is tilted towards the foal. To do this the mare flexes the opposite hind leg and straightens the nearside one. Individuals differ in their degree of cooperation with the foal, younger mares being less cooperative than older ones. Some mares are quite ticklish and this is the reason for their non-cooperation.

In other cases the maternal instincts may be such that, especially at first, the mare moves around and even resents the approach of the foal. Holding such a mare by a headcollar and manoeuvring her into a suitable position may be helpful to the foal. If a mare is ticklish and/or resentful, a tranquilliser may be administered under veterinary supervision. Some Thoroughbred studfarms routinely inject every mare foaling for the first time with a tranquilliser after the birth.

We may also mimic the help of the mare by gently pushing the hindquarters of the foal when it is attempting to suck. This support is often displayed by mares: they will turn their heads and lick or nudge the hindquarters of the foal.

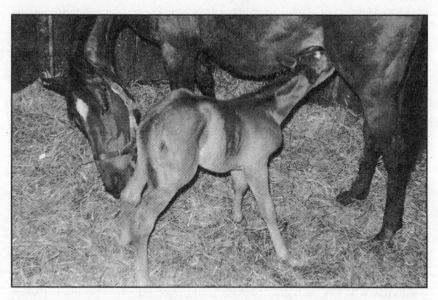

Figure 1   A mare nudging her foal

Assistance in which the front part of the foal is held, as, for example, the head being supported and the lips applied to the teats, may be less helpful or even counterproductive if the foal fights against the restraint. The judgement here must be whether the foal has been given time to attach itself or whether it really requires some assistance because the first suck has been delayed beyond the normal period of, say, three hours.

If this is the case, we should identify the reasons before giving assistance. For example, if the foal is weak, veterinary assistance should be called because the foal may have an underlying disease. The veterinarian will usually administer colostrum through a stomach tube in this instance.

In other cases the foal may be dazed. This may be because it has been frightened for example, by the mare being antagonistic – or confused as a result of an innate dysfunction of neurological coordination, or because happenings in its environment have interfered with the natural process of bonding.

The innate dysfunction may be due to the foal's having suffered oxygen lack or to some circulatory disturbance which is causing pressure in the brain and interfering with the pathways of nervous coordination. This is a veterinary matter and the foal should be treated accordingly. The vet will probably administer drugs that reduce the pressure in the brain at the same time as giving the foal its first feed through a stomach tube.

If the foal has been confused by environmental factors, patience is required, but it may be advisable for the vet to feed the foal through a stomach tube in order to make sure that it receives a full dose of colostrum. An alternative approach is to use a bottle and artificial teat. The foal is fed either standing up or lying on the floor and is then allowed to establish its own relationship with the mare during the course of the next few hours.

The one disadvantage of this approach is that it may cause the foal to seek the artificial teat rather than that of the mare. However, one feed with a bottle is unlikely to lead to this type of misconception.

Perhaps the most important advice in respect of preventing a foal from becoming confused is to be aware of the possibility that human interference may in itself cause this confusion. Because the foal is attracted to dark undersurfaces, it is preferable for attendants to wear light-coloured clothes – white rather than brown overalls, for example. Some foals have become attached to attendants wearing dark overalls, and in the New Forest a pony foal is on record as having become attached to a tree rather than to its mother.

Sounds may also be important to the foal's appreciation of its environment and for this reason any extraneous noise, especially loud sounds, should be avoided in the foaling box.

Finally, the environment of the foaling box should be controlled to avoid dust, too much humidity or undue warmth. The ideal conditions are a minimum amount of dust, especially that emanating from straw and hay, a humidity of 60-90% and an air temperature of 20°C (68°F) plus or minus 3°C (6°F).

The passing of meconium is essential to the wellbeing of the foal. Some individuals have problems in expelling all of this material and may suffer discomfort and colic as a result.

Measures to aid evacuation of meconium are therefore usually routine. Some people like to give castor oil or some other preparation by mouth soon after birth; others may give a concentrated oily solution of vitamins A and D.

There is no harm in any of these procedures providing the medicaments are administered in a scrupulously clean condition. However, care should be taken when selecting a drug to be given in the first forty-eight hours, because during this period the gut is particularly permeable and substances which are not harmful to older foals may be absorbed and cause problems. This has occurred in the USA where administration of an iron preparation to newborn foals was found to be the cause of illness and death.

Enemas and injections of oil into the rectum are also common practices to assist the evacuation of meconium. More recently phosphate buffered solutions (phosphate enema, sodium acid phosphate, sodium phosphate) used for infants have found favour.

The enemas may be administered at any time after birth, although I suggest that they should not be given until the foal has sucked from the mare. At this time it is more tolerant of handling, and there is the added advantage that the enema will coincide with the gastrocolic reflex that stimulates the hind part of the gut when food enters the stomach.

It is important to appreciate that the method of giving enemas and the frequency at which they are given may cause problems. If the nozzle of the tube inserted into the rectum contains any firm or sharp edges or if the instrument is used roughly, this may cause bruising of the anus or even in exceptional circumstances rupture of the rectum. Application requires very gentle handling and the instrument must have a soft, non-abrasive nozzle.

If enemas are given too frequently or in too great a quantity they may cause the rectum to balloon and in itself delay successful evacuation of the meconium.

The loosebox in which the foal is kept should be maintained as free from dust as possible at all times. Straw bedding should be mucked out or rearranged when the foal is at grass or, if this is not possible, it should be moved with the mare temporarily to another box. Foals are particularly susceptible to inhaling dust and this initiates infection of the lungs.

The loosebox should be kept at about 10°C (50°F). Temperatures above or below this are not harmful but cold environments challenge the foal and it has to burn more food just to keep its body temperature normal. At higher temperatures the foal may suffer problems of metabolism associated with keeping its body cool.

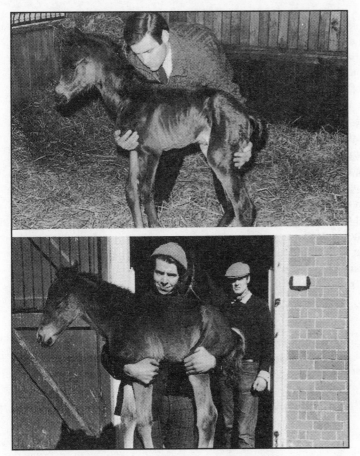

Figure 2   How to pick up and carry a foal correctly

The foal's ability to maintain the balance of heat produced and heat lost (thermoregulation) is compromised if the atmosphere is humid. Humidity may be measured or guessed because there is condensation on the wall. This condensation is most likely to be due to poor insulation of the walls so that the walls are cold relative to the warm, moist atmosphere in the box. Incidentally, condensation may make the foal more susceptible to infection of the lungs.

Steps should be taken to avoid placing the foal in draughts because this may cause excessive heat loss and chilling.

Exercise is as important to the young foal as it is to the mare. Foals and their dams should be confined to their looseboxes for minimum periods. The mare should be exercised up to the time of foaling and, together with her foal, allowed out in a paddock or placed in a large yard or barn when the foal is two days old.

Although facilities and weather conditions may combine to make this impracticable, the problem of restricting a foal to a loosebox and then allowing it freedom may cause it to gallop, and the unaccustomed stress may result in a fractured sesamoid or other injury to the limbs.

In these unfavourable circumstances, therefore, special measures should be taken when the foal is first turned out after several days or weeks of confinement. These measures may include giving the mare her freedom for fifteen to thirty minutes prior to letting her foal join her. This is intended to take the steam out of the mare so that she does not gallop with her foal on first experiencing freedom.

Another approach which might be combined with this is to walk the mare in the paddock for some time prior to letting her loose with her foal. It is the mare and not the foal which usually causes the problem when first freed after a long confinement.

Care of the feet should start at about age two months. If there is abnormal conformation, attention should be paid prior to this but under veterinary supervision (see Chapter 19).

28
CONDITIONS OF THE NEWBORN FOAL

In considering conditions of the foal it is helpful to take account of age, whether or not the condition is infective, and to recognise that although newborn foals are growing they may still be affected by the in between status of life within and outside the uterus. All these considerations apply to conditions which are unique to the age and status of the individual; they also modify those conditions experienced in older and adult horses.

For example, meconium colic is unique in that it is related to the passage of the first dung; once this is passed by about the end of the second day after foaling, the individual will never suffer this particular form of colic again. It is, therefore, a condition peculiar to the first few days of newborn life. Further, it is a non-infective condition, that is, it is not related to microbes and may be distinguished therefore from septicaemic or infective diseases.

Meconium colic is one of a category of conditions with their origins in foetal life or arising from abnormal happenings of birth. One of the major characteristics of these conditions is that the first symptoms appear during the first three or four days after foaling, and often within the first twenty-four hours.

There is logic, therefore, in describing these conditions separately to those developing later. We may also distinguish conditions which are peculiar to the period up to four or five months, that is, up to the time of weaning. These conditions, such as summer pneumonia caused by the microbe *Rhodococcus equi* (p. 478), do not affect older foals or adults, nor are they found in the first few days after foaling.

However, infections do not fit exactly into the categories of the newborn period, the older foal or adulthood. They are ubiquitous and cross the boundaries of definition. For example, infectious disease of the newly born may start *in utero* with symptoms appearing in the first day or two, or even as early as a few hours after birth. However, the same microbe may be present in the environment of the newborn and enter the body through the umbilical stump. Here, they grow in the blood clot formed in the remnants of the umbilical arteries and vein, thus acting as a focus for infection at an older age. This is a classic route for the spread of microbes causing joint ill (infective arthritis) that occurs in foals aged one to three months.

Another route of infection is inhalation of microbes into the lungs or swallowing them in feed. These may result respectively in pneumonia or diarrhoea. These infections occur in both the very early and the later periods and are also responsible for infectious disease in weaned and older foals, yearlings and adults.

A very important consideration in the young foal is its immune status. We discuss in Chapter 27 the way in which immunity is transferred passively to the foal by way of the protective substances (antibodies) in the colostrum. Some individuals do not receive sufficient quantities due to the mare's running milk or for other reasons described above (see p. 431). These individuals are at risk because microbes gaining entrance to the body are not killed by the protective substances and are therefore capable of setting up infection.

This is an example of a failure related to events of the first twelve hours after foaling being the prime cause of diseases which do not appear until the foal is older.

The passive immunity lasts for about six weeks and is then replaced by active immunity gained by the foal's responding to the challenge of infecting microbes in the same manner as an adult responds to infection. However, in the interval between the waning resistance afforded by the antibodies supplied from the mare and the acquisition of new antibodies produced by the foal, infection is more likely to occur. This is one reason why foals aged about six weeks commonly suffer from infectious disease.

Notwithstanding the blurring of definitions, especially of infectious disease, it is convenient to describe conditions of the foal as those occurring in the neonatal or newborn period and those suffered beyond this period and up to the time of weaning.

Conditions of the Newborn (Adaptive) Period (the First Four Days)

The relationship between neonatal conditions and the pre- and intra-natal environment of the foetus is complex. Before birth the foetus may be affected by viral or bacterial infection – e.g. equid herpesvirus 1 (rhinopneumonitis) or *Actinobacillus equuli* – by developmental abnormality, or by placentitis due to hypoxia (shortage of oxygen) or unknown causes. These factors may cause retarded growth, malnourishment or functional immaturity of foetal organs. In these cases the stresses normally imposed by birth and the newborn environment may become disproportionately great. Alternatively, the birth may be abnormal and cause chemical or physical damage to a previously normal, well-developed foetus.

Pre- and intra-natal disturbances account for non-infective conditions such as stillbirth, prematurity and immaturity, developmental abnormalities and states which we will describe under the neonatal maladjustment syndrome (i.e. barkers, wanderers, dummies and convulsive foals).

The term 'stress' applies to abnormal changes in the environment of the foetus at any stage of gestation or birth. It may be acute or chronic, according to the degree of interference produced in the physiological stability of the foetus. Acute stress early in gestation produces foetal death and abortion; in late gestation or during birth it causes stillbirth, delayed onset of respiration, convulsions and other behavioural abnormalities.

Once delivered, the foetus is subjected to extrinsic factors, the most challenging of which are an air environment, gravity, relatively low surrounding temperature, the presence of micro-organisms and the need for alimentation (digestion) and excretion unassisted by the placenta.

No set of conditions which have such diverse, yet interrelated, causes can be classified in other than a broad framework into which further definitions may be introduced as knowledge becomes available. Such a framework is shown in Table 1.

Table 1 Classification of Neonatal Conditions

Infective conditions	
Group I:	Fever, lethargy and reduced strength of the suck reflex
Non-infective conditions	
Group II:	Gross disturbances in behaviour
Group III:	Developmental abnormalities
Group IV:	Immunological reactions between maternal and foetal tissues

Group I: Infective Conditions (Sleepy Foal Disease, Septicaemia, Meningitis)

This group comprises infective conditions characterised by fever, lethargy and reduced strength of suck reflex.

Cause and incidence

Causal organisms include *Streptococcus pyogenes* var. *equi* (*Streptococcus zooepidemicus*), *Escherichia coli*, *Actinobacillus equuli* (*Bacterium viscosum equi*, *Shigella equirulus*), *Staphylococcus aureus*, *Salmonella typhimurium*,

Klebsiella pneumoniae, equid herpesvirus 1 (EHV-1) and cyto-megalovirus, in approximate order of incidence. About 1% of foals are affected, but incidence varies according to geographical area, climate, management and the type and virulence of infecting organisms. In any particular locality the predominant challenging organisms may change from year to year. About 50% of all foal deaths are due to infection.

Predisposing causes
Predisposing factors are chronic uterine endometritis, overcrowding and continual use of foaling boxes, prematurity, artificial severance and ligation of the cord, loss of colostrum before birth and failure to absorb specific antibodies.

Transmission
Prenatal infection may occur by haematogenous spread (i.e. through the blood) or through the amniotic fluid; postnatal infection occurs via the umbilicus or the alimentary tract. It is not usually possible to determine in any particular case whether infection occurred pre- or postnatally. Most of the causal organisms inhabit the alimentary or genital tract of the mare and are a cause of abortion and/or infection of the placenta.

Acute signs of septicaemia may be present within twelve hours of birth and in these cases it is difficult to see how overwhelming infection could begin postnatally. However, to establish a prenatal origin of infection the organism must be recovered from the placenta and/or genital tract of the mare immediately after birth.

Sources of postnatal infection are faeces, contaminated bedding, soil, the mammary region of the mare, feeding utensils, and the hands and clothes of the attendants. Equine infectious anaemia (EIA) may be transmitted through colostrum.

Manner of spread
Localisation in various tissues depends on the nature of the causal organism. *Actinobacillus equuli* has a predilection for kidneys, adrenal glands and brain, and *Sta. aureus* and *S. typhimurium* for articular and periarticular structures including epiphyses. *Str. pyogenes*, *E. coli* and *Klebseilla pneumoniae* are ubiquitous, occurring in lungs, peritoneum, pleura, joints and umbilicus. EHV-1 and cytomegalovirus infect primarily liver and lung tissues.

In practice it is rare to find complete localisation and most cases are partly septicaemic (i.e. blood-borne) and generalised. Traditional classifications have, however, been based on clinical signs and these are often related to the organs most severely affected, for example, joint ill, meningitis, diarrhoea and sleepy foal disease (nephritis). For this reason a summary of the predilections of causal organisms is presented in Table 2, together with a summary of predominant signs, but none of these subdivisions is likely to be found alone in any particular instance.

Table 2 Causes and Symptoms of Infective Conditions

Condition	Synonyms	Characteristics	Aetiology
Generalized infection	Diarrhoea Scours Pleurisy Pneumonia Peritonitis	Fever at 39° C and persisting Diarrhoea Increased respiratory rate, with rales Dehydration, retraction of eyeballs	*Escherichia coli* *Streptococcus* species
Hepatitis	Virus abortion Rhinopneumonitis	Convulsions Lethargy Mild jaundice Leucopenia	Equid herpesvirus 1 Cytomegalovirus
Nephritis	Viscosum Shigellosis Sleepy foal disease Sleeper	Initial fever to 39° C, becoming subnormal Sleepiness Diminished strength of suck Diarrhoea, mild colic Convulsions Uraemia; protein cells in urine Variable leucocytosis	*Actinobacillus equnli*
Meningitis	Convulsions	Fever to 39° C and persisting Convulsions	*Streptococcus* species *Escherichia coli* *Actinobacillus equali*
Encephalitis		Gross disturbances of behaviour Leucocytosis	
Infective arthritis	Joint ill Navel ill	Fever to 39° C and persisting Lameness	*Streptococcus* species *Salmonella typhimurium*
Tenosynovitis		Painful swelling round joints Increasing leucocytosis	*Staphylococcus* species *Escherichia coli*

Symptoms

Although many signs are related directly to the site of infection, in most cases foals show lethargy, reduced strength of the suck reflex and inability to stand and hold the sucking position. Symptoms may appear at any time up to the end of the fourth day after birth but are most common on the second day. They start as slight dullness and a reluctance to feed.

The reduced amount sucked from the mammary glands leaves the udder distended, and milk may drip from the teats so that it stains the face and muzzle of the foal as it makes half-hearted attempts to suck. The rectal temperature at this stage may be normal or slightly raised to 38.9° (102°F).

After several hours, depending on the severity of the condition, the foal becomes increasingly lethargic, disinclined to suck and exhibits definite signs of illness. Rectal temperature may rise to 41°C (106°F), although in many cases it remains below 38.9°C (102°F), especially if the foal becomes comatose; terminally the temperature may become subnormal.

Temperature should be recorded at least every six hours to establish the presence of transitory rises which have diagnostic significance and may be missed by less frequent recordings.

Buccal mucous membranes may become pale, injected or greyish. The conjunctiva may be pale or injected (livid) and the sclera (white of the eye) tinged with jaundice.

Increasing heart and respiratory rates may be present and signs of dehydration include loss of mobility of the skin and retracted eyeballs. Convulsions and extensor rigidity (stiffness) are common neurological signs. A foetid, evil-smelling diarrhoea may develop and be associated with signs of colic, such as rolling or lying in awkward attitudes, such as on the back with the head turned backwards or with a foreleg hung over the poll.

Lameness and painful swelling around the joints are associated with periarticular or articular infections, and rales or dullness over the lung area can be detected in bronchitis and pneumonia.

It is possible to distinguish peracute, acute and chronic cases, but premonitory signs are usually noted by watching carefully. In some instances, however, death occurs suddenly.

Diagnosis
Septicaemia should be suspected if a foal makes half-hearted attempts to suck and after a few swallows of milk lets its head fall down and, with eyelids half closed, allows milk to dribble from its mouth. The foal may also go lame, suffer from diarrhoea or show signs of dehydration. The rectal temperature is greater than 3 8.8°C (102°F). Increasing white blood cell and blood urea counts and the presence of protein in the urine confirm the diagnosis, but a complete diagnosis can only be made when an organism is isolated from body tissues or fluids.

Treatment
Antibiotics should be given immediately infection is suspected, because delay may make this condition less amenable to treatment. For this reason all newborn foals should be observed hourly if managerial conditions allow.

In the absence of laboratory isolation of the causal organism, the choice of a therapeutic agent is subjective (e.g. neomycin sulphate, amikacin, ampicillin, cloxacillin or trimethoprim and sulphadiazine in chloromycetin or amoxycillin). Therapy must be evaluated against the response obtained and treatment continued for at least forty-eight hours after symptoms have subsided.

Dam's plasma or whole blood, cross-matched against the foal's red cells, may be injected into one of the foal's jugular veins using a syringe or transfusion apparatus.

Prevention
Antibiotics can be given during the first few days after birth. The choice of drug and the length of time it should be given is subjective. A regimen of trimethoprim and sulphadiazine, intramuscular neomycin and oral framycetin represent approaches used in practice, but the decision to introduce a preventive programme and the choice of drug are matters for veterinary advice, taking into account local circumstances.

Antibiotic therapy may be supplemented by about 400 ml of donor colostrum fed from a bottle and artificial teat or by stomach tube if gammaglobulin blood levels are below an arbitrarily defined level of 4 g/litre.

Group II: Gross Behavioural Disturbances

This consists of non-infective conditions characterised by gross disturbances in behaviour. We recognise three categories: neonatal maladjustment syndrome (NMS), prematurity and dysmaturity (immaturity) and meconium retention (Table 3).

NEONATAL MALADJUSTMENT SYNDROME (NMS)
(BARKER, WANDERER, DUMMY OR CONVULSIVE SYNDROME)

The term neonatal maladjustment syndrome (NMS) has been coined to include all the conditions listed above. Future research will undoubtedly require the classification to be modified further, but for the present it appears appropriate.

Cause and incidence
The cause of this condition is not fully understood but it is essentially the result of brain haemorrhage or swelling around the nerve cells of the brain due to waterlogging (oedema). The haemorrhages may result from low oxygen concentrations (hypoxia) in the blood and episodes of low and/or high blood pressure surges in the blood circulating through the brain.

Such combinations (hypoxia and alternating low and high blood pressure)

Table 3 Causes and Symptoms of Gross Behavioural Disturbances

Conditions	Synonyms	Characteristics	Aetiology
Neonatal maladjust -ment syndrome (NMS)	Barkers Wanderers Dummies Convulsions	Full-term gestation Onset within first 24 hours: often normal until onset Complete loss of suck reflex and ability to nurse Apparent blindness Convulsions, hypertonus, spasms Coma Hypothermia Acidaemia, hypercapnia	Asphyxia Birth trauma Foetal stress
	Respiratory distress	Low PaO_2 breathing air and 100% oxygen Respiratory rate and minute volume increased Tidal volume decreased	
Prematurity		30–320 days gestation Signs apparent at birth Weakness, delay in first standing Low birth weight Reduced strength of sucking, ability to suck and ability to maintain body temperature Tendency to colic after feeding 'Bedsores' Discoloured tongue, silky skin PaO_2 low breathing air; increased breathing 100% oxygen	foetal stress
Dysmaturity	Immaturity	More than 320 days gestation but appearance and signs of prematurity Emaciation, dehydration Diarrhoea Susceptibility to infection	Foetal stress Placentitis
Meconium retention	Stoppage Ileus	Signs from birth to third day Straining, colic, lying in awkward postures Generally not off suck and in good health Abdominal tympany	Unknown

PaO_2 = arterial oxygen pressure.

may result from exaggeration of the normal effects of the birth process and also from damage to the chest (e.g. fractured ribs), leading to damage of the heart muscle and consequent impairment of the circulation.

Damage to the brain causes convulsions and severe behavioural problems, which in turn lead to disturbances in the balance of organ function on which stability of fluid electrolyte and gaseous exchange is based. These disturbances lead in turn to further neurological problems as they cause further bleeding and waterlogging of the brain.

Symptoms

Behavioural signs usually occur during the first twenty-four hours of life, most commonly during the first hours. The foal may appear normal at first, but becomes affected by convulsions of a jerky (clonic) or general type.

There is a complete loss of the suck reflex and the ability to nurse, although both faculties were present originally. The foal may be unable to stand or may make violent and aimless galloping movements with its limbs; at the same time it may dash its head against the floor. Head and neck and increased extensor tone may be present, the limbs extended and the tall held upright.

Convulsions may be followed by or may alternate with periods of coma. Signs of irritability are manifest by continual chewing, grinding the teeth, sneezing and wandering aimlessly round the box. When able to stand, the foal may appear blind and walk into or press against walls or other objects.

The affected foal may show exaggerated response to handling and restraint. Normal reflex behaviour may continue after stimulation has been removed and certain patterns of behaviour may become displaced.

For example, a foal may suck a teat on a bottle whether or not it is receiving milk, and continue to suck until the teat is removed from its mouth, when it goes into a deep sleep. Some foals exhibit determined sucking motions with the head extended and directed downwards, but seem unable to adopt a sucking attitude under the mare and fight violently against being held in that position. Affected foals often lie in awkward positions and have a tendency to go into a deep sleep when laid on the ground.

Not every case is affected by all the behavioural signs described. Some foals do not convulse, but show loss of suck reflex and wandering; others may be able to suck at a bottle but lose the ability to suck from or even recognise their mothers.

The rectal temperature depends on the activity of the foal. It rises to 41.1°C (106°F) and is accompanied by profuse sweating during convulsions, and falls during coma to 35°C (95°F), remaining within normal limits in mild cases or during convalescence.

Prominent symptoms of respiratory distress (rapid breathing rate) and circulatory failure (jugular pulse and venous engorgement) are commonly associated with this condition.

Course of condition
Signs of NMS may continue for several hours or it may take up to thirty days for the foal to be capable of sucking and following its mother. When recovery occurs it is usually complete. Convulsive foals recover in a definite sequence, first exhibiting coma and then the ability to get up and stand. Auditory and visual awareness return before the ability to suck and recognise the mare.

Diagnosis
Pathognomic (diagnostic) signs of NMS are sudden. There is complete loss of the suck reflex and of visual and other senses, including the ability to seek or follow the mare. Respiratory distress is defined by an increase in the respiratory rate, small amounts of air being inhaled at each breath, and low levels of oxygen in the blood.

Treatment
Symptomatic and supportive treatment is required, aimed at allowing time for the foal to re-establish its bodily means of adapting to the newborn environment. For example, if it is unable to suck, it must be fed through a stomach tube until it learns and is able to do so in the normal manner.

  Behaviour and convulsions   A foal unable to get up or stand unaided should be kept under close observation with, if practicable, an attendant always in the box to prevent it from exhausting itself in its attempts to stand.

  The attendant should sit with the foal's head resting on his/her lap, the animal being restrained in the recumbent position by placing a hand on the undersurface of its head, so that in periods of struggling the muzzle can be raised. At the same time the upper foreleg is held so that the attendant can lean back and avoid being kicked by the hind legs.

  It is helpful for a second person to grasp the tail of a foal which is convulsing or struggling violently, to keep the foal's body at right angles to the person at the head. The legs should not be held together since this may exacerbate the foal's struggles. If the foal is on its own, a soft surface such as a rug should be provided.

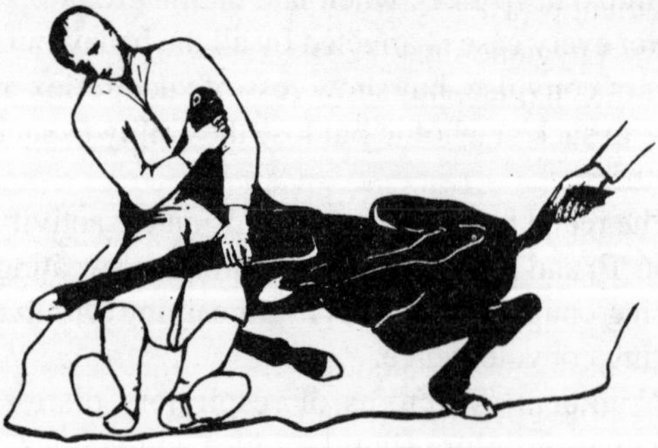

Figure 1   Handling a convulsing foal

Convulsions can be controlled by various types of anticonvulsant drugs including barbiturate and diazapines.

Once the convulsions have been brought under control, the foal accepts restraint and sleeps on a rug or the lap of an attendant with only an occasional movement. It is helpful to reduce the usual stable noises. Vigorous restraint should be avoided wherever possible to minimise the risk of cardiac failure.

Feeding   In the absence of a suck reflex the foal should be fed through a rubber or plastic stomach tube with an outer diameter of about 1 cm and a blunt distal end. The tube should be lubricated with water or liquid paraffin and may be passed with the foal either standing or recumbent.

The end of the tube should not be passed beyond the entrance to the thorax. Before withdrawal it should be flushed with normal saline to prevent milk being deposited in the nasal passages. If the suck reflex is present, a bottle with an artificial lamb's or calf's teat may be used if the foal has lost the ability to suck from the mare.

Clinical experience suggests that a foal up to one week old should be fed according to the following principles:

1. In the first three days after birth the quantity and frequency of feeding are important.
2. Where a normal suck reflex is present, the foal's appetite is a rough guide to the quantity of fluid necessary. If adequate quantities are given, the foal should sleep readily after feeding and yet appear hungry at a subsequent feed.
3. Mare's milk or reconstituted dried milk may be fed at the rate of 150-200 ml/kg bodyweight/day, divided into a minimum of ten equal feeds. A foal of 50 kg bodyweight would then be fed 7-10 litres/day.

Digestive upsets associated with the explosive growth of pathological coliform bacteria are less serious when small feeds are given frequently. The dry matter of liquid diets should be somewhere between 15 and 20%, which is approximately double that of skimmed cow's milk. A number of proprietary dried milk preparations are available and these should be reconstituted using sufficient powder to provide a 50-kg foal with about 4000 kilocalories a day.
4. Strict hygiene should be practised and it is important to feed at 38°C (100°F) or below, but never above.

The advice given here provides a rough guide to the approach to feeding foals that cannot feed for themselves from the mare. However, it should be emphasised that the proper course for the reader is to seek the advice of his/her veterinarian whenever a sick foal is encountered. Cases differ both in the terms of diagnosis and their requirements, so general advice does not necessarily hold good for the particular.

Hypothermia   Body temperature represents the balance of heat produced by metabolism and heat loss by radiation, conduction, convection and evaporation. In the foal the basis of heat production is shivering and muscular activity in movement. A normal foal can maintain its temperature against very low surrounding temperatures, but one suffering from coma and hypoxia, which prevent normal oxygen metabolism, requires special measures.

Mildly affected cases of NMS can be kept warm by fitting a woollen pullover over the body. Severely affected foals require ambient temperatures of 26.6-32.2°C (80-90°F). Radiant heat sources are the most effective, but if these are not available the foal may be covered with a washable electric blanket or rug. Hot-air blowers have some effect, but they create draughts and thereby increase heat loss by evaporation.

As a general measure box walls, ceilings and windows should be adequately insulated to reduce loss of radiation. It has been estimated that most heat is lost in other species by this route.

Homeostasis (blood content stability)   For clinical purposes it may be assumed that foals affected by convulsions, severe diarrhoea or those that fail to establish a normal respiratory rhythm suffer from acidic blood.

Cardiac failure   Cardiac embarrassment can be recognized by a heart rate greater than 120 beats/minute at rest, a marked jugular pulse and evidence of venous engorgement.

Prevention

There are no specific measures which can be taken to prevent NMS. As far as possible the cord should be left intact after birth until the placental circulation has ceased and a respiratory rhythm is established. Any action liable to place increased stress on the foal when it is getting to its feet and sucking for the first time should be avoided. During the first two hours after birth, the foal should be handled as little as possible.

ASPHYXIA NEONATORUM (FAILURE TO BREATHE AFTER BIRTH)

There is evidence in several species that the foetus makes episodic breathing movements *in utero* associated with rapid eye movement sleep (REMS). The significance of this activity is unknown at the present time, but it may form part of neuromuscular preparation for extra-uterine existence.

The stimuli for the first breath and subsequent rhythmic respiratory movements following delivery are tactile, cold and chemical, that is, decreasing arterial oxygen pressure (PaO_2) and increasing arterial carbon dioxide pressure (PaO_2).

The foal may gasp as the chest is being delivered, but the onset of respiration and the establishment of rhythmic movements of the chest and abdomen usually occur within 30 seconds of the hips passing out of the birth canal.

Alterations in blood gases may assume pathological proportions because of undue pressure on the umbilical cord during second-stage labour before the thorax has been completely delivered. Pressure may be caused by the cord being squeezed by the abdomen as it passes through the maternal pelvis, by posterior presentation or by an unusually large chest relative to the maternal pelvis. Other causes of pathological asphyxia are prematurity, inflammation of the placenta or prolonged manipulation to correct abnormal labour (dystocia). In theory changes in maternal uterine bloodflow during birth may affect gaseous placental exchange to the detriment of the foetus, but as yet there is no evidence to support this. A further aspect which must be considered is that a foetus which has already been subjected to stress during development may be detrimentally affected by the usual asphyxial processes. These are physiological to a normal foetus.

Resuscitation
The newborn foal may be delivered with no signs of breathing (primary apnoea) but the gasping which follows will expand the lungs and, provided the airways are clear, spontaneous rhythmic breathing will be established. Respiratory stimulants are therefore unnecessary and all that is required is to ensure that the nostrils are not obstructed. In terminal apnoea (prolonged shortness of breath) the respiratory centre does not respond to stimulants and resuscitation is essential.

Since it is not possible to distinguish primary from secondary apnoea in a newly delivered foal, any individual that fails to establish a respiratory rhythm within 30-60 seconds should be resuscitated in the following manner. The foal's head should be extended and the nostrils cleared of amnion and mucus. The operator should kneel between the foal's head and forelegs, placing the right hand under the foal's muzzle, and inflate the lungs either by inserting a rubber tube attached to an oxygen cylinder into the upper nostril and allowing gas to flow at a rate of approximately 5 litres/ minute, or by applying the mouth to the upper nostril.

In both these methods the under nostril is closed with the right hand while the left hand is free to seal the upper nostril around the rubber tube or mouth. The lungs are inflated by positive pressure, but care must be taken not to overinflate. It is necessary to move the chest only a perceptible amount to cause a substantial rise in arterial oxygen pressure. After inflating by either method both nostrils are released to allow exhalation of carbon dioxide. This inflating should be maintained at the rate of about twenty-five a minute until a spontaneous rhythm is established.

Endotracheal intubation provides a more efficient means of lung inflation because it avoids accidental inflation of the stomach, but once the foal is conscious the tube must be withdrawn to prevent excessive struggling.

Depending on the course of the condition, which is related to the amount of hypoxia, acidity of the blood and consequent cerebral damage, the foal should be further sedated and any convulsions controlled by phenytoin and by gentle restraint.

STILLBIRTH

Many cases of stillbirth are presumably the consequence of cord obstruction or placental disturbance during second-stage labour, causing the foal to be born without any signs of breathing. In the absence of adequate measures of resuscitation, death is recorded as a stillbirth.

PREMATURITY, IMMATURITY AND DYSMATURITY

Considerable confusion surrounds the terms 'prematurity', 'immaturity' and 'dysmaturity'. In human medicine the term 'small for dates' has been used to acknowledge the fact that maturity is a relative state and that quality rather than length of gestation is the major factor. A pregnancy ending close to the average length may, in any species, result in an undersize, weak and at-risk individual. The term 'prematurity' signifies a shortened pregnancy, usually taken as a foal born within 320 days of the last mating. 'Immaturity' and 'dysmaturity' are interchangeable terms. 'Dysmaturity' describes foals that are small for dates and suffering from deprivation due to placental dysfunction or insufficiency. Newborn maturity implies the ability to adapt to the extra-uterine environment, but the definition must be qualified by the extent to which the environment nowadays can be artificially altered.

In horses, the wide size variation between breeds – even within a breed – makes birthweight a somewhat unreliable parameter against which to measure maturity.

Programming fetal development
In recent years groups of medical researchers have been becoming increasingly interested in the effects of the development of microstructure during fetal life and conditions in the newborn and later life. It has been found that each organ of the body is programmed in its development to a stage which is complete at or soon after birth. For example, the number of glomeruli in the kidney is laid down so that the total number in each kidney is present at birth and will not increase subsequently. The same applies to such microstructures as the terminal airways in the lung.

The effect of what is termed intrauterine growth retardation (IUGR) is that the numbers present at birth may be less than in the affected individual than normal.

Again, an example may help understanding. It has been shown that infants suffering from sudden cot death often have a reduced density (number per gram) of terminal airways in the lung and glomeruli in the kidney which makes them susceptible to the effects of challenges, such as infection, which would not be the case normally.

The relationship between IUGR and conditions in later life have now been established through surveys based largely on the birthweight of infants in relation to heart conditions, high blood pressure and other conditions in adult life. Experiments have shown that other species, such as the sheep, suffer the same cause and effect relationship, i.e. permanent functional sub capacity as the result of manipulation of the fetal environment at various stages of development. Feeding sheep on a low then a high plane of nutrition during pregnancy may cause increase to blood pressure in the individual throughout its postnatal life.

Many of these relationships are subtle and not appreciated in terms of illness but merely in a sub functional capacity that is only apparent when the individual is challenged in above average conditions of the environment or of performance.

This connection between fetal development and subsequent performance status in later life is of particular interest with respect to horses because of the demands made on them for athletic performance. Work is currently in progress in the collaborative study between this author's group and Dr Paul Sibbons at Northwick Park Hospital, Harrow. Preliminary results suggest that horses may be somewhat different to other species in that structural development continues in many organs after birth for at least 6 months *postpartum*. The aim of the study is to identify whether or not intrauterine growth retardation in the horse could limit the individuals capacity to perform and, even, be related to such conditions as EIPH (exercise induced pulmonary haemorrhage). It is too early to reach any conclusions in this edition, but perhaps at the next.

The point of importance is that there is undoubtedly a relationship between conditions that occur during fetal life that may have subtle or profound effects on the individual after birth; from slight limitations in performance to an inability to survive or to become markedly unsound.

Group III: Developmental Abnormalities

These are composed of developmental deformities. Hyperflexion (contracture) of the forelimbs is the most common abnormality and this condition is described in Chapter 19.

Table 4 Developmental Abnormalities Seen in the First Weeks of Life

Conditions	Synonyms	Characteristics
Hyperflexion of limbs	Contracted tendons	Range from uprightness of fore- or hind legs to knuckling over at the fetlock and/or inability to extend knee joints
Hypoflexion of limbs	Weakness Down on pasterns	Laxity of ligaments Muscle hypotonia
Parrot jaw	Overshot jaw Parrot mouth	Upper and lower incisors overlapping by degrees varying from 1 mm to 3 cm, molars also overshoot at front and back
Umbilical urachal fistula	Pervious urachus	Wet cord stump, maybe dripping Often necrotic tissue present on both sides of abdominal wall
Congenital abnormalities of genito-urinary tract		
Patent bladder	Ruptured bladder	Signs appear two to three days after birth: may be confused with meconium
colic		
Deviation and shortening of the maxillary bones and asymmetry of the mandibles	Squiffy face	Often the tongue is held to one side and the foal has difficulty in sucking
Atresia coli Anal agenesis	Incomplete alimentary tract	Signs of meconium colic becoming increasingly severe and unremitting
Cleft palate		Regurgitation of milk down nostrils soon after or during feeding
Microphthalmia	Button eyes	Blindness
Scrotal hernia		Soft swelling in scrotum due to descent of abdominal contents. Appears in first few days or immediately following birth; often resolves spontaneously but may become strangulated
Cardiac septal defects Persistent truncus		Sudden death, fainting and/or respiratory embarrassment with rapid heart rate and murmurs
Hare lip		
Hydrocephalus		Excessively dome-shaped forehead
Omphalocele	Hernia	Open abdominal floor
Absence of urachus Megavesica		Dystocia due to size of bladder. If delivered, foal may suffer from acute maladjustment, usually fatal
Ectopic lung		Respiratory embarrassment if in chest and swelling if on ventral aspect of neck

Inherited abnormalities, (e.g. parrot jaw) are the result of dominant or recessive genes in the individual's makeup or are caused by damage to chromosomes at the time of fertilisation of the egg. Many defective individuals are aborted early in pregnancy, as is the case in other mammals.

Drugs given to the mare, especially in the period of the first month or two following conception when the foetus is developing rapidly, may be the cause of deformities such as cleft palate.

Later in pregnancy, illness of the mare, the administration of drugs, infection and damage to the placenta may cause deformities such as hyperflexion or hypoflexion (weakness) of the fore- and hind limbs, absence of parts of the gut or other faults in development.

The position in which the foal lies in the uterus may cause some deformities, especially those affecting the skeleton (e.g. skewing of the spine and deviation from the midline in the limbs).

The developmental abnormalities commonly encountered in foals in the first week of life are shown in Table 4.

Group IV: Immunological Reactions between Maternal and Foetal Tissues

This group is composed of immunological conditions, such as haemolytic disease or combined immunodeficiency of Arabian horses (see p. 738).

HAEMOLYTIC DISEASE

Haemolytic disease is the result of differences in inherited structure of foetal and maternal red blood cells. The foetal cells contain antigens not present in maternal cells. That is, the mother has not inherited these blood cell types from her parents, whereas the foetus has inherited them from its father.

Red cells cross from the foetal into the maternal bloodstream and provoke an antibody response in the mare similar to that stimulated by the administration of vaccine. The antibodies become concentrated in the colostrum and absorbed from the foal's stomach after it has sucked for the first time. They circulate in the foal's bloodstream, attach themselves to the surface of the foal's red cells and cause them to clump and break down (haemolysis).

The ability of these antibodies to be absorbed through the lining of the gut is limited to the first twelve to twenty-four hours after birth. This enables us to prevent the occurrence of haemolytic disease if we can diagnose that a mare is likely to give birth to an affected foal. This can be achieved by testing blood samples two to three times over a period of weeks prior to the expected date of foaling.

Symptoms

Affected foals become sleepy and may yawn repeatedly. If exerted or excited, their breathing and heart rates increase very markedly and the pulse may be observed in the jugular furrow of the neck.

Jaundice develops in the whites of the eyes and on the visible mucous membranes of the mouth and vagina in the case of fillies. Urine becomes red in colour.

Symptoms may appear on the first, but more often on the second, day after foaling. The severity of the case varies depending on the number of red cells destroyed.

If the case is very acute the first symptoms may be collapse and the foal becomes moribund. Less severe cases show symptoms described above.

Diagnosis

The diagnosis is made on symptoms and laboratory examination of the blood. Profound anaemia and haemolysis, together with the detection of antibodies, confirms the diagnosis.

Treatment

The damaged red cells must be replaced and this is achieved by administering a blood transfusion. The best source of red cells is the mare's blood, but these have to be washed free of the mare's serum so as not to introduce further antibody into the foal. This is, of course, a veterinary decision and treatment.

When a mare has been diagnosed as having been sensitised to her foetal foal's red cells, the foal should be muzzled for up to thirty-six hours after birth and the mare's udder stripped of colostrum. It is important that the foal should receive another mare's colostrum in the first feed and then reconstituted dried milk and subsequent feeds until it is aged about thirty-six hours.

Infectious Diseases

Infection is a subject with which all readers will be familiar because it affects both themselves and their horse.

The story of infection is one of a battle between two sides: the microbes or parasites and the horse. The reactions of the horse to the presence of the infecting agent are the symptoms of the disease. These symptoms are typical of diseases such as influenza, metritis (infection of the uterus) and virus abortion. The chapters are written to enable the reader to associate a particular disease with a particular microbe.

Causes and symptoms are described, and the reader may thereby gain an understanding of each condition likely to be encountered. Recognition of symptoms is important at the early stages of disease so that professional advice may be sought in time for treatment to be effective.

An understanding of the way in which infectious disease develops is also important for the practice of good management to ensure that logical and effective control measures are established. The same principles of control apply to parasitism. It is important therefore for the reader to understand how microbes and parasites spread from one individual to another, and how they spread throughout the body and, finally, the manner in which they leave the body to infect others.

This section consists of chapters that describe:

* The bacteria, viruses and other microbes that infect horses;

* In detail, the main bacterial diseases;

* Diseases caused by viruses and protozoa;

* Parasites that infest horses.

29
THE CAUSES OF INFECTIOUS DISEASES

Infectious diseases are caused by living organisms, most of which are very small. In fact, they are so small that individually they cannot be seen by the human eye unaided. We call them micro-organisms or microbes because we need a microscope in order to see them. There are many different kinds of micro-organisms, which are grouped according to how they grow and reproduce. These groups are called viruses, bacteria, mycoplasma, chlamydia, rickettsia and fungi.

Two other groups of organisms must also be included when considering the causes of infectious disease, and these are protozoa and parasites. They are not always quite as small as micro-organisms.

Infection implies that a micro-organism has become established in the body's tissues or on its surface and reproduces itself at the body's expense. It may live outside (extracellular) or inside (intracellular) the body's cells. Its presence causes damage (alteration of function) and death (necrosis) of the cells, and this results in the symptoms of disease usually characteristic of the particular organism involved.

The terms 'virulence' and 'pathogenecity' are used to describe the ability of an organism to enter the body, set up disease and cause symptoms. A pathogen is an organism capable of causing disease; a virulent pathogen is one which readily sets up infection and produces severe symptoms. A venereal pathogen is one transmitted at coitus from male to female or the reverse.

Such organisms enter the body by way of one of several routes: through the mouth (by being swallowed); through the nostrils (by being inhaled); through the skin (by way of wounds, injected by insects, or directly, for example, certain worms burrow through the skin); through the urinogenital tract; or through the conjunctiva of the eyelids.

Identification of the organism causing an infectious disease determines the treatment and prognosis of the disease and the likelihood of spread to other horses.

Bacteria

Bacteria, probably the best-studied group of infective agents, are usually single-celled organisms which occur in a wide variety of forms. They are distinguished from other unicellular organisms such as protozoa in that they contain no nucleus, but they have a special nuclear apparatus with only a single strand of the genetic material DNA (deoxyribonucleic acid). They can be found free-living in soil and water or within a host - a plant or an animal. They have a rigid cell wall which supports and protects them, and most can be cultured on laboratory media.

Bacteria were observed directly as early as 1683 by a Dutch lens maker, Antonine van Leeuwenhoek, but problems of isolation and cultivation took another two hundred years to solve, despite suggestions by von Plenciz, in 1762, that these very small organisms might be the specific cause of certain diseases.

Louis Pasteur is the person whom everyone thinks of as the founder of bacteriology and this claim is certainly true, but there were many others working in the field between 1870 and 1885 who are remembered every day as names of bacteria: Neisser, Loeffler, Welch, Klebs and Shiga, to name but a few.

Pasteur studied the infectious nature of disease and how it was passed from host to host, which were not necessarily of the same species. He demonstrated the cause of anthrax and how to protect against the disease by vaccination. However, this principle had already been demonstrated by Jenner who, in 1796, showed that infection with the mild disease called cowpox conferred a high degree of protection against the virulent smallpox infection.

Pasteur also showed that there were some infective particles much smaller than those which could be seen by the new magnifying instrument, the microscope. When passed through the filters which retained bacteria these particles were able to produce disease. These filterable agents were called viruses.

A further important discovery was made by Joseph Lister, who was Professor of Surgery at Glasgow Royal Infirmary. He was both interested and concerned in postoperative sepsis, which caused high fatality in hospital patients at that time. He applied Pasteur's observations to the problem and showed that sepsis could be prevented by the use of carbolic acid, which killed bacteria in the wounds and in the air. Antiseptic techniques were introduced in 1867.

Normal flora

In the healthy horse (and man) bacteria live on the skin, in the mouth, around the teeth, in the upper respiratory tract, in the genital tract of the female, and on the external genitalia of the male; they also exist in very large numbers in the gut, particularly in the large intestine. These bacteria constitute what is called the normal flora. They play an important role in the gut in helping to break down food, especially in herbivores, forming a finely balanced, mutually advantageous relationship with the host.

Table 1   Bacteria Associated with the Normal Flora

Site	Bacteria
Mouth, nose and respiratory tract	*Acinetobacter* species *Bacillus* species *Bacteroides* species *Fusobacterium* species *Micrococcus* species *Moraxella* species *Pasteurella* species *Staphylococcus* species *Streptococcus* species *Veillonella* species
Gastro-intestinal tract	*Anaerobic cocci* *Bacteroides* species *Clostridium* species *Enterobacter* species *Escherichia coli* *Klebsiella* species *Proteus* species *Pseudomonas aeruginosa* *Rhodococcus (Corynebacterium) equi* *Streptococcus faecalis*
Mare's genital tract	*Bacteroides fragilis* *Micrococcus* species *Staphylococcus* species *Streptococcus* species
External clitoris	*Bacteroides* species *Bacillus* species *Clostridium* species *Corynebacterium* species *Fusobacterium* species *Proteus* species *Pseudomonas* species *Veillonella* species

The bacteria in the normal flora do not, on the whole, produce disease in the host, except under special circumstances (see below), but it is common to find potential pathogens among them. If these bacteria are present and the horse is not showing symptoms of the disease, such an organism is said to be 'carried' and the host is called the 'carrier'.

The normal flora are established soon after birth and certainly within the first few days of life, transmitted from the mother and the surroundings. It is thought that the normal flora are able to protect the host to a certain extent from infection by pathogens. For example, the bacteria present on the horse's external genitalia may protect the individual from becoming infected with venereal microbes (for example, *Klebsiella* or *Pseudomonas* – see p. 483).

Types of bacterial infections

Bacterial infections can be divided into three groups, according to the manner in which the organism gains entry to the host, in this case the horse. Group 1 includes infections caused by physical breakdown of the skin, which then allows bacteria from the outside to gain entry to the body. Group II includes infections caused by access of bacteria to sensitive tissue within the body, for example, via the respiratory, alimentary or genital tract or the conjunctiva. Group III consists of infections caused by bacteria present within the normal flora.

Having entered the host, bacteria seek out a site or situation where they are able to grow and produce substances called toxins and other metabolites responsible for the clinical symptoms that characterise the particular disease.

Group 1: Infections caused by the physical breakdown of the skin

Skin is an efficient barrier to infection, but once it is breached, bacteria invade susceptible tissue. For example, streptococci and staphylococci may be present in eczematous sores on the skin following abrasions from harness or wounds caused by splinters or other foreign bodies. Minor skin infections are an everyday occurrence.

Wound infections usually result from an accident, but occasionally surgical wounds break down and allow infection to become established. The microbes which infect wounds are opportunist: they are those which happen to be there at the time. Organisms of faecal origin and those which live or survive in the soil are prevalent in infections of the foot and cuts and wounds on the legs.

This is particularly important if wounds are deep and dirty. Dirt represents dust, soil and faecal material, all rich in microbial flora. Many of these organisms grow in the absence of oxygen. One such organism is the bacterium which causes tetanus, *Clostridium tetani* (see p. 475). This microbe is present in soil and faeces but is normally unable to penetrate the skin. However, when in a deep or dirty wound, it can grow in the absence of oxygen, producing its toxin with often fatal results.

When one considers the origin of this type of infection it is unlikely that only one bacterial species is causing the infection; many different types of organisms are normally involved. For example, twelve different bacterial species have been identified from an equine foot abscess. This is very important when treatment is being considered because different organisms require different treatment.

Another source of infection is the skin itself. Bacteria which live on the skin can cause infection if the skin is broken and they are able to penetrate the underlying tissue. Abscesses are a very important form of sepsis because they often form deep in the body and are walled off by a barrier of inflammatory reaction (see Chapter 37). This often makes them difficult to treat by antibiotics alone and surgical drainage may be necessary.

Table 2 Bacteria Associated with Wounds and Abscesses

Aerobes	*Escherichia coli*
	Proteus species
	Pseudomonas aeruginosa
	Staphylococcus aureus
	Streptococcus zooepidemicus
Anaerobes	*Bacteroides fragilis*
	B. melaninogenicus
	Clostridium perfringens
	C. septicum
	C. tetani
	Peptococcus species
	Peptostreptococcus species

A list of bacteria which might be expected to be isolated from wound infections is given in Table 2. The terms 'aerobe' and 'anaerobe' refer to the ability of the bacteria to grow in conditions where oxygen is present (aerobe) and where it is absent (anaerobe).

Animal bites are another source of wound infection. Here the bacteria associated with the teeth of the biting animal are the chief source of infection, plus those on the skin of the bitten horse as shown in Table 3.

Burns may also become infected and, again, it is the opportunist microbes which get in first. The bacterium *Pseudomonas aeruginosa* is often associated with burns.

Table 3 Bacteria Associated with Bites and Burns

Bacteroides species
Escherichia coli
Fusobacterium species
Pasteurella species
Pseudomonas aeruginosa
Staphylococcus species
Streptococcus zooepidemicus

Group II: Infections caused by access of bacteria to sensitive tissue within the body

In this group microbes are transmitted from one infected individual to another healthy animal, either directly or indirectly. A common method of host-to-host transmission is by aerosol. Very fine droplets of water or particles of dust containing microbes are inhaled and, because they are so small, they penetrate to the nasopharynx and even to the lungs.

Aerosol transmission is most common with viruses. However, certain bacteria, such as *Bordetella bronciseptica* and *Rhodococcus equi* (formerly called *Corynebacterium equi* – see p. 481), which cause respiratory infection, and *Streptococcus equi*, the causative agent of strangles (see p. 474), can be transmitted by aerosol. Strangles can also be transmitted by direct contact, horse to horse, or by indirect contact, that is, a horse can be infected from a contaminated stable, horsebox or even paddock which has recently been used by an infected animal.

Whether infection is by inhalation of contaminated dust particles or by ingestion by licking or using contaminated water buckets, etc., is irrelevant to the disease process (see Table 4).

The best example of transmission of bacteria by direct contact is venereal disease. The bacterium which causes contagious equine metritis (CEM – see p. 481) is a true venereal pathogen - in the natural environment it is only transmitted from mare to stallion and stallion to mare at coitus, or from an infected mare to her foal at birth or to her foal at foot.

The bacterium, formerly called *Haemophilus equigenitalis* and now called *Taylorella equigenitalis*, but usually referred to as CEM or CEMO, does not survive outside the host for any length of time, probably not more than an hour or so. The stallion does not become infected in the sense of suffering from a disease (as in venereal disease in humans), but if he mates an infected mare and picks up the microbe, it can become established as part of the normal genital flora, where it can survive for years. It only becomes a problem when the stallion subsequently infects a mare at mating.

Both colt and filly foals can be contaminated by an infected dam at birth or soon after; and the microbe may be carried in the normal flora until the animal goes to stud. It is then that the colt foal, now a stallion, infects his mares at mating and the filly, now a mare, passes the organism she has been carrying to the stallion who mates her. He may then infect the next mare which he mates.

Fortunately this cycle can be broken because, although the bacterium can be carried for years, most carriers clear themselves in time. But to control this serious disease any animal thought to be infected, or which has been on stud premises where there has been an infection, should be examined by a vet and, if found to be a carrier, should be treated.

It should be remembered that, although the most serious outbreaks of CEM have been in the Thoroughbred, it can infect all breeds of horses, ponies and donkeys.

It will only be kept under control by identification of infected animals. Veterinary treatment of those infected and all possible carriers is important and meticulous stud hygiene on infected premises should be followed (see Chapter 39).

The bacteria *Streptococcus zooepidemicus, Klebsiella pneumoniae* and *Pseudomonas aeruginosa* cause other diseases in the horse but can be transmitted from stallion to mare or mare to mare via the stallion at mating. They are important because they cause metritis in the mare and, unlike CEM, can infect the accessory glands of the stallion.

Table 4 Aerosol and Indirectly Transmitted Respiratory Bacterial Pathogens

Bordetella bronchiseptica
Enterobacter agglomerans
Klebsiella pneumoniae
Mycobacterium avium
M. bovis
M. tuberculosis
Pasteurella pneumotropica
Streptococcus equi
S. pneumoniae
S. zooepidemicus

Table 5 Bacteria Responsible for Venereal and Venereally Transmitted Disease

Klebsiella pneumoniae (certain capsule types only)
Pseudomonas aeruginosa
Streptococcus zooepidemicus
Taylorella equigenitalis (CEMO)

Two other bacteria, *Rhodococcus equi* and *Actinobacillus equuli*, cause disease in foals, but the route of infection is uncertain. The organisms can be isolated from soil but also from the gut of normal, healthy animals, and the dam may be the source of infection.

Rhodococcus equi is the cause of pneumonia in foals, sometimes called summer pneumonia (see p. 478). The bacteria can survive for years in the soil and can be isolated from garden soil which has had no known contact with horses. *Actinobacillus equuli* is the causative organism of shigellosis or sleepy foal disease, a highly fatal septicaemia of newborn foals. Postnatal infection is thought to be via the navel. The foal may be infected *in utero*, though the mare is not clinically infected.

The diseases caused by *Brucella abortus,* brucellosis, and *Mycobacterium bovis,* tuberculosis, are now rare in horses in this country but both can be transmitted from cattle to the horse. Man can also infect horses with tuberculosis caused by *Mycobacterium tuberculosis*, which is very similar to *M. bovis*; the disease is indistinguishable. There is also tuberculosis in birds caused by *M. avium*, but transmission to horses is thought to be very rare. Glanders is another bacterial disease of historic interest. It was identified by Loeffler in 1882 and is caused by an organism now called *Pseudomonas mallei.* The last reported case in the United Kingdom occurred in 1928.

Table 6   Directly and Indirectly Transmitted Bacterial Diseases

Bacteria	Disease
Actinobacillus equuli	Shigellosis
Bacillus anthracis	Anthrax
Brucella species	Brucellosis
Corynebacterium pseudotuberculosis	Ulcerative lymphangitis
Dermatophilus species	Rain scald
Mycobacterium avium	
M. bovis	Tuberculosis
M. tuberculosis	
Pseudomonas mallei	Glanders
Rhodococcus (Corynebacterium) equi	Pneumonia in foals
Salmonella abortus equi	Septicaemia in foals; abortion in mares
Streptococcus equi	Strangles
S. zooepidemicus	Common cause of inflammatory infection

Group III: Infections caused by bacteria present within the normal flora
This type of infection is called endogenous. It is not really an infection as such, because the bacteria are already present in the body, but the outcome is a disease which has to be resolved. It is not caused by a change in pathogenicity of the organism but by a change in the condition of the host. Such changes may be caused by stress, trauma or infection by other agents.

Stress covers many situations, from malnutrition, overwork and heavy worm burden to being transported; and what stresses one animal may have no effect on another. Stress causes the natural defence mechanisms of the host to be impaired, resistance is said to be lowered, and pathogenic bacteria already present are able to outgrow the normal flora and disease follows.

Table 7 Endogenous Infections – potential pathogens which, when present in the normal gut flora, may be responsible for diarrhoea

Campylobacter jejuni (formerly called *Vibrio jejuni*)
Clostridium perfringens
Escherichia coli
Salmonella species
Yersinia enterocolitica

Diarrhoea is a common clinical symptom of such a situation. Species of *Salmonella*, *Campylobacter* and *Clostridia* and *Escherichia coli* are the most common bacteria responsible. Diarrhoeic diseases can be caused for many other reasons, and viruses and even protozoa can be the causative agents. Disturbance of the normal gut flora by the indiscriminate use of antibiotics can have a similar effect, caused by the overgrowth of undesirable bacteria present within the gut flora.

Familiarity breeds contempt. Because antibiotics are so freely available it is sometimes forgotten how powerful they can be. Antibiotics cannot distinguish between pathogen and normal flora and they kill all bacteria sensitive to them. Upsetting the gut flora of a horse can be fatal.

Antibiotics may have other adverse side effects. Some cause serious damage to nerves, kidney function and so on, and dosage is critical. They should never be used on any animal without veterinary advice.

Another group of endogenous infections are those associated with internal injuries and deep-seated pathological changes such as tumours. The bacteria associated with such conditions are as secondary invaders and usually originate from the gut.

There are also examples of endogenous abscesses. These include dental abscesses originating from the normal flora of the mouth, peritonitis and intra-abdominal abscesses where the bacteria originate from the gut, and pelvic abscesses where the bacteria may be of gut or genital origin.

Yet another way in which bacteria carried in the normal flora are able to cause infection is if tissue is damaged by another infective agent, such as a virus, allowing the bacteria access. Bacteria present in the respiratory tract do not penetrate the epithelial lining cells, although they may attach to the outside, but viruses are able to damage the integrity of the cell wall, and are usually followed by secondary bacterial infections. *Streptococcus pneumoniae*, as the name suggests, can cause serious respiratory disease but is carried in the normal flora of horses, especially in young horses, and has only been shown to cause problems after virus infection.

Table 8   Bacteria Associated with Dental Abscesses

Aerobes	*Staphylococcus* species
	Streptococcus species
Anaerobes	*Bacteroides* species
	Fusobacterium species
	Peptococcus species
	Peptostreptococcus species

Table 9   Bacteria Associated with Deep-Seated Abscesses

Anaerobic cocci
Bacteroides species
Clostridium species
Escherichia coli
Fusobacterium species
Staphylococcus aureus
Streptococcus species

There are two diseases of horses which are not caused directly by a bacterium but by its product (toxin). These are botulism (see p. 477) and tetanus (see p. 475). Both microbes are inhabitants of soil and plant material. As organisms grow, toxin is produced. It is the ingestion of preformed toxin in one (botulism) and the production of toxin from the microbe in an abscess within the body in the other (tetanus) that cause fatal disease.

Viruses
Viruses are sub-microscopic organisms. This means that they cannot be seen when under an ordinary light microscope but require the even higher

magnification that can only be achieved by using an electron microscope.

They have a central core of a single strand of genetic material, either DNA or RNA (ribonucleic acid), which is surrounded by a protein coat. They have the basic material required to replicate themselves but can only do so inside a living cell. They require tissue culture or animal inoculation for culture in the laboratory. They are described in detail in Chapter 31.

Many viral conditions – influenza, arteritis, rhinopneumonitis (equid herpesvirus) are caused by viruses being inhaled into the respiratory tract and setting up infection by that route.

Mycoplasma, rickettsia and chlamydia

Mycoplasma, rickettsia and chlamydia are organisms which are neither bacteria nor viruses but come somewhere in between the two.

Mycoplasma are the smallest free-living organisms. They do not have a rigid cell wall and are therefore very vulnerable to environmental changes. They can be grown in the laboratory on special media. They have been shown to be pathogenic in animals and are responsible for bovine pneumonia. They have been isolated from the respiratory tract of horses and may be involved in mixed viral-bacterial-type infection.

Rickettsia and chlamydia can only live and grow in an animal host cell. They require tissue culture or animal inoculations for culture in the laboratory. Rickettsia are only found associated with lice, fleas, ticks and mites, which are responsible for their spread. Chlamydia are pathogenic for man and other animals, causing serious diseases such as trachoma and psittacosis. They have been isolated from the eye and nose of the horse, but have not, as yet, been proved to be associated with infective disease.

Fungi

Fungi are physically larger than bacteria. Most can be grown on laboratory media. The organisms come in two forms: single-celled round or oval yeasts and the multicellular, mycelial forms. A mycellum is just like a plant's rooting system with lots of branches.

Fungi are very important in the environment. They are responsible for much of the breakdown of decaying plant material because, unlike bacteria, they produce an enzyme which is able to digest cellulose. Of the many fungi which have been identified, only a few cause disease. The majority live in the soil or on plant material. They reproduce themselves by spores. These are very small water-resistant structures which are dispersed into the atmosphere in very large numbers. The mould found on cheese and bread is a fungal growth caused by spores carried in the air.

Fungi are not only larger than bacteria but have one fundamental difference in the cell nucleus. Together with all animals and plants except bacteria and viruses, fungi have two strands of DNA forming their genetic material (chromosomes).

Because fungal spores are so widespread in nature their isolation from clinical material is not always significant, and to be certain that a fungus is causing a disease it is necessary to establish that the fungus is present within the tissue.

Fungal spores penetrate into the tissues of the host where they germinate and form a seat of infection. *Aspergillus* is the most common pathogenic species in the horse, causing infection of mucous membrane and serious infections in the guttural pouch (see p. 64). Spores can cause an allergic reaction, as in chronic obstructive pulmonary disease (see p. 82), without causing an infection.

Some fungi, particularly yeasts, are present in the normal gut flora, where they can become a problem if the flora are upset, particularly by the use of antibiotics. Yeasts are not sensitive to bacterial antibiotics and can overgrow the bacterial populations in the gut.

Yeast infections are not common in the horse, although species of *Candida* can cause infection of the oral and intestinal mucosa in foals and have occasionally caused genital infections in both mares and stallions. *Cryptococcus neoformans* infection is more serious. It starts as a subacute or chronic infection, usually in the form of a nasal granuloma, but may extend to other parts of the body.

The most important and common fungal infections in the horse are the dermatophyte skin infections and ringworm (see p. 139). There are many different fungal species which cause ringworm in the horse but the two most important are *Trichophyton* and *Microsporum. Microsporum canis* infects not only the horse but humans, dogs, cats and many other animals. This is important when considering transmission, which is by contact. *Trichophyton equinum* is the common cause of ringworm in horses and donkeys, occasionally in dogs and rarely in humans.

Protozoa
Protozoa are much larger than bacteria. They have two strands of DNA genetic material, and although they are only single-celled, the cell has a very complex structure. Protozoa are grouped according to their shape and life style. One group has a tail-like projection or a form of membrane which provides mobility. In this group are found trypanosomes and leishmania. Another group comprises those protozoa with a complex life cycle which includes two different hosts, such as an arthropod (e.g. a tick) and a vertebrate (e.g. a horse). One example is the piroplasm which causes tickborne babesia (see p. 504).

Parasites
A parasite is an animal or plant that lives in or on another (the host) from which it obtains nourishment. Therefore bacteria, viruses, fungi, etc., can all be

referred to as parasites and often are, but the parasites to be considered here are much bigger and more complex than any micro-organism.

The most successful parasites live at the expense of the individual host but do not kill it. The degree of dependence and the degree of harm inflicted vary widely with different parasites, a pathogenic parasite being one which damages the tissues of the host to cause disease.

Parasites can be divided into three categories: helminths, (worms), arthropods, (joint-limbed parasites), and protozoa (see above).

Helminths can be subdivided into trematodes (flukes), which are usually dorsoventrally flattened and often leaf-like in outline; cestodes (tapeworms), which are also dorsoventrally flattened, but which have a ribbon-like body made up of segments; and nematodes (roundworms), which are elongated and cylindrical in shape, and taper at each extremity.

Arthropods consist of insects and arachnids. Insects (lice and flies) have a body which is divided into a head, a thorax and an abdomen, three pairs of legs and usually one pair of wings, although lice, which belong to this category, are wingless. Arachnids (ticks and mites) often have a sac-like body with mouthparts at the anterior end and four pairs of legs in the adult stage. Ticks may reach 1 cm or so in length, but mites are usually microscopic and cannot be seen by the naked eye.

The life cycle of a parasite is said to be either direct or indirect. In the direct life cycle the parasite is transferred from horse to horse without the intervention of another organism. However, there may be a period during which the parasite exists as a free-living stage outside the host in the environment, on pasture, for example, while being transferred from horse to horse. In the indirect life cycle the parasite requires two or more different hosts. One host acts as the definitive host, in which the sexually mature, egg-producing stages of the parasite are found. The other acts as the intermediate host, in which the parasite develops but does not reach sexual maturity. The intermediate host is essential to the parasite's life cycle. The most common intermediate hosts are flies and ticks, although for some parasites the horse itself will act as an intermediate host.

Having experienced a first infection with some parasite species, the horse may develop the ability to kill all or some of the parasites invading in a second or subsequent infection. This is known as the protective immune response and it is the main reason why adult horses tend to be less susceptible to infection by certain parasites than foals or yearlings. However, sometimes an exaggerated, allergic type of immune response can occur and the horse becomes hypersensitive to the parasitic infection. This hypersensitivity may itself cause lesions and disease.

A variety of drugs are used to kill or suppress the development of parasites. These are called anthelmintics, insecticides, acaricides and antiprotozoals and are used to treat helminths, insects, arachnids and protozoa respectively.

The same drugs often kill both insects and arachnids.

A few parasites have developed resistance to the effects of the specific parasiticide used to control them. This means that the population of parasites which previously was killed by a certain dose of that particular drug is no longer killed by that dose and the parasites remain alive in or on the horse after treatment with the drug. Resistance to certain anthelmintics by the small strongyles (cyattastomes) is currently of major concern.

30
DISEASES CAUSED BY BACTERIA

Introduction

Microorganisms are ubiquitous in the environment. Many bacteria normally inhabit the external surfaces (skin, eyes) and internal surfaces (upper respiratory tract, alimentary tract, genital tract) of all species. The natural defence mechanisms (components of the immune system) of the body and local antimicrobial factors combine to prevent opportunistic bacteria from becoming pathogenic and exerting deleterious effects. In the horse, many different microorganisms participate in fermenting soluble and insoluble plant material in the large intestine to produce energy and protein for absorption and utilisation. If active defence mechanisms become compromised, suppressed, do not develop, or, as in the case of newborn foals, there is failure of passive transfer of colostral antibodies, then opportunistic bacteria in the environment can adhere to surface cells, invade tissues, multiply and induce pathogenic effects.

Many organisms are associated with disease in a range of species, eg., the gram negative *Escherichia coli* and *Salmonella sp.,* and the gram positive *Staphylococcus aureus* and *Clostridium sp.* However, the horse is more susceptible to the effects of certain bacteria than other species, eg., tetanus resulting from the toxins elaborated by *Clostridium tetani.* Several microorganisms have adapted to the horse including *Streptococcus equi* subspecies *equi* (hereinafter called *Streptococcus equi*), the cause of strangles, and the contagious equine metritis organism, *Taylorella equigenitalis.* Requirements for optimal growth (pH, moisture, temperature, oxygen tension, substrates) vary with different bacteria. *Streptococci* and *Staphylococci* require oxygen (aerobic) and are plentiful on the skin and in the oral cavity. *Taylorella equigenitalis* is more fastidious, requiring a microaerophilic (low oxygen tension) atmosphere. Spore-forming *Clostridia sp.* grow in the absence of air (anaerobic), and are of particular concern in skin and tissue injuries, eg., *Clostridium tetani, Clostridium botulinum,* and can invade damaged intestinal mucosal barriers, eg. *Clostridium difficile, Clostridium perfringens*. Tissue injuries, oral and dental lesions tend to be colonised by a mixed bacterial population, whereas some bacteria target a specific organ, eg., *Bacillus piliformis* in the liver of young foals. Newborn foals are dependent upon passive immunity acquired from the mare's colostrum. If this is poor quality or inadequate the foal is more susceptible to bacterial infection, and may develop a systemic illness (septicaemia). Clinical signs will reflect involvement of multiple organ systems concurrently, or indicate localisation in the respiratory or alimentary tracts, central nervous system, joints or active sites of bone growth.

The extent of disease exhibited depends upon the host's immune status and genetic make up, the challenge dose of the organisms (or of the derived products) and environmental factors. The young, old, debilitated, and animals that are immune-suppressed are at higher risk. Some organisms produce exotoxins that bind to cell receptors. Signs of disease relate to effects induced by the bound toxin; specific therapy is directed at dealing with circulating (unbound) toxin and countering further release. Hence, use of antitoxin in tetanus does nothing for the existing signs, but together with wound lavage and penicillin administration may limit further toxin production and release. Endotoxins (lipopolysaccharides) are part of the cell wall of effete gram negative enteric bacteria. Endotoxin is present in the gut of healthy horses. However, rapid growth and subsequent death of large numbers of enteric bacteria result in high intestinal lumen concentrations. If the mucosal barrier is impaired, overwhelming absorption can lead to systemic endotoxaemia. Consequences include the dramatic cardiovascular and gastrointestinal signs manifest by horses with acute abdominal crises, acute diarrhoea or acute laminitis.

Diagnosis of bacterial infections is based on clinical signs, history, appropriate laboratory data, and confirmed by isolating specific bacteria on culture from discharges, faeces, urine or blood. A negative culture does not preclude the presence of a pathogenic bacterial species. The sample collected or the microbiological culture conditions may have been inadequate for growth. Anaerobic bacteria have assumed greater significance in equine infections with improved sample handling and specific culture methods and toxin assays. *Clostridium difficile* has been associated with acute colitis in horses, and this organism and *Clostridium perfringens* have been incriminated in haemorrhagic necrotising enteritis in young foals. Pathogen isolation improves the likelihood that more specific therapy can be applied. Identification of bacteria and the investigation of disease outbreaks are being enhanced through molecular techniques, eg., polymerase chain reaction (PCR) to amplify the DNA of antigens. PCR is considered a more sensitive and rapid method to identify *Salmonella sp.* in equine diarrhoea than culturing 5-7 consecutive daily faecal samples, thus having a positive impact on management and isolation strategies.

Antibiotics remain the mainstay of treating bacterial diseases. Knowledge of the organism and its sensitivity pattern is vital. However, in acute infections, particularly systemic disease in newborn foals, intravenous antibiotic administration should be initiated immediately at doses and frequency to achieve effective plasma and tissue concentrations against the most probable organisms. Much data is available to guide the clinician in drug selection and dosing schedule. Antibiotics must be used judiciously in light of the growing concern regarding antibiotic resistance in human pathogens that may restrict veterinary use in the foreseeable future. *Pseudomonas* and *Klebsiella* species, enteric bacteria present in the environment, can prove very difficult to treat in equine joint and tendon sheath infections because of antibiotic resistance, necessitating use of highly selective, expensive drugs. Furthermore, such antibiotic resistant bacteria can contaminate the facilities raising the potential for nosocomial infection outbreaks in clinics and hospitals. Molecular analysis is employed to track the isolate from a clinical case to the immediate environment and its subsequent spread to other animals. Consequently, infectious disease control measures must be kept under constant review, clinical facilities may have to be closed for disinfection, and inevitably, costs formanaging critical care patients will increase.

Serum or plasma containing specific antitoxin can be used as part of the therapy for several Clostridial diseases. The response is better if given early in the course of the disease after a presumptive diagnosis is made if the cost of the product can be warranted. In areas where shaker foal syndrome (toxicoinfectious botulism) is a problem, use of *Clostridium botulinum* antitoxin will markedly increase survivability.

Supportive care is critical to the outcome of bacterial infections. The horse owner must appreciate the time and effort necessary to provide nutrition and nursing care to augment the initial aggressive therapy to restore and sustain fluid and electrolyte balance in many acute infectious conditions. The care is compounded if the animal becomes recumbent and has to be hoisted in slings, turned from side to side or kept in sternal recumbency.

Preventive measures against bacterial infection should be implemented by horse owners. Unfortunately, vaccines are not available to protect against most bacterial diseases of the horse. Tetanus is preventable. An inexpensive aluminium hydroxide adjuvanted toxoid is protective once the initial doses are given. Booster doses are recommended on an annual basis, although this may be an unnecessary frequency for most horses. Recovery from tetanus does not make the horse immune from another bout unless protected by toxoid. Strangles vaccines are available in many countries, although not in the UK. The M-protein extract and inactivated *Streptococcus equi* whole cell vaccines are associated with adverse reactions at injection sites, milder clinical signs and short lived immunity. A live attenuated vaccine based on a non-encapsulated mutant of *Streptococcus equi* is available in the USA, given by the intranasal route. Some safety issues remain a concern. Other live attenuated mutant *Streptococcus equi* vaccines are under review. In the near future, a strangles vaccine that is safe and has proven efficacy can be expected to become available.

This chapter highlights the more important specific infectious diseases of horses caused by bacteria. Conditions present in the UK, or of potential concern, are outlined in the table. Glanders, anthrax, and infections associated with *Mycobacterium tuberculosis, Mycobacterium avium* and *Brucella abortus* are not included.

STREPTOCOCCUS EQUI (STRANGLES)

Strangles is a contagious disease of the upper respiratory tract, primarily of younger horses, although animals of any age can be affected. It is caused by *Streptococcus equi* which is not a normal resident of the equine respiratory tract. Infection occurs through contact with purulent material from affected or carrier animals. The disease is characterised by acute pharyngitis and rhinitis followed by abscessation of the regional lymph nodes which may rupture and discharge thick, creamy pus. Strangles can be sporadic or can become a severe problem in some situations. Population density and mobility are important risk factors. Carrier animals are important in inter-epizootic maintenance of *Streptococcus equi*, and in initiating new outbreaks. Incubation period can be as short as three to six days, or extending to 12 to 14 days. Most affected horses develop immunity.

Clinical signs
Affected animals have a fever, a nasal discharge at first watery which becomes mucopurulent, and a poor appetite. Head carriage may be stiffer than normal, swallowing may be difficult and a soft cough heard. Submandibular and retropharyngeal (underneath and behind the lower jaw) lymph node enlargement may become so hard and painful to impair breathing (hence the name 'strangles') by compressing the pharynx. The animal may be depressed and off feed. Lymph nodes may rupture in 10 to 14 days (or require lancing) releasing thick, creamy pus. Nasal discharges and pus contaminate the environment increasing the risk to other horses. Usually the horse recovers rapidly once the swellings rupture.

Several potential complications may follow the clinical course of strangles. Internal abscessation (metastatic or 'bastard' strangles) may involve any lymph node, particularly in the thorax and abdomen, and can be difficult to diagnose and treat. Empyaema (pus) of the guttural pouches is diagnosed relatively frequently. Other complications include septicaemia, respiratory distress, laryngeal hemiplegia, endocarditis, myocarditis, suppurative bronchopneumonia and myopathies. Purpura haemorrhagica, an immune reaction to the streptococcal antigen, is characterised by fever, depression, progressive oedema of the lower limbs, the ventral body wall, occasionally the throat and head, and in some cases, petechial haemorrhages.

Diagnosis of strangles is based on clinical signs and culture of the nasal discharge, draining lymph nodes, or guttural pouch exudates. Lymph node enlargement under the jaw is not definitive for strangles, and can be a feature of many viral respiratory diseases, particularly equid herpesvirus infection in foals and young horses.

Treatment
Affected horses should be isolated from other horses. Strict hygiene measures should be adopted as the organism can be transmitted on hands, clothes and utensils. Nursing care is important. The nostrils should be cleaned, hot packs applied to the swellings and soft, easily swallowed feed provided. Antibiotics are used in early cases before abscessation, in severe cases, and particularly when complications are apparent. Penicillin is the drug of choice administered by intramuscular or intravenous injection. Antibiotics are not indicated when mature abscesses are close to rupture or should be lanced. Tracheostomy may be required to alleviate acute respiratory distress.

Prevention
The organism can be shed from draining abscesses for up to four weeks and remain viable in the environment for another one month or longer. Contamination is a problem. The affected horse should be in isolation. Ideally, in contact animals should be isolated and observed for clinical signs. Antibiotic therapy may be justified if they develop early signs. Vaccines are available in some countries but not in the UK. The immunity conferred is short lived, although the incidence and severity of disease may be reduced (in the face of an outbreak).

CLOSTRIDIUM TETANI (TETANUS)

Tetanus is a highly fatal infectious disease of all domestic animals caused by the toxins of *Clostridium tetani*. It is characterised by hyperaesthesia to stimuli, painful (tetanic) muscular spasms and progressive muscle stiffness. Horses are the most susceptible species. The organism enters through wounds, the umbilicus of the newborn foal, or from the alimentary tract where it is a normal inhabitant. Clostridial growth requires low oxygen tension and devitalized (damaged) tissue favours spore germination. A puncture wound in the foot is a common portal of entry. The organism is ubiquitous in the soil.

Clinical signs
Incubation period varies between one to three weeks, and may range from several days to several weeks depending upon site of entry. There is a general increase in muscle stiffness accompanied by spasms and paralysis of the voluntary muscles. Jaw movement is restricted ('lockjaw'). All four limbs

are stiff, and the animal may adopt a 'saw-horse' posture with the tail held out stiffly behind. The third eyelid is prolapsed (across the medial half of the eye). The expression is anxious and alert with erect ear carriage, eyelid retraction and flared nostrils. Responses to external stimuli are exaggerated.

Initially the animal may continue to eat and drink but spasms of the muscles of mastication and swallowing make this more difficult. Saliva drips from the mouth, and water or food may be regurgitated from the nostrils. Inability to posture appropriately for urination or defecation may cause retention of urine and faeces. The animal may fall down and be unable to rise. The head is drawn back and the limbs are held in extension. Sweating can be profuse and the body temperature rises. Spontaneous convulsions may occur and death results from respiratory compromise. Severe cases progress rapidly and can end fatally in five to ten days. In others, clinical signs may be apparent for up to six weeks. Mild cases may recover gradually over a period of weeks or months. Diagnosis is based on the classic clinical signs and history.

Treatment
Therapy should be directed at preventing further toxin absorption by neutralizing circulating toxin, aggressive wound lavage (if applicable), control of muscle spasms and supportive nursing care. Administration of tetanus antitoxin will not reverse clinical signs. It is unable to cross the blood-brain barrier or penetrate nervous tissue to combine with toxin already in transit to the central nervous system. The objective is to neutralize circulating toxin outside the nervous system. Intrathecal administration, injecting antitoxin into the fluid space around the spinal cord and brain stem, under general anaesthesia may be effective in some cases. Tetanus toxoid should be given at a separate site because protective immunity is not induced by the natural disease.

High doses of penicillin should be given for a minimum of seven days. Hyperexcitability, muscle spasms and convulsions may be managed by use of tranquillisers, sedatives, or general anaesthesia. Muscle relaxants may be helpful. However, central muscle relaxants can cause paralysis of respiratory muscles in adults and should be avoided. Attention to feed and water intake is vital. Intravenous fluid and electrolyte therapy may be required if the animal is unable to eat or drink. The animal should be kept in a quiet, dark stall with padded walls and thick bedding. A recumbent animal has a poor prognosis. Demands on caregivers are onerous in attempts to maintain an adult horse in a standing position with a sling or sternal recumbency with hay bales in addition to sustaining medical and nutritional support. A recovered horse is not immune from tetanus.

Prevention
Tetanus can be prevented by immunization with potent aluminium hydroxide adjuvanted toxoids. The schedule involves two doses given intramuscularly

four to six weeks apart, followed by revaccination after one year, and subsequently every one to three years. Pregnant mares are given a booster one month before foaling to ensure colostral antibody protection for the newborn foal. Foals of mares, unvaccinated in the last month of gestation, and foals with insufficient passive transfer of immunity should receive tetanus antitoxin at birth. This may provide protection for up to 3 months. Foals should be vaccinated at approximately three, four, and six months of age and receive a booster after one year. If the vaccination history of a horse that has been injured or had surgery is unknown or non-existent, tetanus antitoxin should be administered together with toxoid at a separate site.

CLOSTRIDIUM BOTULINUM
(BOTULISM, FORAGE POISONING, TOXICOINFECTIOUS BOTULISM, SHAKER FOAL SYNDROME)

Botulism is caused by the toxin of *Clostridium botulinum*. Horses are among the most susceptible species. The toxin may be produced in silage or vacuum-packed moist hay, contaminated by decaying matter containing the organism. *Clostridium botulinum* is a gram positive, spore-forming obligate anaerobe that reproduces in decaying animal or plant matter. Under favourable conditions of warmth and humidity spores multiply and produce a highly lethal toxin. There are eight distinct toxins, of which seven are neurotoxins, A, B, C1, D, E, F and G. Ingestion of the preformed toxin is the major route of infection in adults. The foal disorder results from toxin production by bacteria in the intestinal tract. Types B and C cause forage poisoning. Type B toxin is responsible for greater than 80% of equine cases in the USA.

Clinical signs
Rapidity of onset, and severity of clinical signs are related to the type and amount of toxin to which the animal is exposed. Most affected foals are between three and twelve weeks of age. Presenting signs include impaired suckling, inability to swallow, decreased eyelid and tail tone and dilated pupils. There is progressive muscular weakness and tremors, leading to collapse, recumbency and inability to rise. Adults may exhibit mild motor weakness to early total paralysis of the entire voluntary, and much of the involuntary, musculature. Muscle tremors over the shoulders and flanks are evident after exertion. Tongue tone, mastication and swallowing are all affected. The gait is weak, shuffling and unsteady. The animal may fall and have difficulty rising. Death results from respiratory paralysis.

Presumptive diagnosis is based on clinical signs and history, eg., previous foals on farm, feeding silage or spoiled feedstuffs (adults). Laboratory diagnosis to detect toxin is frequently unrewarding.

Treatment

The availability of polyvalent equine antitoxin plasma in the USA has improved the prognosis, particularly if the condition is recognized in the early stages. However, the plasma has no impact once the toxin is bound at the neuromuscular junction; it helps to remove circulating toxin and limits progression of the disease. Optimal nursing care and nutritional support are critical. Recumbency carries a poor prognosis. Antimicrobial therapy does not affect the course, other than for wound botulism where bacteria are within the body, or to counter secondary problems, eg. aspiration pneumonia in foals.

Prevention

Protect feedstuffs from rodent contamination and spoilage when stored. Silage should be avoided. A type B toxoid vaccination is available. However, it is rarely used owing to the sporadic nature of the disease and does not prevent other types of botulism.

RHODOCOCCUS EQUI
(CHRONIC BRONCHOPNEUMONIA, SUMMER PNEUMONIA)

This condition usually affects foals aged two to six months. The respiratory form is the most common disorder although abdominal lymphadenopathy and enterocolitis may occur with, or independent of pneumonia. *Rhodococcus equi* gains entry to the body through inhalation or ingestion from the soil or faeces. The disease is present in most countries and is endemic in regions of the USA and Australia. In the UK it is sporadic, and usually affects only a single animal although it can be a problem on some farms. Adult horses can be affected.

Clinical signs

The condition is insidious in onset. Foals rarely show definitive signs until abscesses and associated bronchopneumonia are well established. Signs include rapid and laboured breathing, cough, nasal discharge, a persistent, slightly elevated temperature, poor appetite and weight loss as the disease progresses. Loud, moist rales or rattles are auscultable as respiratory embarrassment increases. Diagnosis can be difficult especially in an isolated case. Non specific signs such as weight loss or failure to grow may reflect abdominal involvement, with signs of colic or diarrhoea in the later stages. The organism can be cultured from trans tracheal washings or at post mortem from samples of lung, lymph node or bowel. Positive culture or PCR of faeces does not necessarily confirm infection. Radiography or ultrasonography can be helpful to diagnose the condition, and determine the extent of lung and/or abdominal involvement. Nodular lung lesions, especially solitary lesions, and lymphadenopathy are characteristic in foals. Prognosis is grave in cases with multiple lung abscesses and regional consolidation of the lungs.

Treatment

Rhodococcus equi is an intracellular organism that provokes an inflammatory reaction characterised by thick walled abscesses containing caseous pus. Successful treatment is difficult. The objective is to achieve high anti-microbial concentrations in abscesses within diseased tissues. Antibiotic penetration into cells and through thick, fibrous tissue is vital. The combination of erythromycin and rifampin is recommended. Twice daily oral therapy may need to be maintained for a prolonged period of time, and is expensive. Erythromycin causes gastrointestinal irritation and can induce mild to severe diarrhoea and colic.

Prevention

Rhodococcus equi is a ubiquitous organism found wherever horses are kept. Thus isolation of the bacterium from faeces is not indicative of infection. Specific factors that may precipitate the disease on some farms are not clearly understood. A dry, dusty atmosphere may be important, is difficult to moderate, and may explain the low incidence in the UK. There is no vaccine.

SALMONELLOSIS

Salmonellosis is associated with acute enterocolitis and diarrhoea in the horse. However, equine diarrhoea is a multifactorial disorder and *salmonella* infection, while severe, probably accounts for a relatively small proportion of cases. Horses of all ages and under every management condition may be affected although the young, old, debilitated and immunosuppressed are the most susceptible. There are over 2000 *Salmonella* serotypes. A small number have been implicated in equine disease. *Salmonella typhimurium* is the most common serotype identified from clinical cases.

Salmonella infection in horses is manifest in several different syndromes depending upon the virulence of the serotype, the infectious dose, host susceptibility and environmental factors. These include inapparent infection; depression, fever, anorexia and neutropaenia without diarrhoea or colitis; enterocolitis with diarrhoea; peracute circulatory shock in adults and septi-caemia in foals with or without concurrent enterocolitis.

Clinical salmonellosis is frequently associated with stressful conditions such as hospitalization, transportation, general anaesthesia, surgery, antibiotic or anthelmintic therapy, changes in feed or management, and weaning. These events may precipitate changes in food intake, intestinal motility and in the normal intestinal microflora allowing overgrowth of opportunistic *Salmonella sp.* present in the intestinal tract of many healthy horses.

Clinical signs

Acute diarrhoea can occur at any age but is most prevalent in young performance horses. Presenting signs include fever, depression, abdominal pain and dark red mucous membranes. Diarrhoea which may not appear for two to four days, is watery, projectile, foul smelling, and may persist for up to four weeks despite therapy. The peracute shock like syndrome is more likely to occur in adult horses. Death can ensue six to twelve hours after first signs appear; diarrhoea may not be evident. Very young foals may develop septicaemia. Older foals may have severe enteritis followed by localization of the organism in joints, the growth plates of bones, lungs, kidneys or central nervous system. Chronic diarrhoea is rarely attributed to *salmonella* infection, although diarrhoea may persist during protracted recovery from an acute episode.

Those cases presenting with mild to severe abdominal pain can be confused with impaction colic or even an acute intestinal obstruction. Diarrhoea may not be evident for several hours. However, the horse is depressed and may have a fever. The white cell count will be reduced markedly, a feature of endotoxaemia. Complications of clinical salmonellosis include laminitis, thrombosed veins, liver and kidney dysfunction that requires continued critical care and supportive therapy.

Confirmation of *salmonella* infection depends upon isolating the organism from faeces. At least five consecutive faecal samples should be cultured on enriched media, as *salmonella* are shed inconsistently even during the acute phase. A rectal biopsy may improve the culture sensitivity. Intestinal wall and content samples should be cultured at necropsy. The polymerase chain reaction (PCR) to identify DNA of *Salmonella sp.* in faeces appears preferable to culture in sensitivity and rapidity of diagnosis. As many normal horses can shed salmonellae, isolation or PCR identification is not indicative of causation unless clinical signs are present.

Treatment

The major objective in treating diarrhoeal disease in the horse is to restore and maintain fluid and electrolyte balance. In the adult this necessitates intravenous administration of large volumes of fluids for 24 to 72 hours or longer. Added plasma or colloids may be vital in severe cases to counter intestinal protein loss. Water, with and without electrolytes, should be available. Prognosis is better for an animal that maintains or regains appetite. Faecal consistency will be restored in most cases without recourse to antidiarrhoeal agents. Use of antibiotics is contentious in diarrhoea attributable to *Salmonella sp.* Foals with septicaemia or enterocolitis should receive intravenous antibiotics to prevent localisation. Oral antibiotics should not be used.

Prevention

Salmonellosis is a highly infectious disease, and the build up of contamination in the environment of an affected horse can place in contact animals at risk. Ideally, suspected or confirmed cases should be isolated, and strict hygiene and sanitation measures observed. Many serotypes, including *Salmonella typhimurium* are zoonotic. As some normal animals excrete the organism intermittently, screening of all animals potentially in contact at a farm would be unsatisfactory (and expensive) as a control method. Such positive shedders are not true carriers. There is no commercial vaccine. Autogenous vaccines have been used with reported success on individual premises where a problem had been encountered.

Venereal Disease

Sexually transmitted (venereal) disease may affect both males and females. In horses, apart from equine coital exanthema, caused by a herpes virus, the stallion is usually a carrier while mares exhibit clinical signs. Bacteria causing venereal diseases include *Taylorella equigenitalis,* and certain strains of *Klebsiella pneumoniae* and *Pseudomonas aeruginosa.*

These organisms can induce disease in the mare's genital tract. *Taylorella equigenitalis* is a true venereal pathogen causing disease only in the genital tract, whereas *Klebsiella* and *Pseudomonas* can induce infection elsewhere including joints, the respiratory tract, skin and wounds. *Pseudomonas aeruginosa* is pathogenic in the eye associated with severe corneal ulceration. *Streptococcus sp.* and *Escherichia coli* may be transmitted sexually but do not assume the same clinical significance. Venereal disease is usually transmitted during natural service, but can be spread by handlers or clinicians. unless strict standards of hygiene are implemented and maintained.

TAYLORELLA EQUIGENITALIS
(CONTAGIOUS EQUINE METRITIS, CEM)

CEM is a contagious venereal infection of mares caused by *Taylorella equigenitalis*, first identified following an epidemic of metritis in the UK in the 1970s. The organism is carried on the external genitalia of stallions and transmitted at mating to susceptible mares. The disease is self limiting and usually clears with sexual rest after about three months. Some animals may take longer to recover and require treatment. Others can remain as carriers,

Table 1

Infectious diseases of horses caused by bacteria

Disease/bacteria	Presence/age	Features	Prevention
Strangles *Streptococcus equi subspecies equi*	Frequent; all ages, 4m to 2 years predominate	Upper respiratory tract; lymph node abscesses, purulent discharges. Response to therapy, abscess drainage. Carriers. Complications possible	Isolation, strict hygiene. No vaccine in UK. Several vaccines USA (safety, efficacy issues)
Tetanus *Clostridium tetani*	Uncommon; all ages	Neuromuscular; hyperaesthesia muscle spasms, stiffness, convulsions. Early therapy crucial to outcome	Preventable disease. Toxoid inexpensive. Yearly booster
Botulism *Clostridium botulinum*	Rare; suckling foals; Adult–forage poisoning wound botulism	Neuromuscular; weakness, paralysis. Therapy early and before recumbency. Antitoxin available	Avoid silage, spoiled feed. Wound attention. Toxoid (type B) in USA
Bronchopneumonia *Rhodococcus equi*	Rare; sporadic in foals 2-6 months old; Adult – occasional	Lower respiratory tract; onset insidious poor growth rate, lung abscesses. Abdominal tract involvement. Response to early prolonged therapy	No vaccine. Confirm culture, PCR
Salmonellosis *Salmonella serotypes* esp. *S. typhimurium*	Single case, sporadic outbreak; young, old, immune compromised	Enteric disease; diarrhoea, colic, shock septicaemia, joint/bone infection foals. Aggressive intensive care therapy. Hyperimmune serum	Isolation, strict hygiene. No commercial vaccine. Confirm cultures, PCR
Clostridiosis *Clostridium difficile*	Probable, rare; in USA foals 2-5 days old. Adults several countries	Enteric disease; mild diarrhoea to severe haemorrhagic enteritis in foals; colitis in adults	None. Diagnosis – toxin assay faeces; culture difficult

Disease / Organism	Occurrence	Clinical features	Control
Clostridium perfringens	Probable, rare; in USA foals <10 days old	Enteric disease; diarrhoea, severe colic haemorrhagic enteritis, peritonitis Hyperimmune serum C,D antitoxins	Toxoid (C,D) immunise brood mares
Proliferative enteropathy *Lawsonia intracellularis*	Potential, probable; foals 4–7 months old Canada, USA	Enteric disease; depression, rapid severe weight loss, pot bellied, ventral oedema diarrhoea, colic. Response to oral erythromycin/rifampin therapy	Unknown Diagnosis-PCR
Tyzzer's disease *Bacillus piliformis*	Rare; sporadic, foals under 2 months old	Acute hepatic disease; sudden death icterus, neurological signs	None
Leptospirosis *Leptospira interrogans serovars*	Frequent intraocular inflammation; rare other forms; all ages	Multisystem; abortion, renal disease foals and adults. Ocular; recurrent uveitis (immune-mediated)	None
Contagious equine metritis (CEM) *Taylorella equigenitalis*	Notifiable; sporadic; breeding females stallions carriers	Venereal disease; mares return to heat acute endometritis, males unaffected Therapy effective, sexual rest; clitoral contamination may require surgery	Code of Practice Breeding farm hygiene Monitoring, surveillance
Klebsiella metritis *Klebsiella pneumonia* capsule types 1,(2),5	Occasional case or outbreak; breeding mares	Venereal disease; endometritis; male accessory gland infection potential Therapy local and/or systemic; sexual rest	Improved breeding hygiene; surveillance
Pseudomonas metritis *Pseudomonas aeruginosa*	Occasional case, can become endemic; breeding mares	Venereal disease; endometritis reduced fertility, difficult to eliminate Therapy local and systemic; persistent infection clitoris and sinuses-surgery. sexual rest, clean/treat stallion's penis	Improved breeding hygiene, surveillance

harbouring the organism but showing no clinical signs. Colt foals born to infected mares may be carriers and thus are potentially capable of inducing disease later in life if used for breeding.

Clinical signs

The mare exhibits signs of genital tract inflammation, vaginal discharge, and lowered fertility. The exudate is seen at the vulvar lips, on the perineum, tail hairs and inside of the hocks. Affected mares may return to heat unexpectedly, often with shortened inter-heat intervals, but usually breed successfully once the infection has been eliminated. Stallions do not show clinical signs. Diagnosis is confirmed by isolation of the organism from the mare's genital tract or from the penis and sheath of the stallion.

Treatment

Resolution may occur spontaneously. However, infected mares (those identified) may be treated with antibiotics (penicillin or synthetic penicillins) by intrauterine infusion and/or systemic therapy over a seven to ten day period. In a small proportion of cases unresponsive to therapy, the organism has been found to persist in smegma in the clitoral sinuses. The clitoris and sinuses can be cleaned with antibiotic or antiseptic washes and packed with antibiotic cream, although complete elimination of the organism can prove difficult. Surgical removal of the sinuses or clitoris may be necessary to overcome the problem. The stallion's sheath and penis should be washed with antiseptics and antibiotic cream applied daily for a prescribed time. Care should be exercised as some antiseptic solutions can cause irritation of the sensitive tissues. The stallion is not returned to breeding until a series of culture samples taken from several tissue sites over a set time frame remain negative on culture.

Prevention

CEM is a notifiable disease in the UK and in many other countries. A Code of Practice for the control of CEM developed with veterinary, scientific and Thoroughbred industry input has been implemented since 1976 for all horse breeding activities. This has proved very successful in limiting the disease to sporadic cases, and ensured the continued international movement of horses for breeding purposes.

31
DISEASES CAUSED BY VIRUSES

Viruses usually cause specific diseases such as influenza. Unfortunately the diagnosis of viral disease is complicated in practice because there may be evidence of the presence of a virus but no symptoms. Further, viruses may affect the body in an almost symptomless way and be followed by a bacterial infection which develops as a direct result of the virus, as, for example, when young horses are affected by one of a variety of viruses (herpes-, rhino- or picornavirus) and subsequently develop a cough or catarrhal nasal discharge (snotty nose). The following viral diseases are therefore described from the clinical viewpoint, that is, based on the typical symptoms displayed in each case.

EQUINE INFLUENZA ('FLU')

Background
A disease clinically indistinguishable from influenza was described in horses as long ago as 1732 and many similar references have been made since. In the 1930s German researchers comparing epidemic coughing in young racehorses with the then recently isolated swine influenza virus, showed for the first time that the disease was due to a filterable virus and that it was reproducible experimentally. An equine influenza virus (H7N7 subtype, formerly termed type-1 equine influenza virus) was isolated for the first time from coughing horses in Prague, Czechoslovakia, in 1956. Retrospective serological surveys demonstrated that the virus had been the cause of disease in many areas of the world and monitoring of epidemic respiratory disease demonstrated that this virus continued to be responsible for disease outbreaks in predominantly young horses in many countries between 1957 and 1963. In January 1963 there was an outbreak of rapidly spreading respiratory disease among horses at several racetracks in Miami, USA. A characteristic of this outbreak that differentiated it from earlier outbreaks was that it affected all ages rather than mainly young horses

and was caused by a novel (H3N8, formerly type-2) equine influenza virus, which subsequently led to an equine flu pandemic. A serological survey in the UK in 1963 demonstrated that British horses were completely susceptible to the new virus and an epidemic was predicted. Indeed, H3N8 (type-2) influenza was first seen in February 1965 on two studs in Sussex with the arrival of mares from France, where the disease had been present for about one month. Since the end of the 1970s H7N7 (type-1) equine influenza has not been confirmed anywhere in the world but type-2 viruses continue to cause disease in most years in many parts of the world. In 1979 in the UK there was a widespread epidemic of H3N8 subtype (type-2) influenza, initially among unvaccinated horses and later in vaccinated animals. Laboratory examination of isolates has since confirmed that equine influenza viruses are continually evolving (a phenomenon called 'antigenic drift'), in a manner similar to, although not as rapidly as, human influenza viruses. The continued occurrence of outbreaks among vaccinated as well as unvaccinated populations of horses and the emergence of a highly fatal 'bird-flu' in horses in China in 1989, have reinforced the need for on-going epidemiological surveillance of this disease in horses. Laboratory virus characterisation has recently recognised two divergent lineages of H3N8 (type-2) viruses, so-called 'American-like' and European-like' strains, and experimental infections have confirmed field observations that there is a need for inclusion of representative of both lineages if future vaccines are to remain effective.

Clinical signs
The characteristic sign of equine influenza in fully susceptible horses is a rapidly spreading, harsh, dry cough, which may persist for up to three weeks in some individuals. High fever (rectal temperature in excess of 40.5°C/102°F), loss of appetite and associated depression are other features of the illness and usually last four to five days in most animals. A watery discharge from the nose may be present early in the disease and in most cases this soon becomes thick and pus-like due to secondary bacterial infection. There may also be muscle stiffness and constipation. Signs spread very rapidly to most if not all unvaccinated individuals in a stabled population, although vaccinated horses generally show much less severe signs, if any at all. Most cases recover completely, but complications of bacterial pneumonia, pleurisy and/or damage to the heart muscle sometimes occur, especially if precautions to minimise the effects of the disease are not taken, and may be fatal in a few cases. Some horses may show rapid weight loss with loss of appetite and high fever.

Diagnosis
Although the characteristic harsh cough and very rapid spread of signs may be highly suggestive of influenza among horses, confirmation of the diagnosis requires laboratory testing of appropriate samples. Blood samples can be used for detecting the presence and amount of specific antibody to influenza

viruses (a technique referred to as serology). Rapid and large rises in antibody are produced after horses are infected (and after vaccination) and this is used to diagnose viral infections. This diagnosis requires that horses are bled twice, firstly shortly after the onset of signs and then again at least two weeks later. Both samples are tested for antibody and a significant (four-fold or greater) rise in antibody level indicates that the horse was infected (or vaccinated) around the time of the first sample. Influenza viruses may be isolated in the early stage of the disease from nose and throat swabs. Influenza is traditionally isolated by inoculation in embryonated hens' eggs but isolation in tissue culture cells is also possible.

The adoption of more widespread vaccination has made the diagnosis of influenza infection less straightforward, with clinical signs being less severe, acute blood samples already possessing moderate levels of serum antibody and the quantities of live virus retrievable from the respiratory tract being greatly reduced. The development of a sensitive and rapid enzyme linked immunosorbent assay (ELISA) for the detection of influenza in swab samples has greatly improved the ability to diagnose influenza in both unvaccinated and vaccinated horses.

Treatment
Although antiviral drugs that reduce the effects and duration of infection when it occurs are becoming more widely available in human medicine, these have not been used very much in horses and expense does not justify such therapy, especially because prevention by vaccination is more practical and effective.

Advice on the most effective treatment for affected horses should be sought from your veterinary surgeon immediately. Treatment of fever by anti-inflammatory drugs and secondary bacterial infections, including pneumonia by antibiotics, may be required. A very important contribution to recovery of horses affected with influenza is rest and the provision of fresh air as avoiding dust helps minimise the risk of bacterial infections. Affected horses should be walked for short periods in order to maintain proper circulation of the limbs. This approach should be adopted for at least the period of fever and coughing, followed by a period of gradually increasing exercise, rather than a sudden return to fast or strenuous work.

Prevention (Vaccination)
Vaccination is the administration of a modified form of a disease-causing agent (vaccine) to the immune system of a horse, in order to increase the animal's ability to resist infection. Vaccination should provide protection against the disease whilst at the same time not producing signs of general illness or localised adverse reaction.

In the UK the need for an accurate experimental model for equine influenza infection in order to develop and test effective vaccine was recognised. Models have been developed in susceptible ponies using different routes of administration and infectious doses; these have shown thatvaccines are effective in preventing infection and have since been used in the licensing of effective equine influenza vaccines in the UK. Vaccines currently used in horses in the UK (Table 1) are officially regulated in order to ensure that they are both effective as well as safe. It is important to remember that vaccination, whilst being an effective part of a disease control strategy, is no substitute for good animal husbandry.

Table 1: UK equine influenza vaccines

Vaccine Name	Vaccine Type	Virus Strains
Equip F	Immune stimulating Complex (ISCOM)	A/eq(H7N7)/Newmarket/77 A/eq(H3N8)/Brentwood/79 A/eq(H3N8)/Borlange/91
Duvaxyn IE Plus	Carbomer adjuvanted	A/eq(H7N7)/Prague/56 A/eq(H3N8)/Miami/63 A/eq(H3N8)/Suffolk/89
Prevac Pro	Aluminium hydroxide adjuvanted	A/eq(H7N7)/Prague/56 A/eq(H3N8)/Newmarket1/93 A/eq(H3N8)/Newmarket2/93

Note: Vaccines listed may vary from those currently available due to updating of strains or changing of adjuvants

The manufacturers' recommendations for timing between vaccine doses are broadly similar for all influenza vaccines and include a primary course of two vaccinations administered four to six weeks apart followed by a first booster dose given six months after the primary course and subsequent boosters every 12 months thereafter. It is important that influenza vaccines are periodically updated with relevant strains of circulating viruses because the virus is continually evolving and with time older strains may become increasingly ineffective.

From March 1981 following the loss of racing because of an equine flu epidemic in 1979, The Jockey Club in the UK made influenza vaccination mandatory for all horses running at British racecourses and this is still the case today.

Jockey Club Rules on influenza vaccination:
1st vaccination of the primary course is given on day one;
2nd vaccination of the primary course is given between 21 and 92 days (three weeks to three months) after the 1st vaccination;
3rd vaccination (1st booster) is given between 150 and 215 days after the 2nd injection (five to seven months);
  Subsequent booster vaccinations are given at intervals of no more than 12 months (annually);
  No horse is permitted to race unless vaccinated seven or more days previously and the primary course has been completed.
  A predicted need in 1987 for vaccines to be periodically updated was proved correct when in 1989 there were outbreaks of influenza among recently vaccinated horses. This subsequently led to an update of strains in UK vaccines. Surveillance of the disease continues and periodic updating of vaccines takes place when appropriate.
  There are many factors that influence the effectiveness of vaccines in individual horses. In order to maximise vaccine response, only healthy horses should be vaccinated and every effort should be made to minimise stress for several days following vaccination. Vaccination of foals may be affected by colostrum, the first milk produced by mares immediately after foaling, which contains high levels of antibodies which help fight infections. When colostrum is absorbed in the first few hours of life this provides protective immunity in the foal (so-called 'passive transfer of immunity') against a wide range of diseases. The absorbed antibody is referred to as 'maternally derived antibody' or MDA. Blood testing foals at one to two days of age can measure the level of MDA and appropriate measures can be taken to address any failure of transfer of this antibody. MDA can interfere with vaccination by neutralising the vaccine antigen, and therefore the timing of primary vaccination should coincide with falling levels of MDA. The earliest that foals should be vaccinated is at six months of age unless a failure of transfer of MDA requires that it be started sooner.
  Vaccines contain a component, known as adjuvant, which enhances the intensity and the length of the immune response of the horse to the antigen component. The effectiveness and safety of different vaccines depends on the type of adjuvant used and the way that the antigen is prepared. In some species of animals, vaccines contain modified live antigen (termed 'attenuated'). However, all current UK horse vaccines contain inactivated antigens which, because they are killed, cannot revert to a disease-producing form which is a possibility with live-attenuated vaccines.

EQUID HERPESVIRUSES 1 AND 4
(EHV-1 AND EHV-4) (SNOTTY NOSE, STABLE COUGH,
VIRUS ABORTION, RHINOPNEUMONITIS)

The two closely related herpesviruses Equineherpes virus 1 and 4, EHV-1 and EHV-4, (formerly termed EHV-1 subtypes 1 [abortion strain] and 2 [respiratory strain]) both cause respiratory disease. EHV-1 is also an important cause of single or multiple abortions ('abortion storms'), and can occasionally cause inco-ordination or paralysis. EHV-4 is a rare cause of single abortions and has not been conclusively shown to cause nervous disease. Abortion caused by either virus characteristically occurs between seven months and full term, although it can occasionally be as early as four months. In horses under the age of two years, herpesvirus infections are characterised by catarrh or nasal discharge (snotty or dirty nose) and an intermittent cough infrequently associated with fever. In older individuals a mild watery nasal discharge may be the only sign of infection.

Cause
Both EHV-1 and EHV-4 are essentially infections of the respiratory system, causing inflammation of the nasal cavity, pharynx, airways and lungs (rhinitis, pharyngitis, bronchitis and pneumonitis). The passage of the virus into the foetus, thereby causing abortion, is a comparatively infrequent happening and the virus cannot be considered to be primarily of an aborting nature. Paralysis of the hind limbs and sometimes the front limbs is another incidental form of EHV-1 infection, affecting horses of all ages, but is less common than abortion.

Symptoms
Abortion (usually caused by EHV-1). The abortion form of the disease starts with the virus being inhaled, circulating in the bloodstream within lymphocytes, infecting blood vessels within the uterus and crossing the placenta to enter the body of the foetus. Here it causes characteristic signs of damage (lesions) in the liver, lungs and other organs of the unborn foal. As the foetus becomes ill, the mare expels the contents of the uterus (i.e. her foetus and its membranes) in a sudden unheralded event. If the foal becomes infected close to foaling then it may be born alive, but is weak and typically dies within a few days. Such congenitally infected foals may shed large amounts of virus and present a considerable risk to in-contact pregnant mares.

The incubation period between infection of the mare and abortion is very variable. It may be as little as seven days or as much as a hundred days. The explanation for this variation is unknown although it may depend on the immune status of the mare, the strain of virus, and the stage of pregnancy when the virus enters the mare's body.

For a fuller description of the disease see p. 397

The foetus and foetal fluids are heavily contaminated with virus and are a source of infection to in-contact animals, unless they are removed quickly and the local environment disinfected. To achieve a rapid diagnosis and thereby limit further spread of infection it is vital to contact your vet after any abortion so that a specialist laboratory can examine the foetus and placenta. Since EHV-1 usually causes characteristic damage to the foetus, and rapid tests for the virus are available, it is often possible to confirm the diagnosis and institute control procedures within 24 hours of the abortion. Detailed information on measures that studfarms should take following an EHV-1 abortion is available in the Horserace Betting Levy Board Code of Practice, which is available through your vet.

Depending on the time of the initial infection, a mare may remain infectious for several weeks after the abortion, shedding virus from the respiratory tract or harbouring virus in the blood. Mares may also shed virus from the respiratory tract prior to abortion, with no symptoms of respiratory disease.

There is no effective treatment. Control of the infection must be based on sensible management practices and vaccination. Inactivated vaccines (Pneumabort K and Duvaxyn 1/4) for use in the prevention of abortion are available.

Pregnant mares should be vaccinated in the fifth, seventh and ninth months of pregnancy, and it is recommended that young stock on studfarms should also be vaccinated because they are a potential source of infection. Although vaccination may not protect the individual from abortion, it reduces the amount of virus shed if an animal does become infected and thereby reduces the spread of the infection and the likelihood of abortion storms occurring. Since herpesvirus infections are very common in young stock it is also important to try and minimise contact between this type of horse and mares in late pregnancy if possible.

Respiratory disease (caused by either EHV-1 or EHV-4). A watery discharge from the nose starts about three days after infection. It may cause a sore tract to appear at the junction of the nose and muzzle where the nasal discharge runs over the area. At this stage the affected individual may suffer a slight fever and an occasional cough. After about a week a secondary bacterial infection may occur and the nasal discharge becomes pus-like (purulent), the cough may increase and pneumonic signs develop (i.e. increased rate and effort of breathing). Rales and moist crackling sounds may be heard on listening to the lungs through a stethoscope.

Pharyngitis develops and an increase in the lymphoid (tonsillar) tissue in the pharynx may be seen by means of an endoscope. These symptoms (lymphoid hyperplasia) are particularly prevalent in horses of two years old or less.

Diagnosis can be achieved only be recovering the virus in material collected from the windpipe or pharynx during the early stages of the disease. Once the secondary infection has developed it is probable that the virus can no longer be obtained by these means.

Confirmation of the disease can be made by serological tests on blood serum. This consists of measuring antibody levels (titres) at the onset of the symptoms (acute phase) and again two to three weeks later (convalescent phase). A four-fold increase or more in antibody levels indicates that the virus has challenged the individual.

It is possible by both these means of diagnosis (growth of virus and serology) to establish whether the infection is caused by EHV-1 or EHV-4. The polymerase chain reaction (PCR) test, which detects viral DNA, is now beginning to replace diagnosis by growth of virus as results can be obtained much more quickly (one day rather than eight days or more).

Course of condition
Affected horses show symptoms to a greater or lesser extent according to the age of and the degree of immunity possessed by the particular individual. Immunity is short-lived, so repeated attacks may occur, although the older the animal the less likely that severe secondary infection occurs.

A four-year-old or older animal will probably only present the initial signs of increased nasal watery discharge rather than suffering the snotty-nose condition. However, younger individuals may suffer the secondary effects for weeks or months following an initial infection.

The infection may be latent (i.e. no symptoms) for long periods and subsequently episodes of symptoms occur following stress or other precipitating factors, many of which are as yet poorly understood. Research has demonstrated that the majority of horses in the United Kingdom are carriers of EHV-1 and EHV-4, with the viruses persisting in nerve ganglia and lymph glands. This type of latent infection is a common method by which herpesviruses persist in populations, as exemplified by cold sores in humans. Since stress can cause this type of latent infection to flare up, resulting in further shedding of virus, it is important to avoid all unnecessary stresses in mares in late pregnancy (e.g. mixing of groups or long journeys to studfarms).

Treatment
The principles for treatment and management of virus respiratory infections outlined under equine influenza also apply for equid herpesvirus 1 and 4 infections (see above).

Preventative measures
Vaccination against EHV-1 is undertaken principally to prevent the potentially large economic loss due to abortion in mares. The value of vaccines in the prevention of respiratory infections is not fully known and booster vaccinations may be required at three to six monthly intervals in order to maintain effective immunity against the disease. On account of this many vets doubt the value of vaccination against EHV-1 infection other than in pregnant mares

where vaccination does prevent multiple abortion storms, although not protecting against single abortions. It is best to discuss this with your own vet, who will advise you according to the horse's age, the type of work for which it is required and the risk of infection.

Hind-limb inco-ordination and paralysis (caused by EHV-1). The paralytic form of the disease is capricious in onset. It is not clear why some individuals suffer this debilitating condition whereas most do not. However, the paralytic form often occurs in several individuals, and it is suspected that certain strains of EHV-1 have a special attraction for the nervous system. Current opinion is that the nervous form is due to the virus causing inflammation and clot formation in blood vessels supplying nervous tissue ('equine stroke'), possibly as the result of some immunological or allergic response of the individual to virus circulating in the bloodstream.

Symptoms include loss of co-ordination and paralysis of the hind-limbs (sometimes also of the forelimbs). Incontinence (failure to hold urine in the bladder) may be a feature. Cases of the paralytic form show symptoms similar to horses which have broken backs or suffered other major skeletal injuries (see Chapter 18).

Recovery occurs providing sufficient time is given and the paralysis not such as to leave the individual unable to get to its feet or otherwise so disadvantaged that survival is virtually impossible.

Treatment
Injection of corticosteroids and supportive measures, such as suspending an individual in a sling or supporting it with straw bales in the standing position to avoid the risk of its lying down and being unable to get to its feet.

EQUID HERPESVIRUS 3 (EHV-3) (COITAL EXANTHEMA, SPOTS)

This venereal disease is characterised by small blisters which develop on the vulva of mares and penis of stallions and break to form small deep ulcers. It is caused by equid herpesvirus 3, a virus distinct from equid herpesvirus 1 or 4 (see above).

Symptoms
The vesicles (blisters) are not usually visible before they burst, and the first symptoms seen are the ulcers, with their distinctive circular outline and craters varying up to about 0.5 cm in diameter. In the mare the ulcers occur on the vulval lips and sometimes on the vulva itself. In the stallion the ulcers may occur on any part of the penis. Usually the infection can be identified on both the stallion and one or more of the mares with which he has mated during the previous ten days.

However, the condition can occur in mares without any recent history of mating. It seems that mares may be infected either by the virus remaining dormant in the body for long periods until activated by some unknown trigger or that infection occurs through ingestion or inhalation without any sexual contact.

Treatment
Treatment is not really necessary, although mild antiseptic lotions or cortisone and antibiotic ointments may be applied. Healing of the ulcers takes about ten days, and mares and stallions are not usually infectious after a lapse of about two weeks. Sexual rest is therefore important because, if mating is continued, the ulcers may fail to heal and become wider and deeper and fresh crops of blisters and ulcers develop.

EQUINE VIRAL ARTERITIS (PINK EYE)

Equine viral arteritis is a systemic infection of horses and donkeys caused by equine arteritis virus (EAV), the prototype member of the family *Arteriviridae*, which includes another important virus in veterinary science, porcine reproductive and respiratory syndrome virus (PRRSV).

Symptoms
The virus can grow in many types of cells of the body but mainly in white blood cells and small arteries. This causes a reduction in white blood cell numbers and oedema or hemorrhage in different organs. The result of the infection is variable depending on virus strain, age of animal and environmental factors. Thus, affected animals may or may not develop one or a combination of the following clinical signs: fever, loss of appetite, depression, conjunctivitis ('pink eye'), swelling of the limbs, sheath and scrotum, runny nose, urticarial skin rash and lymph node swelling. The clinical signs presented and their severity vary widely between outbreaks. Furthermore, on many occasions EAV causes infections without symptoms or symptoms that can be very similar to other viral infections. For this reason confirmation by a laboratory is essential for all suspected EAV cases. After infection the animal develops immunity and becomes seropositive (antibodies to the virus can be detected in the serum). These antibodies can last for many years. Of particular importance is the capacity of EAV to cause abortion in pregnant mares and to establish persistent infection in stallions. The virus is transmitted by nasal secretions or other body fluids during the acute phase of the disease, and venereally through semen of infected stallions. These animals can carry the virus for many years and despite not showing signs of illness they transmit the infection through their semen. Both natural and artificial insemination are very effective in disease

transmission. This is why detection of persistently infected stallions is crucial to prevent the spread of EAV.

Treatment
No specific antiviral treatment is currently available. Natural cases of EAV are rarely fatal in adult horses but antipyretic, anti-inflammatory and diuretic therapy can help to alleviate the symptoms of severe cases. The use of corticosteroids is not advisable as it may enhance the potential of establishment of persistent infection.

Prevention
Because of the asymptomatic nature of persistent shedding stallions and the efficiency of the venereal route of infection, preventive measures are directed mainly at breeding activities. These measures are based on periodically testing of all the animals within a premises (and most importantly, those coming to it) to isolate those carrying the virus. It is recommended that mares, stallions and teasers should be serologically tested each year at the beginning of the breeding season. Mating should not commence until results are available. Throughout the year, all cases of respiratory disease or pyrexia in stallions should be subjected to a full virological investigation. Animals returning from abroad, e.g. from stud or international competition, should also be isolated and tested on their return. When a seropositive stallion is detected, a semen sample should be collected and sent to a competent laboratory to determine whether it is a virus shedder or not. Until this is known, the stallion should remain in strict isolation. If there is any possibility that abortion has been caused by EAV, the entire foetus and placenta should be submitted for examination, along with blood samples from the mare.

Outbreak Control
If EVA is confirmed, seek veterinary advice immediately. In the UK, the Divisional Veterinary Manager (DVM) of DEFRA must be notified. All mating, teasing, semen collection and movement on and off the premises must be stopped. Owners of horses which have left the premises and any recipients of semens must be informed.

All clinical cases and their in-contacts must be isolated and samples submitted for virus detection. All horses on the premise should undergo serological screening. Blood testing should be repeated at 14 day intervals until the outbreak is over. Seropositive horses should be kept in isolation for one month and any stallions or teasers which remain seropositive must undergo semen testing before mating activities are resumed. Pregnant mares should be isolated for at least a month after active infection is over.

Movement on and off the premises, mating activities and semen collection should only be resumed following veterinary advice.

Vaccination

It is important to emphasise that vaccination should not be considered a substitute for the preventive measures described above but another part of disease prevention programmes.

A killed whole virus adjuvanted vaccine (Artervac; Willows Francis) has been available in the UK and Ireland since 1993. This has been shown to give significant protection against experimental infection with EAV, but little is yet known about duration of immunity. As vaccinated horses will become seropositive, it is important to test blood immediately before the first vaccination to show that they were previously seronegative. Accurate serological and vaccination records are essential for breeding and export purposes.

A live attenuated vaccine (Arvac; Fort Dodge) is available in the USA. Vaccinated animals do shed the virus and may become clinically ill, but the vaccine does not induce semen shedding in stallions. This vaccine is not recommended for pregnant mares.

Animals receiving these vaccines become seropositive and even a negative serological test prior to vaccination does not prove that infection, with subsequent virus shedding, has not occurred after vaccination. Current EAV vaccine research focuses on the development of a safe 'marker' vaccine which will be suitable for widespread use, without compromising disease surveillance via serological screening. In other words, with this vaccine it would be possible with a single blood test to determine whether the horse, vaccinated or not, has experienced EAV in the past.

EQUINE RHINOVIRUS 1 (ERV-1, COLD VIRUS)

ERV-1 can cause upper respiratory tract disease, characterised by an increase in temperature (pyrexia), copious nasal discharge and enlarged submaxillary lymph glands. It can also infect individuals without causing any overt clinical signs of disease. Infection normally results in long-term immunity.

OTHER EQUINE PICORNAVIRUSES (COLD VIRUSES)

Equine rhinovirus 2 and 3 and acid stable picornavirus have occasionally been recovered from cases of mild respiratory disease but are generally regarded as apathogenic. Picornaviruses can often be recovered from the oral cavity of apparently healthy horses.

There are no vaccines available for prevention of equine picornavirus infections.

ADENOVIRUS (COLD VIRUS)

Adenovirus has been recovered from the respiratory tract of horses affected by mild respiratory disease. Soft faeces are sometimes a characteristic of adenovirus infections. This virus is generally regarded as apathogenic except in Arab foals with combined immunodeficiency disease (see p. 738). In these individuals the virus produces a generalised infection which alone or in association with other micro-organisms leads to death.

EQUINE INFECTIOUS ANAEMIA (SWAMP FEVER)

Cause
The virus is present in the blood and is transmitted from an affected to a non-infected individual by way of insect bites or by the use of contaminated hypodermic needles or other implements with which blood may be involved, for example, tooth rasps. The virus may also be transmitted from a mare to her foal in milk, and under certain conditions ingestion of the virus may be responsible for spread of infection.

Symptoms
Symptoms include fever, which may be constant or intermittent, anaemia accompanied by depression, profound weakness to the point of incoordination and marked loss of condition. Fever rises and falls precipitously and may vary considerably within the space of an hour. Jaundice and soft swellings of the abdomen, prepuce (in colts and geldings) and legs develop, and there are small pinhead-sized haemorrhages on the lining of the tongue and on the mucous membrane of the nose.

Symptoms vary in intensity and there may be periods of remission when the individual appears quite healthy. A definitive diagnosis is made using a blood test named after Dr Coggins.

No specific treatment is available, although supportive measures, including blood transfusions and iron therapy, may be used. In the UK the disease is notifiable and, apart from an outbreak in the 1970s, the condition is not known to be present here. The disease has been found in certain areas of the USA, Canada, France, West Germany and South America, as well as in numerous other countries.

Preventive measures
Use of the Coggins blood test to identify affected individuals and carriers of the virus enables measures of control to be introduced whereby healthy horses are segregated from indirect contact with affected individuals. Because the chief means of spread is through biting flies, the spread of the

disease is seasonal, and measures to reduce the fly population may help. However, the optimal means of eradication of the disease is the slaughter of affected animals or confining them to premises at some distance from unaffected horses. The greater the seasonal or climatic risk of biting flies being present, the greater the distance that must be introduced between healthy and affected animals.

VIRAL ENCEPHALOMYELITIS (EASTERN, WESTERN AND VENEZUELAN-ENCEPHALOMYELITIS – EE, WE AND VE)

An infectious disease affecting horses and communicable to man, which is characterised by symptoms of paralysis, inco-ordination and loss of consciousness.

Cause
The disease is caused by an arbovirus, of which three strains are known, Eastern, Western and Venezuelan. These are distinct and vary in their ability to cause disease, although the symptoms are similar with all three viruses.

Symptoms
The disease is restricted mainly to North and South America. The incubation period is one to three weeks. Initially there is fever accompanied by loss of appetite and depression. However, the reaction may be so mild that it goes unobserved. Nervous signs develop later and include exaggerated response to sound and touch, and transient periods of excitement and restlessness with apparent blindness.

An affected individual may stand with the head low and appear to be asleep, perhaps with a half-chewed mouthful of food hanging from the lips. This dummy-like effect is illustrated by the reaction of some individuals if food is placed in their mouth but not otherwise.

Paralysis follows these initial symptoms. There is an inability to hold up the head, the lower lip becomes pendulous and the tongue may hang out. Unnatural postures are adopted, such as standing with the weight balanced on the forelegs with the legs crossed. Head pressing or leaning back on the halter is often seen.

The course of the condition is progressive and many affected horses do not recover, usually becoming recumbent and completely paralysed before death ensues.

Treatment
There is no specific treatment although supportive measures may be undertaken to enable the affected individual to survive sufficiently long for recovery to take place.

Preventive measures

Control is based on a programme of identifying and destroying or segregating affected individuals, taking steps to avoid contact with mosquitoes, which spread the virus.

Vaccination may be practised in areas where the disease is likely to occur. Vaccination should take place well before the anticipated season of infection occurs – i.e. the summer months. Two doses of vaccine are given ten days apart, followed by annual revaccination, which is necessary because effective immunity in response to the vaccine does not appear to last beyond a year in all individuals.

ROTAVIRUS INFECTION

Rotavirus infection in young foals (four days to five months old) causes diarrhoea. Infections are rarely lethal unless they occur in association with bacterial pathogens such as *Salmonella typhimurium* and toxinogenic strains of *Escherichia coli*.

The virus damages the lining of the intestinal tract. The villi (minute folds) on the surface of the lining become damaged. Thus, a foal which has suffered from rotavirus may fail to absorb nutrients satisfactorily, a problem which may sometimes last for the rest of the individual's life.

In severe cases affected foals go off suck and develop a profuse diarrhoea. They become depressed, lose condition and experience temperatures up to 41°C (105°C). Duration of diarrhoea can vary between two and twelve days.

Rotavirus can be detected in scours shortly after the onset of the disease and occasionally has been detected in the faeces of healthy individuals, indicating that the inapparent-carrier state exists and is likely to be important in the spread of this infection. There are no vaccines available for foal rotavirus although products have been developed for use in calves.

RABIES

A highly fatal viral infection of the central nervous system affecting all warm-blooded animals and transmitted by bites from affected individuals.

Cause

Rabies is caused by a rhabdovirus which has an affinity for nerve cells. However, it is susceptible to most standard disinfectants and is killed in dried saliva in a few hours.

Symptoms

Horses show excitement and mania. Their uncontrolled actions may be violent and include galloping blindly, suddenly falling and rolling. They may chew at their skin. Death usually ensues within days.

The disease is notifiable but it occurs infrequently in horses even in countries where the disease is prevalent. The disease is not present in the UK or Eire. If cases occurred, they would be destroyed on humane grounds and to prevent serious risks to man and others.

32
DISEASES CAUSED
BY PROTOZOA

Protozoa exist as single cells that are part of the animal kingdom. A number of different protozoa infect horses. Some of these are very important causes of disease in tropical and subtropical countries, *Trypansoma* and *Babesia* species. On the whole they affect horses less in temperate countries. Although protozoa have a simple, single-celled structure, their life-cycles can be exceedingly complex and can differ markedly from one species to the next.

SARCOCYSTIS NEURONA
(EQUINE PROTOZOAL MYELOENCEPHALITIS [EPM])

Most cases of equine protozoal myeloencephalitis (EPM) in horses have been associated with *Sarcocystis neurona* in North and South America. In addition a few cases have been ascribed to *Neospora caninum* and a possible new species, *N. hughesi*, described in California.

Life-cycle and epidemiology
Sarcocystis spp. have predators as the definitive host that pass the infection in their faeces to prey that act as the second host, the intermediate host. Development takes place in these and the life cycle is completed when the infected prey is eaten by the predator. The only definitive host described for *S. neurona* is the opossum and the geographical range of EPM matches the presence of opossums. The parasites multiply in the intestine of the opossum and large numbers of very small, translucent infective sporocysts will be excreted in the faeces. The life-cycle continues when these are eaten by an intermediate host. The normal intermediate hosts of *S. neurona* are armadillos and skunks but the parasites also does infect the horse. The life-cycle of

related species, i.e. *S. cruzi* and *S. tenella* has been characterised. These parasites use ruminants as their intermediate hosts and in these multiply asexually by merogony (multiple fission), first in the walls of arterioles and then in the walls of capillaries in many organs of the body, followed by monocytes and finally parasites move to the muscles to form cysts. These become filled with sausage-shaped bradyzoites that are infective when the intermediate host is preyed on by the definitive host. However, for *S. neurona* horses are aberrant and dead-end hosts as only the non-infective meronts have been found. The meronts and merozoites are described only in the central nervous system where they have been described in neurons, in the endothelial cells of capillaries and phagocytic cells as well as free. They seem to undergo asexual division repeatedly in the central nervous system.

Clinical signs
These are greatly varied and almost every neurological sign is possible. EPM commonly starts insidiously as spinal cord disease manifesting as mild lameness and limb weakness progressing through incoordination, ataxia, head shaking, bucking, and muscle atrophy of various muscle groups but particularly the gluteals or biceps. Brain signs may be depression and paralysis of muscles of the head and neck. The condition, without treatment, progresses steadily or intermittently. Some cases start acutely with sudden recumbency developing in a few hours.

Diagnosis
Up to 50% (and focally up to 80%) of horses in the USA have been exposed to infection. Many of these never develop disease although if levels of exposure in a herd are high disease is more likely. Therefore, the usefulness of detecting antibodies in serum is limited although absence of antibodies has merit in ruling out EPM. Separation of the parasite proteins and detection by immunoblot (available commercially) of the 22.5, 13 and 10.5 kDa bands with a horse's serum antibodies differentiates *S. neurona* infection from the other *Sarcocystis* spp. of horses. Detection of antibody produced within the CNS in the cerebrospinal fluid has greater specificity and sensitivity. However, the significance of antibodies in the CSF of a clinically normal horse is still in question. It is suggested that some young horses might have experienced a subclinical infection and eliminated the infection but would remain CSF antibody positive for some time. Others may remain positive producing clinical signs at a later time.

Histologically, lesions occur in the CNS and may be microscopic or visible grossly. There is perivascular cuffing, multifocal cell infiltrates and a non-suppurative encephalitis. Intracellular meronts containing merozoites and free merozoites may be visible. If merozoites in a meront are seen in a rosette formation then this is characteristic for *Sarcocystis* compared with other protozoa in the brain. Merozoites and meronts are more likely to be visible when stained with labelled antibody.

Treatment and control

Sulphonamide (usually sulphadiazine or sulphamethoxazole) plus pyrimethamine treatments (but without trimethoprim with which they are often formulated) have been adapted from use for toxoplasmosis. Newer drugs now used for *Toxoplasma* treatment in humans might be more effective but have not been tested. Diclazuril, toltrazuril and nitazoxanide have been used. Treatment must be prolonged preferably until the horse is CSF antibody negative. Some horses, for reasons as yet unknown, do not become negative even with prolonged treatment. With shorter treatment, i.e. 90 days, as many as 50% of horses may remain antibody positive and 25% may later relapse. Side effects, provided trimethoprim is not included, are usually mild. One reported is a mild anaemia. Occasional severe neutropaenia and thrombocytopaenia have required temporary suspension of treatment. Caution must be shown in treatment of pregnant mares. Non-steroidal anti-inflammatories, DMSO and anti-oxidant therapies may help reduce the inflammatory damage in the brain particularly as this might be exacerbated temporarily by death of the parasites. Brief corticosteroid therapy has been used but must not be prolonged as it could increase parasite numbers. It is thought the use of corticosteroid therapy for unrelated reasons can increase the risk for young horses showing clincal signs of EPM.

Opossum control, prevention of their access to feed stores and even fencing to exclude them from paddocks seems appropriate.

NEOSPORA CANINUM

This parasite causes disease in cattle and dogs. It is passed from an infected mother repeatedly to her progeny. In some infected cows *N. caninum* manifests particularly as an abortion. Congenitally infected young dogs infected from their mothers and occasionally older dogs show neuromuscular deficits. The majority of animals born infected do not immediately show signs of disease but themselves may abort or produce congenitally infected progeny later in life. This vertical transfer from mother to young appears to be a main method of transmission but recently the dog has been shown to be a definitive host passing sporocyts in its faeces, so horizontal transmission from dogs' faeces is possible.

A few cases of EPM due to *N. caninum* or *N. hughesi* have been documented in the USA. As *N. caninum* appears to occur world-wide there is potential for disease occasionally in horses elsewhere in the world. *Neospora caninum* can be differentiated from *S. neurona* serologically, by the presence of rhoptries in the merozoite, multiplication by endodyogeny and by the fact they occur in clusters. They also have different antigens and so can be distinguished serologically or in the tissues using labelled antibodies.

SARCOCYSTIS FAYERI, SARCOCYSTIS BERTRAMI

These *Sarcocystis* spp. occur in horses throughout the world but are not normally associated with disease. They complete their life-cycle in the horse so that after merogony the parasites move to the muscles and form cysts. The cysts are small and can only be detected histologically, particularly in the oesophagus. Some surveys have revealed infection in as many as 50-70% of horses. The life-cycle of these *Sarcocystis* spp. is completed when dogs eat infected muscle. The infection is seen therefore where dogs are fed raw horse-meat, i.e. usually hounds (foxhounds and beagles). These pass cysts in their faeces, and horses grazing land where hounds are exercised have the highest risk of infection. Rarely, muscular weakness in horses has been associated with large numbers of cysts dying in the muscles and the inflammatory reaction they provoke.

BABESIA CABALLI, BABESIA (THEILERIA) EQUI (BABESIOSIS, BILIARY FEVER, PIROPLASMOSIS)

Both *Babesia caballi* and *Theileria equi* are parasites of the red blood cells in horses. Babesiosis is widespread in Asia, the former Soviet Union, Southern Europe, Africa, Central, South and parts of North America, the Caribbean, and occasionally is seen in imported horses in other countries.

Life-cycle
A variety of ticks act as the intermediate host transmitting the *Babesia* parasites from one horse to another (see p. 562 for tick life-cycle). The tick picks up the infection when it sucks blood. *Babesia caballi* then multiplies in the tissues of the tick as it develops on the ground to its next life-cycle stage and/or the *Babesia* passes through the egg of the tick to the next generation of ticks. When in its next stage of development the tick feeds on a new horse, the *Babesia* will move to the mouthparts and are injected into the horse. The *Babesia* parasites then infect and multiply in the red blood cells in the circulation of the horse. *Theileria equi* passes only from larva to nymph and nymph to adult tick and not onto the next generation. It multiplies in lymphocytes in the lymph nodes before it enters the red cells. Mechanical transmission of both these parasites by syringe has occurred so the same needle or syringe should not be used to inject or bleed different horses.

Clinical signs
Babesiosis can be quite severe in horses and 10% or more of those infected may die. About ten to twenty days after the horse has become infected the first clinical signs are seen. *Babesia caballi* is the less pathogenic of the two

parasites and may present only as fever and anaemia. Severe babesiosis or theileriosis can begin as marked depression, with fever and loss of appetite. Colic may be seen. This is followed by a massive destruction of the red blood cells so that the horse becomes anaemic, showing very pale mucous membranes in the mouth and eyes. These later become yellow with jaundice. The urine may be stained red with haemoglobin from the destroyed red blood cells. The animal becomes constipated and passes very hard, small balls of faeces, which may be coloured with yellow, sticky bile coloured mucus. In some horses oedematous, fluid swelling of the head, legs, lower abdomen and chest occurs, and in a few cases the central nervous system is affected so there may be paralysis of the hind legs. Severely affected horses may die within a few days of the onset of symptoms. The disease may also run a longer course lasting several weeks in which the horse rapidly loses condition. Subsequent recovery can take months. After the horse has recovered from the illness the parasite remains in its red blood cells, although at very low levels so that no illness is seen. The parasite may remain in the horse for years and sometimes relapses occur, most commonly after some form of stress, such as travel, surgery, etc. Carrier horses can be severely affected by, for example, strenuous exercise.

Diagnosis
In blood smears, *B. caballi* appears as dark-stained rings and pear-shaped bodies often in pairs in the red blood cells. *Theieria equi* is smaller and often *B. Theileria* in the red cell form a Maltese cross. Serological tests for antibodies are available and may detect infection earlier after infection than blood smears. They are very useful in detecting carrier animals that may have an undetectable parasitaemia. A number of serological tests are used. The complement fixation test, an indirect fluorescent antibody test and more recently an ELISA all have been developed. PCR also is used at least experimentally to detect low levels of infection and to classify the parasites.

Treatment
Imidocarb is the drug most commonly used for *Babesia* but it does have some side effects and may not eliminate the infection, leaving the horse as a carrier. Diminazine diaceturate also is effective againt red cell stages but it also has side effects. Imidocarb is less effective against *T. equi*. For this latter parasite administration of parvaquone or buparvaquone with imidocarb in the very early stages of disease can increase efficacy. To aid its recovery, an acutely ill animal could be given a blood transfusion to replace the red blood cells being destroyed by the parasite.

Preventive measures
It is very difficult to control infection with *Babesia* in horses. Reducing both

the population of the tick intermediate hosts and number of infected hosts can reduce the possibility of transmission and so decrease the number of cases. Regular spraying or dipping in acaricide will reduce the number of ticks considerably but will not eliminate them. If the horses are stabled and groomed, then daily removal of the ticks reduces the likelihood of infection as the ticks do not often start injecting *Babesia* as soon as they attach. Unfortunately the tick can transmit *Babesia* at all stages of its life-cycle, and larvae in particular can be less than 1 mm long, attach anywhere on the body and so are likely to go unnoticed. It may be necessary for horses to be tested and declared free from *Babesia* before they can be imported into certain countries. The complement fixation test was widely established for diagnosis and to declare horses free of infection for transport internationally. However, it does not necessarily detect carriers and can give some false positives.

Trypanosomes

These leaf-shaped protozoan parasites live in the plasma of horses and cause a variety of serious diseases – dourine, surra, mal de caderas, nagana. Most of these trypanosomes are transmitted from horse to horse by biting flies. Many are transmitted only by the tsetse fly (*Glossina*) and so are largely restricted to sub-Saharan Africa. However, *Trypanosoma vivax* and *Trypanosoma evansi* can be transmitted mechanically by flies (especially horse flies and also stable flies). The trypanosome contaminates the mouthparts of the fly as it sucks blood and is then carried on the mouthparts to be injected into the next horse. *Trypanosoma equiperdum* is spread by the venereal route. These three species therefore are more widespread with potential to establish should they be imported into a country.

TRYPANOSOMA EQUIPERDUM (DOURINE)

Trypanosoma equiperdum occurs in Africa, Central and South America, the Middle East and parts of Asia. The parasites are in the urethra of stallions and vaginal discharge of mares and are spread at service. Dourine produces a swelling of the external genitalia two to four weeks or longer after a mare has been served by an infected stallion or vice versa. In the stallion the scrotum and sheath become filled with fluid and swollen, and the swelling may extend along the belly. In the mare the vulva becomes swollen and reddened, and there may be a discharge. Soon after, but only in some animals, circular areas of swelling, like plaques, 2-10 cm in diameter, appear in the skin over the body. These are called 'dollar spots' as they often look as if a coin has been inserted under the skin. These appear, last a few hours to days, and then disappear, frequently to reappear. The final stage in the disease is neurological, beginning as incoordination leading to paralysis. Presenting animals most commonly show incoordination of the hind legs (80%), swelling of the genitalia (50%) and emaciation (40%). Without treatment most horses will die. There are some animals, however, in which the course of the disease will take several years or in which few signs of disease are ever seen. Trypanosomes may be detected in the genital exudates, blood and skin plaques. A complement fixation test is effective if no other *Trypanosoma* spp. are present in the animal.

There are some reported successes after treatment with trypanocidal drugs but the drugs do have side effects. In many countries *T. equiperdum* is a reportable disease and horses may have to be tested and declared free from *T. equiperdum* before they can be imported.

TRYPANOSOMA EVANSI (TRYPANOSOMA VIVAX) (SURRA, MAL DE CADERAS)

Trypanosoma evansi causes a highly fatal disease (surra or mal de caderas – sick hips) of horses in parts of Asia, North Africa and Central and South America. The organism is carried mechanically between horses on the mouthparts of biting flies like tabanids and stable flies (p. 549). Surra is nearly always fatal to horses if left untreated, death occurring within a few days to months and as long as six months later, depending on the severity of the infection. The affected horse may have a temperature, become weak, lose weight very rapidly and develop fluid, oedematous swellings and scabs on the legs, belly, chest and neck, become staggery and eventually collapse.

TRYPANOSOMA BRUCEI, TRYPANOSOMA CONGOLENSE

These cause nagana (to be in low or depressed spirits) in all types of animals, including horses. The infection is confined to tropical Africa where the intermediate host tsetse fly exists. The infections are severe in horses with lethargy, weakness and anaemia leading to progressive loss of weight, fluid swelling of the lower part of the body, depression and sometimes nervous signs. The disease will last for a few weeks to months, until the horse dies.

BESNOITIA BENNETTI

This protozoan has been reported in the skin of horses in southern France, Africa and Mexico. Over a period of months cysts, like those of *Sarcocystis*, develop in the skin. The skin becomes thickened, hard and scaling and looks scurfy and loses its hair. Gradually the horse loses weight and becomes weak. Little more is known about this parasite, although it is assumed that, like *Sarcocystis*, it requires a wild or domestic carnivore to transmit the infection.

EIMERIA LEUCKARTI

This *Eimeria* produces very large, thick walled, 80 x 60 µm, dark brown oocysts in the faeces. These do not float in the salt solutions commonly used to detect gastrointestinal parasite eggs in faeces so infection usually goes unnoticed. Sedimentation techniques are required. Parasites sometimes have been observed with pathology in the lamina propria of the intestine but there is no conclusive evidence that *E. leuckarti* induces disease in foals. The few surveys for this coccidian parasite often demonstrate infection in up to 50% of foals while the parasite is found only occasionally in adult horses. Generally foals seem to pass oocysts beginning from two to five weeks or much later after turn out to pasture and pass oocysts intermittently for several months. This epidemiology suggests that infection passes from foals in one year to those in the next (viz a viz *Parascaris equorum* page 530) with the thick-shelled oocyst being very resistant to environmental changes.

GIARDIA SPP.

A recent study has suggested that infection with *Giardia* may be common. It multiplies on the surface of the epithelium of the duodenum and small intestine and in the lumen of the intestine. An increase in cyst output in the faeces of mares after parturition has been related to subsequent infection in the foals. Cysts can be detected in faeces using a commercial test kit of fluoresceinated antibodies that detect the small, oval cysts in faeces. Cysts will also float following centrifugation of faeces in concentrated zinc sulphate solution. Either technique may require repeating as cysts can be shed intermittently. Rarely, diarrhoea has been associated with *Giardia* infection but there is very limited evidence associating *Giardia* with disease in horses.

CRYPTOSPORIDIUM PARVUM

Cryptosporidium parvum is ubiquitous but again an increase in oocyst output in the faeces of lactating mares has been correlated with infection in foals. The parasite multiplies just under the membrane of intestinal epithelial cells in the posterior small intestine. In immunocompromised foals (i.e. combined immunodeficient Arab foals) it causes a severe, persistent diarrhoea. In normal foals or experimentally infected foals high oocyst output has been associated with diarrhoea lasting a week or two. Most foals and horses show no symptoms. *Cryptosporidium parvum* infects most mammalian species including horses and horses undoubtedly can acquire it from other animals, particularly artificially fed calves that can be heavily infected. Currently, different strains and genotypes of *C. parvum* are being identified so the relevance of equine infections for man remains unresolved. Nonetheless, it must be assumed that horses are a source of infection for man in whom it can be a severe infection in the immunocompromised and causes disease also particularly in children. Man more commonly can obtain infection from water (even commercial supplies) and other animals. Special staining or fluorescent antibody staining of oocysts in faeces identifies infection. An ELISA assay that detects products of the parasite in faeces of cattle and humans is available but it has not been tested for its efficacy in diagnosis of infection in horses.

PARASITIC CONDITIONS

HELMINTHS (WORMS)

Helminths, the large class of parasitic worms, include the various forms of roundworms (nematodes), tapeworms (cestodes) and flukes (trematodes).

Nematodes (Roundworms)

Life-cycle

The life-cycles of the different nematodes have several similar features. The basic life-cycle can be seen in some of the nematodes, such as the strongyles and cyathostomes that live in the gastrointestinal tract. In general, eggs (but sometimes first-stage larvae) are passed in the faeces of horses and then three life stages take place outside the host. A first-stage larva, which is a microscopic roundworm, develops inside the egg-shell and then escapes by hatching. It develops in the manure to a second- and then an infective, third-stage larva, and only this third-stage larva can infect horses, usually by ingestion with grass. The third-stage, in addition to its own cuticle (skin) on the surface retains the shed cuticle of the second-stage larva. The presence of these two protective layers means that the third-stage is relatively resistant to adverse conditions. They can survive on pasture overwinter but do die quickly in hot or dry weather. The eggs and earlier larval stages of these worms do not survive well. All these stages are microscopic and not visible to the naked eye. A variation with some nematodes is that the first-, second- and third-stage larva all remain within the egg-shell, and the horse becomes infected by eating the egg containing the infective larva. The infective larva then hatches from the egg inside the host. The advantage for the parasite is that, while in the egg shell, it is relatively or greatly protected from adverse environmental conditions so that the larva within the egg can remain alive for months and even years. An additional variation is that these three life-cycle stages can take place within another host called an intermediate host, i.e. within the body of a fly. The fly might eat the nematode while it, the fly, is developing in horse manure, or the adult fly might either lap up the larva in the horse's secretions or when biting and sucking blood. The infective third-stage larva that develops in the fly then may be eaten by the horse or the fly might inject the larva through the skin of the horse. When the infective larva has entered the horse, irrespective of the route of entry, it passes through two more life-cycle stages. The third-stage larva develops to the fourth-stage, which in turn develops to the fifth- or adult-stage male or female worm and eggs and larvae are produced once more. The parasites in the horse may undergo a complex migration through the body before the adult stage develops or they may develop in the organ of entry such as the gastrointestinal tract.

STRONGYLUS SPP., CYATHOSTOMES (STRONGYLES, REDWORMS)

These are very important parasites of horses and the adults are found in the large intestine of horses throughout the world. There are more than 50 different worms in this group so, for ease of description, they can be divided into two groups. First there are the large strongyles, the *Strongylus* species (*S. vulgaris, S. edentatus, S. equinus*). Adults of these are 1.5-5cm long and grey to red in colour. Secondly, there are a large number of different species of small strongyles or the cyathostomes (i.e. *Cylicodontophorus, Cylicostephanus, Cylicocyclus, Cyathostomum* species). These reach 1-1.5cm long in the adult stage and are white or red in colour. Both the large strongyles and the cyathostomes cause disease in horses but in different ways.

Life-cycle in the horse
When the large *Strongylus* species larvae are eaten, the immature stages migrate quite extensively in the horse's body before they return to the large intestine to mature to egg-laying adults. *Strongylus vulgaris* larvae migrate into the intestinal wall to moult here to the fourth-stage and then they migrate in the walls of the small and large arteries supplying blood to the intestine, until they reach the junction of the anterior mesenteric artery and the aorta. Here the larvae remain for three to four months before they moult to the fifth-stage and migrate back down to the large intestine. They form nodules in the wall of the large intestine emerging some six weeks later to mature to adults. The adult worms begin to lay eggs about six months after the horse became infected. *Strongylus edentatus* larvae migrate in the liver and then the inner wall of the flank before they return to the intestine while *S. equinus* migrates

in the liver, pancreas and abdominal cavity. These become adult at about 8-12 months. An additional large strongyle, *Triodontophorus* species, has a life-cycle more like that of the cyathostomes and is included with that group in its life-cycle and in the disease it causes.

Figure 1
Two large *Strongylus* spp. and two cyathostomes on the wall of the caecum

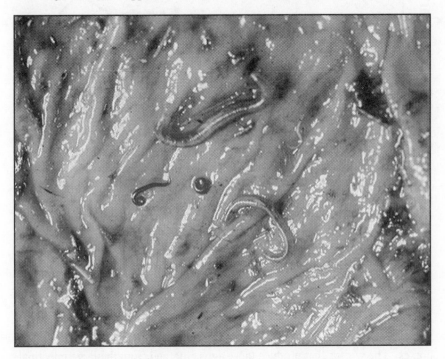

The life-cycles of the cyathostomes or small strongyles in horses are much simpler. When eaten these larvae migrate no farther than the wall of the large intestine. After about four to six weeks they break out of the wall of the intestine into the lumen and begin to lay eggs as little as five weeks later, but commonly about two to four months after infection. However, the cyathostomes also can prolong the time they spend in the wall of the intestine, so some larvae eaten in the autumn do not emerge to become egg-laying adults until the following spring. In this way the small strongyles survive the adverse winter conditions outside by being inside the horse. The same probably is true in subtropical/tropical climates, where the larvae may prolong their development in the horse in the hot or dry season and probably recommence their development when the cool or rainy season begins.

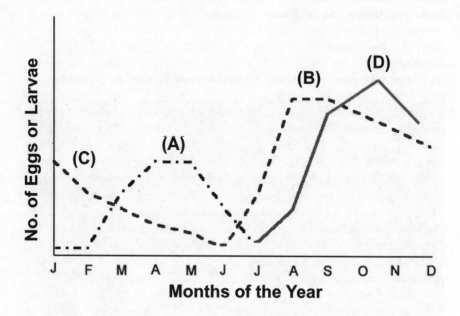

Figure 2 Pattern of cyathostome faecal egg production by the horses and pattern of resultant infective larvae on pasture in the course of a year in a northern temperate climate.
A) Spring rise in faecal egg counts in mares, youngstock and some adult horses. The worms that produce these eggs emerged from the large intestinal mucosa in Feb/Mar to continue development to adults and in the process could have induced cyathostomosis Type II in some horses.
B) Summer/autumn peak of infective larvae on pasture that develops from the spring rise in faecal eggs. When ingested by the horses some larvae will develop directly into adult worms this year (see D), others will inhibit and create next year's spring rise in faecal egg counts.
C) Overwintered infective larvae on pasture – these have survived over winter from the previous year's peak of larvae on pasture. Ingestion of these will contribute to the autumn peak in faecal egg counts (see D).
D) Faecal eggs produced by the peak of adult worms that have been acquired from ingestion of the overwintered larvae and from some of the summer peak of infective larvae on pasture (B). These worms contribute to cyathostomosis Type I.

Life-cycle on pasture

The life-cycle of all the strongyles outside the horse is similar. Most information is available for pastures in temperate climates and for the cyathostome larvae and most of the following description describes development in the northern temperate climate in Britain.

Immature worms that have overwintered in the horse develop to adults in early spring (approx. February/March/April). Eggs from these are passed in the faeces of infected horses, and a peak of eggs is passed in the spring and early summer, called the 'spring rise in faecal egg counts'. It is these eggs that are pivotal in perpetuation of the life-cycle of the worms. In warm, moist conditions the first-, second- and third-stage larvae develop in the faecal ball. To infect horses the infective larvae must migrate from the manure out onto the grass so that they can be eaten. This migration occurs in wet, warm weather, particularly after rain. If the weather stays dry the larvae will remain in the faecal ball where they are relatively protected from adverse conditions.

For the purposes of control of strongyle infections in horses, it is important to understand both the rates at which the parasites develop to the infective third-stage and the ability of the infective stages to survive on the grass. The development of the eggs to infective larvae requires a degree of moisture as well as temperatures of over approximately 10°-15° C but under 30°-35° C. The rate of development is slowest at the lower temperatures, taking several weeks, but once developed, the infective third-stage larvae can remain alive and available to infect horses for weeks or months at low temperatures. At the higher temperatures infective larvae develop in a few days, but they remain alive for only a few days to a week or two in very hot weather. The parasites are also killed by dry conditions.

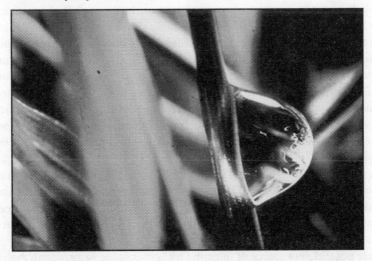

Figure 3   Infective strongyle larvae migrating in moisture up a blade of grass

Thus, in temperate climates such as Northern Europe the spring rise in faecal egg counts initiates the year's development. As spring and summer progress these eggs develop to infective third-stage larvae and the rate of development of these eggs increases from needing several weeks in the spring to about a week in midsummer. As a result large numbers of infective larvae develop together and are present from around mid-July onwards. With wet weather these larvae will migrate from the faeces onto the grass to be eaten by horses in the second half of summer through the autumn. It should be noted that while foals, yearlings and younger horses pass the highest numbers of eggs some adult horses remain susceptible and pass eggs throughout their life to contribute to the spring rise each year. Also, aged, debilitated horses may lose their resistance and show increased levels of infection.

Once eaten in the second half of summer and autumn by the horse the route of development of the worms depends in part on the species of the worm.

1) The infective larvae of the large strongyles, *S. vulgaris*, *S. edentatus* and *S. equinus*, migrate in the tissues of the body of the horse for several months returning to the large intestine to finally mature and lay eggs from the following spring.

2) Some of the infective larvae of the cyathostomes will develop in the large intestinal wall and emerge to become adults to pass eggs some two to four months later in early winter. However, these eggs are unimportant to the life-cycle as conditions outside are too cold for development and survival of the egg. Gradually the worms cease laying eggs overwinter and die.

3) Some of the infective third-stage larvae of the cyathostomes after they penetrate the intestinal wall suspend their development in the third-stage. These third-stage larvae remain inhibited or dormant over the winter. In early spring (February/March) they resume development through fourth-stage to adults and start laying eggs a few weeks later to produce the spring rise in faecal egg counts. So it is these inhibited larvae that are the most important in the perpetuation of the life-cycle of the worms. It should be noted that not all the inhibited larvae will resume development in the spring. Some larvae will remain inhibited and resume development at any time up to a year or two later. Equally, the conditions that induce the larvae to undergo inhibition inside the horse are unknown. By analogy with related parasites of cattle possibly a cold chill induced by the declining temperatures in autumn is responsible. Alternately, or in addition, the presence of the accumulating numbers of adult worms could provide negative feedback signals inducing the incoming third-stage larvae to inhibit. This then seems to mean that removing the adult worms with an anthelmintic can allow some of the inhibited worms to develop.

There is a different source of infection for horses at the beginning of the year. The infective third-stage larvae survive well over winter on pasture in temperate climates. Their numbers do decrease with time so that by June there are relatively few surviving from last year or these have been diluted by the new season's growth of grass. Nonetheless, there are still considerable numbers of infective larvae available to grazing horses in the spring. When ingested these larvae develop directly through their life-cycle to become egg-laying adults as little as two to four months later. While the earliest eggs laid could develop and contribute to the rise in infective larvae on pasture in the summer, most eggs laid by these worms will be passed in the autumn and so will not contribute to the life-cycle of the parasites.

Far less is known about transmission in hotter climates. Without rain early development of the eggs will not occur. As temperatures increase summer can become too hot, even if there is rain, for survival causing poor survival of those infective larvae that do develop. This occurs at summer temperatures above a minimum of about 28°C. Conversely, the now warmer and longer spring and autumn can allow development of larvae in two periods, one in spring and one in autumn. Further, the winter in some subtropical/tropical climates allows successful, albeit possibly slow, development of eggs and prolonged survival of L3 provided there is not prolonged frost. Thus, in these tropical/subtropical areas, cool season transmission with increased faecal egg counts beginning in the autumn, October/November in northern areas and April in southern areas, followed by high levels of development to infective larvae produces infection on pasture continuing through winter and into spring. The cool season then becomes the pivotal part of the life-cycle of the worms. The larvae do not survive long as summer approaches because of the high temperatures. Another variation in climatic effects on the infective stages of the strongyles is the division of the year into hot/dry and wet periods. Transmission occurs in the hot wet periods even though survival will not be long in the heat, with the hot/dry summer inimicable to larval survival.

Clinical signs
It is the immature stages of the large strongyle parasites that cause damage and disease while they are migrating in the body. The presence of a number of *S. vulgaris* in the arteries migrating up to the anterior mesenteric artery can induce fever, depression, inappetance and abdominal discomfort and colic may be seen 2-3 weeks after infection. This response therefore is most likely to be seen in the second half of summer when the horses will be exposed to the greatest number of infective larvae. The mechanisms by which the migrating larvae induce this reaction remain unknown although release of parasite products and the inflammatory response to them might induce intestinal motility disturbances. Within the lumen of the anterior mesenteric artery *S. vulgaris* causes clots and narrowing of the lumen and inflammation and thickening of the arterial wall.

Again there may be colic but frequently infected animals are depressed, tucked up, inappetant and unthrifty over the winter months. Migration back to the intestine in late winter/spring again may induce signs of colic with damage and clots particularly in the ileo-caeco-colic artery.

The artery will heal considerably when the larvae leave but a degree of damage will always remain. Also, repeated infections produce permanent damage, with thickening and hardening or, rarely, thinning and ballooning of the wall. However, horses do develop protection against reinfection with *S. vulgaris* so that disease is most commonly seen in foals and yearlings. It must be remembered though that under a very good parasite control programme horses may not be exposed to infection and could remain relatively unprotected to infection sometime in the future.

Strongylus edentatus and *S. equinus* migrate for some time in the liver and can cause fibrosis and hardening of the liver. Both parasites might induce adhesions of the intestines to each other and to the abdominal wall, and clinical signs of colic and unthriftiness. *Strongylus equinus* may cause pancreatitis. These signs now tend to be rare. Somewhat more common is the fact that *S. edentatus,* when resident in the abdominal wall, in some horses may cause inflammation of the abdominal wall and, rarely, rupture of the inflamed arteries producing a large internal clot and severe colic.

Disease due to the cyathostomes occurs mainly at two times of the year although ill thrift and occasionally severe disease can be recorded in horses at other times of year. The first form of disease is seen in the autumn/early winter of the year in northern temperate climates and is called Type I cyathostomosis. Affected horses may produce soft or diarrhoeic faeces, often intermittently, with loss of condition, sometimes oedema and thickening of the limbs and sometimes colic and even deaths. The disease probably is multifactorial. The cyathostome larvae penetrating into, developing in and leaving the large intestinal wall in late summer must cause a host inflammatory response. This will be compounded by the accumulating adult cyathostomes. Antigens produced by these, plus the damage induced by some adult worms grazing on the mucosa, also would induce a host inflammatory response. Finally, larvae of *S. vulgaris* will be migrating up to the anterior mesenteric artery at this time and these are known to induce abdominal discomfort, fever, inappetance, etc.

The second time disease is seen is in late winter/early spring. It is called Type II cyathostomosis. At this time the infective larvae eaten the previous autumn, that underwent inhibition over winter in the horse, emerge to continue development to adults.

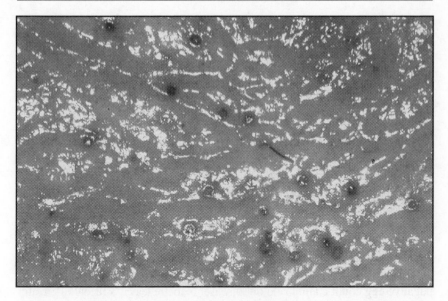

Figure 4   Encysted cyathostome larvae resuming their development in the spring to break out of the wall of the large intestine

They emerge relatively simultaneously from the wall of the large intestine and, if a large number of worms are present, this massive emergence breaks down the intestinal wall. Also a marked host inflammatory response can occur and there can be massive infiltration of eosinophils and other cells and oedema of the wall in some horses. The emergence can cause acute, severe diarrhoea, possibly containing blood, that can be fatal. Other or less severely affected animals may show one or more of a longer course of diarrhoea, loss of appetite, severe loss of weight, oedema and thickened limbs. Type II cyathostomosis is most likely to be severest in foals and yearlings under-going their first and second winters, respectively, after a summers grazing. Age resistance, possibly immune resistance to infection does develop in some horses so cyathostomosis Type II is most frequent in horses less than five years old. However, other horses remain relatively susceptible to infection throughout their lives. These horses not only contribute to contamination of the pastures but could suffer from Type I or Type II cyathostomosis even as adults. While many horses without suitable control programmes can be infected with large numbers of cyathostome larvae frequently there may be only modest changes to the intestinal mucosa. Why in some horses there is a marked response and acute Type II with sudden onset diarrhoea, emaciation and possibly death over two to three weeks is not known. Possibly there are differences in the immune, allergic response of the individual horses to the antigens of the parasites.

Diagnosis

Heavy infections with adult small strongyles (Type I cyathostomosis) causing diarrhoea, loss of condition and even death in horses in the late summer and autumn can be diagnosed by counting the numbers of eggs in the faeces. While faecal egg counts may not directly correlate with levels of infection, they are a good indicator of the severity of the infection. In general, counts of 500-1,000 eggs per gram are considered indicative of subclinical disease. The horses may be 'poor doers' or not perform as well as might be expected. Counts of over 1,000-2,000 eggs per gram must be considered serious with the potential for serious disease, colic, etc..

Diagnosis of of the migration of *Strongylus* spp. and of Type II cyathostomosis is much more difficult. Unfortunately most of the clinical signs of the disease (colic, poor condition, diarrhoea, etc.) due to the *Strongylus* spp. migrating in the winter/spring or due to the cyathostomes emerging in the spring are caused by the immature stages. These are not yet laying eggs so that diagnosis cannot be made directly by faecal egg counts. Thus, a low or negative egg count cannot rule out disease. Nonetheless if a faecal egg count were positive then it could help to indicate a history of exposure to infection although it cannot conclusively diagnose disease. A number of blood parameters, an increase in the number of eosinophils or IgG(T), both frequently raised in parasitic infections, or a decrease in plasma albumen or fructosamine lost into the intestine because of leakage are useful indicators. However, these are non-specific responses and so are not reliable as diagnostic tests. If faeces were collected and washed and sieved large numbers of worms might be present and also they might be found on the glove after a rectal examination. These are useful if present but not if absent. Examination of a biopsy of the bowel mucosa would reveal large numbers of worms and a marked host inflammatory eosinophil response to them. Very useful will be the history of grazing and managemental and anthelmintic measures applied over the year. Do these indicate that perpetuation of the life-cycle was possible? However, repeated prophylactic anthelmintic treatment is not guaranteed to rule out disease due to the strongyles/cyathostomes. The parasites may have developed resistance to and so will tolerate therapeutic doses of the drugs without being killed.

Treatment and prevention

It is far more satisfactory to institute a regular anthelmintic treatment and/or management programme to control infection and prevent disease due to the large strongyles and cyathostomes than it is to treat the disease after the damage has already been done. Also, while the adult worms are killed readily by anthelmintics, the larval stages involved in or actually causing disease are much less susceptible to being killed.

A number of anthelmintics (Table 1) are effective against the adult *Strongylus* spp. and the adult cyathostomes. These therefore are useful in control

Table 1 Anthelmintics available for horses. (Not all these products are available in every country and nor will all the indications be approved for use in any one country)

	Strongylus spp adults (1)	Migrating Strongylus (5)	Cyathostome adults	Encysted cyathostomes (2)	P. equorum (3,5)	O. equi	Anoplocephala spp. (4)	Gasterophilus spp
Febantel	++		++		++	++		
Thiabendazole	++		++		88mg/kg	++		
Mebendazole	+ - ++		+		++	++		
Fenbendazole	++		++		++	++		
Fenbendazole 5-day 10mg/kg	++	++	++	++	++	++		
Oxfendazole	++		++		++			
Oxibendazole	++		++		++	++		
Pyrantel	+ - ++		++		++	+	++ double dose Other regimens	
Ivermectin	++	++	++	+/-	++	++		++
Moxidectin	++	++	++	++	++	++		++
Dichlorvos	+ - ++		+ - ++		++	++		++ (>1 mth.) (6)
Piperazine	+/-		++		++	+/-		
Levamisole/piperazone	+ - ++		++		++	+		

1 Efficacy against *S. edentatus* adults tends to be lower than against *S. vulgaris* adults.
2 In foals and yearlings heavily infected with *P. equorum* avoid using fast-acting drugs such as those containing piperazine or the organophosphates as they kill the worms too fast with the potential of forming a bolus of dead worms passing down the gut.
3 Ivermectin – 34-42% effective (mainly late L4 and L5); moxidectin – 70-80% effective (late L3, L4 and L5); fenbendazole five-day – 90-95% (early L3 90%, late L3, L4 and L5).
4 Pyrantel normal dose also about 80% effective.
5 Low daily doses of pyrantel help prevent tapeworms and migrating *P. equo rum* and *S. vulgaris*.
6 Dichlorvos does not kill bots during their first month in the mouth of the horse.

programmes designed to prevent egg production. They also are useful in treatment of cyathostomosis Type I in the autumn in northern temperate climates. It should be noted that there is a tendency, however, for the anthelmintics to be less effective against adult *S. edentatus* than *S. vulgaris*.

There are a few anthelmintics that will kill the migrating *Strongylus* spp. Migrating larval stages of *S. vulgaris* causing colic or severe ill thrift in the winter months are susceptible to ivermectin or moxidectin or fenbendazole at an increased dose rate (30-60 mg/kg) or as the 5-day regimen. Resolution of lesions in the anterior mesenteric artery does occur provided repeated and permanent damage has not occurred.

Again there are a few anthelmintics that have effect against either the inhibited or the developing stages of the cyathostomes in the mucosa of the large intestine. Ivermectin does have some effect but only against the oldest of the developing worms. Moxidectin has greater effect killing most of the developing third-, fourth- and fifth-stages. Fenbendazole five-day has been shown to kill these and as many as 90% of the inhibited early third-stages. As a result these latter two drugs should be used to treat cyathostomosis Type II. As the disease is associated with marked inflammatory pathology in the intestinal mucosa and loss of fluids, anti-inflammatory corticosteroid therapy and fluid therapy also are necessary. Nonetheless, the prediction of a successful recovery is poor, as many as 50-60% of affected horses may die despite treatment.

As a result prevention definitely is preferable to 'fire-engine' therapy to cure strongylosis and cyathostomosis. Currently two main types of control programme are in operation, 'pick-up-faeces' and anthelmintic control. Both control programmes are designed to prevent the pastures becoming infected with the infective stages of the worms and so consequently should prevent infection in grazing horses.

The first, and certainly a most effective although labour-intensive, programme is purely managemental and consists simply of regular removal of the manure from the paddocks either manually or by vacuum or sweeper machines. The manure must be removed at least twice a week during the warm summer months when the parasites are developing very rapidly, but slightly less frequent removal would suffice in the colder months. This measure on its own has been shown to very effective at removing the eggs from the pasture and so vastly reducing the numbers of infective larvae on pasture. Furthermore, as horses avoid grazing near areas of grass contaminated with manure the grass here tends to grow roughly and rankly (the zone of repugnance). Removing the manure prevents this and so has the advantage of increasing the amount of grazing and improving the pastures. Pick-up-faeces should also reduce the numbers of other parasites available to the horses on pasture, i.e. *P. equorum* and *Anoplocephala perfoliata*. The collected faecal material preferably should be composted away from the grazing as, if the muck heap is on the edge of pastures there could be some development of larvae in the surface layers. Either the surface layer should be covered rapidly with additional manure or it should be turned inwards weekly to create the heat and lack of oxygen required to kill the parasites. Potentially, covering the pile with plastic sheeting will have a similar effect and this is known to increase the rate of composting for sale of the product.

Before a pick-up-faeces programme is begun however, the horses should be treated with a cleansing dose of a highly effective anthelmintic, i.e. they should be treated with moxidectin or fenbendazole 5-day, else they could carry large numbers of worms for many months after institution of the programme. All horses entering the property should also be so treated. Also, treatment of the resident horses for bots should be considered or, far preferably, bot eggs should be cut from the horses to prevent the use of drugs all together. Finally, *P. equorum* must continue to be targeted. While a 'pick-up-faeces' programme will remove the vast majority of the eggs, this worm is extremely prolific, each producing some hundred thousand eggs a day, and the eggs are very sticky. Thus eggs will stick to floors and grass and soil and even small amounts of faeces that remain uncollected could contain many eggs. As the eggs can remain alive for a few years' egg numbers could accumulate. Therefore, both foals, and possibly yearlings, must be treated to control *P. equorum* or a grazing management programme instituted to prevent infection.

The second method of control is designed to reduce greatly the number of eggs being passed in the faeces of horses out onto the grass. The adult worms are killed with an anthelmintic. This will greatly reduce the number of eggs being excreted for a period of weeks. The time after anthelmintic treatment when eggs are again passed is the egg reappearance period (ERP). The length of this depends on the age of the parasite stages in the horse that are killed and so the ERP is shortest for those that kill only adult and near adult stages, longer for those that kill fourth-stages and longest for those that kill third-stages. Thus the ERP for pyrantel tends to be about 4-6 weeks, that for the benzimidazoles about 4-6 weeks, ivermectin as much as 8 weeks or more and moxidectin and fenbendazole five-day some 12-15 weeks or more. The treatment of horses at the time of ERP for that drug will markedly reduce egg output and so the number of infective stages that can develop on the pasture. In order to reduce the number of treatments that must be given, the anthelmintics should be given at the time that is most strategically important in the life-cycle. Thus, in northern temperate climates anthelmintic treatments should begin in February and continue at the ERP for that particular drug through to about August/September. In hotter climates with cool season transmission treatments should start at the end of summer through the cool season to prevent the cool, winter season transmission.

A modification of the anthelmintic treatment programme is to identify and treat only infected horses, i.e. target infected horses. In northern temperate climates this targeting will begin in February. All horses in the herd will undergo faecal egg counts at about two-week intervals. Those horses showing a faecal egg count of over 100-200 eggs per gram of faeces will be treated, those with numbers lower than 100-200 eggs per gram remain untreated at that examination. These examinations must continue until about July/August although at an increasing interval. Among the herd of horses some horses will have to be treated several times depending on the ERP of the drug used. Other horses will not require treatment at all. In the autumn/early winter (October/early November) the horses should be re-examined to ensure efficacy of the programme. In the first year of such a programme counts could well have increased at this time due to the ingestion of larvae overwintered from the previous year. Although these eggs are unimportant for control as they will not develop to the infective stage, infected horses with a clinically significant egg count must be treated. As the programme continues each year, the counts in October will reflect the efficacy of the programme and the horses should remain with very low counts. Gradually, horses will be identified as susceptible, regularly producing egg counts greater than 200 eggs per gram and examinations will concentrate on these. Others will be designated as resistant (either due to their genetic make up and/or immune capability) and will rarely require treatment. Nonetheless, these resistant horses must not be ignored as they may well lose their resistance for a variety of reasons that include increasing age and concurrent disease. The advantage of this targeting method of control is that there are always some horses and therefore some worms, even though at low levels, that remain unexposed to treatment and so this should help prevent the development of resistance to anthelmintics (see below). It is essential that all horses entering the property should be dosed on arrival with moxidectin and quarantined indoors for three to seven days to prevent potentially drug resistant eggs, or eggs at all reaching the pastures.

Preferably these horses should have a pick-up-faeces programme or have egg counts monitored regularly for sometime after their arrival, particularly their first winter and spring, or longer bearing in mind that a few cyathostomes could remain inhibited within the horse for a year or more.

Whatever control programme is instituted an important part is monitoring the programme. Faecal egg counts from some or all the horses should be examined at times when peak faecal egg counts are expected for that particular climatic region. Egg counts in October in a northern temperate climate, if high, would indicate a failure in control. A faecal egg count reduction test on the horses (egg counts before and about 10 days after treatment with the drug used that year) should be carried out. This would indicate whether the failure has been due to the anthelmintic used that year (a reduction of >95% is needed to show that the anthelmintic is still effective). Remedial 'fire engine' therapy with an anthelmintic effective against all stages then will be required, this given immediately and possibly again the following January/February to remove any accumulated, overwintering larval stages. It must be noted too that a figure of 100-200 eggs per gram at the moment is relatively arbitrary so the programme must be monitored with care to determine the level in a particular region, climate, etc..

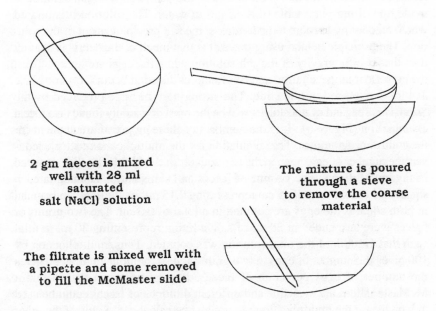

2 gm faeces is mixed well with 28 ml saturated salt (NaCl) solution

The mixture is poured through a sieve to remove the coarse material

The filtrate is mixed well with a pipette and some removed to fill the McMaster slide

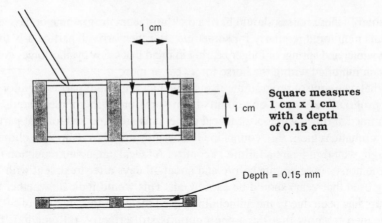

1 cm

Square measures
1 cm x 1 cm
with a depth
of 0.15 cm

1 cm

Depth = 0.15 mm

The eggs are counted in the squares on both sides of the
McMaster slide.
Each egg multiplied by a factor of 50 gives the number of
eggs/gm of faeces.

Figure 5   Faecal egg counts are relatively easy to perform and although a
microscope is required it need not be sophisticated and requires only 100X
magnification. The technique is presented in Figure 5 and requires mainly
kitchen equipment but it also requires a McMaster slide. The salt solution is
made by boiling plain table or rock salt in water. The solution is saturated
when, on cooling to room temperature, some salt precipitates out of the solution. The principle behind using this salt is that much of the debris is heavier
than the specific gravity of the salt solution while the eggs are lighter. Thus,
the eggs float in the solution and can found in the chamber in the same plane
as the lines etched on the slide. The strongyle-type eggs produced by the
Strongylus spp. and cyathostomes will be the most commonly found on a faecal
examination (Figure 6). It is the numbers of these eggs that are counted for
the control programmes. The calculation for the multiplication factor to convert the number of eggs seen in the two squares of the McMaster slide depicted
in Figure 5 follows. The volume of faeces and salt solution counted in each
square is 1 cm x 1 cm x 0.15 cm representing 0.15 ml. As the eggs are counted
in both squares the eggs are counted in a total of 0.3 ml. The two grams of
faeces were suspended in 28 ml of salt solution representing 30 ml in total
such that 1/100th of the total solution was counted. Thus, multiplication by
100 gives the number of eggs in two grams and so multiplication by 50 gives
the number of eggs per gram of faeces. It must be noted that different
McMaster slides are available and different dilutions of faeces could be used
in which case the multiplication factor must be calculated. Some of the other
eggs that will be seen and that are counted separately are presented in
Figure 6.

Figure 6   Eggs commonly found on faecal examination of horses.

(A) A strongyle-type egg

(B) An *Anoplocephala* spp. egg

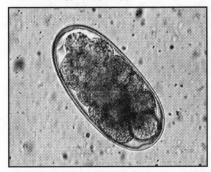
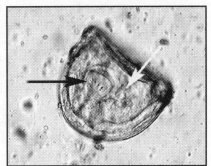

(C) A *Parascaris equorum* egg

(D) An *Oxyuris equi* egg

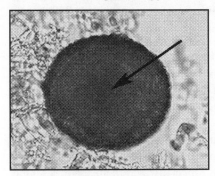
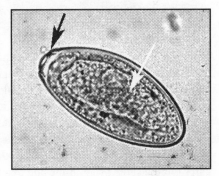

(A) A strongyle-type egg. This egg is produced by the large *Strongylus* spp., by all the different cyathostomes and by *T. axei*. It contains a morula of eight or more cells when passed in the faeces and is mainly brown in colour. Often 90-120 μm long

(B) An *Anoplocephala* spp. egg. This egg is characterised by containing the six-hooked infective stage, the oncosphere (black arrow). The oncosphere lies in the base of a pear-shaped apparatus although on this photograph the prongs forming the top of the pear (white arrow) are barely visible. The egg is grey in colour and can be D-shaped as here or square in shape and about 70-80 μm in diameter

(C) A *Parascaris equorum* egg. This egg is dark brown, about 80-100 μm round and it is very difficult to see the single cell, the ovum (arrowed), through the thick, dark brown, sticky wall

(D) An *Oxyuris equi* egg. These sometimes fall from the perineum into the faeces. This yellow egg, around 80 μm long, has an operculum (cap) (black arrow) at one end. The larva (white arrow) can be seen within the egg

Other techniques aid control. The grazing can be rotated with horses grazing pastures one year (or half year) and sheep or cattle grazing the following year and preferably for two years. The ruminants will eat the equine infective larvae but there is likely be transmission to the horses of *T. axei* (p. 531). Pastures should not be harrowed except in very hot/dry weather or extremely cold weather. In a northern temperate climate such as Britain the weather is rarely suitable to rapidly kill the larvae once they are spread from their faecal refuge onto the grass. The paddock would need to remain free of horses for many months after the harrowing. Reduced stocking densities are helpful so that horses do not have to graze the grass in the zone of repugnance where the highest numbers of infective larvae are found. An area for continued investigation is use of the nematophagous (worm-eating) fungi. Spores of these fungi when fed to horses are excreted in the faeces and the fungi then grow in the manure. The fungus then traps and uses the nematode larvae as a source of food. Some, such as *Duddingtonia flagrans*, have been tested on horses. This has been shown to reduce the numbers of larvae developing in faeces, to reduce the numbers of infective third-stage larvae on pasture and to reduce the number of worms present in grazing horses. While the effect is not absolute this would be a non-anthelmintic adjunct to a control programme. Also, the fungi would have no effect against *P. equorum* in eggs that still would need to be targeted in youngstock. There is potential that fungi could be marketed in feed or in supplement blocks if their use passed the relevant licensing authorities in each country.

A number of factors must be borne in mind when instituting a control programme. Climate and management are important. These mean that a programme must be prepared individually for each different stable. Everyone must carry out the same programme and this is especially a problem at liveries. One person picking up faeces is pointless unless only their own horse(s) graze that paddock and the horse(s) eat grass nowhere else on the property. In particular, horses are taken to areas frequented by other horses (other stables, showgrounds, even roadside verges on which horses are ridden regularly) and they are at risk of becoming infected even by eating small amounts of grass. Equally, horses visiting a property could deposit their worm eggs and also these might be eggs from drug resistant worms (see below). Do not import other people's worms or give your own. This can be achieved by picking up faeces and not grazing elsewhere. Studs must be particularly careful. Visiting mares must not be allowed to deposit eggs on pastures that are then going to be grazed by youngstock. The mares must be treated and quarantined, or housed and faeces disposed of carefully or there must be a very efficient pick-up-faeces programme. Whichever method is used to control the strongyles, particular attention must be paid to the foals and yearlings. Young animals are highly susceptible to infection and so disease and they can pass very large numbers of eggs in their faeces. Also, anthelmintic treatment does not produce as big a reduction in the number of eggs passed by foals and yearlings compared with older horses. Managemental control by twice weekly removal of faeces for paddocks grazed by youngstock is essential. Finally, a highly effective control programme started from scratch could over several years reduce the nematodes so markedly that the horses lose or are unable to develop immunity to *Strongylus* and the cyathostomes. These horses would be highly susceptible when subsequently exposed (i.e. if sold). A very useful development would be specific tests to monitor the acquired resistance of the horses.

Anthelmintic resistance in *Strongylus* spp. and the cyathostomes
Anthelmintic resistance by the worms has been a problem mainly with the cyathostomes and only rarely has been described in the large *Strongylus* spp.. It is an important problem that will arise in the anthelmintic treatment control programmes. The worms are capable of developing resistance to the effects of the anthelmintics. This means that a dose of anthelmintic that was effective in killing the worms no longer is able to do so as the worms resist its effects and these resistant worms remain in the horse after treatment. Also, resistant worms can shorten their egg reappearance period. The resistance is genetic and arises by spontaneous mutation but once one population of worms has developed a resistant gene then that resistant gene can be spread all over to other stables and countries by movement of horses. Initially within the horses there will be a very few resistant worms and many worms that still carry the genes of susceptibility to the drug. When wormed with that particular anthelmintic to which they carry the gene then the susceptible worms will be killed and only the resistant worms will remain. It is only these resistant worms that will produce eggs thus contaminating the pastures with resistant progeny. This will continue until essentially all the worms in the population are resistant to the anthelmintic. In the early stages of resistance development the horses will appear normal and unless faecal egg counts are performed no evidence of resistance will be seen. Gradually as more of the worm population remains in the horse the horses will not 'do as well' but as parasites are very insidious creatures it can be difficult to detect this clinically. Finally, obvious signs of disease will develop as primarily Type I or Type II cyathostomosis and horses will lose weight, show colic, etc. Once this has occurred the drug has failed completely and essentially can never be used again. Furthermore no other drug in that group can be used. Thus parasites resistant to the benzimidazoles will be resistant to all of febantel, thiabendazole, mebendazole, fenbendazole normal dose, oxfendazole and now oxibendazole. While a higher or longer dose, i.e. fenbendazole 5-day, will break this resistance this effect is only temporary as the worms will develop resistance to this larger dose. Also, when parasites become resistant to either ivermectin or moxidectin they will develop resistance to both of these anthelmintics and resistance to pyrantel will result in resistance to levamisole where it also is available. This is why it is important to note the generic name

of the drug and not purchase drugs on the basis of their Trade name.

Resistance to the benzimidazole anthelmintics now has been detected at high frequency in horses in all countries of the world. This is because these drugs were the first very safe drugs developed, they were developed early and they have been used very frequently. However, resistance to the second group pyrantel/levamisole now is being detected. It seems inevitable that resistance will develop sooner or later, if not already started, to the third group of drugs, namely ivermectin and moxidectin as it is known that resistance has developed among sheep parasites to these drugs. These three groups are the only groups of drugs available. It should be noted that on some sheep farms in some areas of the world, the worms in the sheep have developed resistance to all the groups of drugs available (and more groups are available for sheep) and sheep farming as an enterprise had to cease on the properties. The same could happen to horse stables. There is very recent evidence of a newly discovered anthelmintic that does show efficacy in the treatment of worms in horses but it will take a long time to determine whether this product will reach the market as it goes through all the testing for safety, etc..

Although resistance is deemed inevitable, there are various methods that are recommended to reduce the rate at which resistance develops although considerable information yet is required as to the full validity of each method. It is essential that, before an anthelmintic treatment programme is begun, the worms are tested for the presence of resistance. If the worms are resistant to a drug, then it is pointless to use this drug or any related drug to treat the horses. Use of the drug will only worsen the situation. Currently, resistance can only be detected by a faecal egg count reduction test. Unfortunately, this is relatively insensitive. However, in the near future it is hoped that new laboratory based tests will become widely available. Initially these will test the developing egg and L1 stages either in the laboratory or elsewhere using the test in kit form. Finally it is hoped that tests that will detect the actual resistance gene in individual worms will become available although this certainly is not expected in the near future.

The recommendations to reduce the rate at which resistance develops include:

1) Use as few anthelmintic treatments as possible each year (indeed an effective 'pick-up-faeces' programme does not need anthelmintic treatments (although see the possible special considerations above).

2) Rotate the group of anthelmintic slowly, usually yearly, making the change in the spring of each year when the population of worms changes over in a northern temperate climate. This means perhaps that a benzimidazole (if no resistance is apparent) should be used in year one, pyrantel/levamisole in year two, and ivermectin/moxidectin in year three. Bot eggs should be removed manually although this may not be necessary in the year ivermectin/moxidectin is used.

3) Avoid underdosing. Preferably find access to a weighscale.
4) Avoid introducing resistant worms in visiting or newly purchased horses.
5) Monitor for resistance by submitting samples for faecal egg counts.

Finally, consider the advice given to you. A major source of information is commercial advertising targeting a drug or drugs at particular parasites at certain times of year. Obviously the advertising is intended to sell the product and while it is likely to be technically and factually correct it could be unbalanced or misleading in the context of the overall picture of a control programme. Advertising may have influenced even articles in journals and veterinary advice itself.

TRICHOSTRONGYLUS AXEI

These very small, 6-mm-long, slender worms occur in sheep, cattle and goats in every country of the world. They can also be found in the stomach of horses. Horses usually become infected when they graze with sheep and cattle, but once infected they may transmit the infection among themselves. The life-cycle of *T. axei* on the ground is similar to that of the horse strongyles, infection of horses occurring mainly in the second half of summer in temperate climates. Once eaten, the larvae become adult, egg-laying females in three weeks. Usually *T. axei* is not pathogenic in horses and causes no disease, so no measures need be applied to control the infection. Heavily infected horses could show gastritis, inappetance and weight loss. Diagnosis is difficult since the eggs laid by *T. axei* are virtually identical to those produced by the *Strongylus* and cyathostome spp. Development of eggs to third-stage larvae in the laboratory does, however, allow morphological differentiation of *T. axei* from *Strongylus* and cyathostome spp. If horses are grazing with ruminants it could be important to do this in control programmes aimed at the *Strongylus* and cyathostome spp. that are based on strongyle-type faecal egg counts. This because the prepatent period of *T. axei* is much shorter and the early reappearance of *T. axei* eggs in the faeces might be mistaken for a breakdown in control of the more important *Strongylus* and cyathostome spp.

PARASCARIS EQUORUM (LARGE ROUNDWORM)

These long, robust roundworms, cream/pink in colour up to 50 cm long, are found in the small intestine. Large numbers may be found in foals, yearlings also are infected, while adult horses carry few or no worms.

Life-cycle

Eggs passed in the faeces develop on the ground to infective larvae retained within the egg's very thick shell. When foals eat infective eggs, the microscopic larvae hatch, and migrate through the intestinal wall and via the blood to the liver, heart and lungs. In the lungs the larvae break out into the air spaces and migrate up the trachea to be swallowed. All the larvae are in the intestine by 25 days. Adults start laying eggs two to three months after infection and each female passes thousands of eggs a day.

Young foals can become infected repeatedly and several hundred to a thousand adult *P. equorum* can develop in their intestines, but these worms are lost gradually over six to nine months. Foals gradually develop a protective immune response so that, on each reinfection, an increasing proportion of the invading larvae is killed and cannot develop to adult worms. Therefore the infection is most common in foals up to six to nine months of age and to a lesser extent in yearlings. Occasionally adult horses will be infected with a few adult ascarids but these normally are unimportant.

Development of eggs takes two to three weeks or much longer, depending on the weather. In warmer climates (and in stables) eggs passed by foals can develop quite rapidly and are the source of infection for the same and other foals born that year. In temperate climates, development occurs in the summer months and ceases in autumn through winter to begin again in the spring. As the majority of worms are found in foals, *P. equorum* infection therefore is passed from the foals born and infected in one spring to the foals of the next year. The infective eggs, protected by their thick shells, are very long-lived and remain alive at least a year and probably two or three. The eggs of *P. equorum* have a very sticky coat. Thus, the eggs passed by foals in one year will stick to and remain alive on the walls, floors and equipment in stables and particularly on the pastures. They act as the source of infection for the foals born in the next year's foaling season. Egg numbers are reduced by filtering down to lower levels in the soil if paddocks have well drained, gravel/sand soils.

Clinical signs

Occasionally, if a foal is exposed to a large number of eggs over a short period of time, then coughing and respiratory distress can result one to three weeks later as the larvae migrate through the lungs. More usually the foal eats eggs over a longer period of time, and then the adult worms in the intestines cause loss of appetite, dullness, unthriftiness and diarrhoea. The foal will not grow as well as expected and may have a potbelly and staring coat. Very occasionally large numbers of worms coiled and tangled in the intestines can block it physically. A few worms cause no harm to foals, or adult horses.

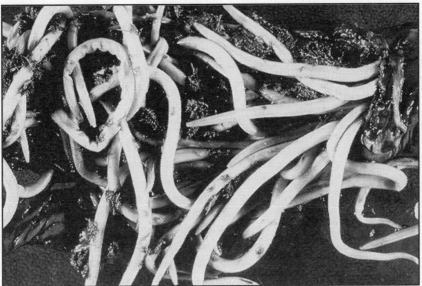

Figure 7   A very heavy burden of *Parascaris equorum* in the small intestine

Diagnosis

The thick- and rough-shelled, brown eggs can be found on faecal examination. As the female worms are prolific egg layers, only large numbers of eggs will be significant clinically.

Treatment

The majority of anthelmintics developed to treat the strongyle nematodes in horses are 90-99% effective against adult *P. equorum* (see Table 1). Ivermectin and 5-day fenbendazole are very effective at killing lung larvae.

Control

Disease can be prevented but eradication of *P. equorum* essentially is impossible. Since the thick-shelled eggs are very long-lived on pastures and in stables, as well as being very resistant to disinfectants, etc., control of *P. equorum* infections by good hygiene is very difficult. Only prolonged dry heat is lethal. Many thousands of eggs are passed and they are very sticky, so while a pick-up-faeces control programme will reduce numbers markedly, it will not remove all of the eggs from surfaces. Prophylactic treatment of foals (and yearlings) with anthelmintic at intervals of one to two months until they reach six to nine months of age substantially reduces burdens but again does not totally prevent egg output. The use of different stables and pastures for the foals each year will reduce levels of infection substantially, but some of the eggs will survive more than a year in temperate climates, so this procedure is not absolute in practice.

DICTYOCAULUS ARNFIELDI (LUNGWORMS)

These white, 3.5-cm-long, slender worms live in the air passages (bronchi and bronchioles) of the lungs. Although lungworms are probably found in many areas of the world, usually only a small proportion of horses are infected or show signs of disease.

Life-cycle
Eggs containing a larva are laid in the air passage, coughed up and swallowed and passed in the faeces. In the summer months the larvae hatch and develop quite rapidly to the infective stage. When eaten with grass by horses, the larvae migrate through the intestinal wall and via the circulation to the lungs, where they break out into the air passages to develop to adults. In many horses, particularly adult horses, the development of the worms is stopped when they reach the stage of immature adults. Consequently the worms rarely mature to lay eggs. Younger horses sometimes carry worms laying eggs so that transmission within a herd of horses is possible. Most commonly however, horses become infected from donkeys when they graze land in common with donkeys or mules. Up to 70% of donkeys may be infected with lungworms, but show no clinical signs of disease.

Clinical signs
Presence of the worms and death of the worms in the lungs and bronchioles causes an inflammatory response and heavy infections can cause respiratory disease. It is not known how many horses are infected with lungworm nor what proportion of those infected actually show any clinical signs of disease. Infected foals usually show no signs of disease. Some infected adult horses will have a chronic cough, particularly during exercise, and an increased respiratory rate, and these signs can persist for a long time.

Diagnosis
Diagnosis is difficult since usually, in horses infected with lungworm and displaying a chronic cough, the parasites have developed only to immature adults. Therefore eggs will not be passed in the faeces and no other reliable diagnostic test is available. If lungworm eggs were found in the faeces of other, younger horses or donkeys grazing the same pasture, then this would warrant treatment for lungworm. Tracheal and bronchial washings may reveal the presence of high numbers of eosinophils. However, while this might indicate lungworm, eosinophils are also present in allergic respiratory conditions. Occasionally worms or eggs may be seen in the aspirate.

Treatment

The horses can be treated with ivermectin or with moxidectin or with increased doses of fenbendazole.

Preventive measures

All the horses (and donkeys, mules, asses) in the stable should be treated to prevent continued transmission of the infection. Horses should not be grazed with donkeys, nor should they be grazed near paddocks where donkeys are grazed as the infective larvae might be transferred quite a distance.

OXYURIS EQUI (PINWORMS)

Found in the large intestine of horses throughout the world, the males are small, but females reach 5-10 cm long. They are white grey in colour with a long tail tapering to a point, hence the name pinworm.

Life-cycle and epidemiology

The female worms live in the large intestine but, when mature and filled with eggs, they move down the gut, crawl out through the anus and lay clusters of yellowish eggs in a sticky mass on the skin around the anus under the tail. The eggs develop to an infective larva within the egg in a few days. The eggs later fall off or are rubbed off onto bedding, into feed troughs, and so on, and horses are reinfected when they eat eggs with fodder and bedding. If the eggs fall off in paddocks they can dehydrate and die quite rapidly, so pinworm infections are most intense in stabled horses.

Clinical signs

Female worms laying eggs and the eggs stuck in gelatinous masses around the anus are irritating. Heavily infected horses rub their tails, breaking hairs producing an unkempt rat-tail. If the horse rubs its tail on rough or protruding objects within the stable it can break the skin, producing sores.

Diagnosis

Occasionally a whitish female pinworm with its pointed tail is passed on the surface of faeces. Sometimes, but not routinely, eggs can be found on faecal examination. A rubbed tail might suggest an infection. Confirmation requires detection of eggs. These can be seen microscopically on a piece of clear sticky tape that has been applied to the skin around the anus and then pulled off, or in yellowish masses that have been scraped off. The horse must be restrained properly during these procedures.

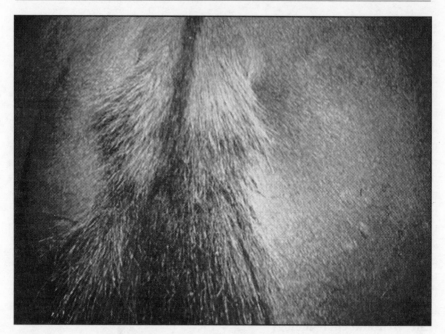

Figure 8   Rubbed 'rat-tail' due to the irritation caused by *Oxyuris equi*

Treatment
All the drugs listed in Table 1 are effective for the treatment of pinworms.

Preventive measures
Measures are not usually applied specifically for the control of pinworms. Any anthelmintic treatment programme for the *Strongylus* spp. and cyathostomes will control infection with *O. equi* also. In fact, the presence of *O. equi* may suggest that a strongyle control programme is not being applied properly or at all and the complete worming programme should be reviewed. However, if the worms are being controlled by twice weekly removal of manure from the paddocks, then *O. equi* could develop in horses stabled for all or part of the day. Eggs can be removed by cleaning the perianal area with a damp cloth when grooming, so breaking the cycle.

STRONGYLOIDES WESTERI (THREADWORM)

This is a very small, fine worm found in the intestine of foals. It occurs throughout the world.

Life-cycle

Strongyloides westeri has a very complicated life-cycle. The mare passes the infection in her milk to her foal when the foal is only a few days old. The worms develop very rapidly in the foal and eggs will be passed in its faeces by the time it is ten-days-old. In warm, moist conditions these eggs develop in as little as twenty-four hours to infective third-stage larvae to reinfect the foal. In addition, in very warm, damp conditions, in the wet bedding of dirty stables, for example, the parasites can multiply their numbers outside the host in a non-parasitic form of the life-cycle. The larvae develop to free-living males and females. These in turn produce eggs and infective larvae. This increases greatly the number of parasites available to infect the foal. Horses become infected either by eating the infective larvae or, alternatively, the larvae can penetrate through the horses' skin. In foals the larvae migrate via the circulatory system through the liver and lungs, are coughed up and swallowed and develop as adults in the intestine. In adult horses, by contrast, the larvae usually migrate into the body tissues, where they remain without any further development to adult worms. Only in the mare do these larvae reactivate, and when she begins to produce milk the larvae migrate to the udder to be transferred in the milk to her foal.

Clinical signs

Strongyloides westeri used to be considered a relatively common and important cause of diarrhoea in very young foals. Much of this diarrhoea now is thought to be due to overconsumption of milk (nine-day scours) and to bacterial or viral infection, so that the importance of *S. westeri* has fallen. Nevertheless in some heavily infected foals, particularly those kept in relatively unhygienic conditions, damage to the intestine caused by the worms will result in yellowish to bloody, fluid faeces. Particularly heavy infections might well develop in immunocompromised foals.

Diagnosis

Thousands of thin-shelled eggs already containing a first-stage larva will be present in the faeces. Only very large numbers of eggs will be significant.

Treatment

The foals can be treated with the normal dose of ivermectin, moxidectin or thiabendazole or with increased doses of oxibendazole or fenbendazole.

Preventive measures

Control usually is not attempted, but on stud farms, where heavy infections in foals occasionally can be encountered, the mares can be treated with ivermectin just before they foal to reduce the number of larvae passed in their milk to the foal. Clean, very dry bedding will prevent the parasites increasing their numbers by the free-living part of the life-cycle.

HABRONEMA AND *DRASCHIA* (SUMMER SORES)

Adult worms of *Habronema muscae, H. majus* and *Draschia megastoma*, all white and 1-2 cm long, are found in the stomach of horses and do not usually cause problems. The infective third-stage larvae can be deposited on wounds in the skin, where they cause summer sores.

Life-cycle

The life-cycle is indirect, using flies (the housefly and stable fly) as intermediate hosts. Infection of horses therefore takes place in the summer months when the flies abound. Eggs containing larvae that soon hatch or larvae themselves are passed in faeces. These are eaten by the larval (maggot) stages of *Musca* and *Stomoxys* flies, which also are growing in the manure. When the adult fly emerges it contains the infective third-stage worm larvae, and these move to the mouthparts. When the fly imbibes fluid from the lips and nostrils of the horse, the larvae crawl out of the fly's mouthparts and are swallowed by the horse. While *Stomoxys* flies usually scarify the skin to suck blood, the worm larvae block their mouthparts and affected flies begin to lap fluids, so transmitting the larvae. Horses can also eat dead infected flies in food and water. The adult worms then grow to maturity in the stomach. Flies also feed on other surfaces such as wounds and the conjunctiva, sheath or penis, and in response to the moisture the larvae again will crawl out of the fly's mouthparts and infect the wound. The *Habronema* or *Draschia* larvae cannot develop any further in the wound but they do cause summer sores.

Clinical signs

Habronema adult worms commonly cause little harm living on the surface of the stomach. Possibly there may be a gastritis and excess mucus production. *Draschia megastoma* does cause fibrous nodules containing several worms but again usually causes no signs.

Summer sores can be serious. The sores are seen in the summer months when the flies are active, and carrying the worm larvae and the fly host means that sores are much more likely in warm climates and are relatively rare in temperate climates. They occur on those parts of the body most likely to be injured (legs, head, withers). The presence of the *Habronema* or *Draschia* larvae in a skin wound causes ulcers containing an exuberant growth of soft reddish-brown granulation tissue, which protrudes from the wound. Continual reinfection of the sore can cause a quite extensive lesion. The summer sore may be very irritating to the horse, which rubs it, causing it to bleed. *Habronema* lesions on the conjunctiva appear as red/pink raised lesions containing yellow/white inclusions. They may ulcerate and also can damage the cornea of the eye. The wounds attract the flies, but, for some reason, although many horses are exposed to infected flies, only a few develop summer sores.

This predisposition of certain animals may be related to their developing a hypersensitivity reaction to the *Habronema* larvae, and often the condition will recur annually in these horses.

Diagnosis
Usually a diagnosis of the presence of adult worms in the stomach of horses is never made, because very few eggs or larvae are passed in the faeces and they are very difficult to see. The lesions of summer sores are fairly characteristic. A biopsy reveals areas of fibrous tissue plus necrosis and yellow/white inclusions of caseous or calcified material plus many eosinophils and occasionally sections of larvae. An extensive scraping of the wound if digested with KOH may reveal fragments of larvae or a whole larva up to several cm in length.

Treatment
The most effective drugs against adult worms will be ivermectin and moxidectin. Summer sores are difficult to treat although the same drugs do resolve many summer sore lesions. They will kill the larvae in the wound and treatment is effective in about 70% of uncomplicated cases, but sometimes causes side effects. Occasionally pain or swelling at the site of injection or oedema and pruritus possibly due to the hypersensitivity response of the horse to the death of larvae is seen. This can be controlled with corticosteroids and these alone through their action on the hypersensitivity reaction have been known to resolve uncomplicated lesions. Alternatively surgery or cryosurgery to clean the wound of diseased tissue can treat the lesions. The wound must be covered after treatment to prevent renewed fly attack and rapid reinfection.

Preventive measures
Regular treatment of all horses for their adult worms should reduce the incidence of summer sores. Horses which have developed lesions in previous years must be carefully monitored. The intermediate fly hosts should be killed in manure piles where they breed (see p. 548) and fly repellent should be applied to all wounds in the fly season. This also will help to prevent myiasis caused by blowflies (see p. 553).

THELAZIA LACRYMALIS

This white worm about 1-2 cm long lives in the conjunctival sac and lachrymal duct. It occurs in Europe, North America and some other parts of the world.

The worm lays first-stage larvae and these are ingested by lapping *Musca* spp. flies. In these the infective third-stage larvae develop and these crawl back into a horse's eye when the fly is feeding. Usually the adult worm causes no, harm remaining alive for several years. The young, developing worm does move around the conjuctiva and its serrated surface can irritate the eye. Therefore, in summer when the flies are active young worms may produce excess lachrymation and conjunctivitis. Treatment can be by simple removal of the worms under local anaesthetic. Ivermectin and moxidectin now supply a simpler method of treatment.

ONCHOCERCA CERVICALIS (FILARIAL WORMS, ONCHOCERCOSIS)

Onchocerca cervicalis infects the neck, skin and occasionally the eyes of horses. It is found throughout the world. Another species, *O. reticulata*, infects the tendons and suspensory ligaments, usually of the front legs.

Life-cycle
Adult *O. cervicalis* live in the ligamentum nuchae, the main ligament in the neck. The adult female worms lay first-stage larvae (called microfilariae) that migrate to the skin. The microfilariae congregate particularly in the skin on the lower abdomen and chest. From here a biting *Culicoides* midge picks them up when it feeds on the horse. The microfilariae develop to infective third-stage larvae in the body of the midge. When the midge bites another horse the larvae are injected and they migrate to the ligamentum nuchae to mature.

Clinical signs
Adult *O. reticulata* in nodules, tendons or suspensory ligaments sometimes cause swelling or lameness in the front legs. Adult *O. cervicalis* seem to cause no problems but the microfilariae of *O. cervicalis* can cause skin lesions. Furthermore, while a high proportion of horses carries *O. cervicalis* microfilariae in their skin, the majority never show any signs. In a small proportion of horses skin lesions are seen. Lesions are associated with the horse's hypersensitive immune reaction to the microfilariae in the skin although why some horses, and not the majority of those infected react remains unknown. Initially hair is lost, possibly with scurf or crusting, along the ventral part of the belly and chest and sometimes on the head and other parts of the body, in horses that are 2- to 4-years-old or more. The lesions are very irritating, and the horse will bite, kick and scratch at itself, causing further damage, ulceration and chronic thickening. The microfilariae also occur in the eye. They cause pink/red raised lesions on the conjunctiva and corneal depigmentation and are thought to be one of the causes of periodic ophthalmia (see p. 180) in horses producing conjunctivitis, lachrymation and other ocular signs.

Diagnosis

As many horses with microfilariae show no signs, a positive diagnosis of *O. cervicalis* microfilariae as the causative agent is difficult to make. However, unlike many insect-induced lesions, onchocercosis is non-seasonal and the site of lesions, ventrum with perhaps forehead lesions is helpful. A small piece of skin can be taken as a biopsy. When minced in saline large numbers of microfilariae may indicate disease but there is no true correlation between severity and numbers. Cell infiltrates, particularly eosinophils and tissue lysis near microfilariae may suggest that the horse is hypersensitive to the microfilariae.

Treatment

No drug will kill *Onchocerca* adults. Those few horses that develop the skin lesions can be treated with ivermectin or moxidectin, preferably early in the course of the disease, to kill the microfilariae in the skin. In some there may be a temporary exacerbation in lesions. A fluid oedematous swelling may appear ventrally along the belly, chest and neck, with swelling of the face. This is in response to the dead and dying microfilariae and can be treated with corticosteroids. Systemic and local ocular corticosteroid treatment is required if ocular lesions are present. Ivermectin (injected) does prevent reproduction in the adult worms for a few months, but these are not killed. Therefore, microfilariae production will resume and repeated treatments may be required. Control is not usually attempted but measures against *Culicoides* midges to reduce transmission may be helpful (see p. 551).

PARAFILARIA MULTIPAPILLOSA (BLOODY SWEAT)

This parasite found in Russia, Asia and Eastern Europe is reported elsewhere and has been imported into Britain. *Haematobia* and *Musca* flies seem to be intermediate hosts and as the related parasite in cattle has established in and is transmitted in Sweden by *M. autumnalis*, the face fly, imported horses that develop lesions must be treated. The adult female worm grows coiled in a nodule under the skin. Mainly in the spring and summer months the female worm pierces through the skin and lays her microfilariae. These exude in a bloody fluid that drips down the skin, attracting the flies in which development and transmission to the next horse occur. The nodules usually appear suddenly, break open, bleed, leaving matted hair, and then heal up, but a succession of female worms may pierce the skin for 2-3 years. The worms usually cause no major problem but being on the sides, shoulders and neck they interfere with the saddlery. Little is known about treatment, although ivermectin is very effective against *Parafilaria* in cattle.

SETERIA EQUINA

This long, white, roundworm occurs in the peritoneal cavity of horses in areas where its intermediate hosts, mosquitoes, are plentiful. It causes no harm although rarely it is found in unusual sites such as the eye. It lays small larvae or microfilariae that circulate in the blood so they sometimes might be found on a blood smear.

HALICOCEPHALOBUS GINGIVALIS (MICRONEMA DELETRIX)

Up to 40 cases of this infection have been described in various places throughout the world. This worm is very closely related to *Strongyloides* but normally is free-living in soil and humus. Often the lesion is sited in the bones of the face suggesting entry through damaged mucosa in the mouth. Some located at other sites (prepuce, eye, etc.) suggest entry though a wound. In the bones such as the mandible, maxilla or femur, or in the tissues, the worms lay larvae and multiply. Development of many worms induces production of pink host inflammatory granulomatous tissue. This forms as many nodules around the worms. These can be spread to other tissues particularly brain but also kidneys, lymph nodes, lungs, etc. where again masses of granulomata surrounding worms develop. The spread may occur both via the blood and lymphatics and, to the brain, possibly via nerve tracts from the jaw. The lesions must be and can be differentiated from tumours by the presence of the worms. There is no conclusive evidence for effective treatment but ivermectin must be tried. Even with aggressive treatment resolution of any but localised cases seems unlikely.

Other free-living nematodes have been identified occasionally in horses. *Pelodora (Rhabditis) strongyloides* lives in soil and decaying material. They may penetrate the skin and the host response to them produces papules, pustules, ulcers, loss of hair, etc.. Cleaning up the unsanitary environment may result in cure. In addition, administration of ivermectin should be helpful. Another free-living worm, *Cephalobus*, has been described in the mammary gland.

Cestodes (Tapeworms, Flatworms)

The cestodes (or tapeworms) all have an indirect life-cycle that requires two hosts. The adult, sexually mature tapeworm lives in the intestines of animals. These are the definitive host. In the intestines the adult tapeworm grows continuously from its head, producing a ribbon-like body made up of a large number of segments. The whole body is dorso-ventrally flattened and usually white to grey in colour. The segments at the end of the tapeworm contain the eggs. Segments break off and release some eggs in the intestine so both segments and eggs are shed daily in the faeces of the definitive host. The eggs do not need to undergo any further development once they have been passed in the faeces onto the ground. They are immediately infective for and are eaten by the second host in the life-cycle, the intermediate host. An often fluid-filled cyst is formed in the internal organs of the intermediate host, and one or more future head(s) of the tapeworm develop in the cyst. The life-cycle is completed when the definitive host eats the intermediate host containing the cyst. The tapeworm head(s) in the cyst attach to the wall of the definitive host's intestine and from them the adult tapeworms grow. Horses may act as the definitive host for some species of tapeworms and carry the adult tapeworm in their intestines. Horses also can act as the intermediate host for other species of tapeworms and carry the cysts in their body.

ANOPLOCEPHALA PERFOLIATA, ANOPLOCEPHALA MAGNA, PARANOPLOCEPHALA MAMMILANA (TAPEWORM)

These greyish-white, flat, segmented worms are found in the intestines of horses of all ages and throughout the world. *Anoplocephala perfoliata* is the most common of these species. It lives as an adult tapeworm mainly in the caecum, where some tend to cluster around the ileo-caecal valve that divides the small and large intestines. They also occur in the terminal small intestine and occasionally colon. The adult worms are wedge-shaped in outline, finely segmented and up to 8 cm long and 4 cm wide but commonly they reach only about 5 cm long. *Anoplocephala magna* is ribbon-like, up to 80 cm long, and is found in the small intestine of horses. *Paranoplocephala mammilana* is reported only occasionally.

Life-cycle
The adult tapeworms in the horse continually grow segments containing eggs. Segments and eggs are passed in the faeces onto the pasture. Free-living oribatid mites that live in the matt of the grass eat the eggs. The tapeworm develops as a microscopic cyst in the body of the mite. Horses become infected while grazing when they eat mites containing cysts that climb onto blades of grass in the daytime. Horses begin to pass segments after 6 - 10 weeks or longer. Generally highest levels of infection in horses are seen in the second half of the summer.

Clinical signs

Frequently, adult tapeworms are of little significance to the horse. However, *A. perfoliata* clustered in close proximity at the ileo-caecal valve can produce small ulcers, oedema, fibrosis, granulation and thickening of the mucosa. Their presence around the ileo-caecal valve is considered important as ileo-caecal colic can account for 15% of all surgical colic cases and *A. perfoliata* is suggested to be involved in a proportion of these. Initially, some surgical colics to correct ileo-caecal intussusception, where the posterior small intestine inverts and passes through the ileo-caecal valve, were considered due to large numbers of *A. perfoliata* in the caecum. More recently, a statistical association has been shown between high numbers of *A. perfoliata* and a proportion of ileal impaction or spasmodic colic cases. Possibly the worms interfere with motility of the ileo-caecal valve. What, however, initiates the *A. perfoliata* associated colic remains uncertain. Certainly a number of post mortem studies have shown that high worm burdens correlated with damage to the caecal mucosa. On the other hand, studies have reported no history of acute abdominal distress in heavily infected horses. Thus the reasons why an individual horse develops problems due to *A. perfoliata* remain unknown. Even less is known concerning *A. magna*. In large numbers they possibly might cause abdominal discomfort, possibly inappetance. Very occasionally rupture of the small intestine has been attributed to *A. magna* but probably erroneously.

Diagnosis

These worms usually have been noted only on a routine post-mortem examination carried out for other reasons. Also, it is difficult to find eggs in the faeces of known infected horses. Combinations of sedimentation of faeces and then flotation in solutions of high specific gravity may detect only 30-50% of infected horses. However, some studies have shown increased efficacy (80%) of egg detection in horses with greater than 100 worms, i.e. those more likely to be at risk of colic. Recently an ELISA assay has been developed commercially. It detects antibodies to a purified antigen of *A. perfoliata* and there was a statistical relationship between increased binding of antibody and high levels of infection. This requires more extensive testing in the field but it seems likely to be a useful test.

Treatment and prevention

Anoplocephala perfoliata can be treated with double the normal dose rate of pyrantel. Even at the normal dose rate pyrantel does have very good efficacy although this is not as great as double dose in removing tapeworms. Therefore, pyrantel in the year it is used with an additional double dose will reduce tapeworm burdens when used in a yearly rotation with other drugs for the treatment of the strongyles/cyathostomes. It should be noted that ivermectin and moxidectin do not kill tapeworms. Because the life-cycle of the tapeworms involves a free-living mite that is ubiquitous on pastures, eradication of infection is not possible. However, although never tested, a good 'pick-up-faeces' programme to control the strongyles/cyathostomes should also control tapeworms. It seems highly likely that the faeces will be removed before many mites have time to become infected.

ECHINOCOCCUS GRANULOSUS (HYDATID CYST)

The tapeworm *E. granulosus* uses the horse as its intermediate host and the dog as its definitive host. The tapeworm is quite common in horses in Great Britain and Ireland but rare in the USA and Australia except that it has been seen in imported horses and horses in contact (even years previously) with imported hounds. The very small, 2-6-mm-long adult tapeworms live in the intestines of dogs and eggs are passed in dog faeces. Dogs show no signs of the infection. Horses become infected by eating the eggs, and a cyst, called a hydatid cyst, develops, most commonly in the horse's liver. Dogs become infected with adult tapeworms when they are fed raw horse liver. This life-cycle makes the infection common in packs of foxhounds and beagles, which are fed horsemeat in the kennels. These dogs then contaminate fields with the eggs in their faeces, with the result that hydatid cysts are most common in hunters and horses grazing fields where the hounds are exercised.

Even though the cyst(s) can grow slowly over years to a large size in the horse's liver and can contain several litres of fluid, and sometimes more than one cyst is present, they usually cause no clinical problems. Normally, they are noted only incidentally on a post-mortem examination carried out for another reason or in a knacker's yard. Occasionally cysts may occur in other body sites and produce clinical signs, but this is rare and the signs diverse depending on the organ infected. In man, rupture of a related type of cyst can cause systemic anaphylaxis (a more severe form of asthma) and collapse. Theoretically the same could occur in an athletic horse that falls and ruptures a cyst. There is no treatment for the cysts in horses. The only way they can be prevented is to prevent the infection in the dogs. These should be fed only well-cooked horse viscera (heat kills the cyst); alternatively dogs can be treated every six weeks with the anti-tapeworm drug praziquantel to kill the tapeworms.

A second type or strain of *E. granulosus* exists. This tapeworm again infects dogs, particularly sheepdogs or any dog that is fed or can scavenge raw sheep meat, as the main intermediate host for this strain of *E. granulosus* is sheep, in which the cysts are found in the liver and lungs. This strain of *E. granulosus* is far more important than the horse strain as man can become infected by it. A human who accidentally ingests eggs from dogs develops one or more hydatid cysts in the body (in the liver, lungs, brain, bone, etc.). The infection in man can have serious consequences and government-sponsored schemes to control and eradicate the sheep strain of *E. granulosus* from sheep and dogs are in operation in several countries. The sheep strain, which has a dog–sheep (or man) cycle, does not seem to infect horses; nor do humans seem to become infected with the dog–horse *E. granulosus* tapeworm. Thus the infection in horses is not of significance to human health.

TAENIA HYDATIGENA

Also a dog-sheep tapeworm this can reach a metre long in the dog's intestine again usually causing no harm. White segments about one cm long and eggs are passed in dog faeces. The cyst migrates through the liver, with fibrosis when the lesion heals, on its way to the peritoneal cavity. The cyst commonly is 2-3 cm in diameter but may reach 5-10 cms with a single head inside. In sheep rearing areas where dogs can scavenge or are fed raw sheep, the grazing horses also can become infected. The cyst is only an incidental finding and causes no harm.

Trematodes (Flukes)

Flukes have a complicated life-cycle involving a snail intermediate host. Eggs passed in the faeces of the host develop in a warm, moist environment and the larval stage, called a miracidium, hatches into water. The miracidium swims in the water until it finds and penetrates the tissues of a snail. The miracidium multiplies asexually in the snail and eventually the next free-living life-cycle stages, the cercariae, are released from the snail. These produce a thick cyst wall around themselves for protection and encyst on plants or in mud. Horses become infected by eating these metacercariae with herbage.

GASTRODISCUS AEGYPTIACUS

This fluke is found in the large intestine of horses, but also of pigs and warthogs, and mainly in Africa. It has a typical trematode life-cycle involving a water snail. Horses gain most of their infection in the dry season. This is because the snails occur in permanent water but their habitat extends peripherally in the rains. When the waters recede concentrations of metacercariae are found on herbage and as this is the most palatable grazing in the dry, horses will gather near the water and become infected. Heavy infections can cause a bloody diarrhoea and rapid loss of weight. Diagnosis can be a problem since it is the immature stages developing in the intestine and before they become egg-laying adults that cause the most harm. The clinical signs, season of the year, type of grazing with suitable habitats for the snails and knowledge of previous outbreaks of disease due to *Gastrodiscus* in the area would warrant treatment. Chronic, long-lived cases will show large, clear *Gastrodiscus* eggs in their faeces. Resorantel or oxyclozanide have been used for treatment but praziquantel should be safer and more effective. Permanent control would be to supply water in clean troughs and to fence off permanent water plus the extended habitats of the snails, or to kill the snails with molluscicides. Since this is usually impracticable, treating the horses to eliminate any infection they might be carrying at the end of the dry season can reduce the number of eggs available to infect the snails.

FASCIOLA HEPATICA (LIVER FLUKE)

Fasciola hepatica is an important infection in ruminants in areas throughout the world where the geographical conditions are suitable for multiplication of its intermediate hosts, which are mud snails. The snails require soil saturation with slow moving water. They live permanently in the mud at the edge of water on the banks of streams, etc., and on low lying, marshy ground or meadows and around water seepings from sandy areas near marshes. The snails prefer slightly acid pH. In some areas snail habitats can be recognised by rushes, in other areas snails can be found on clay-peat soils, although snails do not like the acidity of peat alone. The reservoir habitats of the snails are those with relatively permanent water. Then, in wet weather, extension habitats can develop when snails flood out to multiply greatly on poached pastures, even gateways, so markedly extending the area and amount of infection. In arid areas snails and parasites can develop in irrigation ditches to infect animals grazing irrigated pastures. In all the areas snails can survive dry weather by aestivating under the mud.

If the ruminants on a farm are infected then horses grazing with or after them on poorly drained/marshy pastures are equally likely to be infected by the metacercariae on the herbage. This infection can cause abdominal pain, anaemia, inappetance and poor performance in horses. Diagnosis requires the detection of the yellow, bile-stained *F. hepatica* eggs in the faeces of the horse but faecal examination is very insensitive. Even techniques that examine large quantities of faeces may not find the eggs. Other serological tests are still experimental. Triclabendazole is a highly effective drug for treatment. If, however, populations of *F. hepatica* in ruminants on the property have developed resistance to triclabendazole this drug cannot be used. Praziquantel also has been used in horses as have the older drugs oxyclozanide and rafoxanide. The horses should be removed from the contaminated pasture and retreated about three months later. Horses should not be grazed with or after ruminants on flukey pastures.

ARTHROPODS

This large group of organisms (arthropod meaning jointed legs) includes flies, lice, ticks and mites. A number of these cause diseases, particularly lesions on the skin of horses producing worry, irritation and loss of condition.

Biting and Nuisance Flies

A number of different flies will attack horses. The flies breed in the warm, summer months, and this is the time when fly attack occurs. They are more prominent and troublesome in tropical and subtropical countries than in countries with a temperate climate, although even in temperate climates fly attack can be severe. There are four stages in the life-cycle of flies. The adult females lay hundreds of eggs. From these hatch larvae or maggots, usually white, segmented and somewhat circular, increasing in breadth from front to back. They grow from about 1 mm to 10 mm in length depending on fly species. The larvae then pupate, frequently inside a hardened, protective pupal case. During the pupal stage the tissues of the larva dissolve and are re-formed to produce the adult fly. Once developed, the adult fly emerges from the pupa and is on the wing to attack horses. Different species of biting and nuisance flies have different preferred breeding places in which their larvae develop. These range from fresh manure to compost piles, mud and even water. Therefore, to control flies adequately in a stable, it is important to know which species of flies are present. Their size, colour, patterns of veins on their wings and structure of their mouthparts can readily differentiate most flies.

Some adult flies, the nuisance flies, have mouthparts for lapping fluids and are annoying when they feed on the secretions around the eyes, nose, etc.. Other flies, the biting flies, have mouthparts that can scarify or penetrate through the horse's skin so they can feed on blood. This can be annoying and may be painful. Also, while feeding, the fly injects saliva into the skin. Some horses develop hypersensitivity reactions to the injected materials and develop skin lesions. Flies also transmit other diseases either mechanically, by physically carrying the organism on their mouthparts from horse to horse, or as an intermediate host, essential in the life-cycle of the transmitted parasite as the parasite multiplies or develops in the fly.

MUSCA DOMESTICA, MUSCA SORBENS, MUSCA AUTUM-NALIS, ETC. (HOUSE FLIES, FACE FLIES)

These are yellow-grey, lapping, nuisance flies which feed on the secretions around horses' eyes, nose, vulva and prepuce, and on wounds. They are common in stables as they prefer to breed in horse manure. The flies irritate the horse when they are present in any numbers, causing it to shake its head and swish its tail. Some visit for short periods (*M. domestica*), others stay on the face (*M. autumnalis*). Their irritation to the eye can cause excess tear formation, attracting other flies that further damage the eye. Good sanitation can control *M. domestica* as it prefers to breed in horse manure. Manure and wet bedding should be removed regularly and packed tightly into a compost heap (preferably a container with a back and two solid sides into which bedding and manure can be heaped). The heat generated by the wet, fermenting manure and bedding will kill any flies developing in the manure. The surface of the pile, where it is cooler, can be sprayed with an insecticide to kill the flies or the surface turned in every few days. Timed space sprays of insecticide in barns can kill adult flies. Fly veils attached to the browband can help to protect horses' eyes. *Musca autumnalis* is more of a problem in that it breeds in fresh bovine manure. They can be controlled along with the *Haematobia* spp. below. Browbands of a synthetic plastic impregnated with insecticide can be attached to halters and bridles and worn permanently by the horse. The insecticide spreads over the surface of the horse's body to repel and kill flies. Each band will remain active, releasing insecticide and repelling flies, for several weeks. The insecticidal bands are more effective at killing *M. autumnalis* that rests on the horse for long periods than *M. domestica* or *S. calcitrans*. In paddocks horses will congregate in the fumes from burning smudge pots to protect themselves from many of the flies described here. *Musca domestica* can transmit *Habronema* spp. (page 538) to horses. The muscids can transmit *Thelazia* (page 539) and *Parafilaria* (page 541) species between horses.

STOMOXYS CALCITRANS (STABLE FLIES)

These biting flies also are common in stables, as they like to breed in wet bedding contaminated with horse urine and manure or in calf barns. During the day greyish-coloured flies with spots on their abdomen can be seen resting on sunny walls and windows. Their bites can be quite painful and they will bite a horse several times or switch between horses to complete their feeding. They can be extremely annoying to the horse, that will stamp, kick and switch its tail. The bite site may bleed after the fly has fed and often leaves a small nodule and central crust particularly over the neck and chest but also back and legs. Some horses can develop marked crustiness on the back, chest, neck and legs when bitten by many flies or when they are hypersensitive to bites. The flies also will bite humans, and dogs that frequent stables may have crusts particularly around the edge and on the bends of their ears where the flies bite. Stable flies also transmit a number of diseases to horses – for example, *Trypanosoma* (see Chapter 32) that they transmit by carrying on their mouthparts and *Habronema* and *Draschia* spp. (see p. 538) for which they are intermediate hosts. The sanitation at manure piles and the space sprays used for *M. domestica* will have effect in controlling stable flies. The sunny walls of barns and stables can be sprayed with an insecticide, i.e. a pyrethroid (every few days to weeks, depending on the length of activity of the insecticide). The flies absorb the drug by contact and are killed. The flies don't often enter dark stables.

HAEMATOBIA IRRITANS, HAEMATOBIA STIMULANS (HORN FLIES)

These small, dark grey flies are normally associated with bovines as they breed in fresh bovine manure, but their painful bites can be very irritating to horses grazing with or near cattle. The flies often cluster on the horse's ventral abdomen and may cause a summer dermatitis. The flies cause nodules with crusts, perhaps ulcers, on the belly. The flies often stay in the same area for quite some time after feeding, causing the horse to become very agitated and repeatedly stamp its feet and kick at its belly. There will be loss of hair, thickening and even wounds if the horses are very irritated. Symptomatic treatment and then a thick coat of Vaseline and insecticide over the lesion will provide a barrier to prevent more flies biting. The flies can be controlled on a farm by feeding the cattle insecticides or insect growth hormones (these latter stop the development of the fly at the larval stage). These are excreted in the faeces and so kill the developing flies. Alternatively, because flies spend a long time on the host, long acting repellents and insecticides sprayed onto the animals will kill the flies.

TABANUS, HAEMATOBIA, HYBOMITRA, CHRYSOPS (HORSE-, DEER-FLIES, BUFFALO GNATS)

The flies are recognised easily by their large size (ranging from 0.5 to 2.5 cm) and brownish colour; they often have brightly coloured eyes. They breed in muddy soil and are most commonly seen flying on hot, sultry days near damp areas, i.e. near woods and along streams, although some species are active over damp pastures. Horse flies cut into the skin and suck up the pool of blood that wells up. Their mouthparts are very coarse so the bite is very painful and makes horses restless. There is a lesion with central ulcer and bleeding to form a crust that can attract other flies, i.e. *Musca*. The horses rub and bite at themselves to remove the flies, and as the flies need to feed for several minutes they will then repeatedly return to the same horse or to one very close by to finish feeding. The horses will try to move away from the flies or even stampede and will stop feeding and lose weight if continually attacked. The horse flies transmit equine infectious anaemia (EIA – see p. 497) between horses and also *Trypanosoma evansi*, carrying the virus or protozoa, respectively, mechanically on their mouthparts. Since the flies will not normally move far to complete their feeding, separation of horses and separation of paddocks to prevent the flies feeding in quick succession on different horses will reduce transmission of EIA.

SIMULIUM (BLACK FLIES)

These are small, black, hump-backed flies. Their larvae develop on stones and vegetation in fairly fast-running water in streams and rivers. Adult flies emerge to attack animals, particularly those grazing near water on warm, sultry days, being more common morning and evening in hot climates. Black flies can be a particular problem in hot weather after floods and are active mainly in spring/early summer. Their bite is painful and they also inject a toxin, leaving behind a small, painful, fluid-filled necrotic blister or nodule. Only small numbers of these flies are present in the UK but swarms of them occur in hotter climates near rivers. If the flies swarm and hundreds of them bite a horse they can inject enough toxin to kill the animal. In smaller numbers there is chronic damage to the skin from self-excoriation. Some black flies, i.e. *Simulium equinum*, particularly like feeding in, and can accumulate in the ears causing head shaking and scabs inside the ears. Others feed on the neck, chest and abdomen. Animals must be stabled when flies are active. The insect growth hormone, methoprene, and the biological control agent, *Bacillus therunginensis* (the spore of this latter bacterium contains a toxin that lyses the intestine of black fly larvae) can be applied locally to rivers in problem areas. These have been formulated to kill black fly larvae in rivers in large areas in West Africa where they transmit river blindness to man.

RECURRENT SEASONAL DERMATITIS DUE TO *CULICOIDES* (MIDGES, PUNKIES, NO-SEE-UMS, SWEET ITCH, QUEENSLAND ITCH, KASEN, SUMMER ECZEMA)

Midges are minute flies, perhaps most important for their transmission of African horse sickness. They breed in wet, muddy areas in fresh or salt marshes, along coasts and the estuaries of rivers, streams, and around lakes, ponds, or in wet, decaying compost, leaves, etc. The flies are active, usually as swarms, biting horses principally in the early morning and late afternoon; if it is humid and cool but greater than 10°C they may remain active through the day and also through warm nights. They cease activity only in cold weather.

When the flies are biting the horses will be very uneasy and restless with tail swishing and rubbing, and they may huddle together to escape the flies. A proportion of horses, particularly, but not only, those that are outdoors all the time, develop an allergic, hypersensitivity reaction to the midge bites called sweet itch. Prevalence of sweet itch in surveys has ranged from 3% in British horses, 22-26% in Israel and British Columbia and up to 60% in Queensland. There does seem to be a familial incidence correlating more with the dam than the sire and associated with the major histocompatibility complex genes. Icelandic horses, particularly those imported into Scandinavia, have shown higher prevalence with a possible increased susceptibility in Shire horses also. There is also increased prevalence with extended times of fly activity.

Horses commonly begin to react to the bites between one to four years of age, the earlier age probably associated with greater and longer activity of the midges. Initially the hypersensitivity reactions and dermatitis develop seasonally in the warm weather and subside in the winter, hence recurrent, seasonal dermatitis. However, the self-excoriation and chronic damage may result in permanent lesions. A large number of species of midges attack horses and several species have been associated with sweet itch. As each prefers to feed at certain sites on the horse the site of lesions corresponds to this. Commonly midges that cause sweet itch feed along the dorsal surface (forehead, withers, back, rump, and base of tail) and these are the areas where the lesions are seen. In other geographic regions horses may also have lesions on the ventrum, groin, chest, ears or lesions may be only at these sites.

The lesions are due to an allergic hypersensitivity response with horses showing a pruritic immediate Type I response starting some minutes after the bite and a delayed Type IV response that can last several days after the bite. The allergic reaction to the fly bites starts as very small, itchy nodules with erect hairs, and the horse will rub and bite at it. Initially the hair is lost, crusts are seen. The horse may rub itself for prolonged periods against trees or posts, and may mutilate itself. Rump, tail, withers and mane usually are affected first and there may be a rat-tail. Eventually the whole dorsal area of the horse can become reddened, with crusts and scaly material over the surface and no hair. The mane and tail regrow sparsely each season.

The time of the year (summer), initial seasonality and the distribution of the skin lesions on the horse (dorsal but varying in some locations) suggest that the damage is caused by an allergic reaction to the bites of the midges. However, diagnosis is difficult since other allergies and other skin parasites cause similar types of lesion. A veterinarian may be able to obtain an extract of the midges, although this is not available commercially. If the horse reacts to a small injection of this extract over twenty-four hours with an irritating lesion and nodule, then it is allergic to the fly bites. Application of ointments containing corticosteroids or short-term, low dose corticosteroids will reduce the severity of the lesions by reducing the itchiness of the reaction. However, this will only alleviate the problem temporarily. The only way to prevent the lesions in hypersensitive horses is to protect them from the bites of *Culicoides* midges each year.

To protect them from the midges, which is particularly important if the horse is allergic to midge bites, horses can be stabled from evening through to morning or all day if the weather is cool. The midges tend not to enter the darkness of stables. Burning smudge pots around the stables in the morning and particularly in the evening will reduce the numbers of midges. Repellents (i.e. pyrethroids) on animals being exercised are helpful. Drainage of habitats can reduce the problem.

MYIASIS (BLOWFLIES, SCREW-WORM FLIES)

Myiasis is a condition found throughout the world where blowflies and screw-worm flies are attracted to and lay their eggs in wounds. These include the green-bottle (*Lucilia*), blue-bottle (*Calliphora*) and black blowflies (*Phormia*) throughout the world and screwworm flies (*Callitroga* and *Chyrysomia*) in Central and South America, Asia and Africa. The immature larval stages (maggots) that look very like those of the biting and nuisance flies, hatch from the eggs. These larvae however, invade the living tissues of a wound and grow to about 1 cm long, feeding by dissolving the tissues. The larvae of the blowflies can also live in carcasses and so are very difficult to eradicate.

The maggots growing, moving and tunnelling into the wound are irritating, and the horse will stamp, kick and swish its tail. A horse affected by these larvae often can be recognised early on by its restlessness. The wound becomes necrotic and will begin to ooze a foul-smelling brownish or reddish-stained fluid. The screw-worm fly is particularly unpleasant; its larvae cause very serious lesions. Untreated cases of blowfly strike or screw-worms may die from toxaemia and septicaemia. Close examination will reveal the infected wound in which maggots can be seen.

The wound must be cleaned thoroughly and as many maggots as possible removed manually and collected for identification. The wound must then be treated with an insecticide to kill any remaining larvae, as often these cannot be reached, are too small to be easily visible or are hidden in pockets and tunnels. The surface of the wound then must be covered or treated with a fly repellent to stop the adult flies being reattracted to the wound. All wounds found on horses in the warm summer months when blowflies are active should be treated with a fly repellent to prevent the adult flies laying their eggs on the wound. In hotter climates, where numerous flies, particularly screw-worm flies are present, it may be useful to spray groups of horses routinely with an insecticide or repellent every few days to weeks. The frequency of treatment will depend on the length of activity of the insecticide used and the number of flies present. The importance of screw-worm fly myiasis in cattle is such that in some countries tremendous efforts have or are being made to eradicate the fly or to prevent it from entering the country. In these areas screw-worm fly myiasis is notifiable and any suspect maggots must be preserved in alcohol and sent to government laboratories for identification.

GASTEROPHILUS INTESTINALIS, GASTEROPHILUS NASALIS (BOTFLIES)

The larval stages (bots) of these flies are found throughout the world in the stomach of horses. The majority of horses are infected. Usually *Gasterophilus intestinalis* is the commonest bot. In some countries *Gasterophilus nasalis* is more abundant but it is not found in colder climates, such as central and northern England and Scotland. Other species occur in various areas. The adult flies have yellow and dark bands on their bodies and look like bees except they have only one pair of wings. The female bot fly has an ovipositer curving down from her abdomen with which she attaches her eggs to the horse, and this can be mistaken for a sting. The larval bots are yellow to pink in colour, reach 1-2cm in length and are made up of broad segments. They have a pair of large black hooks at their anterior end with which they attach to the wall of the horse's stomach.

Life-cycle
Bot flies attach their eggs to the hairs of the horse with the exception of *G. pecorum* that lays its eggs on plants. *Gasterophilus intestinalis* female flies attach yellow eggs to the longer hairs on the forelegs, shoulders, neck and mane. After a few days the first-stage larvae are ready to hatch and they are stimulated to do so by the moisture, warmth and friction of the horse's tongue and lips when biting itself. On stimulation the larvae escape from the eggs and penetrate into the horse's mouth. Here they burrow into the tissues of the tongue and into the peridontal spaces for a month before they are swallowed. The second- and third-stage larvae then attach to the stomach wall. In all the larvae spend nine months in the horse. At the end of this time they release their hold and are passed in the faeces to develop for one month in the soil to the adult stage. The life-cycle of *G. nasalis* is similar to that of *G. intestinalis* except that the yellow eggs are laid on long hairs of the head. These eggs do not require stimulation to hatch; instead the larvae hatch spontaneously and

then enter the horse's mouth. Larvae of some other species attach temporarily by their hooks to the wall of the rectum as they leave the host. The adult flies lay their eggs on horses in late summer and autumn in temperate climates, but the flies are active for longer – during spring, summer and autumn – in warmer climates. Cold and frost kill the adult flies, so in winter the entire population of bots is present as larvae inside the horse. This is important for the institution of control measures.

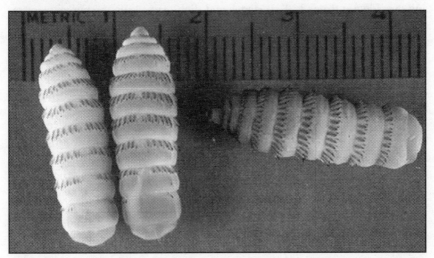

Figure 9   *Gasterophilus intestinalis* larvae from the stomach

Clinical signs
Generally bots are not of major importance. Egg-laying female flies, especially those laying eggs on the head, may annoy and upset the horse as they hover near the animal and dart in to lay their eggs. Rarely, larvae migrating through the skin may cause dermatitis. Larvae migrating in the tongue and peridontal spaces do produce tunnels and microabscesses that may temporarily put the horse off its food and occasionally cause sores. The larvae in the stomach make circular, crater-like depressions surrounded by fibrosis where they are attached to the wall. *Gasterophilus intestinalis* larvae attach to the non-glandular cardiac region. Clusters of *G. nasalis* larvae occur in the pyloric stomach, pyloric sphincter and the very first part of the duodenum. Although never studied, large numbers of larvae in the stomach and their lesions over a large part of the stomach must cause some discomfort, which could be very important in performance horses. Rarely, fatalities are described due to perforation of the stomach wall but as bots are common it is difficult to prove blame. Occasionally *G. nasalis* could perhaps interfere with the pyloric sphincter valve and affect passage of food. If the larvae temporarily attach to the wall of the rectum, they can cause discomfort and sometimes straining, as if the horse is trying to pass faeces.

Diagnosis

There are no tests to diagnose the presence of the larvae in horses other than endoscopy. If eggs have been seen on the horses in the summer and autumn, this will indicate that the animals are infected.

Treatment and control

A number of drugs are available to kill bot larvae. In particular, the ivermectin and moxidectin drugs kill all stages and dichlorvos kills the parasites once they have reached the stomach (Table 1). The horses should be treated in early winter after the flies have been killed by the first frosts of the autumn. It is important at this time to cut all the eggs of *G. intestinalis* from the hairs as the larvae which have not yet been stimulated to hatch can remain alive in the eggs on the hairs for several months and so continue to infect the horse after treatment.

It is far preferable not to use drugs to control or treat bots. These could interfere with the rotation of drugs for control of the far more important strongyle and cyathostome infections. Instead the eggs should be cut or shaved off the hairs every one to three days while grooming.

Lice

HAEMATOPINUS ASINI, DAMALINIA (BOVICOLA) EQUI (LICE, LOUSINESS)

Horses are affected by both sucking (or piercing) and chewing lice, *H. asini* and *D. equi* respectively. These flattened, wingless, six-legged insects live on the surface of the horse's skin. *Haematopinus asini* are large and dark being 3-5 mm long and normally dark yellow/brown in colour, although they become bluer when filled with blood. They have pointed heads and penetrate the skin with their mouthparts to suck blood and tissue fluids. They are most common on the long-haired parts of the body such as the mane, tail and fetlocks but can spread over the whole body. *Damalinia equi* are smaller, 2 mm long, and light yellow/brown in colour, and they feed on scurf and surface cells. They are found most commonly along the back and flanks but may spread over the whole body.

The whole life-cycle takes place on the horse. The lice attach eggs (nits), about 0.5 mm long and white in colour, to the hairs. Small immature lice (nymphs), which closely resemble the adults, emerge from the eggs in about ten days and gradually develop to mature adults in three weeks. The lice are transmitted by direct contact from horse to horse but, if warm and damp, they will survive hours to a few days on inanimate objects, and so can be transferred on saddlery and stable equipment.

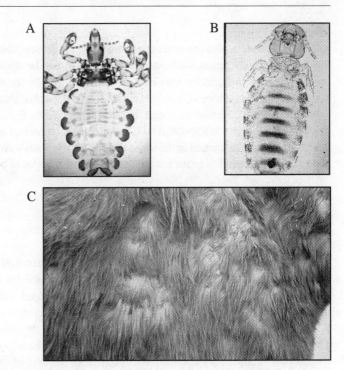

Figures 10 a, b, c Lice
A. *Haematopinus asini*, showing the long pointed head of a sucking louse;
B. *Damalinia (Bovicola) equi* showing the blunt head of a chewing louse;
C. Damage to the hair on the shoulder where the horse has rubbed itself due
    to the irritation of an infection with *Damalinia equi*.

Clinical signs
Louse populations build up in the cold months under the protection of the
horse's long coat. Heaviest infections occur in winter and spring and lice can
be found in very large numbers on ill-kempt, poorly fed horses, often those
out on pasture. There is dandruff in the coat, and as the lice are very irritating,
the horse will bite and rub itself, pulling out the hair and even causing self-
mutilation. The horse will feed poorly and its condition will deteriorate. A very
large number of sucking lice can remove a significant amount of blood so that
the mucous membranes of the horse may become pale.

Diagnosis
The poor condition and ragged, ill-kempt coat are highly suggestive of lice
infection. The large, dark brown- or bluish-coloured sucking lice are easily
visible to the naked eye. The chewing lice live close to the skin and may be
very difficult to see amongst the dandruff, but close scrutiny will reveal the
tiny lice moving away from light and their white eggs.

Treatment

A variety of insecticides are available to treat lice on horses. These are usually in the form of dusts, sprays or washes and they must be applied thoroughly. Ivermectin and moxidectin can be used orally but only for the sucking lice. Treatment should be repeated in two weeks to kill those lice that were present as eggs at the time of the first treatment and so not affected by the insecticide. These lice will have hatched out and will be killed by the second treatment. All the horses in a stable should be treated at the same time as they probably are infected with at least a few lice even if they are not showing the clinical signs of a heavy infection.

Mites

The mites that are the most important are the mange mites. These are microscopic parasites of the skin. They all have a similar life-cycle. A six-legged larva hatches from an egg and develops to an eight-legged, sexually immature nymph. Finally the sexually mature male and female mites are formed. The whole life-cycle takes about two weeks from egg to adult laying eggs. Transmission of the mites from one horse to another is by close contact, whereupon the mites are transferred directly from the skin of the infected horse to the skin of the uninfected horse. However, the mites also can survive a few days (*Sarcoptes*), a few weeks (*Psoroptes*) or longer (*Chorioptes*) off the horse if the environment is warm and damp, and so can be transferred between horses on saddlery and equipment.

SARCOPTES SCABIEI (SARCOPTIC MANGE, SCABIES)

These mites burrow in tunnels in the surface layers of the skin and the lesions they produce can be quite severe in horses. The lesions usually begin on the head and neck but spread over the body if the horse remains untreated. The infected horse develops a hypersensitivity reaction to the mites and their waste products in the skin. This hypersensitivity reaction takes some time to develop and the lesions are first seen some two to five weeks after the horse contracted the infection. Initially, small, highly irritating nodules appear on the head and neck. The horse will begin to rub and scratch itself on objects to relieve the irritation. The skin damage progresses, with possibly sores, loss of hair and crust formation and later thickened, often very thickened, scaly skin develops. The irritation can be intense and the horse will lose condition and even starve. Sarcoptic mange in horses has public health significance, as humans handling and riding infected horses can pick up the mites on their skin and develop the highly irritating lesions of scabies; the infection on humans will die out once contact with infected horses ceases.

Diagnosis is made by identification of the mites in a skin scraping. The scraping must be deep enough to cause bleeding and extensive enough to find the mites as sometimes only very few seem to be present. The material is then digested in 10% potassium hydroxide that dissolves and breaks up skin tissue so making the mites more visible under the microscope. A skin biopsy examined histologically would reveal eosinophils, possibly tunnels and occasionally mites and eggs.

As the mites live in tunnels burrowed into the skin, treatment can be difficult. Any acaricide creams or washes must be well rubbed or scrubbed in and several treatments at a ten-day interval are required. It helps to wash the lesions first with soap. This will remove surface grease and soften the skin, allowing better penetration of the acaricide down into the skin to the mites. Ivermectin injected into the horse will be effective but side affects must be considered. Ivermectin will require at least two doses at a weekly interval. As the infection can be transferred to man any humans handling or treating infected horses should wear protective gloves. All in contact horses could be incubating the infection and should be treated. Equipment and premises should be treated or not used for several days.

Figure 11
Sarcoptes scabiei female

Figure 12
Sarcoptes scabiei male

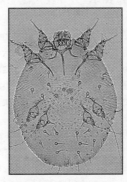
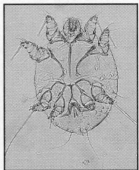

CHORIOPTES EQUI (LEG MANGE)

This still is a common form of mange of horses throughout the world. The mites live on the surface of the skin and are found mainly on the back of the pasterns and on the fetlocks, although they can spread up and cause discrete lesions on the legs or even on the belly and groin.

The mites feed on tissue fluid. The hypersensitivity reaction to the mite antigens results in exudation of tissue fluids. The fluid that oozes to the surface dries and forms crusts over reddened, inflamed skin. The lesions are itchy, so the horse will stamp and kick at itself, and the hair is lost. Shod horses could damage the backs of their forelegs badly. Infections tend to be more severe in horses with feathers. Nonetheless, many infections are subclinical particularly in the summer months, as the short hair and light are detrimental to mite development.

There may be an inverse correlation between numbers of mites and lesions. Possibly the hypersensitivity reaction is destroying the mites although whether the exuded tissue fluids will feed the mites or the immunoglobulins within the fluid help to kill the mites is not known. Care should be taken not to miss the mites on examination. A skin scraping taken from a lesion will reveal the mites with their characteristic structure when examined microscopically after the skin tissues have been digested with KOH.

A limited number of acaricide washes are available. These are applied as a leg bath and to any other affected part of the body. The horse is treated at ten-day intervals to make certain that any parasites that were present as eggs or in the environment and hence not susceptible to the first treatment are killed. There are reports that *C. equi* has developed resistance to some acaricides and that these are no longer effective. If marked improvement is not apparent within a week of the first treatment, the treatment should be started again using a different type of acaricide.

PSOROPTES EQUI (PSOROPTIC MANGE, EAR MITES)

In the UK and elsewhere *Psoroptes* mites have been reported occasionally in the ears of horses, although it is probable that they are more common but cause no signs. The mites occasionally cause an excessive production of wax in the ear, sometimes in the form of a thick brown exudate. The horse can become very sensitive around its ears, resent bridling or become a head-shaker. The infected ear may droop.

Psoroptic mange on the body is uncommon but more severe. The lesions can be quite extensive. Initially the mites multiply and lesions first develop at the base of the mane and tail and under the forelock, but then can spread over the body. Irritating papules may be seen first. The mites feed on fluid exuded from the hypersensitive, very reddened and inflamed skin. The fluid oozes out to form crusts on the surface and the mites keep moving to the periphery to avoid the lesion so extending the lesion. The hair is lost and the horse will constantly rub, scratch and bite itself, even to the extent of self-mutilation.

In a quiet or sedated horse examination of the ear with an auroscope may be possible. When magnified, the small white mites will be visible very deep in the ear moving about on the surface of the wax. Alternatively a swab of the secretions in the ear can be taken and examined for mites microscopically. A skin scraping will diagnose body mange. It must be taken from the very edge of the lesion at the junction with normal skin. Treatment is as for sarcoptic mange.

The relationship between *Psoroptes* mites on horses and those on other species such as cattle remains to be fully determined. Until determined transfer of mites particularly from cattle in common grazing must be considered possible.

DEMODEX EQUI
(DEMODECTIC MANGE, NODULAR MANGE)

Only rarely are cases of demodectic mange seen. The mites live deep in the hair follicle at the root of the hair and sebaceous glands and are transferred from the mare to her nursing foal. Probably all horses are infected with the mites but only a few ever show any signs of the infection. Information from other host species would suggest that signs will appear only if the horse is immunocompromised or immunosuppressed perhaps with long term gluco-corticoid treatment or by stress. Two types of lesion can be seen. In the first the skin becomes thickened and scaly and the hair is lost over the head, neck and withers. In the second the horse develops pea-sized or larger nodules over the neck, shoulder and face. If the nodules are squeezed, a creamy, cheesy material can be extruded. Both forms may become secondarily infected with bacteria. Diagnosis is made on several deep scrapings of the skin (squeezing the skin at the same time to help expel the mites from deep in the follicles) or by extracting the cheesy material from the nodules usually with KOH digestion. Many cigar-shaped mites will be seen micro-scopically in this material. The underlying cause for multiplication of the mites should be sought and treated also. There is really no effective treatment. Some animals may recover spontaneously without any treatment if the underlying cause is corrected. Various washes such as fenchlorphos can be scrubbed in well at frequent intervals. This must he done under veterinary supervision as there can be side effects. Injected ivermectin can be considered with consideration to potential side affects. Nodules in the saddle area could be excised surgically.

TROMBICULA (HEEL BUGS, HARVEST MITES)

The *Trombicula* species mites, commonly known as harvest mites, scrub-itch mites or chiggers, live in the soil on low-lying pasture, scrubland or arable land. They are most common on sandy or chalky soils. The larval mites are normally parasites of small rodents, but they may attack horses, particularly in the late summer and autumn after the corn harvest. The larval stages attach around the heel and pasterns, hence the name, heel bug, but also may occur on the head and chest. The mites attach to the skin, produce a cement tunnel through which they suck fluid, and hypersensitivity develops. Exudated fluid crusts over reddened skin. When the crusts are removed the mites can be seen as very small orange or red dots embedded in the skin. The mites are extremely irritating and the horse may damage itself by scratching, kicking at itself and stamping but it also can remove the mites by this scratching although the secretions of the mite remain and con-tinue to be extremely irritating. The mites are easily killed using a leg bath of one of the acaricides plus local symptomatic therapy to relieve the intense pruritis.

Only keeping horses away from the land where the harvest mites are common in the autumn can prevent the infection. Repellents such as benzyl benzoate can be applied to the heels and pasterns for some control. In parts of Southeast Asia where these mites transmit scrub typhus to man, large areas of ground can be dusted or sprayed with acaricide.

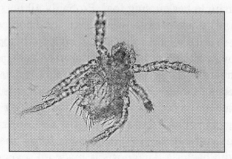

Figure 12
Trombicula autumnalis,
the harvest mite

Ticks

Ticks have, at the anterior end, some simple mouthparts attached to a rounded body bearing three or four pairs of legs. The adult female tick lays eggs from which hatch six-legged larvae, 1-2 mm long. The next stage is the eight-legged nymph, which is slightly larger than the larva. The nymphs in turn develop into the adult males or females, which again have eight legs but which are now sexually mature and 0.5 cm or more in length when fed. Each life-cycle stage feeds once. With some ticks all the stages (larva, nymph, adult) feed on one host and it is only the adult female tick which, when fed, drops to the ground to lay eggs in protected places (in cracks and crevices or under stones). Alternatively, each life-cycle stage can feed on a host and then drop off; it moults on the ground and then has then to find another host for its next life-cycle stage. The tick pushes its mouthparts through the skin and anchors itself for about two to ten days, or occasionally much longer, and sucks blood. They inject saliva and various cements and induce a hypersensitivity reaction at the site of the bite. This may develop into a pustule, ulcer or nodule. As it feeds, the tick swells and becomes a blood-filled, leathery bag, usually grey or yellow-brown in colour. Many ticks are brown or grey but some species may be ornate, with white, green or other coloured enamelled markings on the dorsal or anterior-dorsal surface. The ticks attach particularly in and around the ears, the perineal, inguinal and axillary regions and legs and face.

OTOBIUS MEGNINI (SPINOSE EAR TICK)

This is a pink or blue-grey, leathery tick found in America, Southern Africa and Asia. It will infect the ears of many different animals including the horse.

Only the larval and nymphal stages will infect animals. The larvae attach and climb to the ears inside which they feed. They feed for one to several months and become almost spherical before the nymphs drop off the horse. The adult ticks live and lay eggs in sheltered spots such as cracks in poles, crevices in walls, under mangers and under the bark of trees. Because of this, spinose ear ticks are found only on stabled and corralled horses where parasite and host are in close proximity.

The horses can be sensitive about the head, shake their heads and rub their ears. The ear may droop. Clusters of ticks often are easily visible. If only a few are present then a swab can be rubbed firmly over the skin in the ear canal; some ticks will be dislodged and can be seen on the swab. Infected ears should be treated with acaricide. Routine monthly treatment will reduce the numbers leaving the horse to lay their eggs in stables and paddocks. Where horses are becoming heavily infected, the wood and walls of the stable, etc., should be sprayed with an acaricide.

RHIPICEPHALUS, DERMACENTOR AND OTHER TICKS AND TICK PARALYSIS

A large number of other species of tick will feed on horses, attaching themselves to the body, in the ears and under the tail leaving sores and scabs. Occasionally hypersensitive wheals occur. Heavily infected animals are irritated and will lose condition. The occasional tick on a horse can be removed manually or treated individually. In heavy infections in tropical countries horses can be sprayed with an acaricide or dipped like cattle. These ticks may breed around the building but also under scrub and stones on pasture. Changing pasture and leaving pasture without animals for three months in hot, dry weather will reduce tick numbers substantially.

There are a few ticks that cause tick paralysis in animals, including horses. Foals are the most susceptible, but even adult horses can be affected by the presence of forty or more female ticks. A toxin injected into the animal by the adult female tick as she is feeding brings about the paralysis. It usually starts as a paralysis of the hind legs which moves progressively forward until paralysis of the muscles of respiration and the heart cause death. Searching the horse for and removing all the ticks can treat a case of tick paralysis. If the paralysis has not progressed too far, it will reverse itself when the ticks are removed. The most important ticks which cause paralysis and the areas where tick paralysis is most common are: *Ixodes holocyclus* in eastern Australia *Ixodes rubicundus* in Southern Africa, particularly the Karoo; and *Dermacentor andersoni* in north-western USA and western Canada. There are other ticks, which cause paralysis, and occasionally the condition is found in other countries including Western Europe. Ticks are most important, however, for their transmission of parasites to horses. *Rhipicephalus, Dermacentor* and *Hyalomma* spp. ticks transmit the protozoans *Babesia* and *Theileria* and *Ixodes* ticks the spirochaete, *Borellia burgdorferi*.

Medical and Surgical Matters

This section should provide the reader with the basic concepts of veterinary practice. As with previous sections, it may be read in order to gain a better understanding of the subjects as a whole, or used for reference.

* The section starts with a description of how medicines are administered and summarises those which are currently available.

* Then a chapter covers the causes, course, treatment and prevention of inflammation.

* Poisoning is a risk and worry for owners and those responsible for horses. A chapter on this subject is therefore appropriate to this section.

* Preventive medicine is a most important subject on the grounds that prevention is better than cure. Some ideas are put forward regarding this subject, particularly in relation to the studfarm.

* Casting and anaesthesia are a very necessary adjunct nowadays to surgery, and these subjects are accordingly covered in this section.

* Also covered is the topic of castration and the conditions arising from it.

* Wounds and their management are discussed in another chapter, and advice on the first-aid kit is given.

* Finally in this section, growths, or as they are often known, tumours or neoplasias, are described.

34
ROUTES OF ADMINISTRATION
OF MEDICINES

The route of administration of a medicine depends on many factors, including the nature of the disease or injury, the drug being used, the temperament of the patient, the ease of administration of the chosen drug, as well as the nature of the drug itself.

Most drugs can only be administered by certain routes: for example, penicillin is not used orally in horses but may be given intramuscularly or intravenously or applied locally to treat wound infections.

Sometimes different formulations of the same drug are available and each must be administered by a different route. It is important that the person responsible for administering the drug is fully familiar with the chosen route; if not, he or she should use another method of treatment.

The severity of the disease determines the speed required for the onset of drug action and this also influences the choice of drug formulation and the route of administration. For severe infections or other emergency situations it is important to achieve high circulating blood levels of a drug as quickly as possible, and in such cases the intravenous route is often used initially and levels maintained either by further intravenous or by intramuscular or oral treatment. Drugs may be used topically, i.e. applied to the skin, if a local effect is all that is required.

Regardless of the route of administration, the required dose should be calculated accurately before treatment begins.

Oral route

There are several ways to administer drugs to horse by mouth. Powders may be mixed into food or made into a paste with honey or molasses which is applied to the tongue. Some drugs are soluble and can be administered in the horse's drinking water.

In these cases the amount of water used to dissolve the drug should be limited and no more given until the dosage is ingested, unless it appears unlikely that the horse will drink any of the medicated water. In the latter instance another method should be used. A separate supply of clean water should always be made available.

Balls or boluses (rounded masses of medication) used to be popular forms of drug presentation but are now seldom used. Prepared pastes are available as vehicles for anthelmintics, antibiotics and anti-inflammatory drugs, as well as for electrolyte, vitamin and mineral preparations. These are often presented in syringes so that the drug can be deposited on the back of the horse's tongue by simply depressing the plunger with the syringe placed well into the horse's mouth.

Drenches or drinks which are administered by bottle are occasionally used, but there is a danger of choking the horse if the head is held too high or the medicine given too quickly. The use of a stomach tube overcomes these problems (see below).

Stomach tube
This method of administering drugs is a technique for veterinarians rather than lay people because of the distinct risk of placing the tube in the trachea (windpipe) rather than the oesophagus (gullet).

The use of a rubber or plastic tube allows the administration of a large volume of fluid or medicine directly into the stomach or into the lower part of the oesophagus. It bypasses the mouth, pharynx and much of the oesophagus, so that drugs which may be irritant to these areas can safely be given. It can be used to ensure accurate dosage of drugs such as anthelmintics and anti-inflammatory preparations, for the administration of drugs required to have a local action on the stomach or intestines (e.g. kaolin), or for feeding either debilitated animals or very young or weak foals.

There are many different tube diameter and length combinations available but as a rough guide the following may be used:

	External diameter	Length
Foal	9.5mm	210cm
Medium	16mm	270cm
Large	19mm	300cm

The tube is passed by the veterinarians up the lower part of the nostril, through the pharynx and into the oesophagus. The horse will often have to swallow to allow the tube into the oesophagus. The tip of the tube should be passed to just below the level of the cardiac sphincter (the opening between the oesophagus and stomach), although it may fall short of this point. In foals, the tube should not enter the stomach.

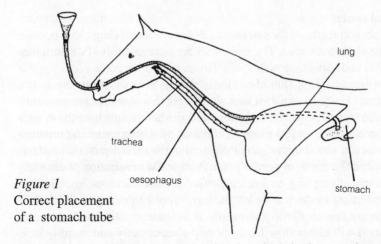

Figure 1
Correct placement
of a stomach tube

Great care should be taken to ensure that the tube is in the oesophagus and not the trachea because deposition of fluid or drugs into the trachea and lungs can result in severe pneumonia or drowning and death of the horse.

There are five ways to check for correct placement of the tube in the oesophagus.

1   The tube can often be seen or felt on the left side of the neck almost in the jugular groove as it passes down the oesophagus.

2   By placing the fingers over the top of the larynx, the tube can be palpated in the very proximal (upper) oesophagus. This may not be possible in horses which are tense or heavily muscled.

3   'Rattling' the trachea will often result in being able to hear the tube if it has accidentally passed into the trachea.

4   If the tube is in the trachea, it is normally easy to blow down the tube and the horse's breath can be felt at the outer end of the tube when it exhales. If the tube is correctly inserted into the oesophagus there is resistance to the operator's attempts to blow into the tube and a bubble of gas can often be seen passing back up the oesophagus after the tube has been blown down.

5   Air cannot be sucked from the oesophagus.

A funnel or pump can be attached to the free end of the tube to administer the treatment. If a pump is used, it is important not to pump too quickly as this may result in overdistension of the stomach and cause pain or rupture. A pump should not be used in foals.

Parenteral routes

There are several methods for parenteral administration of drugs, that is, other than via the alimentary tract. The main ones are intravenously (IV), intramuscularly (IM) and subcutaneously (SC). No matter which route is chosen, the needle, syringe and drug should be sterile and the skin should be clean. It is preferred that the site be swabbed with alcohol but this is not always necessary.

The needle should be placed in the required site before attaching the syringe or administration set, and its position checked by noting either the presence or the absence of blood in the hub of the needle, the nature and colour of any bloodflow and the depth of needle point. Accidental penetration of an artery or vein when attempting an intramuscular or subcutaneous injection, or correct placement of the needle for the intravenous injection, will result in blood entering the needle. If the needle is of wide enough diameter, dark venous blood will either flow freely or drip continuously and steadily from the needle hub when the needle is in a vein. Arterial blood is bright red and either flows in spurts or in a strong stream.

Blood from smaller vessels or through small-diameter needles may only appear in the hub of the needle or come in slow drips. It is important to know whether the drug is suitable for intravenous, intramuscular or subcutaneous administration before proceeding as some drugs which are safe intramuscularly, for example, may cause severe reactions if given intravenously or subcutaneously.

Intravenous administration

This route is used for rapid onset of drug action, for administering large volumes of fluids or drugs either quickly or slowly, or because it is the only safe or convenient route for administration of certain drug formulations. For administration of irritant or large-volume solutions a catheter may be used instead of a needle. A catheter is similar to a needle except that it is made of soft non-irritant material and is blunt-ended so it can remain in the blood vessel for long periods without causing damage.

The jugular vein is most commonly used because of its large diameter, length and superficial position in the neck. Other veins of the limbs may be used for long-term fluid administration or if the jugular vein is inaccessible for any reason.

Care must be taken to ensure the needle or catheter is placed well *into* and not through the vein. Venous blood should flow from the needle or be able to be aspirated into the syringe to ensure placement is correct before giving the drug.

Accidental intra-arterial or perivascular (around the vein) administration of certain drugs not only reduces their effectiveness but may have severe tissue-damaging or even fatal consequences. Some drugs, if given intravenously, must be given slowly to avoid side effects, while others must be given very rapidly, as a bolus. It is important to know the properties of the drug before administration.

Intramuscular administration

This route is commonly used for administration of drugs as a continuation of therapy and to prolong the action of the drug. The drug usually requires a longer period to take effect than with intravenous treatment.

Such injections may be made into any large muscle mass, the most usual sites being the rump or gluteal region, the neck or the pectoral (chest) region. Occasionally the back of the thigh (semitendinosis, semimembranosis muscles) is used.

Proximity to joints, blood vessels or large fat deposits should be avoided because placement of drugs near these structures may result in damage or interference with drug absorption from the site. Always ensure there is no blood coming back down the needle after positioning it in the muscle by withdrawing the plunger on the attached syringe slightly before depressing it to deliver the drug.

Subcutaneous administration

This involves placement of the drug or fluid just under the skin and is achieved by pinching up a fold of loose skin, e.g. on the neck, and placing the needle so that its tip comes to lie in the space created under the fold of skin. This route is used for some vaccines, for fluid administration in certain cases, and for some drugs which cannot be given by other routes.

Occasionally treatment is given via the intraperitoneal (into abdominal cavity) or intrathoracic (into thoracic cavities) routes, but these are specialised methods of treatment and should not be undertaken by inexperienced persons.

Inhalation

The inhalation of steam or vapours can aid in treatment of respiratory disease. Eucalyptus oil, oil of turpentine or camphor may be added to boiling water in a clean bucket and the horse's head held over the bucket for ten to fifteen minutes. Do not cover the horse's head completely because horses usually resent the resulting interference with respiration.

An alternative method is to use a nosebag or sack in which a sponge or bran soaked in the medicated solution has been placed. Nebulizers, which deliver micro-droplets of drugs, are available for use with drugs such as cromoglycolate and corticosteroids which are used in the prevention and treatment of allergic respiratory disease (chronic obstructive pulmonary disease or heaves – see p.82)

Enema

This method allows administration of large volumes of fluids with or without added drugs to aid evacuation of the rectum and colon or to aid in treatment or prevention of dehydration. The rectum should first be cleared of faeces (droppings) using a well-lubricated gloved hand. A lubricated flexible tube is then inserted into the rectum and *gently* passed forward. A pump can be attached to the free end of the tube and the warm fluid slowly pumped into the rectum. No force should be used in an attempt to push the tube farther forward but it may be able to be advanced after the rectum has been distended with fluid. A stomach tube is suitable for this purpose.

Retention of meconium (first faeces) is common in foals and can result in severe pain and signs of colic. Enemas of warm soapy water, paraffin or commercially available solutions which contain sodium phosphate can be used to help lubricate the offending meconium and aid in its evacuation. Extreme care should be taken when positioning the tube in a foal's rectum as the tissues are delicate, often dry and sticky, and the rectum is only small and narrow. Do not use any force but gently advance the tube, if necessary, while pumping the fluid in. A soft tube with no hard or sharp edges is essential for safety.

Intravaginal or intrauterine administration

Treatment of metritis, vaginitis, retention of foetal membranes or induction of luteolysis often requires the administration of fluids into the vagina or uterus. For vaginal or uterine infections and to prevent infection in cases of membrane retention, antibiotics may be added to the fluid. The perineum (the skin around the vulva and anus) is washed and a gloved hand is used to introduce a catheter either through the cervix into the uterus or into the front of the vagina; the fluid is then pumped or poured in. The fluid used must be sterile and preferably warmed to just below body temperature to prevent the introduction of infection and unnecessary irritation.

Pessaries are tablets designed for use in the uterus or vagina and which contain antibiotics. Some pessaries foam after contact with the normal tissue fluids to assist the distribution of the contained drug(s). These are not often used nowadays as they may result in local irritation of the lining of the uterus.

Topical administration or application

Substances can be applied to surfaces such as the skin, mucous membranes, eyes, hooves, etc., when an effect is only required locally or, in some instances, as a method of administering systemically acting substances, that is, substances which have a general, as opposed to a local, effect. These substances include antibiotics, anti-inflammatory agents, local anaesthetics and astringents, and may be applied as creams, ointments, powders, pastes or solutions. It is important that these preparations are used correctly to be effective.

Some substances, e.g. liniments, have to be rubbed well into the skin to be properly absorbed, whereas others should only be applied lightly. Some should not be used near broken skin as they can be toxic if absorbed into the circulation. To be effective, eye creams and ointments must be placed onto the eye or into the conjunctival sac and not just around the eyelid margins.

35
VETERINARY MEDICINES

New legislation has resulted in a marked reduction in the number of medicines available to veterinary surgeons and restrictions in their use. A 'cascade' system allows equine veterinary surgeons limited use of human medicines and preparations meant for use in other species, but such medicines are often expensive and in inappropriate formulation for use in the horse. This has meant that treatment options for veterinary surgeons and horse owners are diminishing. However, there is still a reasonably large number of drugs available to veterinarians, many of which are also easily obtained by owners, for treatment of disease and injury in horses. You, as a horse owner, should be familiar with the use and effects of the most commonly used medicines, but it is unwise to undertake treatment with unprescribed drugs without consulting your vet.

The following notes are not exhaustive but serve as a guide to the most commonly used and/or readily available medicines.

Acetylpromazine   This is one of a group of antihistamines used as tranquillisers and sedatives in the horse. The group also includes chlorpromazine and promethazine. They are useful in fractious horses but may be inadequate if restraint is necessary for handling when clipping, shoeing or for treatment such as stitching (suturing). The animal must still be handled quietly after tranquillisation because overstimulation will result in the horses overcoming the calming effects of the drug.

These drugs also have an analgesic effect and may help to reduce the muscle spasm and pain associated with azoturia. One of the side effects, however, is a decrease in blood pressure, and consequently these drugs should not be used in shocked or debilitated animals.

Acetylpromazine is used orally, intramuscularly or intravenously. Accidental intra-arterial administration results in convulsions and death.

Acridine dyes (acriflavine, aminocrine, proflavine)   These dyes have bacteriostatic (microbe-inhibiting) properties and are used in wound powders, solutions or emulsions for skin and wound disinfection and antisepsis. A gel containing acriflavine (0.1%) is often used as a burn treatment; however, it may encourage excessive granulation tissue (proud flesh).

Adrenaline   Adrenaline is commonly found in solutions of local anaesthetic agents where it helps to prolong the effect of the anaesthetic. It may be used on its own to control minor haemorrhage when applied topically to a wound. When used systemically, it causes an increase in heart rate and strength, and thus helps to reverse hypotension (low blood pressure) often encountered in anaphylactic shock, i.e. severe allergic reaction.

Aloes (anthracene purgatives)   Aloes is one of a group of substances – the anthracenes – used as purgatives. Other related drugs include Atlan and Danthron. They have an irritant and stimulatory effect on the large intestine and aid passage of material through the gut. There is a complex absorption – recirculation cycle associated with the metabolism of the anthracenes and this delays the onset of purgation for up to eighteen hours after administration. The dosage is 8-20g given by mouth or through a stomach tube.

These substances are most often used as physics (laxatives) or in the treatment of colic associated with impaction of food material or straw in the large intestine. In the latter instance the impacting mass should be lubricated by the administration, by stomach tube, of 2-6 litres of liquid paraffin or faecal softening agents such as dioctyl sodium succinate.

Overdosage or injudicious use of the anthracenes can cause severe diarrhoea (superpurgation) or even death. Purgatives must not be given to any animal with suspected enteritis, peritonitis, intestinal torsion or debilitation conditions.

These substances are now difficult to obtain and they have been largely replaced by Magnesium sulphate.

Anabolic steroids   This is a group of substances which includes trenbolone, testosterone and nandrolone. Their effects include the acceleration of recovery of weight lost due to debility or undernutrition; an increase in muscular development and tone; the speeding up of tissue regeneration to help the resolution of bone and tissue injuries; assisting in recovery from infectious diseases; and increasing the efficiency of protein utilisation. These hormones should not be used without a specific need or for long periods because sudden withdrawal after prolonged administration often results in a marked loss of condition in the treated animal. They may produce male-type behaviour in some fillies and mares. Their use is now banned in performance horses or animals which may enter the human food chain.

Anodynes (colic mixtures)   These are largely outdated medicines which were used to relieve pain in colic. The use of injectable spasmolytics and analgesics such as hyoscine and dipyrone or flunixin meglumine, pethidine and other morphine derivatives has reduced the use of orally administered anodynes. Chloral hydrate is still used orally and/or intravenously. It has a sedative effect and helps in flatulent colic. If given orally, it must be mixed with a large volume of water or oil (paraffin or linseed) to avoid severe irritation to the mouth (if given by bottle) or stomach. Chlorodyne is also given orally in the treatment of colic, either alone or mixed with chloral hydrate.

If no response is seen after dosage or if the colic symptoms become worse, a vet must be called.

The dosage is 15-45g chloral hydrate given orally in 1-2 litres water or liquid paraffin; or 15g chloral hydrate and 15ml chlorodyne with aloes in a vehicle of linseed oil.

Antibacterials and antibiotics These substances are used to destroy (bacteriocidal) or inhibit (bacteriostatic) the growth of bacteria and other disease-causing organisms. There is a large number of these agents and any attempt to cover them all in this book would be impossible and unnecessary. Drugs are constantly being developed and others which were previously only available to doctors are being made available to veterinarians. Many of them are unsuitable for use in the horse because of their side effects, and consequently we often fall back on the basics such as penicillin and sulphonamides.

Briefly, there are several main groups of antibiotics and antibacterial agents.

1. The penicillins, e.g. benzyl penicillin, ampicillin, carbenicillin, cloxacillin and amoxycillin.
2. Aminoglycosides, including gentamycin, streptomycin and neomycin.
3. Tetracyclines.
4. Macrolides, e.g. erythromycin, lincomycin.
5. Cephalosporins.
6. Sulphonamides.

Combinations of drugs are often used either to broaden the range of treatment or to enhance the effectiveness of one or other of the constituents. The effective combinations are fairly standardised, and random mixing should not be undertaken.

The choice of antibiotics or antibacterial agent is essentially based on culturing the infecting organism and observing its susceptibility to various drugs in the laboratory. Veterinary experience, based on recognition of symptoms and the nature of the disease, can enable the most appropriate choice of antibiotic to be made when laboratory facilities are unavailable or can allow treatment to begin before laboratory results are obtained.

Antibiotics can be administered by injections, by mouth or topically, the route depending on the drug used and the nature of the infection (see Chapter 33).

Antihistamines   This is a class of drugs which interfere with the action of histamine, a substance released in the body which causes pruritis (itchiness), urticaria (rash) and bronchoconstriction (narrowing of the small airways). Some antihistamines (see **Acetylpromazine** above) are also used as tranquillisers. The effectiveness of these drugs as antihistamines in the horse is questionable, although they have been suggested for the treatment of conditions including sweet itch, laminitis, azoturia, and allergic skin and respiratory diseases such as chronic obstructive pulmonary disease.

Aspirin   This drug is infrequently used as an anti-inflammatory analgesic (pain-relieving) agent in the treatment of muscle or joint injury and arthritis. It is also occasionally used as an antipyretic agent (i.e. to decrease fever) in animals with an elevated temperature. Long-term usage is accompanied by the risk of gastric (stomach) irritation and haemorrhage.

Atropine   Atropine is a belladonna alkaloid. It is used topically in eye preparations to relieve pain and spasm of the iris by dilating the pupil. It has a long action of several days. It is occasionally used systemically, being given subcutaneously as a premedicant prior to general anaesthesia and in the treatment of organophosphorous poisoning. It causes a slowing of intestinal motility and reduces the production of saliva and digestive enzymes. Poisoning can occur through overdosage or through ingestion of the belladonna plant from which atropine is derived.

Boric acid (boracic acid)   This is used as a wound dressing either alone, as a 4% solution, or combined with zinc oxide and iodoform for application to wounds. It is also often incorporated in poultices.

Camphor   This is a volatile oil, like turpentine and mustard oil. All these substances cause mild local irritation and pain relief when applied to areas of inflammation, sprains, etc. They are called rubefacients or mild blisters and are used as liniments. They should be applied with friction. They are on the list of 'banned substances' and should not be used in horses which are to compete.

Caustics   These are substances which destroy excess granulation tissue and minor superficial tumours. They cause death of cells and precipitation of protein to form a scab, which must be removed prior to reapplication of the caustic agent. This group of substances includes copper sulphate, phenol, antimony trichloride and silver nitrate.

The skin surrounding the excess granulation tissue or tumour should be protected by a covering of Vaseline or other ointment and the caustic carefully applied to the lesion only. The area should be lightly bandaged if possible, and re-examined and cleaned twenty-four to forty-eight hours later. If necessary the caustic can be reapplied at this time.

Chalk (calcium carbonate)   Prepared chalk is a valuable antacid and protectant in the treatment of diarrhoea. It is usually combined with kaolin.

Chloral hydrate   This drug is less frequently used now than in the past due to the development of modern sedatives and analgesics, although it is still sometimes used for the treatment of colic and prior to induction of general anaesthesia (see **Anodynes** above). Given orally, it produces a sedative effect approximately half an hour after administration and can be useful when clipping or shoeing fractious horses. It must be given well diluted (a dosage of 15-45g in 1-2 litres water). Chloral hydrate is also used as a general anaesthetic agent. It is given intravenously, normally in combination with magnesium sulphate and pentobarbitone.

Chlorhexidine   Chlorhexidine is a very effective antiseptic agent. It is found in powders or creams at a 1% concentration, and for preoperative skin preparations as a 0.5% alcoholic or 1% aqueous solution.

Clenbuterol   Clenbuterol is used to relieve spasm of the small airways in chronic obstructive pulmonary disease (allergic respiratory disease), chronic bronchitis and influenza. It is available as an injectable solution or as granules which are mixed into food.

Codeine   Codeine is used as a cough suppressant in animals with respiratory disease and as a constipant and analgesic in horses with diarrhoea. It is given orally, either as a solution by stomach tube or drench, or mixed with honey or molasses into a paste to be applied to the tongue.

Copper sulphate   This blue salt is used as an astringent and caustic agent in the reduction of granulation tissue (see **Caustics** above). It can be applied as a 2-4% solution paste or as the dry crystal, care being taken not to damage the epithelium around the edge of the wound.

The area should be covered lightly for twenty-four hours, after which time the scab should be removed and the area washed and dried. Treatment can be repeated, if necessary either immediately or twenty-four hours later.

Copper sulphate solution (1-2%) or ointment/paste (5%) is also useful as an antifungal treatment for ringworm.

Corticosteriods (cortisone)   Cortisone is a steroid hormone (see p. 166) produced by the adrenal gland. It and many similar synthetic substances influence metabolism, healing, allergic reactions, kidney function and the body's electrolyte balance. The major application of corticosteroids is in the control and reduction of inflammation associated with skin, muscle and joint conditions. Unfortunately the anti-inflammatory effects cannot be utilised without some of the side effects influencing tissue healing, hormonal balances, and so on. The use of certain corticosteroids can significantly increase the risk of laminitis. Consequently corticosteroids should only be used as prescribed by a vet.

Commonly used corticosteroids include betamethasone, dexamethasone, prednisolone, triamcinolone and hydrocortisone (cortisol). They may be used intravenously, intramuscularly, intra-articularly (into the joint space), locally or topically (e.g. in the eye or on the skin).

Cough mixture   A cough is a symptom of disease, not a disease itself. In many cases coughing is due to or worsened by irritants such as dust in the stable. Consequently any horse with a cough should have its feed dampened and its hay soaked. Paper, shavings or another form of dust-free bedding should be provided. Orally administered preparations usually contain a mixture of expectorants and cough sedatives or suppressants. Potassium iodide, sodium iodide and codeine are common constituents of cough mixtures. Etamiphylline is a stimulant which improves respiratory function; it should only be administered under veterinary supervision.

Dichlorvos   Dichlorvos is used in the treatment of stomach bots (see p. 554).

Dimethyl sulphoxide (DMSO)   Dimethyl sulphoxide is used topically to reduce pain, pruritis (itching) and inflammation and to promote healing. It is rapidly absorbed through the skin and can be used as a carrier to help transport other substances, such as phenylbutazone, through the skin. It is useful in the treatment of muscoloskeletal injuries, some skin disorders and joint problems. The area to be treated should be cleaned first and the solution of DMSO applied with a brush. Always use gloves when using any solution of DMSO.

Diuretics   Diuretics are drugs which cause the excretion of larger than normal volumes of urine. They are useful in the treatment of oedema due to protein loss, as, for example in liver or intestinal disease, and also in cases of parasitism, inflammation, heart disease and allergy. They are also administered in some cases of azoturia and shock to help maintain kidney function. Drugs commonly used include furosemide and hydrochlorothiazide.

Electrolytes Electrolytes are salts of various kinds such as sodium chloride (common salt), sodium acetate, sodium bicarbonate (baking soda), potassium chloride and lactate. Combinations of electrolytes in solution are useful in supportive therapy in cases of diarrhoea, excessive sweating, exhaustion and dehydration, when loss of electrolytes from the body may have occurred. Commercially prepared electrolyte mixtures are available as powders or syrups for dilution in drinking water, mixing with feed or for administration by drench or stomach tube. Occasionally vitamins, minerals and glucose may also be included in these mixtures. Such preparations must be diluted and administered according to manufacturers' recommendations.

In severe cases of diarrhoea, dehydration or other debilitating conditions, electrolyte solutions can be administered intravenously by a veterinarian. These solutions are specially prepared and sterile and this form of therapy should not be undertaken by unqualified people.

Eucalyptus oil   This is used as a liniment and mild counter-irritant for application to sprains and superficial contusions. It may also be used as an inhalant to help relieve catarrh, a few drops of eucalyptus oil being added to boiling water.

Eye lotions   In the absence of veterinary advice in cases of conjunctivitis or following a blow to the eye, any of the following can be used with the assurance that, if not beneficial, they will not aggravate the condition:

10g boric acid in 250ml purified, freshly boiled water, which is allowed to cool;
10g sodium bicarbonate in 10ml purified water; or
10g sodium chloride (regular table salt) in 110ml purified water.

If no improvement is seen in twenty-four hours, veterinary advice should be sought.

Ferric/ferrous compounds   Many iron preparations act as astringents, both internally and externally. Ferrous sulphate is used as an intestinal astringent agent, often with kaolin or chalk. Excessive use may result in gastric irritation, constipation or diarrhoea. Iron compounds are also used as haematinics (substances which stimulate red blood cell formation) in the treatment of anaemias. Ferric chloride is used as a topically applied solution to control minor haemorrhage.

Flunixin meglumine   Flunixin meglumine is an anti-inflammatory and antipyretic (temperature-reducing) analgesic used for the treatment of inflammation and pain associated with musculoskeletal disorders and some forms of colic. The recommended dose is 1.1mg per kilogramme bodyweight either orally or by intramuscular or intravenous injection daily for up to five days.

Fomentation   A fomentation is, strictly speaking, the application to the skin of heat and moisture by some vehicle such as flannel. In stable parlance, bathing any part with warm water is called 'fomenting'.

Fomentation over large surfaces are best applied by dipping a blanket or other woollen cloth in hot water, wringing it moderately dry, applying it to the part, and then covering it with a waterproof sheet or dry blanket. When the underneath blanket loses most of its heat, it should be changed for another blanket, care being taken that animal does not get chilled during the interval. The fomentations should not be hotter than the hand can comfortably bear.

Griseofulvin/antifungal agents   Griseofulvin is most often used as an antifungal agent in the treatment of ringworm. Although administered orally, it accumulates in the layers of the skin. Dosage of 10mg per kilogramme body-weight daily should be continued for at least one week.

Other antifungal agents are used topically. These include emilconazade (used as a 0.2% solution) and benzyldazic acid (used as a 0.5% solution). One of these solutions should be applied very two or three days for three or four applications, and then again after an interval of approximately two weeks. Scabs, mud and debris should be removed prior to treatment to ensure total coverage of the affected area(s).

Hyoscine (hyoscine-n-butyl bromide)   This is an antispasmodic with smooth-muscle relaxant properties, used in the treatment of diarrhoea and colic. It is related chemically to atropine (see above) but has more specific actions on the gut with fewer side effects. It is available as an injection for intravenous use.

Iodine   Iodine has antiseptic and irritant actions. Strong iodine solution is used as a rubiefacient and mild blister. Weak solution of iodine contains potassium iodide and iodine, and is used as an antiseptic and mild irritant to help relieve inflammation. Aqueous Solution of Iodine (Lugol's iodine) was frequently used for uterine irrigation but can be very irritant and has lost favour.

Iodine is often found in combination with surface-active agents as iodophors, which are non-irritant, non-staining and have cleansing and antibacterial properties. These are used for pre-surgical skin preparation, the cleansing of wounds and, in very dilute form, for flushing wound cavities or cleansing sites. An example is povidone iodine.

Some iodine salts (sodium iodide, potassium iodide) are used systemically in the treatment of a number of chronic or abscess-forming infections because they appear to reduce or penetrate the fibrous tissue associated with these conditions which often interferes with or prevents adequate penetration of administered drugs.

Magnesium sulphate (Epsom salts)   This is commonly used as a laxative and, at higher doses, a purgative in horses. It acts to increase the amount of water in the food material passing through the intestine, thus increasing the fluidity and volume of the intestinal contents. It must not be used in dehydrated animals as it may exacerbate the condition. The normal dose for purgation is 30-60g in food or administered through a stomach tube.

Mefenamic acid/meclofenamic acid   These are related anti-inflammatory agents, with antipyretc and analgesic actions. They are more powerful than phenylbutazone and are used in the treatment of musculoskeletal disorders. Meclofenamic acid is available as granules for administration in feed.

Naproxen   Naproxen is an anti-inflammatory agent useful in the treatment of pain and lameness associated with soft-tissue disorders such as muscle sprain and inflammation.

Opium, morphine and related drugs   This group includes codeine, pethidine and other morphine derivatives. Their effects on the body are numerous and widespread but they are most valuable for their analgesic, spasmolytic and cough-suppressant actions.

Morphine is commonly used with kaolin in the treatment of diarrhoea. It decreases intestinal mobility and helps reduce pain. Codeine is also useful in diarrhoea.

Pethidine is a commonly used analgesic, although it has only a short duration of action and has been replaced by new, longer-lasting painkillers such as flunixin meglumine. It is occasionally combined with tranquillisers such as acetylpromazine to enhance the degree of tranquillisation.

With all these drugs, central nervous system depression is a major feature. Consequently they must be used with care and are only available to vets.

Peroxide (hydrogen peroxide)   Hydrogen peroxide is used as a 10-50% solution for antisepsis and deodorization of tissues. It has a cleansing effect and is useful in deep wounds and abscesses, especially in the foot. Its foaming action is associated with the release of oxygen, which has a mechanical cleaning effect and lasts as long as the solution is active.

Phenylbutazone   Phenylbutazone is one of the most frequently used and abused drugs available for use in the horse. It is a non-steroidal anti-inflammatory drug (NSAID) which is also an analgesic as a result of its anti-inflammatory action.

It is widely used in horses for reducing pain and inflammation in the treatment of traumatic or inflammatory musculoskeletal disorders and lameness. It is also used to prevent or reduce post-operative swelling and pain, and in some infectious conditions such as ulcerative lymphangitis.

It is available as a powder for mixing with feed, as a paste for oral administration, as a solution for intravenous injection, and in some topically applied medicaments, in combination with dimethyl sulphoxide. The intravenous form is *very* irritant if accidentally administered into muscle or around the vein. If given intra-arterially it causes death.

The recommended dosage for a 450kg (1000lb) horse is 2g both morning and evening on day one of treatment, then 1g morning and evening for four days, then 1g daily or on alternative days. *Ponies do not tolerate phenylbutazone as well as larger horses and are more susceptible to its toxic effects.* Consequently lower dosages must be used, i.e. 1g per 225kg (500lb) daily for four days, followed by 0.5-1g every other day.

Long term use or use in very sensitive horses can cause irritation of the lining of the stomach and intestine and occasionally severe intestinal malfunction. Blood and bone marrow abnormalities may sometimes be associated with phenylbutazone therapy.

Poultices   These are valuable as soothing applications and for cleansing wounds, in which case they should be combined with a mild antiseptic to discourage growth of microbes which would be favoured by the moist warmth of the poultice.

Poultices can be applied to the feet with the aid of a boot or bandage, and can be bandaged or 'plastered' onto limbs or body.

The most commonly used poultices include: antiphlogistine, which is available as a paste; kaolin, which is available as a powder or paste; Proprietary boric-acid-impregnated dressing which should be wetted with warm to hot water before application.

Poultices have a drawing action on wounds and are most useful in cases of puncture or infected wounds. They are also useful in the treatment of bruised sole and in cases of pus in the foot, as they tend to soften the sole and draw the bruise or infection, allowing easier drainage, thus alleviating pain. The hoof should be dry bandaged or otherwise protected after removal of the poultice to allow the horn and wall to dry and harden before the shoe is replaced and the animal put back into work.

Sodium bicarbonate (baking soda)   'Bicarb' is used to reduce gastric acidity following grain engorgement or associated with high intake of soluble carbohydrate. It can be given orally in feed or drinking water. It is believed to help in reducing acidosis associated with exhaustive exercise or azoturia.

Sterile solutions of sodium bicarbonate (usually 1.5%) are used intravenously to treat acidosis associated with colic, respiratory depression or other metabolic disturbances.

Sulphonamides   The sulphonamides are antibacterial compounds used both topically and internally for the prevention and treatment of non-specific infections. Sulphanilamide is a common constituent of wound powders and dressings. It is also given orally as a powder in the feed, or mixed with honey or molasses to form a paste which can be applied to the back of the tongue. Dosage is 40-60g daily for a 500kg adult horse.

The sulphonamides are bacteriostatic, that is, they prevent the multiplication of some bacteria but do not destroy them. Combination with trimethoprim to form potentiated sulphonamides enhances the effectiveness of both sulphonamide and trimethoprim and produces a bacteriocidal (microbe-killing) action for the treatment of established infections.

Sulphur   Sulphur has, for many years, been used as a treatment for skin diseases of bacterial and parasitic origin. It is frequently found in shampoos, in some skin lotions and in ointments or combined with talc or kaolin in dusting or dispersible powders.

Tannin/tannic acid   This is an astringent used both internally, in cases of diarrhoea, and topically for skin lesions and minor burns. When given orally it helps the formation of a protective coating for irritated or inflamed intestinal lining. Topically, tannic acid may be combined in hydrophilic gels or solutions to sooth minor burns, reduce inflammation and help reduce haemorrhage.

Zinc   Commonly used zinc salts include zinc oxide and zinc carbonate. These are used topically in powders, creams, lotions and liniments. They have stringent, antiseptic and protective actions.

Zinc oxide is combined with castor oil to produce a soothing protective dressing (zinc and castor oil cream), and with cod liver oil as a treatment for conjunctivitis. It can also be combined with lard for application to cracked heels.

Wound powders containing zinc oxide or carbonate usually have a chalk, talc or starch base and may contain sulphanilamide and insecticides.

Zinc sulphate is a stronger astringent and promotes scab formation on wounds. White lotion contains zinc sulphate (4%) and lead acetate (5%) in water and is a cooling, soothing lotion for minor superficial inflammation, bruising and itching.

36

METHODS OF RESTRAINT AND HANDLING

Occasionally, just observing a horse loose in its stable or paddock will give enough information to determine if there is anything wrong with it. Most often, however, a degree of restraint is necessary to allow observation, examination, manipulation, palpation and treatment of a part or the whole of the animal. This not only applies to veterinary procedures but also to farriery, dentistry and all aspects of horse handling and education. Restraint can be achieved either by physical or chemical means or by a combination of both.

Physical restraint
For minor procedures in quiet or very ill animals, manual restraint with either a head collar or a bridle is often adequate: most horses can be injected with antibiotics or a vaccine while being held quietly. For firmer control a Chifney (anti-rearing) bit may be useful.

Further restraint can be achieved by grasping or pinching a fold of loose skin on the neck, just in front of the shoulders. The skin should be held tightly in a closed fist. This method is very effective for horses which tend to wriggle or to pull away and is easily achieved by the person holding the horse's head.

For procedures involving one of the limbs or when trying to prevent a horse kicking, a front leg can be held up so that the animal is standing on three legs. This often requires a second person so that whoever is holding the head can concentrate on keeping the head up and the animal still. Obviously no attempt should be made to pick up another of the horse's legs while one is already being held up in case the horse panics or falls over.

The twitch, consisting of a length of smooth wood with a loop of rope, chain or twine through a hole at one end, is a very useful tool when trying to restrain a horse physically. It is normally applied to the upper lip, although occasionally it is used on one of the horse's ears. The loop of the twitch is passed over one of the operator's hands, while the handle of the twitch is held in the other hand or by the person holding the horse's head. The horse's lip or ear is grasped in the hand with the loop. The loop is then passed over the hand and the twitch handle twisted to tighten the loop onto the chosen part. This will result in the animal standing rigidly and any required procedure can then be carried out. Other types of twitch include a metal hinged 'humane twitch' or a loop connected to a strap which is tied to the headcollar once the twitch has been applied. Care must be taken when using a twitch as many horses 'explode' in response. This situation is particularly dangerous when working at or near the horses head as many of these horses will rear and strike out or lunge forward in response to having a twitch applied. Veterinary procedures which might be made easier and safer to perform with a nose twitch in place include rectal examination, injecting into or around joints and other structures in the legs, or procedures for which the horse must be standing absolutely still.

Casting is an outdated method of restraint which made use of ropes and hobbles, or a rope and a casting harness. Unfortunately it caused a high degree of anxiety and struggling on the part of the horse as its legs were literally pulled out from underneath it.

Casting is rarely used nowadays since the development of effective tranquillisers and local and general anaesthetics. Occasionally it is combined with one or a combination of chemical agents which reduce the animal's struggles and thus the risk of injury to horse and humans.

Chemical restraint
The use of drugs such as sedatives, tranquillisers, local and general anaesthetics and analgesics makes restraint safer for horses and handler. It also simplifies many procedures by making the animal tractable and helping to minimise pain and anxiety.

Tranquillisers and sedatives are given by injection or by mouth. Their effect can vary from mild tranquillisation to profound sedation, depending on the drug being used and the dosage given. Many of these drugs can have a seriously detrimental effect on blood pressure and the central nervous system if given incorrectly or in overdose.

Signs that the drug is taking effect include a dropping of the head, prolapse of the penis in colts and geldings, and a glazed look about the eyes. Profound sedation is marked by a drooping of the upper and lower lips and eyelids, and a rocking motion with the horse occasionally knuckling on one of its fetlocks. The use of certain drugs may result in the horse standing perfectly still without knuckling.

Depending on the drug or combination used, the dosage given, the temperament of the animal and the effects of any other drug or drugs being used, the time for which the animal is effectively tranquillised or sedated will vary greatly, being anything from a few minutes to several hours.

Some drugs have an analgesic (painkilling) action as well as a tranquillising effect. This property makes them very useful for minor procedures which involve potentially painful steps such as stitching superficial wounds. In most cases, however, such procedures will require the use of a local anaesthetic agent, either administered in combination with a tranquilliser or on its own.

Anaesthetic agents
Anaesthesia may be local (involving only a small area), regional (involving a larger region or part of the body) or general (involving the whole body). Drugs used for regional anaesthesia are called local anaesthetics or local anaesthetic agents. Drugs used for general anaesthesia are called general anaesthetic agents or, more loosely, just anaesthetics.

Local and regional anaesthesia
Local and regional anaesthetics can be used on their own, with the animal twitched, or, if necessary, with the animal tranquillised or sedated. Local anaesthesia is used when stitching wounds, lancing haematomas or removing small lumps of skin. In these cases the local anaesthetic is injected along the edges of the wound or an inverted 'L' pattern several centimetres away from the wound and through all affected layers to desensitise the nerves passing to the area to be treated (nerve blocking).

Regional anaesthesia involves desensitising or numbing the nerve or nerves supplying a particular region which is often distant from the site of injection of the anaesthetic solution. This type of nerve block is most often used in the diagnosis of lameness or when treating limb injuries. The local anaesthetic solution is injected into a specific site around a particular nerve, resulting in the desensitisation of part of the limb. Injection over the outer aspect of both sesamoid bones in one limb, for example, will desensitise much of the pastern and foot in that particular limb. If, after desensitisation, a lame horse subsequently goes sound it is almost certain that the lesion is below the level of the nerve block.

Local anaesthesia is also used for standing castrations. The solution is injected into the testicle and cord and under the scrotal skin along the line of incision. Regional anaesthesia is also used for standing procedures involving the abdomen and chest. Laparoscopic examination and treatment of abdominal conditions is becoming more widely available and is most often performed in the standing, sedated patient. Very occasionally colic surgery may also be performed in the standing horse using regional anaesthesia.

Epidural anaesthesia involves the injection of a local anaesthetic agent into the spinal canal around the spinal cord, thus desensitising the nerves within the spinal canal and where they exit into the surrounding tissues. This type of anaesthesia is most often used for obstetrical procedures and surgery in the region of the perineum or tail.

General anaesthesia

General anaesthesia is anaesthesia of the whole body: the animal becomes recumbent, does not move (except for minor involuntary movements), does not feel pain and does not have any recall of the procedure performed. It is mainly used when the procedure is painful or lengthy, when total immobil-isation of the patient is necessary, when the temperament of the patient or the site for surgery is not conducive to local or regional anaesthesia, or when the animal has to be positioned unnaturally – for example, on its back. The types of case which require general anaesthesia in the horse include repair of fractures, castration, treating major wounds, surgery for colic and surgery on the head and upper respiratory passages.

General anaesthesia must be induced and then maintained. Induction is the transition from consciousness to the state of anaesthesia. This state must then be maintained for the duration of the procedure. After this the animal is allowed to wake up or recover.

There are a number of anaesthetic drugs available and these can be classified as injectable or inhalable (volatile or gaseous) anaesthetic agents. Injectable anaesthetics include the barbiturates, the combination of xylazine and ketamine, glyceryl guaiacolate and thiopentone and many others. The drugs are usually injected after premedication of the patient with a tranquil-lizer and the dose rate depends on the weight of the animal. If the patient is severely ill or depressed, the dose rate is reduced accordingly. Using a combination of different tranqullizers and anaesthetic agents may permit a reduction in the required dosage of all the agents used, thus minimising the depressant effects on the patient.

Inhalation anaesthesia with volatile liquids or gases is used almost exclusively for maintaining anaesthesia after induction with an intravenous agent. The major exception to this is when inducing anaesthesia in foals. When very young, foals can be masked down, that is, induced by placing an anaesthetic mask over their nostrils or a nasal tube into a nostril to allow the administration of gaseous anaesthetic until unconsciousness is achieved. After induction in both foals and adults, an endotracheal tube is introduced via the mouth into the trachea and this is connected to an anaesthetic machine which supplies both oxygen and the anaesthetic agent to the patient. The depth of anaesthesia depends upon the concentration of anaesthetic in the oxygen being inhaled by the patient. Once the procedure is completed the concentration of the anaesthetic gas in the mixture is reduced to zero so that the patient is no longer inhaling any anaesthetic, and the horse is allowed to breathe pure oxygen via the machine for at least ten minutes. After this time the horse breathes air via the endotracheal tube until it swallows; the tube is then removed and the animal allowed to recover.

The time taken for the horse to recover until it is able to stand varies with the anaesthetic agent or agents used, the duration of the procedure, and the temperament and condition of the horse. Recovery after prolonged intravenous anaesthesia can be long, and the animal may struggle considerably before being able to stand. Horses anaesthetised in the paddock must not be left unattended until standing and able to walk.

Occasionally it is necessary to have an attendant sitting on the horse's head and neck and covering its eyes to try to reduce the animal's struggles and attempts to stand before it is ready. If necessary, the horse should be supported by its head and tail until it is standing steadily on its feet.

Veterinary practices with surgical facilities usually have a special recovery box with padded walls and floor where the horse is anaesthetised and later allowed to recover. In some cases the same room functions as the operating theatre. In others, the anaesthetised horse is moved by hobbles and winch, in a net or on a mobile table or fork lift to the operating theatre and back again.

Although general anaesthesia simplifies many diagnostic, surgical and manipulative procedures in the horse, it is not without its inherent complications. Most of the problems encountered when anaesthetising horses are associated with its large size and weight. In some cases pressure on the underlying muscles causes muscle cell damage, with associated pain, swelling and release of cell contents, resulting in lameness and in some cases inability to bend or bear weight on one or more of the limbs. This is known as post-operative myopathy. It is most common and most severe in horses held in dorsal recumbency (on their backs) for long periods, although it is not uncommon in horses kept on their sides for a lengthy operation. The affected horse may not be able to stand at all, or may be able to stand but unable to move, or may be able to move only with difficulty after the anaesthetic has worn off. Many of these cases need intensive treatment to recover fully. Occasionally only one or a small group of muscles or nerves is affected and this leads to local paralysis of, for example, the facial nerve or the radial nerve of the forelimb.

Horses are not unlike all other animal species in that some individuals will be particularly sensitive to an anaesthetic agent. All anaesthetic agents cause a drop in blood pressure, respiration and cardiac output. Overdosage in healthy animals or relative overdosage – that is, the administration of normal doses to a sick or otherwise compromised animal or to an animal which is particularly sensitive to a particular drug – will result in severe cardiovascular depression and compromise and in many cases death. On the other hand, there is a very small percentage of horses which, when given an appropriate dosage of an anaesthetic agent, will fail to become anaesthetised or may even go into a stage of excitement. Such animals will usually respond normally to a different drug or combination of drugs.

37
INFLAMMATION

Inflammation is the active response of living tissue to injury and infection. The following description is therefore applicable within the context of this book where diseases caused by infection (pp. 455-563) or injury to parts such as tendons, joints and bone (pp. 203-276) or wounds (pp. 637-646) are discussed. In essence, wherever there is disease or injury suffered by an individual, the inflammatory process is present.

The suffix 'itis' denotes inflammation, e.g. bronchitis = inflammation of the bronchi. It is characterised by the appearance of redness, swelling, heat and pain, and frequently attended by loss of function of the affected part.

The inflammatory process is a non-specific defence mechanism, brought into play by the phagocyte system and initiated in response to chemical messages released by cells and damaged tissues.

The phagocyte system is composed primarily of macrophages and polymorphonuclear leucocytes (types of white blood cell) which ingest and destroy bacteria, particularly foreign material and degenerate cellular tissue. This system is mobilised at the site of injury via the terminal vascular system of capillaries and lymphatic channels.

It should be noted that the inflammatory process may become integrated with the other major body defence – the immune system, which is regarded as a specific defence mechanism.

The immune system attacks invasive bacteria, viruses or toxins with 'killer' lymphocytes and antibodies specifically manufactured to deal with a particular organism which has been recognized as foreign to the host from previous exposure. The phagocyte system primes the immune system with antigens derived from the breakdown of the invasive organisms by the leucocytes.

The inflammatory process occurs in two phases:

1. The immediate response, which is an initial transitory reaction of twenty to thirty minutes' duration induced by any stimulus which damages mast

cells (which are found in connective tissue). It is characterised by increased blood flow to the area and leakage of plasma into the surrounding tissues. This is clinically manifested as redness and heat.

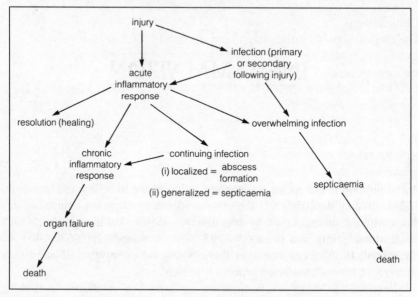

Figure 1   The course of infection arising from an injury

2. The delayed response, which is more severe and prolonged, is characterised by persistence of plasma leakage, stasis of blood flow and possible haemorrhage and emigration of leucocytes and macrophages into the tissues. Clinically this is manifested as swelling and pain.

As a consequence of tissue swelling the lymphatic channels open, thereby increasing lymph flow and drainage, with removal of cell debris, bacteria and waste products. Clinically the lymph nodes which drain the area may become reactive and enlarged.

This basic process occurs in all types of tissue injury, from simple skin penetration by a thorn to that of gross tissue damage associated with trauma or in septic states caused by specific bacterial infection, which may affect any tissue or organ system.

Causes
The causes of inflammation are many and varied, but they may be placed in one of four categories:

1. Mechanical – direct trauma or mechanical overload of a tissue, such as overstretching of a tendon resulting in sprain.

2. Thermal – excessive heat or cold, ultraviolet and infrared light and radiation.
3. Chemical – caustic alkali, acids and blisters.
4. Toxic – plant poisons, bacterial and fungal toxins.

Clinical signs

The clinical signs of inflammation are classically defined as redness (rubor), swelling (tumour), heat (calor) and pain (dolour), as well as loss of function - the signs of celsis.

At this stage, if the reader recalls from personal experience the effects of a bee sting, he or she will be able to appreciate the changes described above.

The redness and heat are associated with increased bloodflow to the area, and swelling and pain are associated with the formation of oedema, as well as with the release of enzymes and vasoactive substances which are involved in mediation of the inflammatory response.

The physical signs of inflammation depend on factors such as the nature and severity of the injury or infection, the tissue or organs affected, species susceptibility to particular micro-organisms, and host adaptations of the inflammatory response, as well as the virulence of the invading organisms, the severity of infection and other complicating factors such as loss of blood supply or tissue anoxia (oxygen starvation).

Inflammatory disease of the musculoskeletal system invariably results in lameness, a symptom which is readily appreciated and directly referable to the organ system involved. However, the clinical signs of inflammation may not always be directly attributable to their source. For example, inflammatory disease of the biliary system of the liver may produce clinical symptoms of jaundice in the skin, the membranes or the appearance of bile pigments in the urine. In this instance some of the symptoms of hepatitis are being manifested indirectly via different organ systems.

Pain is another feature frequently associated with inflammatory disease, and appreciation of the source of pain depends on the presence of pain receptor nerve endings in the affected tissue. Some tissues – for example, the myocardium of the heart and the brain itself – are poorly endowed with pain receptors, and injury here may be poorly appreciated. Inflammation of the myocardium or abdominal viscera may result in awareness of 'referred' pain, which the patient may think arises in a part distant from the actual inflamed area.

Frequently when the body mounts an inflammatory response there will be a systemic (general) reaction which may incorporate, in addition to the local signs, a pyrexic episode (an increase in body temperature), rigors and generalised discomfort, dullness and anorexia (lack or loss of appetite).

Course of inflammation

The course of an inflammation depends on several of the above factors, as well as the ability of the horse to mount a vigorous and successful response to the original challenge. A debilitated subject may not be able to muster sufficient reserves to produce an effective response to bacterial challenge which, under normal circumstances, would not be markedly pathogenic. The hope for the outcome of any inflammatory process is for healing of tissues with restoration of function and without undue secondary complications.

The outcome of the acute inflammatory process falls into one of the following categories:

1. Resolution, whereby the injury heals rapidly without complication, as in a surgical wound which heals by first intention with a minimum of scar tissue.
2. Resolution after extensive tissue damage complicated by wound contamination, bacterial infection and resultant exudation. These wounds are characterised by an exudative inflammatory process, followed by the production of granulation tissue and significant end-stage fibrosis (scar formation). Examples of these are suppuration, abscessation, sinus, fistula, cellulitis, ulceration and necrosis.

   Suppuration refers to the formation of pus by massive exudation and accumulation of leucocytes in response to pyogenic bacteria, e.g. staphylococcus, streptococcus and corynebacteria. These organisms produce toxins and are not readily destroyed by white blood cells. Suppuration may occur in any tissue or on any body surface such as the skin and the pleura.

   Abscessation refers to the formation of abscesses, which are localised collections of pus produced by the deep seeding of infectious bacteria, frequently caused by a penetrating foreign body.

   A **sinus** is a blind discharging channel which may form as the drainage tract from an infected vicinity or established abscess. For example, a bony sequestrum (dead bone) will discharge through a sinus. Other examples are fistulous withers and poll evil, often the result of an injury.

   A **fistula** is a channel from a natural cavity or duct to the exterior, for example, a recto-vaginal fistula.

   Cellulitis is a diffuse spreading inflammation in solid tissues – for example, along muscle or tendon sheaths or subcutaneously. It may be purulent.

   Ulceration consists of lesions formed by superficial necrosis of an epithelial surface leading to exposure of underlying tissue; it has little tendency to heal.

   Necrosis means death of a limited portion of tissue and may be a result of anoxia or loss of blood supply secondary to clot formation. Necrosis includes gangrene, which is termed dry when it is caused by loss of blood circulation, or moist when it is the result of potent toxins produced by bacterial infection.
3. Non-resolution, which consists of:
   (a) acute inflammation in association with extensive fibrosis;

(b) a proliferative cellular response and induction of the immune system in which a delayed hypersensitivity reaction may occur, as, for example, in tuberculosis; or

(c) infective granulomata. These consist of a particular type of abscess which is produced in response to specific bacterial infections.

Treatment

The general principles of treatment of inflamed areas are as follows:

1. The cause should be identified and removed.

2. Circulation to the affected part should be restored and improved, thereby hastening the removal of waste products and supplying nutrients for tissue repair.

3. Collections of pus should be drained and dead tissue removed as soon as possible.

4. The injured area should be rested in the acute phase and may require immobilisation.

5. Local treatment may consist of lavage with antiseptics, saline solution or antibiotic.

If shock or blood loss is apparent, then fluid replacement therapy and administration of corticosteroids may be necessary. Systemic administration of drugs to control pain and inflammation, to reduce oedema and to control bacterial contamination or infection with pyogenic organisms is frequently indicated. Medication with non-steroidal anti-inflammatory drugs, diuretics and antibiotics is employed.

Simple acute inflammation of a traumatic nature involving the musculoskeletal system may be treated initially with cold applications to reduce blood supply to the area and control the formation of oedema. The application of pressure with bandages may be helpful to this end. Subsequently application of heat alternating with cold will be beneficial by stimulating the circulation and the healing process. Local application of enzyme preparations, non-steroidal anti-inflammatory drugs or dimethyl sulphoxide (DMSO) with or without cortisone may be employed for treatment of athletic injuries. Articular inflammatory disease is currently treated with the local introduction of hyaluronic acid into the joint space.

Ultrasonic stimulation of inflamed areas may be beneficial. Recently the use of cold lasers has been claimed to control the inflammatory response and significantly improve the healing rate.

Chronic inflammation is more difficult to deal with, and in addition to the above treatments there may also be a place for the use of counter-irritants, whereby an acute inflammation is set up in the hope that this will result in improved repair.

Preventive measures
The therapeutic administration of non-steroidal and steroid drugs, both systemically and topically, is the most important method of controlling inflammation.

It is not recommended that anti-inflammatory drugs be given as a pro-phylactic measure to healthy horses because, by masking the early signs of inflammation, they may allow a disease process to become well established before it is recognised. This would obviously compromise the prognosis for a complete functional recovery, particularly in the case of injuries of the musculoskeletal system.

Non-steroidal anti-inflammatory drugs are commonly used to enable chronically lame horses to perform, albeit at a reduced capacity. In this way the useful working life of an unsound horse may be prolonged. Steroid drugs may also be beneficial, both prophylactically and therapeutically, in horses with chronic obstructive pulmonary disease; inhibiting or alleviating the inflammatory response in the lungs' airways may render many horses capable of light work.

It is worth stressing the prevention of pulmonary inflammation arising from equine influenza: this may be prevented, or the side effects ameliorated, by prior vaccination.

38
POISONING IN HORSES

A poison is any substance detrimental to health at a specified minimum intake. Poisoning may occur through contact or penetration of the skin, by inhalation or by consumption.

Poisons may be classified as (1) those that are corrosive – these include strong acids and strong alkalis that destroy tissue; (2) irritants, that cause inflammation of tissue; (3) potent fat solvents, that destroy epithelial tissue by dissolving out its fat components; and (4) poisons that interact with metabolism.

In this review those poisons most likely to be encountered by stabled and grazing horses will be discussed.

Routes
The gastro-intestinal tract is by far the most common route for poisons to gain access to the body under natural conditions. In comparison with another and larger group of herbivores, the ruminant, the horse seems to suffer a disadvantage in respect of gastro-intestinal poisoning. A number of poisons are partly, or extensively, destroyed by rumen micro-organisms which decrease the extent of subsequent absorption of the poison from the small intestine. In the case of the horse not only is this facility unavailable, but the acid conditions of the stomach may lead to the solution of materials that are insoluble in neutral solutions.

The stomach of a horse under normal feeding conditions contains fairly large quantities of ingesta, so the effect of stomach fill on the toxicity of a poison is not of great significance. However, it is not possible to make any general statement about the effect of the degree of stomach fill on toxicity because for some poisons a full stomach decreases toxicity, but for others it leads to an increase in toxicity.

Toxicity
Although the toxicity of some poisons is increased by their being metabolised in the body, the toxicity of most is decreased. Many organic poisons are

processed by the liver into forms which are less harmful and more water-soluble. Most of these poisons are then excreted through the kidneys, although some are passed out with the bile, through the bile duct into the intestinal tract. Much of this is reabsorbed. Many volatile poisons are partly disposed of in the expired air. Some poisons are deposited in a relatively inert form in tissues out of the way of normal metabolic processes. This applies to many elemental poisons such as lead, cadmium and strontium.

Bone is a typical site for such deposition. It can be appreciated readily that horses which have malfunctioning livers and kidneys as a result of malnutrition, parasitic infestation, or old age, are less able to dispose of certain poisons than are healthy animals, and old horses therefore succumb to lower intakes. However, during periods of stress and malnutrition heavy metals deposited in bone may be mobilised, causing a crisis long after the initial poisoning occurred.

Repeated small doses of a poison may be expressed in a different way from one massive dose, but generally speaking the toxicity in both cases is roughly proportional to the unit of bodyweight (bwt). Because the horse is a large animal, a much bigger dose is required, generally speaking, to kill it than is required by dogs, cats and sheep. However, for many substances the toxic dose is roughly proportional to $bwt^{0.7}$. Thus a dose that was just toxic in a 500 kg horse would be only four times, and not seven to eight times, the dose per animal that was just toxic in a 70 kg sheep. The young and the old may be more susceptible than the healthy adult, so the dose per unit of bodyweight that causes damage may be less in their cases than in the case of the healthy adult.

Diagnosis

The differentiation of the great variety of causes of poisoning is extremely difficult because symptoms are similar. The most successful solution to this problem is to examine the environment carefully and to determine whether the horse, or pony, has had access to anything that could do it harm.

For this it is necessary to be fully aware of those substances which are hazardous, and therefore the main purpose of this review is to enlighten the reader of the principal causes of poisoning, so that either they may be removed from the environment or measures may be taken to ensure that animals have no access to them.

The most effective way of diagnosing the cause of poisoning is to analyse samples from the stomach contents, faeces, body tissues, feed or other suspected materials that may have been fed to the horse or to which the animal has been exposed. This analysis may have to be performed in specially equipped laboratories, in which specific requirements will have been established as to how the samples should be prepared and dispatched. Certain samples may have to be stored frozen. Advice on these matters should therefore be sought from a vet or other qualified person.

Clinical signs

Signs of poisoning are numerous and, although they differ between poisons, a number are common and frequently encountered. These include loss of appetite, incoordination of gait and lameness, depression, diarrhoea, irregular and laboured breathing, muscular twitching, discoloured urine and unusual smell of the breath and faeces, salivation, thirst, anaemia, icterus (jaundice), blindness, dilation of pupils, colic, and photosensitization expressed as oedematous swellings around the face, eyes, neck and flanks.

Treatment

Appropriate treatment is not easy to ascertain and normally this should be carried out by a veterinarian. Where damage to the skin has occurred, generally speaking little harm can be done by washing the skin with clean water. It may not be a good idea to add soap or detergent to the water as this may increase the penetration of the skin by the poison.

Where poisons have been imbibed, the stomach contents may be washed out by gastric lavage, or a substance may be given that absorbs the toxic material. Such substances include mixtures of activated charcoal, light magnesium oxide, kaolin, tannic acid or charcoal on its own.

Where heavy-metal poisoning has occurred, treatment either orally, or by injection, with sodium versenate or sodium calcium versenate, sometimes described as sodium calcium EDTA, may be used to chelate the metal, which is subsequently excreted, even by the kidney. Demulcents, that are viscid in character, protecting mucous membranes from irritation, are frequently used in the oral treatment of poisoning. These include gum acacia and glycerol.

HEAVY METALS AND OTHER POISONS

Many cases of poisoning by heavy metals and other elements are caused by industrial pollution of grazing areas, often as a result of human carelessness. Others come about through the inquisitive nature of animals themselves, particularly their tendency to chew objects in the environment not intended for eating. There are also some cases of poisoning by elements that, for geographical or geological reasons, have accumulated naturally in the soil.

Selenium Selenium is found in high natural concentrations in some areas of the world. Parts of the USA are well known for their selenium toxicity, and small areas of marginally toxic concentrations occur in Eire. Selenium is readily absorbed by certain plants and consequently ingested by grazing animals. The chronic disease caused by selenium poisoning has been called **alkali**, owing to the alkaline nature of water that is rich in selenium.

Horses with selenium poisoning suffer loss of hair from the mane and tail, develop rings around the hoof below the coronet, become lame owing to erosion of articular surfaces of leg bones and display a deterioration in appetite.

Where very high concentrations of selenium occur in plants, a condition known as **blind staggers** develops. Horses lose weight dramatically, develop a staring coat and wander aimlessly with impaired vision, salivating and showing signs of paralysis.

Treatment may be unsuccessful. If possible, horses should be removed from the area and given a high-protein, high-quality diet. Some improvement has been achieved by the provision of small amounts of arsenic under veterinary supervision.

Arsenic Somewhat similar clinical signs occur with arsenic poisoning, which is usually caused by an animal inadvertently consuming a product that contains the arsenic. Apart from a staggering gait, paralysis, salivation and thirst, there is severe irritation of the intestinal tract, which develops a rose-red inflammation. Gastric lavage is carried out if the signs are detected early enough.

Fluorine Fluorosis caused by excessive fluorine intake is less frequent in horses than in other grazing stock. Some soils and water courses are naturally rich in this element, and in the past industrial contamination of pasture by aerial deposits has been a typical cause.

Fluorine is deposited in bones and teeth, and if ruminants show pitting and discoloration of the teeth, this may be the cause. Where pasture contains an excess of 50mg fluorine per kilogramme dry matter, the danger of toxicity exists.

If grazing horses become lame and their forage is shown to contain large amounts of fluorine, it is wise to remove them from the area. Aluminium oxide added to grain-based diets at a level of 0.5% helps to eliminate fluorine from bone.

Molybdenum and sulphur   **Induced copper deficiency** arising from excess molybdenum in herbage has been suggested as a possible contributory factor in bone disorders of foals and yearlings. In sheep a condition known as swayback is a characteristic copper deficiency syndrome, caused by excessive intakes of molybdenum and sulphur. Signs in sheep occur in the so called teart pastures, which are found in parts of Somerset, Gloucestershire and Warwickshire, where the copper: molybdenum ratio in herbage is less than 6: 1. Induced copper deficiency is caused by copper binding with thiomolybdates either in the gut or in body tissue. The formation of thiomolybdates from sulphur and molybdenum may depend on the presence of rumen microorganisms and it therefore seems that induced copper deficiency in horses is far less likely than in ruminants.

Nevertheless in areas where grazing sheep and cattle are showing typical signs of induced copper deficiency, it is wise to ensure that young horses, in particular, receive adequate copper supplementation. This is achieved by injection at regular intervals, a routine and effective therapy. Copper toxicity in horses does not occur until intake greatly exceeds that causing copper toxicity in ruminants.

Lead Lead is one of the commonest causes of poisoning in cattle, sheep and horses. Signs of toxicity are more frequent in young horses and these include lack of appetite, muscular stiffness and weakness, diarrhoea and, in an acute form, pharyngeal paralysis and regurgitation of food and water.

Lead accumulates in the bones and as little as 80 mg lead per kilogram diet may eventually cause toxic signs, which are sometimes brought on by stress. Natural feeds with 1-10 mg of lead per kilogram cause no problems. However, inquisitive animals will sometimes consume objects in their environment, some of which may be rich in lead. These include putty, linoleum, golf balls, red lead and particularly accumulator battery plates. Lead-based paints are less frequently used today, but they may still be found in old buildings and may be ingested by horses that persistently chew wooden objects.

Vegetation in the vicinity of smelter works and highways may contain as much as 500 mg lead per kilogram dry matter and therefore vegetation may be a significant cause of damage (The exclusion of lead from petrol should decrease this risk.). Lead shot from shotgun rounds indiscriminately used on pasture has been found to be a cause of severe lead toxicity in silage produced from the pasture grass (The replacement of lead in shot should also remove this source of danger). The acidic conditions that develop in the silage clamp encourage the solution of the metallic lead. Furthermore the acid secreted in a horse's stomach will contribute to the solution of lead shot.

Unless lead toxicity is suspected it may be somewhat difficult to diagnose, although lead analysis of faeces, stomach contents and blood will help. Lead accumulates in bone and kidney tissue and therefore can be detected post mortem in many, but by no means all, cases. Veterinary treatment includes administration of sodium calcium EDTA (calcium disodium versenate) at a rate of 75 mg per kilogramme bodyweight daily.

Cadmium Pasture may be contaminated by cadmium, derived from mine workings, waste dumps and sewage sludge, in the form of aerial dust or through water erosion. Pastures in the vicinity of factories using zinc ore may be polluted with cadmium. Cadmium is absorbed by plants to a much greater extent than lead is. Of common pasture species, the daisy *(Bellis perennis)* accumulates 60-80 mg cadmium per kilogramme (thirty times as much as grasses) from contaminated soils.

Signs of cadmium toxicity include reduced food intake, diarrhoea, incoordination, icterus and fatty degeneration of the liver. The only reasonable solution to cadmium toxicity is to remove stock from areas where it may occur.

Mercury Mercury is highly poisonous and the metal is volatile at normal temperatures. In compounds it occurs as mercuric chloride ($HgCl_2$), mercurous chloride (Hg_2Cl_2), calomel and methyl mercuric chloride (CH_3HgCl). Mercuric chloride is less toxic than methyl mercuric chloride and more toxic than mercurous chloride. However, organic mercury compounds generally are said to be less toxic than inorganic compounds and therefore they are used more widely. One such use is as seed dressing in agriculture and, despite the lower toxicity, this is a likely source of poisoning in horses.

Symptoms include violent gastro-enteritis and diarrhoea, nephritis and inflammation of the mouth. There is a loss of appetite, nervousness and incoordination of gait.

Speedy treatment is essential and this includes gastric lavage with saturated sodium bicarbonate solution.

Nitrates, nitrites and oxalates The rapid growth of pasture after high rainfall and the excessive use of nitrogen fertilizers can lead to high concentrations of nitrates in the herbage and contamination of ground water, ditches and streams through the leeching of soils. Although nitrates are only slightly toxic they can be reduced to nitrites before, or generally after, consumption.

High levels of nitrites may accumulate in plants after herbicide treatment and during the making of oat hay, as a result of nitrate reduction, that is encouraged by inclement weather. Where root vegetables, such as mangels (mangolds), are boiled and left in the boiling water, nitrite can accumulate and cause poisoning. Sugarbeet tops are frequently fed to cattle after wilting. The purpose of wilting is to allow oxalates present in the leaves to be converted to insoluble salts, which are less toxic, but the leaves can also contain nitrate in lethal quantities – in fact, as potassium nitrate up to 4.5% of dry matter. Sugarbeet tops are less toxic to ruminants as rumen micro-organisms convert oxalates to bicarbonates.

The toxicity of nitrite is due to the conversion of blood haemoglobin to methaemoglobin and also to the formation of dimethylnitrosamine from dimethylamine plus nitrite under the influence of the intestinal flora. These compounds damage the liver.

Some effective treatment of nitrite toxicity is apparently achieved by giving ascorbic acid (vitamin C) or methylene blue intravenously, which brings about the partial reconversion of methaemoglobin to oxyhaemoglobin.

Oxalate toxicity is most likely in domestic livestock in subtropical areas, where a number of grass species, either grazed or used as hay, contain high levels of oxalates. Oxalates interfere with calcium deposition in bone and also may cause some kidney damage through the formation of calcium oxalate deposits. Toxicity has been prevented in horses by supplementing the diet with dicalcium phosphate ($CaHPO_4$). This brings about a deposition of calcium oxalate in the gut, preventing its absorption. Where there is a large intake of oxalates during grazing, the diet should be supplemented with a cereal concentrate containing 10 per cent dicalcium phosphate at the rate of 1-1.5 kg per day to prevent oxalate poisoning.

Antibiotics and pesticides Most antibiotics used for feeding to farm livestock have little ill effect on horses unless given at therapeutic levels. When this occurs colic might be induced through disruption of the intestinal flora. On the other hand, three antibiotics used agriculturally, and one in particular, are highly toxic in horses.

Monensin, also marketed as Rumensin and Elancoban, can cause death in horses if they mistakingly consume, for more than a very few days, concentrate feed intended for poultry or cattle. Horses present signs of posterior weakness, profuse sweating, occasionally muscular tremors and myoglobinuria (dark brown urine). There can be permanent damage to heart muscle, but toxicity may be arrested in the early stages by removing the stomach contents and then feeding mineral oil. Generally speaking, confirmation of the cause can be achieved by analysis of stomach contents.

Salinomycin, an anticoccidial ionophore, in higher doses than for monensin, causes somewhat similar signs, that may appear immediately, or several months after exposure. Lincomycin is an anti-bacterial drug sometimes included in pig feed. It is less toxic to horses than monensin but can cause liver damage. In all these cases the toxic feed should be removed as soon as possible.

Many pesticides require careful management at stables where horses are kept. Two that have been widely used and to which the horse is susceptible are mentioned here. The molluscicide, metaldehyde, that has in the past been used as slug bait, is palatable to horses and horses are more sensitive to it than are cats or dogs. Warfarin, used against rats, is an anti-coagulant causing bleeding, and intoxicated horses should be treated with vitamin K_1 (1 mg/kg body weight, daily).

Bacteria, bacterial toxins and other diseases from feed Disease caused by pathogenic enterobacteria such as pathogenic species of *Salmonella* cause a chronic diarrhoea in horses that is difficult to eliminate. Sources of these organisms include dead rodents and rodent droppings and badly, or incorrectly, processed animal protein sources. Even properly processed bovine and ovine sources of meat and bone meal may present a route for the transmission of bovine spongiform encephalomalacia. Rodent infestation of cereal grains should be kept to an absolute minimum and there is no need, or justification, to feed horses any form of meat or meat and bone meal.

Feed contaminated by the soil-borne, pathogenic species of *Clostridium* can lead to the proliferation of *C. perfringens* in the intestines of horses, causing a severe gas colic. Large intakes of succulent forages increase the likelihood of this type of infection, which can lead rapidly to death. Only small meals of cut fresh forage or silage should be permitted for horses.

A number of cases of **botulism** (see p. 477-8*)* have occurred in horses as a consequence of the consumption of insufficiently fermented haylage or silage. *C. botulinum* will grow under anaerobic conditions in a silage clamp where the pH is above 4.5, or where the silage contains less than about 35% dry matter. Only a very small quantity of this toxin, present in feed, is required to kill a horse. Botulism is caused in adult horses by the ingestion of toxins produced by *C. botulinum.* By comparison botulism in young animals can be caused by the growth of the organism and production of the toxin within the gut lumen. Persuasive evidence now indicates that equine dysautonomia (grass sickness) may be a toxicoinfection with a neurotoxin produced by *C. botulinum* type C growing in the ileum of horses. It is hoped that an effective vaccine may be developed against this type of *C.botulinum* prevalent in Europe.

It is important that green feed and silage provided for horses should be contaminated as little as possible with soil, and that silage has a sufficiently high proportion of dry matter (preferably over 50%) and a sufficiently low pH (below 4.5*)*. Lush forage and silage should be fed to horses only in small quantities at each meal.

Poisonous seeds contaminating vegetable protein concentrates In the past, cases of poisoning occurred as a consequence of feeding horses imported vegetable protein concentrates that contained highly toxic seeds, including castor seed, croton seed and certain species of tropical peas and beans. This problem does not now occur, although cheap protein concentrates of unknown origin should always be viewed with suspicion.

Miscellaneous farm poisons Concentrated sources of herbicides, insecticides, fungicides, rodenticides and molluscicides should be kept well away from livestock. Horses should not have access to sheep dips, and care should be taken to keep tractor paraffin, diesel oil, sump oil, disinfectants (mainly phenols) and antifreeze (ethylene glycol) well away from feed and horses.

Snake bites and stings by bees, wasps and spiders The horse is very susceptible to bites from venomous snakes. However, because of a horse's size, a bite that would kill a small domestic animal may only injure a horse. Such bites might be recognised by the fang marks in the centre of a swollen area. Where species of poisonous snakes are known to inhabit an area, it is wise to keep a supply of the appropriate serum for immediate use and also to keep a supply of antivenin from the serum of horses that have been immunised.

The horse should be kept quiet to reduce the rate of absorption of the venom and, in addition to serum, it is normally given cortisone or other anti-inflammatory steroids, an antibiotic and possibly anti-tetanus. The latter two are required to counteract bacterial contamination of the fangs and subsequent infection of the wound. Similarly, where known species of poisonous spiders inhabit a particular area, specific antivenin should be kept on hand.

When bee or wasp stings occur, the sting should be removed and an effective antihistamine administered generally and locally around the site of the sting.

Allergies and hypersensitivities Hypersensitive reactions to biting flies (*Culicoides*), causing a pruritic skin disease are common in summer months. Therapeutic approaches are limited to a reduction in exposure and treatment of the clinical signs, using corticosteroids, antihistamines and essential fatty acids. None of these treatments is completely satisfactory.

Moulds and mould toxins (mycotoxicosis) Serious damage to livestock can be caused by many species of mould through their production of toxins. These toxins may be present, either in the feed together with the active mould, or the toxin may be left as a residue in the feed after the mould has been largely destroyed. Two or three species of mould, however, may damage horses by an entirely different mechanism, and that is by inducing a respiratory allergy (see chronic obstructive pulmonary disease, p. 76).

The mould particles and spores are inhaled during the consumption of mouldy hay. They may also be present in the atmosphere of badly contaminated and poorly ventilated stables. Some horses are more likely than others to develop signs. The damage may be partly repaired, or the problem avoided, by ensuring that buildings and hay racks are properly ventilated and that very dusty hay is not used – it should either be soaked before feeding or replaced with properly fermented silage. Dusty, mouldy straw bedding also should be avoided.

The most notorious mould toxin is produced by ergot of rye *(Claviceps purpurea)*. This mould also infects several species of pasture grass, although it is unlikely that horses will become seriously intoxicated during grazing. Horses given 500g ergot showed only transient symptoms and even heavily contaminated pastures are unlikely to contain more than approximately 0.3% ergot. The most likely cause of intoxication by this source is badly infected rye grain.

A number of other mould species found on cereal grain (including *Puccinia graminis)* can cause fatal poisoning in horses, but the most poisonous mould toxin produced in badly stored oil seeds and cereals is aflatoxin, a hepatotoxin produced by *Aspergillus flavus*. The horse seems to be more susceptible to this toxin than most other domestic species of animals.

Stachybotrytoxicosis is associated with hay and straw spoiled by strains of *Stachybotrys alterans*, producing tricothecene toxins that are generally fatal. Facial oedema and inflammation, ulceration of the ocular, oral and nasal mucosae are common features. Bone marrow suppression results in leucopenia and thrombocytopenia with petechiation, or small haemorrhages, of the mucous membranes.

Endophytic fungal toxins Endophytes occur, particularly, in ryegrass (*Lolium*) and fescue (*Festuca*) pastures. The fungi infect other warm season weeds and grasses (including: *Agrostis, Andropogon, Eragrostis, Paspalum, Sporobolu* and *Stipa.*) in none of which are they pathological to the plant.

Infected plants show no signs and the grazing of endophyte (*Acremonium coenophialum*)-infected tall fescue depresses grass dry matter intake and body weight maintenance of horses. Endophytes are transmitted in infected seed and the resulting plants may be more resistant to a range of pests. They grow more vigorously, producing a higher DM yield, and they may be even more drought tolerant and winter hardy.

Fescue toxicosis There are several microbial species growing in plants that are a cause of intoxication in horses. In the U.S.A. widespread reproductive problems in mares grazing tall fescue (*Festuca arundinacea*) pastures have been reported. Signs include increased gestation length, agalactia, foal and mare mortality, tough and thickened placentas, dystocia (abnormal labour at foaling), weak and dysmature foals, increased sweating during warm weather, reduced serum prolactin and progesterone and increased serum oestradiol-17β concentrations. Unlike the effects in many other species, horses consuming infected tall fescue do not exhibit an increased body temperature. The abnormalities in gravid mares are caused by vasoconstrictive ergot peptide alkaloids (pyrrolizidine alkaloids have also been isolated) produced by endophytic fungi, principally *Acremonium coenophialum,*but also by *Balansia epichloe* and *B. henningsiana*, identified in tall fescue. *Acremonium* grass endophytes live their entire life within the aerial parts of their grass host, producing no spores.

Endophyte-infected tall fescue hay is less digestible than endophyte-free hay, and young horses consuming infected pasture grow more slowly than do those on endophyte-free pasture. Advice has been given that domperidone, a dopamine receptor antagonist, is effective in preventing the signs of tall fescue toxicosis in horses without neuroleptic side effects. The minimum effective dose in gravid mares is 1.1 mg/kg BW daily, given orally for 30 days before foaling, or 0.44 mg/kg BW, subcutaneously for 10 days before foaling.

Fescue toxicosis causes increased susceptibility to high environmental temperatures and light intolerance. Recent hot summers in Europe may increase the European frequency of this disease in horses, cattle and sheep. One solution to the risk of endophyte intoxication is to remove horses from pastures where the condition is known to occur.

Fusarium-related mycotoxicosis is increasingly common. This includes mouldy corn poisoning that presents with dullness, head-pressing, aimless walking, circling and blindness. The signs usually develop within eight days of ingesting the toxins and the horse is particularly susceptible. The ailment may be caused by water-soluble fumonisins, causing liver damage and leucoencephalomalacia, a destruction of the white matter of equine cerebral hemispheres. The toxins occur in *F. moniliforme*, growing aggressively on maize both pre- and post-maturity. The fungus also colonises a wide variety of mature plant products and debris and is not necessarily visually apparent (the fungus might be described as an endophyte). The toxins have been detected in a high proportion of maize grain samples grown in Australia, Iowa and South Africa. Concentrations of from 0.1 to 500 mg/kg maize grain have been detected and concentrations of 40 mg/kg, and somewhat less, are considered to be lethal in horses. Weevil infestation of the grain seems to increase the risk of infestation by the fungus. Similar mould toxins can develop when cereal grain is stored in silos at a moisture content above 14%. All such feed stored in bulk should have a moisture content of no more than 13% and the storage facilities should be well ventilated and not subject to any wide daily variations in temperature.

Several other species of fungi grow on forage crops and are a cause of intoxication of grazing animals.

Lupinosis is caused by the ingestion of toxins produced by a fungus growing on lupin plants that causes damage to the liver. The only solution is to remove horses from pasture where lupins are found and to feed hay and concentrates. Another toxin – sporodesmin – is produced by a mould which grows on rye grass and which causes facial eczema in sheep. This toxin has also caused photosensitization reactions in horses in Queensland.

Phototoxicity Sunburn is a photochemical reaction involving the dermis and epidermis caused by exposure to powerful UV rays within the wave band range 290-320 nm. The effects are expressed as erythema, inflammation and tissue damage in uncovered non-pigmented skin.

Photosensitization reactions In bright sunny weather horses with unpigmented skin, and with white or grey coats in particular, may be subject to photosensitization. This causes a form of dermatitis. Dermatitis is frequently preceded by swellings on the muzzle, around the eyes and on various other places of the body. Photosensitization occurs particularly in horses with damaged livers. Unwanted toxic compounds absorbed from the intestine are normally degraded by the liver and excreted, but this process is less reliable in horses with damaged livers.

Photosensitivity is a severe cutaneous reaction that follows penetration of much weaker UV rays, in the range 320-600 nm, than are involved with phototoxicity. The effects are expressed in exposed, non-pigmented dermis and epidermis that contains deposits of photoreactive molecules, derived, either from the circulation, or by topical application. The responses are classified as primary, secondary, photocontact or photo-allergic.

Primary photosensitivity This results from the deposit of sensitizing agents directly into the skin following ingestion or injection. Several pasture plant species can cause the effects, as they contain photodynamic chemicals such as furocoumarins (wild carrot, *Daucus carota*), fagopyrin and photofagopyrin (buckwheat, *Fagopyrum esculentum*), perloline (perennial ryegrass, *Lolium perenne*) and hypericin (St John's wort, *Hypericum perforatum*). Other species and chemicals are also causative and several species of aphids may cause primary photosensitization, following ingestion by horses grazing aphid-infested pastures. Some evidence exists that the ingestion of cereal gluten leads to a photosensitive erythematous reaction in unpigmented skin areas of susceptible horses.

Secondary photosensitivity This results in horses with liver damage and, or, biliary stasis. Photodynamic substances that are normally degraded in the liver and, or, eliminated in the bile, become concentrated in the skin and other organs. The most widespread substance associated with the secondary condition is phylloerythrin, produced by the bacterial breakdown of chlorophyll within the intestines. Phylloerythrin is normally cleared by hepatic conjugation and biliary excretion. A typical cause of liver damage, and increased risk, in grazing horses are the pyrrolizidine alkaloids found in ragwort (*Senecio jacobaea*) and heliotrope (*Heliotropium europeum*). Ragwort infestation is rife in many unkempt meadows and the refuse from cut plants must be removed. Alkaloids contained in blue-green algae (Myxophyceae), causing liver damage, are of concern, especially during hot dry summers when the rate of flow of rivers is reduced. Mycotoxins, such as aflatoxin, produced by *Aspergillus flavus,* discussed elsewhere in this Chapter (p. 603), are also a cause of liver damage.

Photocontact reactions These reactions occur when photodynamic agents contact, and are absorbed by, non-pigmented skin, subsequently exposed to sunlight. Sensitizers occur in members of the Umbelliferae – cow parsley (*Anthriscus sylvestris*), fennels (*Peucedanum*), hogweed (*Heracleum* spp.) and Ranunculaceae – the buttercup family, although the latter may not require the intervention of strong sunlight.

Photo-allergic reactions These are very rare and only occur following repeated cutaneous exposure to certain pharmaceutical products.

Treatment of photosensitization A veterinary surgeon should be contacted immediately in acute, severe cases. If the causative agent is known, or suspected, its consumption, or contact with it, should be stopped. Presenting animals should be removed from pasture, if the causative agent is a plant species in the pasture. Furthermore, care should be taken that implicated species are not present in meadow hay fed to horses. Affected animals should be placed in a dark environment and barrier creams applied to the skin. Anti-inflammatory agents, such as hydrocortisone, together with diuretics, may be of help if applied early. Treatment for liver dysfunction, where this occurs, is also indicated.

TREES AND SHRUBS

Cyanogenetic plants. Several *Prunus* species (e.g. cherry laurel, *Prunus laurocerasus*) contain cyanogenetic glycosides. The hydrogen cyanide released will complex iron in haem and other cytochromes. The intoxicated horse gasps for breath, the blood is cherry red and tissues are anoxic. Veterinary treatment is indicated.

Nuts such as unripe oak acorns (*Quercus* spp.) and beechmast (*Fagus sylvaticus*) are poisonous to horses. Acorns contain large amounts of tannic acid and they cause dullness, inappetence colic, constipation or diarrhoea, haematuria and generalized weakness, although horses may be less susceptible than cattle. Some animals develop a liking for acorns and such horses should not have access to areas where oak trees are present. Treatment includes administration of liquid paraffin or purgatives. Beech nuts cause colic, hyperexcitability, tremors and staggering gait. The nuts contain several poisons, including thiaminase, also found in bracken (*Pteridium aquilinum*) that destroys thiamin (vitamin B_1). Thus treatment with that vitamin is helpful. Beech and oak leaves contain the same principals as the nuts.

Box (*Buxus sempervirens*) contains the alkaloid buxine, causing colic, diarrhoea and seizures.

The bark and seeds of false acacia (*Robina pseudoacacia*) contain two tox-albumins. These cause gastrointestinal irritation with colic and diarrhoea.

All parts of the yew (*Taxus baccata*) are highly toxic to horses. Laburnum (*Laburnum anagyroides*), to which the horse is extremely sensitive, is toxic in all parts, especially the flowers and seeds. Privet (*Ligustrum vulgare*) leaves are said to be toxic, but are clearly less so than yew or laburnum. The rhododendron (*Rhododendron ponticum*), that is quite invasive on acid soils, also presents a risk.

POISONS FOUND IN VEGETABLE PROTEIN SOURCES

Tannins Many common plants contain tannins (weak acids), referred to above, which depress both protein and carbohydrate digestion and cause colic in horses when present in high concentrations in the diet. Autoclaving or pressure cooking destroys these tannins, but when lower temperatures are applied prolonged treatment is required. Brown varieties of sorghum grain are rich in tannins and therefore only the white grain varieties should be used. Field beans *(Vicia faba)*, particularly the coloured-flower varieties, also contain tannins, and again prolonged cooking to a great extent rectifies the problem.

Lectins (proteins) Lectins seem to disrupt the brush borders of the small intestinal villi and hamper the absorption of nutrients. Apparently they also allow the absorption of certain toxic substances that increase tissue breakdown and urinary nitrogen and thus they depress growth in young stock.

Field or horse beans *(Vicia faba)* contain small quantities of lectins, and relatively larger amounts are contained in black grams and kidney, haricot or navy beans *(Phaseolus vulgaris)*. Horse grams, moth beans *(Phaseolus aconitifolius)*, certain pulses, cow peas, lima beans (P. *Lunatus)*, butterbeans and winged beans, groundnuts or peanuts *(Arachis hypogaea)*, soya beans and rice germ also contain these substances. Most rice bran fed to horses has had the germ removed, although some residual activity is normally found.

The susceptibility of lectins to destruction by heat varies with the plant source and therefore the safety of certain vegetable protein sources may not be guaranteed even after cooking. The lectin content of kidney beans is very stable: treatment for two hours at 93° C (199.4° F) is necessary for adequate destruction. Kidney beans are therefore generally unsuitable for nonindustrial processing and should not be fed to horses in normal circumstances. Steam flaking of field beans is more effective in the destruction of the trypsin inhibitor and lectin activities than is micronization at 150° or 100° C (302° or 212° F).

Enzyme inhibitors Many of the vegetable proteins already listed contain substances that depress the digestion of protein and in some cases of carbohydrate. These substances are considered to be somewhat less toxic than lectins and by and large are more susceptible to destruction by wet heat. Where a bean or pea of unknown origin is available, it should only be used in horse feed after prolonged cooking by steaming or boiling.

Lathyrogens The horse is particularly and characteristically affected by lathyrism or poisoning by lathyrogens. This is a condition in which there is a sudden and transient paralysis of the larynx with near suffocation, brought on by exercise. This is associated with a degenerative change in the nerves and muscles of the larynx and profound inflammation of the liver and spleen. A number of pea species of the family *Lathyrus* contain lathyrogenic agents, including the Indian or grass pea *(L. sativus)*, the sweet pea *(L. odoratus)*, the wild winter pea *(L. hirsutus)*, the singletary pea *(L. pusillus)* and the everlasting pea *(L. sylvestris)*. Although the whole plant contains the toxin, the seeds appear to be the most potent source, and the toxin is only partly destroyed by heat.

Gossypol Cotton seeds contain the yellow pigment gossypol which is toxic to horses and which is only partly destroyed by heat. It depresses appetite and protein and iron utilization. Its toxicity can apparently result in death from circulatory failure. Fairly large additions to the diet of iron in the form of ferrous sulphate will partly suppress the adverse effects of gossypol. Owing to differences in temperature achieved during manufacture, expeller meals contain less gossypol activity and are therefore less dangerous than solvent-extracted meals. High-quality cotton-seed meal is palatable to horses and varieties which contain low amounts of gossypol, or which have had the germ removed, can be usefully included in mixed feeds. Cotton-seed meals derived from the safe varieties are generally not available in the UK; feeds containing more than 60 mg free gossypol per kilogramme are unsatisfactory for horses.

Cyanogenetic glycosides (also see trees and shrubs, above) Certain glycosides (sugar compounds) present in lima beans, sorghum leaves, linseed *(Linum usitatissimum)* and cassava (tapioca – *Manihot esculenta)* will generate hydrogen cyanide (HCN) when acted on by specific enzymes contained in the plants. HCN can cause respiratory failure, but as the poison is released by enzyme activity, heat treatment will ensure safety so long as prolonged storage of moist seeds or roots has not led to an accumulation of free HCN. Thus it is important that raw, uncooked materials should be stored in a dry condition. HCN can also react with any thiosulphate present in the material to produce thiocyanate, that is responsible for thyroid enlargement after prolonged feeding.

Linseed is unique in so far as it contains a relatively indigestible mucilage. This can absorb large amounts of water, producing a thick soup during cooking, and its lubricating action regulates faecal excretion and sometimes overcomes constipation, without causing looseness. The cooking of linseed also destroys the enzyme linase, that would otherwise release HCN, if the linseed was merely soaked. For this reason linseed should be added to boiling water rather than to cold water and then boiled. However, HCN is volatile and a proportion of any already present will be driven off by subsequent boiling. UK law states that linseed cake or meal must contain less than 350mg HCN per kilogramme, although this takes no account of the effect of any linase that may be present.

Anti-thyroid substances A large number of vegetable protein sources, particularly those in the genus Brassica, contain thyroactive substances. When consumed persistently, particularly by young stock, these substances can cause goitre. Both the seeds and the vegetative parts of cabbages, rape, mustard and kale are incriminated. The effects of goitrins are not counteracted by additional dietary iodine, although further metabolism of certain of them can release isothiocyanates and thiocyanates. The antithyroid effect of these on young horses can be overcome by additional dietary iodine. Goitrins are released by enzymes contained within the plant and these can be destroyed by heat treatment. However, this is impractical with the vegetative parts of plants.

Kale contains a goitrogenic substance, but the plant is also relatively low in iodine content. The effect of the plant on sheep can be partly overcome by supplementary iodine. Kale also contains a sulphur compound metabolized by rumen bacteria to form dimethyl sulphide, which is said to cause haemolytic anaemia. This particular substance, however, is not likely to be of great significance in horse feed. For the same reasons cruciferous vegetables are not recommended for feeding to young, or lactating, horses in other than small quantities.

Among the brassicas the principal seed byproduct available as a vegetable protein source is rapeseed meal, which contains large amounts of goitrogens. In recent years, varieties of rapeseed have been bred that contain low quantities of goitrogens. These varieties are available generally in North America, the U.K. and the rest of Europe. Rapeseed meal derived from these varieties is suitable for feeding to horses.

Potato poisoning Potato (*Solanum tuberosum*) poisoning and death has been recorded in horses given waste potatoes. Early signs include salivation, diarrhoea, colic, thirst, depression, weak incoordinated movements, paresis (slight or incomplete paralysis), laboured breathing and dehydrated injected (livid) mucous membranes. The cause may be associated with a steroidal glycoalkaloid, solanine, contained in green potatoes. This toxin is not destroyed by cooking, although some of it is partly removed by leeching into boiling water. Evidence shows that the horse seems to be much more susceptible than ruminants and it will succumb to potato poisoning even when no green potatoes are apparent in a batch fed to it. The best course of action is not to feed potatoes of any sort to horses.

Onion poisoning Onions contain a volatile oil (n-propyl disulphide) which can cause severe damage to horses and cattle fed large numbers of waste onions. The signs include inappetence, tachycardia (rapid heart beat), staggering, jaundice, haemoglobinuria and haemolytic anaemia. It is unwise to feed onions and similar vegetables to horses.

Poisonous pasture plants A large number of plant species, available to the grazing animal in various parts of the world, are poisonous. The degree of toxicity varies considerably from species to species.* Many of the toxic substances present in pasture plants are alkaloids, which are organic basic compounds, and their toxic effects on the horse vary widely. Alkaloids are rare in grasses.

One of the commonest causes of poisoning amongst all grazing animals, including horses, in the British Isles is common ragwort (*Senecio jacobaea*), which causes permanent liver damage. Elevated plasma gamma glutamyl transferase activity is a useful early indicator of the damage. Despite claims that horses will not eat this plant, many outbreaks of poisoning have followed the consumption of growing ragwort. Intoxication can also result if ragwort is present in hay as the poison remains stable after the hay has been made.

Horses with ragwort-damaged livers should be given a well-balanced diet, containing good-quality protein supplemented with B vitamins and trace

* For a complete list of plant species thought to be the cause of poisoning in horses, see David Frape, *Equine Nutrition and Feeding*, 2nd Ed. Blackwell Science, Oxford, 1998.

elements. They should not be given access to pasture infested with either ragwort or groundsel *(Senecio vulgaris),* which contains the same toxin as ragwort, but at lower concentrations.

Other plants causing a similar liver condition include heliotrope *(Heliotropium europeum)* and the legume crotalaria, numerous species of which have proved very poisonous to horses in South Africa, America and Australia. One species of this legume causes Kimberley horse disease. In some species the highest concentration of poison is present in the roots, which are normally inaccessible. However, roots of water dropwort *(Oenanthe crocata)* may be unearthed during ditching operations and then be consumed by horses.

Horses usually avoid alkaloid-containing pasture plants unless there is a major shortage of palatable grazing as a result of overgrazing or drought. However, they sometimes develop a predilection for bitter or unusual flavours.

Many leguminous plants contain a variety of poisons. Some have already been mentioned, such as laburnum, but others include broom *(Cytisus scoparius)* and lupin *(Lupinus).* The toxicity of the latter species is principally confined to the seeds and the different strains vary in their potency. Sweet lupin *(L. luteus)* has a low alkaloid content and is grown on poor land as a source of fodder. Occasionally horses eating lupins have died from respiratory paralysis, whereas the chronic and progressive liver damage associated with lupinosis in horses and sheep is caused by an associated fungus growing on the lupins (see p. 605).

A number of pasture legumes, particularly subterranean clover *(Trifolium subterraneum)* grown on light soils, contain appreciable amounts of oestrogens. These substances are known to affect fertility in other domestic livestock, although their influence on the breeding mare has not been determined. The pasture legume marsh bird's-foot trefoil *(Lotus pedunculatus)* is rich in condensed tannins when growing on poor soil. Other related species found in pastures also contain tannins.

A number of plant species containing piperidine alkaloids have been associated with equine uterine malfunction and foetal abnormalities in North America. These genera include milk vetch, or locoweed *(Astragalus* spp. and *Oxytropis* spp.), poison-hemlock *(Conium maculatum),* wild tree tobacco *(Nicotiana glauca)* and lunara lupine *(Lupinus formosus).* Locoweed is also recognized as eliciting irreversible nervous signs in horses. None of the poisonous members of these genera is found in the British Isles. Where they exist in the USA, their growth begins in late summer and they remain green in the winter. They must be grazed for a period before poisoning is obvious.

Some plant poisons remain active after drying during haymaking. These species include horsetails *(Equisetum),* bracken *(Pteridium aquilinum),* hellebores *(Helleborus),* larkspurs *(Delphinium),* poppies *(Papaver),* greater celandine *(Chelidonium majus),* St John's wort *(Hypericum),* pimpernels *(Anagallis),* henbane *(Hyoscyamus niger),* black nightshade *(Solanum nigrum),* foxglove *(Digitalis purpurea),* meadow saffron *(Colchicum autumnale)* and black bryony *(Tamus communis).* Sweet clover, or melilot, *(Melilotus)* contains coumarin, which is broken down to dicoumarol in hay made under bad harvesting conditions or during moulding. Dicoumarol prolongs blood-clotting time. Sweet clover hay made during inclement weather develops mouldy patches and should not be used in horse feeding.

Poor pasture management, including overgrazing by horses, the absence of ruminants and lack of pasture cultivation, the failure to use appropriate fertilizers and to manage pasture as a crop leads to its general decline both in terms of productivity and the ingress and dissemination of poisonous, and therefore unwanted, plants. The reader should acquire the ability to recognize the most important of these species in his or her area. Their spread can be prevented by increased competition from productive pasture species and by preventing them from seeding. The encroachment of bracken may be difficult to counter in areas of marginal land, but today the enormous spread of ragwort is simply a reflection of neglect. The removal of these and other pernicious weeds can be achieved by spraying clumps at the appropriate time with herbicides from a knapsack sprayer or by digging them out before the plants have a chance to seed (several weed species also spread by underground stems). Many other poisonous plants are much less likely than ragwort to cause poisoning of a serious kind and their beauty should be allowed to decorate hedgerows and copses from which the horse can be kept at bay by adequate fencing.

TREATMENT OF POISONING

The veterinary surgeon should be contacted immediately in all severe cases. Early treatment may, nevertheless, be critical. Always retain samples of the suspected toxicant for analysis. In cases where the coat has been contaminated copious washing with water is advised. Detergent should be used only for oily materials, remembering that solubilization can increase absorption and therefore cause greater risk. To reduce this risk application of a vegetable oil to the coat, prior to washing with soap may aid removal, and reduce absorption of an oily contaminant

When a veterinary surgeon is not available, gastrointestinal decontamination may be attempted by administration of up to 4.5 L of a suspension of activated charcoal (200 g/L) in water, as an adsorbent, followed by a laxative half an hour later. Laxatives include sodium sulphate, or magnesium sulphate. Mineral oil (liquid paraffin) may be used, except where fat-soluble intoxicants, such as organophosphorus compounds and chlorinated hydrocarbons are the toxicants, as the absorption of these may be enhanced by this procedure.

39
PREVENTIVE MEDICINE

Preventive medicine is the use of environmental measures and veterinary treatment to control the development and build-up of disease. Preventive medicine and good management are interrelated and inseparable, and they provide a challenge both to stud managers and owners and to veterinarians.

The objectives of preventive medicine are: to keep all animals in good health and condition and to maintain a steady rate of growth and development in young stock; to minimise the possibility of disease entering the studfarm or stables from outside; to minimise the build-up of disease; to identify individuals especially at risk for special care; and to control the spread of infection after an outbreak of infectious disease.

Keeping animals in good health
Housing   Poor housing is stressful to all animals and will result in a build-up of respiratory and intestinal disease. The most important factor is ventilation, which should be variable to provide a maximum flow of air to reduce temperature and a minimum flow of air to reduce humidity; a ratio of 10:1 between maximum and minimum flows is desirable. Horses kept in a dry environment can tolerate very low and very high temperatures, so control of humidity is much more important than control of temperature. However, in providing ventilation it is important to avoid draughts at ground level which will chill stabled animals.

All housing should have ventilation inlets and outlets and the most common method of air circulation uses the 'stack' effect. This relies on the principle of cold air entering through the side inlets, warming as it filters through the building, and rising in the centre to be drawn out through the roof. The roof outlet may be boosted by extractor fans. The minimum requirement for ventilation has been estimated at 1 sq ft per horse outlet and 3 sq ft per horse inlet.

The other major influence on ventilation and air movement in buildings is insulation. Insulation reduces condensation on the side walls and roof and increases air movement through the building. Many buildings can be greatly improved by the appreciation of these basic principles.

Bedding   Bedding should be dry and dust-free. A thick, dry straw bed allows a foal to keep warm when the environmental temperature is low. Dusty straw increases the incidence of chronic obstructive pulmonary disease and a variety of materials have been used as alternatives. Peat moss is dust-free but cold and tends to soften the feet. Wood shavings and chopped paper are clean and dust-free, but not as warm as straw, and the soiled bedding is difficult to dispose of. Processed hemp is commercially available and constitutes a satisfactory bed but is expensive and necessitates regular attention or the quality of the bed deteriorates rapidly. The waste provides a valuable garden compost. Much effort has been allocated to the use of rubber mats but as yet it would be fair to say an entirely satisfactory system has not evolved. On the whole, horses are reluctant to lie down on a surface which is generally cold and wet.

Deep-litter bedding has the advantages of keeping dust to a minimum while, at the same time, reducing labour costs. The disadvantages are that moulds may form in deep-litter straw or wood shavings and cause allergic reactions such as chronic obstructive pulmonary diseases. In addition, deep-littering leads to moist conditions underfoot and may cause thrush unless the feet are cleaned regularly.

Figure 1   A correctly laid bed

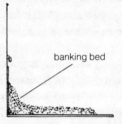

banking bed

Nutrition Nutrient requirements and levels of feeding are discussed in Chapter 44. However, there are a few basic considerations which are of importance in relation to disease.

Clearly, inadequate nutrition, resulting in weight loss and debility, makes animals susceptible to disease of all kinds. However, more frequently there is a tendency to overfeed high-energy and protein feeds to growing horses and this can result in an unusually high level of limb abnormalities in foals and yearlings (see Chapter 19).

Overfeeding also results in damage to the growth plates producing enlargements of the epiphyses (physitis – see p. 214). Such reactions may result in gross deformity of the limbs, such as medial or lateral deviation of the carpus (knee). The importance of severely reducing the total food intake to control such abnormalities cannot be overstressed. The total calcium intake and the ratio of calcium to phosphorus in the diet must be checked and corrected if necessary (see p. 700).

In recent years it has become clear that trace elements also are of importance in the feeding of stud animals. Zinc, copper and selenium have all received attention and may be important in relation to abnormal bone and muscle development.

Pasture management Horses are notoriously bad grazers and all readers will be familiar with the untidy appearance of paddocks persistently grazed by horses; some areas will be grazed to the ground while other areas grow coarse and long. These grazing patterns are controlled by faecal contamination of the pasture rather than by urine excretion. The grazing patterns can only be eradicated by regular removal of droppings or by allowing other herbivores such as cattle or sheep to graze the land. Ploughing and reseeding pastures will not remove established grazing patterns.

Vaccination Vaccination of all stock against commonly occurring diseases is clearly desirable. In the UK and Ireland vaccination is frequently carried out against three common diseases – tetanus, influenza and Equine Herpes Virus. Vaccination against Rotavirus and Equine Viral Arteritis has also recently become available. The principle of all vaccination is to administer an initial course and to follow this with booster doses at various intervals, depending on the nature of the vaccine and the immune response for each product.

Permanent vaccination with tetanus toxoid can be started at any age from three months onwards and consists of a primary vaccination of two doses separated by two to four weeks. A booster vaccination is then given a year later and the manufacturers recommend boosters every other year thereafter.

Pregnant mares are often given a tetanus toxoid booster shortly before foaling to increase the level of tetanus antibodies passed in the colostrum to the newborn foal. To supplement this many foals are given tetanus antitoxin soon after birth to provide temporary cover for three to four weeks. A further dose of antitoxin may be given at a month old.

Tetanus vaccination is often coupled with vaccination against influenza, and several drug companies now produce combinations of influenza and tetanus vaccine.

Vaccination against influenza is highly effective and is now mandatory for all racehorses and for all horses using racecourse premises. The vaccination requirements are strict and tightly enforced. A primary course of two injections, 21-90 days apart, must be followed by a booster 150-215 days later. (Manufacturers may differ as to timing but this does not matter to within a couple of months.) Subsequently a dose may be given annually within twelve months of the last injection. Some manufacturers recommend a further primary vaccination six months after the first booster and annual vaccination thereafter. This vaccine covers against all the commonly occurring strains of influenza (see p. 485). However, it should be remembered that influenza viruses vary periodically and are subject to a phenomenon known as antigenic drift and such variations may result in a breakdown in immunity. (For Jockey Club Rules on vaccination, see p. 489.)

Vaccination again EHV 1 & 4 is available in the form of an inactivated vaccine. The same vaccine can be used to protect against both abortion in brood mares and the respiratory form of the disease in horses in training. In pregnant brood mares three injections are given annually in the fifth, seventh and ninth months of pregnancy. There is little doubt that some animals will abort despite vaccination, but the use of the vaccine does appear to prevent at least the widespread abortion storms which have plagued the breeding industry in the past. In horses in training it is recommended as a primary course of two injections given four to six months apart and thereafter at six-monthly intervals.

Pregnant mares may also have a rotavirus vaccine administered to them. The manufacturers recommend vaccination at eight, nine and ten months gestation. The vaccine is effective by raising the level of protective antibody in mare's milk reducing the incidence of infectious diarrhoea.

The use of vaccines against EVA (equine viral arteritis) is complicated by the difficulty in differentiating between the vaccinated and the naturally exposed animals and particularly entire male carriers. Currently an inactivated vaccine 'Artevac' is available under special licence. The live vaccine 'Arvac'; available in the USA is not licensed for use in the UK.

Teeth All horses should have their teeth examined at least annually to check for the development of abnormally sharp edges on the outside of the upper molar teeth and the insides of the lower molar teeth. These edges can be removed easily by rasping.

Two-, three- and four-year-old animals may be shedding temporary incisor and premolar teeth (caps) and these can be removed by routine dentistry at the time of examination. In older animals the molar teeth must be examined for signs of abnormal wear or overgrowth which requires more vigorous attention. For more details, see Chapter 54.

Feet Good farriery and regular trimming of the feet of all young stock and brood mares is essential. Changes in the shape of the feet can occur very rapidly, and unless the animals are carefully inspected and walked up in hand, important changes may be missed.

It is helpful to record the observations made at these examinations for future reference; changes in diet and levels of exercise can also be recorded. Many studs rely on monthly visits from the farrier, but at certain times of the year, particularly through the grazing summer months, foals and yearlings may benefit from attention at shorter intervals, even down to fortnightly, in order to prevent the development of sandcracks and splits in the walls of the feet (see Chapter 20).

Minimising the introduction of disease

Most disease enters a studfarm or stables through the arrival of an animal which is already infected or one which is a carrier. It is therefore essential to ensure that all animals which join a resident group should be carefully screened for the presence of disease. During this period they should be isolated from the resident animals. Good isolation facilities are therefore necessary.

New arrivals should enter the isolation premises where they can be inspected for overt clinical disease, such as respiratory disease or ringworm. At this time tests can be carried out for any diseases for which special precautions are needed. An example is the collection of dung samples for a worm egg count to enable any necessary worming treatment to be carried out. Animals should be kept in for twenty-four to forty-eight hours after such treatment to ensure that the parasite eggs being expelled from the alimentary tract are not voided onto pasture. If such droppings are allowed to contaminate the pasture, they should be collected within forty-eight hours of being passed.

Screening for more unusual infectious diseases should be carried out before a horse arrives at a stud. In particular, blood samples can be collected from mares from high-risk areas for serum antibody levels against equine infectious anaemia (Coggins test) or equine arteritis. These two diseases do not, under normal circumstances, occur in the UK and their likely route of entry into the country is through the importation of horses from the United States and South America, although both diseases occur in other parts of the world.

It is also advisable to screen all mares for venereal disease, and this can be done by taking a sample for bacterial culture from the clitoris, particularly from the clitoral sinuses based on the upper border of the clitoris. This site harbours the common venereal bacteria. This test may be performed before or immediately upon arrival at the studfarm because evidence of spread other than at mating is minimal. Samples should also be taken from the cervix when the mare is in oestrus. Compliance with the Code of Practice has virtually eliminated CEM in the UK.

Minimising the build-up of disease

Where animals are kept in a stable or an intensive stud environment, the bacterial population will increase. This is not necessarily harmful, although a newborn foal or a debilitated or sick adult will be more susceptible to disease when challenged by large numbers of organisms. Thus, some basic principles should be followed to reduce the build-up of infective microbes.

It is advisable to maintain separate groups of animals so that the interaction and mixing of mares, yearlings and foals are kept to a minimum. Barren and maiden mares should be kept separate from pregnant mares, and mares with foals at foot and yearlings should be kept in separate buildings from adult animals.

The build-up of bacterial contamination in the environment is perhaps most serious in the foaling unit. It is essential that the newborn foal, and particularly its navel, is not exposed to more organisms than necessary in the crucial first twenty-four hours of life.

To achieve this, occupation of the foaling boxes should be kept to a minimum and bedding should be scrupulously clean. Between foalings the box should be cleaned out completely and the floors and walls disinfected, using Ministry of Agriculture-approved disinfectants.

Healthy foals can be removed from the foaling unit, but each foal should then be kept in the one box and moved as little as possible because each time it is moved it is exposed to new microbes, both viral and bacterial, en couraging the outbreak of respiratory disease and diarrhoea.

Parasite control   The biggest single cause of poor growth and intestinal disease is a build-up of roundworm infection. Strongyles (redworms) contaminate horses of all ages, while ascarids (whiteworms) tend to cause unthriftiness in foals (see Chapter 33). The gravity of tape worm infection is not so widely agreed but many authorities consider it a significant cause of colic. At worst the eradication of tape worm cannot be detrimental and can be effected by an annual dose of one of the pyrantel derivatives at double dosage. Parasite control represents the most important form of preventive medicine in any horse establishment where animals are grazing, and paddock management is the first and essential step in any programme of parasite control. The need to alter established grazing patterns has already been discussed (see p. 615 above), particularly the use of sheep and cattle to clear rank patches of grass which horses will not touch. Only one relatively insignificant roundworm infects both cattle and horses, and therefore cattle grazing also reduces significantly the number of infective larvae on paddocks.

It is also important to avoid overgrazing. Ideally the stocking density should not exceed one mare and her foal per hectare. Where stocking densities are high, removal of droppings is a particularly necessary part of pasture management. Paddocks where young foals and yearlings are to be grazed must be cleared of all faecal contamination, the droppings being removed within forty-eight hours of being passed. Fortunately machines for collecting droppings are now available, making this routine chore less arduous.

Regular dosing of animals of all ages with a dewormer (anthelmintic) every four to six weeks is a crucial aspect of worm control. This topic is dealt with in full in Chapter 33.

Identifying individuals at risk
Careful observation of all the animals on the premises will reveal some that have problems which require special attention.

With adult horses, particular problems may be associated with the conformation of the feet or dental irregularities. These abnormalities must be carefully noted and special care taken.

Mares going to stud should be subjected to a veterinary examination by rectal palpation and vaginal examination to establish the normality of the genital tract. Swabs may also be taken from the cervix for bacterial culture and the examination of cells (cytology).

If these tests are unsatisfactory a clearer picture of the condition of the mare's uterus can be achieved by taking a uterine biopsy for histological examination. On the basis of these tests individual mares may be separated from the band for special care using management procedures which minimise the contamination of the reproductive tract at mating.

The newborn foal is especially at risk, both to infectious and non-infectious problems. Considerable physiological and anatomical changes take place in the neonatal period. Detailed knowledge of behaviour of young foals is necessary in order to be able to detect deviation from normal patterns (see chapters 27 and 28).

Following birth, attention to the umbilical cord is important to reduce occurrence of infection through the navel. The cord is usually dressed with antiseptic or antibiotic powder or solution. For discussion of the advantages and disadvantages of this practice, see p. 428.

It is essential that the newborn foal rapidly ingests good-quality colostrum from the mare. Colostrum is the secretion present in the udder at the time of birth and is rich in antibodies. These are absorbed through the intestine of the foal if ingested within twelve hours of birth (see p. 431).

However, the earlier this colostrum is given or sucked by the foal the more certain is its adequate uptake. Mares which run milk before foaling or foals which are slow to suck must be identified and treated accordingly.

A supply of donor colostrum collected from other mares at the time of foaling is very useful. Such colostrum can be kept in a deep freeze for long periods but must be thawed slowly before being fed to a newborn foal. Temperature in excess of 60°C is thought to damage the immunoglobulins present in the colostrum.

Blood samples taken from the foal on the second day of life will give a good indication of the colostral transfer of immunity. It is necessary to measure the globulin and particularly the immunoglobulin level in the serum. At the same time routine haematology may be used to pick up signs of infection or haemolytic disease (neonatal jaundice).

It is usual to give newborn foals an injection of tetanus antitoxin (see p. 476), although this may not be necessary if the mare is vaccinated with tetanus toxoid because antibodies should be transferred in the colostrum. To increase the levels of tetanus and influenza antibodies, pregnant mares should be given a booster influenza and tetanus toxold vaccination four to six weeks before foaling. Primary vaccination against influenza and tetanus may be started at three to six months of age. It is important to remember to give the third influenza vaccination 150-215 days later.

It is common practice to start worming foals at six to eight weeks of age and the anthelmintic may be given as paste or by nasogastric tube. Worming should be continued monthly thereafter. Worm egg counts should be carried out twice a year to ensure that parasite control is adequate.

Young growing horses are highly susceptible to alterations in the conformation of the limbs. Acquired deviations in the forelimbs are common. Lateral deviation from the knees, the development of club feet and going straight through the fetlocks are the most common abnormalities seen (see Chapter 19). It is very important that these changes should be seen as early as possible, at a time when the abnormalities can often be corrected by rapid change in management such as reducing exercise and feed levels. Once the abnormalities have become established they are extremely difficult to correct.

Controlling the spread of infection
The most common epidemic infections to strike groups of horses are the respiratory virus infections, particularly rhinopneumonitis (see p. 490) and influenza (see p. 485), and the bacterial respiratory disease strangles (see p. 474) which has once again become prevalent. Epidemics of venereal disease (see p. 484) may be associated with infections such as *Taylorella equingenitalis* organism, *Klebsiella pneumoniae* and *Pseudomonas aeruginosa*. Ringworm (see p. 139) is a highly contagious disease caused by a variety of fungi and is most commonly seen in stabled horses. It is prudent with racehorses at a race meeting for the trainer to supply his own girths and pads to avoid fungal infection being transferred from one runner to the next. Once an infectious disease has become established in a group of horses it is necessary to introduce control measures to prevent the spread of infection to other animals on the same premises and to other premises. Certain principles should be followed.

1. In the more serious conditions all movement of horses on or off the premises must cease.
2. The affected group of animals must be isolated as far as possible and treated for the infection from which they are suffering.
3. Personnel should not move from this group of affected animals to other animals. The latter must be regarded as 'in contacts' and should be kept under constant observation for any sign of the disease.
4. In the case of venereal infection mating should cease until the situation has been thoroughly investigated and infected animals treated.
5. Vaccination of in-contact but unaffected animals may be considered if an effective vaccine is available. However, once a disease is present in a community it is often too late to vaccinate because of the interval between administration and development of the individual's immune response.

40
SURGERY

The horse is kept primarily for athletic prowess and anything which diminishes its ability to perform successfully will, of necessity, affect adversely its usefulness and value. Thus the demands made of surgery in the horse are very exacting.

The success of any surgical procedure may be qualified as follows: complete success with return to soundness; partial success whereby the horse's eventual soundness is compromised although an improvement in the condition may have been achieved; or failure to restore soundness. Partial success may allow the horse to perform at less demanding levels than before, whereas failure to permit a return to work might not necessarily be deemed a technical failure if surgical intervention has been life-saving. In this respect the salvage of severely injured fillies and occasionally colts by surgical intervention may be undertaken despite a poor prognosis for a functional recovery. These animals may subsequently be used for breeding purposes. However, surgery of this nature would only be undertaken in exceptional circumstances on geldings as they have no value for breeding.

Limitations
Before we embark on a course of surgical treatment we should be realistic in our expectations of surgery. Old or debilitated animals are not suitable candidates for general anaesthesia or major surgery, and those animals with an underlying defect or disability may subsequently develop complications, sometimes insuperable, in the post-operative period.

Another facet to be considered carefully is that of economics. In the case of an animal of relatively little value, all due consideration should be given to the financial cost of surgery and post-operative attention.

We should also be aware that no guarantee of success can be given for the outcome of any operative procedure, even for the treatment of cases in which there is a high success rate. Any number of eventualities or complications may arise, not necessarily associated with the surgery itself, but sometimes as a consequence of the individual animal's temperament or an underlying inherent defect, possibly congenital or acquired, structural or physiological.

Surgical success is ultimately dependent on accurate diagnosis, technical expertise, correct management and realistic but optimistic prognosis. As well as recognition of the disease itself, an understanding of its pathogenesis (natural development) and its relationship to disturbance in function is essential.

Surgical success rate depends on the surgeon's competence and ability to handle tissues and, in addition, the availability of equipment and materials essential to the surgical techniques employed. Surgical success rate is also, to a large extent, affected by case management and therapeutics in the post-operative period whereby complications are dealt with. This frequently depends on anticipating a problem before it arises.

Progress

The field of equine surgery has expanded dramatically over the last twenty-five years due to the great advances made in the biological and technological sciences. Our greater understanding of biological structure and function has given us a new insight into the means of treatment and refinement of established techniques. Technology has risen to the demands made on it by our increased awareness. It produces equipment necessary for basic scientific investigation, which in turn can be used by clinicians for diagnosis and treatment.

The discovery of safe and effective methods of general anaesthesia in the horse has had a profound effect on surgery of the horse, enabling prolonged invasive surgery to be undertaken with the development of more refined techniques. Two prominent examples are orthopaedic and abdominal surgery. The application of the principles of engineering has resulted in very great advances in fracture repair work by the implantation of bone screws and plates as developed on the internal fixation principle. Newer forms of casting materials have major advantages of lightness, great strength, ease of application and water resistance, and have all but superseded the use of plaster of Paris casts.

The advent of antibiotics has made a major contribution to the overall success rate of surgery by the prevention and treatment of post-operative infection. Historically, wound infection was by far the biggest single cause of surgical failure and death. Non-steroidal anti-inflammatory drugs have also made a significant contribution to the control of post-operative tissue reaction and oedema, as well as improving post-operative mobility.

Surgical success rate has climbed in parallel with the development of more refined methods of diagnosis, examples of which are radiography, ultrasonic echography, thermography, nuclear scanning techniques, and the use of the flexible endoscope and the operative arthroscope. In line with these has been the development and advanced treatment methods, including high-power lasers, electromagnetic stimulation of tissue healing, cryotherapy, radio-frequency-induced hypothermia, and the advent of inert synthetic materials which are non-antigenic (in other words, they do not stimulate an immune-type rejection response) and may be permanently implanted in the body with a minimum risk of rejection.

MAJOR SURGICAL TECHNIQUES

In the following section a variety of surgical techniques are described in relation to the different organ systems.

RESPIRATORY TRACT

Surgery is almost entirely confined to the head and neck and involves either the paranasal sinuses and guttural pouches or the airways.

The paranasal sinuses (see p. 60) are not commonly the seat of infection which results in the accumulation of pus. This may arise as a primary infection or secondary to tooth root disease. Cysts may form during the development of the tooth or in the surrounding bone; tumours may also occur at these sites.

Simple infection has a good prognosis and is readily treated by flushing the sinuses using a catheter placed through the overlying skull. Cysts or tumours of the nasal sinuses or nasal passages and ethmoid haematoma, that is, blood blisters around the ethmoid bones which form part of the nasal passages, all require more radical surgery and carry a poorer prognosis because of risk of recurrence. The four rear upper molar teeth have their roots within the maxilliary sinus, and dental disease is treated surgically through the sinus.

The guttural pouches may develop empyema (accumulations of pus) subsequent to infection. Treatment consists of surgical drainage and frequently carries a good prognosis. Fungal infection (mycosis) of the guttural pouch is a much more serious problem as there is a risk of fatal haemorrhage. The condition is caused by the formation of a fungal plaque and erosion of the arterial wall of the internal carotid artery within the guttural pouch. Treatment is by ligation of the artery to prevent haemorrhage. The fungal infection is treated locally.

Laryngeal hemiplegia, usually left-sided, is manifested in the exercised horse as roaring or whistling. Surgical treatment to relieve obstruction to the airflow carries a good prognosis. The standard method of treatment for many years past has been stripping of the laryngeal ventricle (Hobday operation), but this technique has been further refined in the treatment of pronounced hemiplegia by the insertion of a supra-laryngeal prosthesis.

Horses affected with persistent pharyngeal or laryngeal conditions not amenable to surgical treatment may have their respiratory function improved by a tracheostomy operation. In this procedure a fistula is created between the windpipe and the front upper neck and a metal tube inserted. The tubing of animals with respiratory difficulties has a high success rate. However, the management of the fistula is important and complications may arise.

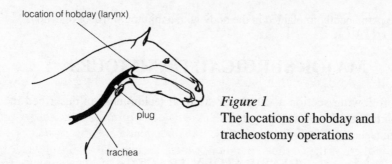

location of hobday (larynx)

plug

trachea

Figure 1
The locations of hobday and
tracheostomy operations

GASTRO-INTESTINAL TRACT

Gastro-intestinal disorders have always been of major importance in the horse. The sheer size and complexity of the organs pose great difficulty for the clinician. Diagnosis of the underlying cause of colic poor access to a large part of the abdomen and the difficulty of handling such heavy, bulky structures pose particular problems for the surgeon.

As practical experience has been gained in operation techniques and improved methods of diagnosis have been developed, there has been a gradual but steady increase in the success rate of the surgical treatment of colic.

The outcome of surgery depends on many factors. Simple obstructions and malpositions, including torsion of the large colon, carry a relatively good prognosis, as does simple resection of fibrous bands.

The prognosis is less favourable in cases where enterotomy (incision into the intestine) is carried out to relieve obstruction, or bowel resection is undertaken to remove devitalized tissue secondary to the loss of its blood supply.

Conditions of the small intestine are usually more acute and frequently fatal unless rapid intervention takes place. Disorders of the large intestine may also be acute in onset, with early death; however, most conditions of the large intestine tend to be of a more chronic nature.

Any situation involving volvulus or torsion of the bowel, with strangulation and loss of blood supply, results in tissue death, leading to absorption of toxins from the devitalised bowel and the development of peritonitis. Any procedure involving resection of devitalised tissue, prolonged manipulation of the bowel, lengthy surgery or late presentation carries a poor prognosis.

Control of shock is essential, both during surgery and in the post-operative period. In the post-operative period paralytic ileus (failure of the gut to establish normal motility) is a major problem, as is the development of peritonitis and post-operative intra-abdominal adhesions. The long-term prognosis may be poor, with significant damage to the blood supply associated with migratory larval worms. This also applies to cases in which extensive adhesions have formed.

URINOGENITAL SURGERY OF THE MARE

CASLICK AND POURET OPERATIONS

There are a number of surgical procedures related to restoring reproductive performance and fertility in mares. The most frequently employed and best known of these is the Caslick operation, which is named after an American veterinarian. This involves suturing the upper part of the vulval lips together, thus reconstituting the valve formed by the vulva and its surrounding tissues, the perineum, which prevents air being sucked into the genital tract (pneumovagina) (see Figure 1 on p. 376).

The operation is performed under local anaesthetic. A small strip of skin is removed from each side of the vulva and the two areas are then brought together by suturing. They heal within about a week of the operation.

The essential object of the operation is to suture the upper part of the vulva so that it is closed to the level of the brim of the pelvis. The results are effective but, because the vulval aperture is artificially reduced, it is necessary to cut the sutured part to open the way for the foal at birth (the approach to this procedure is described on p. 416). After the foal has been born, the wounds on the vulva are resutured to restore the vulval seal.

In recent years an increasing number of individuals, especially older mares, require a further operation to restore the conformation of the vulva and perineum. This operation has been named after the veterinarian who introduced it, Dr Edouard Pouret of France. The Pouret operation involves a more radical approach to restoring the normal conformation. It is required when the Caslick operation has, of necessity, been extended to such a degree that the lower aperture in the vulva is too small for a stallion to penetrate at mating.

The surgery is performed under a combination of spinal and local anaesthesia. A dissection is made between the rectum and the roof of the vagina. This frees the vulva from the pull exerted by the rectum either because it has been drawn forward with age or because of poor conformation. The vulva then returns from its abnormal horizontal inclining position to the normal verticle situation. After the dissection the wound is sutured and heals within two to three weeks.

The advantage of this operation compared with the Caslick is that it reduces the amount of suturing of the vulval lips, thus giving a larger aperture at the lower part of the vulva.

The disadvantage of both the Caslick and the Pouret operations is that they overcome a defect which has an inherited basis. The more the operations are performed, the greater the number of individuals likely to require the procedure. Discerning breeders should reject mares with poor conformation for breeding and thereby improve the fertility of their herd.

OPERATIONS TO OVERCOME URINE POOLING

In some young mares the pooling of the urine on the floor of the vagina occurs as a result of poor perineal conformation or other features which allow the cervix and entrance of the urethra into the floor of the vagina (see p. 379) to be drawn forward, while at the same time the floor of the vagina between these two openings becomes depressed below the pelvis. Urine emerges from the urethra and, instead of being voided posteriorly, drains forward and collects in the pouch formed by the depressed vaginal floor.

Surgery to correct this abnormality includes the Pouret operation, which allows the vagina to move back so that the urethra is restored to its proper position. In addition, plastic surgery to the floor of the vagina around the opening of the urethra can be attempted in order to draw the urethra back into its normal position.

RECTOVAGINAL FISTULA

Tears in the vagina may occur during foaling if the foal's limbs or head are forced through the roof of the vagina into the rectum. The injury is seen most often in mares foaling for the first time and is due to the violent expulsive efforts of the mare in combination with some degree of malalignment of the foal.

The condition can only be rectified by surgery. The technique consists of a first operation in which a shelf is constructed between the rectum and the vagina, followed by a second operation which reconstructs the perineum and vulva. The procedure is usually carried out with the mare tranquillized and placed in stocks, using epidural and local anaesthesia.

CALCULI

The urethra in the male and female can be blocked by a calculus (stone). The surgical procedure to relieve this condition in the mare consists of dilating the urethra with forceps and removing the stone. In the male it may be necessary to cut into the urethra at the level of the pelvic brim as it passes around this area from the bladder to the penis. An incision is made through which the stone is removed.

HERNIA (RUPTURE)

A hernia (rupture) is a protrusion of bowel, omentum or any organ through a natural or an artificial opening in the walls of the cavity within which the organ is contained. Strictly speaking, a hernia is a displacement, perhaps congenital, through a natural opening. However, very often the term is applied to what is correctly referred to as a rupture, i.e. the passage of an organ through an artificial opening.

Rupture of organs such as the lungs or the eyeball do occur, but hernias are generally found in connection with abdominal organs. The protrusion may be bowel, omentum or both. In some cases the bladder is involved and, in other cases, the uterus (womb). In the horse inguinal (scrotal), umbilical and ventral hernias are quite common. Hernias are also encountered in the mesentery (causing colic), the diaphragm and the perineum.

Causes

In congenital cases a natural opening – for example, the umbilicus – is abnormally large. In cases of scrotal or inguinal hernia in newborn foals, there is usually a large opening in the abdominal wall in the groin through which the testes descend (see p. 358 and Figure 3, p. 361) during development.

Hernias acquired after birth are commonly caused by rearing, kicking, jumping or straining; they may also occur when a horse is cast for a surgical operation. Ventral rupture may arise from an external injury, such as staking or being horned by cattle. In the mare an accident producing a hernia may occur at foaling or during the later stages of pregnancy due to the weight of the foetus. In the male it may occur after castration or after an operation for scirrhous cord.

The severity depends on the age of the animal, the condition and size of the opening, whether it is natural (i.e. congenital) or acquired, and the volume of the protrusion. In some cases, for example, small congenital umbilical, ventral and, occasionally, scrotal hernias. recovery takes place spontaneously. If the hernia is due to displacement of part of the bowel, it is quite likely to disappear as the animal becomes older.

In acquired cases hernias do not disappear spontaneously. However, they can often be rectified, but seldom without some form of surgical intervention.

Most congenital cases, when first seen, are reducible. The volume of the swelling varies and may be more pronounced at some times than at others. When the animal lies down, the swelling tends to disappear, only to reappear or increase in volume when the horse gets up.

Umbilical, inguinal and even a few ventral hernias may be reducible when first seen, but over time there is a danger of them becoming irreducible due to the formation of adhesions. Sometimes there is an alteration in the contents of what is termed the sac, that is, the pouch containing the herniated organ. For example, a loop of bowel may become filled with food, which then prevents reduction.

STRANGULATED HERNIA

This is always a serious condition. It is caused by a narrowing of the hernial ring (the mouth of the sac) or by changes occurring in the hernia itself. Changes in pressure alter the blood supply to the herniated tissues, causing swelling, pain, haemorrhage, exudation, peritonitis and, if not relieved, necrosis. In most cases of necrosis death follows. A strangulated hernia requires immediate surgical correction.

VENTRAL HERNIA

Initially the swelling is compressible but may not be very evident. Sometimes a hard swelling may be seen, the result of blood extravasation from haemorrhage arising from the cause of the hernia. In most cases it is compressible, and coughing will produce a vibration. The ring may be felt, but not always. In some cases of ventral hernia the ring may be situated some distance from the swelling. The discovery of the ring may take a little time, because the bowel is flattened as it escapes through the opening and cannot be traced easily.

INGUINAL HERNIA

Hernias coming under this designation are not always easily discernible and there may be no external evidence of their existence. However, if an adult animal is at all restless and shows signs of colic, a rectal examination may reveal the presence of a hernia. In some cases this examination is the only method by which to discover the opening through the abdominal wall. By moving the hand towards the swelling, the part of the intestine will be felt to be very tense; by tracing the course of the tenseness, it is possible to discover the opening through which the hernia has passed.

UMBILICAL HERNIA

If a swelling is noticeable at the navel, nine times out of ten it is a hernia (Figure 2). A hernia in this position is nearly always compressible. By thrusting a finger towards the centre of the swelling, a hole or opening in the abdominal wall, the so-called hernial ring, can be easily detected.

Treatment
It should be remembered that umbilical hernia in foals usually resolves spontaneously with maturity. However, in practice, cases in which the hernial ring is more than 2 cm in diameter should be treated to speed up resolution of an abnormality which may become strangulated.

Traditional methods of treatment involved the use of blisters, skewers, clamps and trusses. Such methods have now been superseded and two methods are commonly used by veterinarians:

Rubber rings Elastrator rings, normally used for docking lambs' tails, may be applied to the skin over the hernial sac. Two or three rings are usually applied in succession.

Care in placement is essential to avoid strangulating a section of bowel or mesentery in the hernial sac. Such a mishap would produce pain, necrosis and death if not corrected rapidly.

The technique is simple and can be performed in the standing position, although sedation may be necessary with fractious foals. The rings should be placed as close to the abdominal wall as possible, in effect holding the contents of the hernial ring, which will then close spontaneously. The necrotic tissue below the rings will shrink and drop off in three to four weeks.

As with any surgical procedure, it is vital that the foal be vaccinated against tetanus or given antitoxin before this treatment is undertaken.

Surgical closure Surgical closure of the hernial ring under general anaesthesia is the method of choice when the defect is too large for the application of rubber rings or when the hernia is irreducible or has strangulated. Modern surgical techniques and anaesthetics render the operation simple and routine.

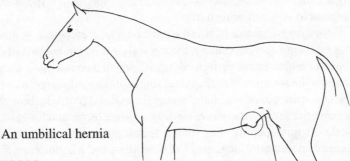

Figure 2   An umbilical hernia

CASTRATION

The removal of the testes, an operation known as castration or gelding, is carried out to render the animal more docile and to facilitate control in the presence of mares. It also renders the animal sterile.

Castration may be performed at any age. The main problems in castrating a foal are the testes are small and more difficult to grasp and the foal is not so used to being handled. Advocates of castration of foals have maintained not only that the operation is quite successful and has no effect in retarding development, but that there are fewer accidents and complications. Nevertheless most authorities would not advocate castration prior to a year of age, and the heavy breeds, especially those like hunters destined for prolonged hard work, are often left until they are three or even four.

When a horse is castrated many of the characteristics of a stallion fail to develop or regress if they have developed. The crest does not appear and the neigh becomes more like that of a mare. Changes in temperament vary with the breed, though most geldings are more docile than stallions. Whether or not a stallion is aggressive often depends on his management – Standardbred stallions are often extremely docile and the author's children ride his pony stallions in hand with aplomb.

Castration can be carried out at any time of year, but the custom is to do it in the spring or autumn. Spring is generally preferred because there are fewer flies about and the animal can be turned out afterwards and so reduce the swelling that is otherwise likely to develop.

The operation must, in the United Kingdom, be performed with adequate anaesthesia or analgesia and must be performed by a veterinarian. It may be carried out with the animal standing (in which case anaesthetic is injected deeply into the testis) or with the animal recumbent. (There are so many good anaesthetic agents available today that there can be little justification for casting the horse with ropes.)

Both methods have their advocates and the choice should be the result of a consultation between owner and veterinarian. The advantage of the standing method is that all the risks of a recumbent animal are avoided. Its disadvantage is that it is more risky to the operator, especially if the animal does not respond to sedation or restraint.

Castration by emasculator is the most popular method today; the older methods involving clamps, cautery, torsion and ligation having almost disappeared.

Most castrations are performed 'open', which means leaving open the wound through the scrotum. If the inguinal ring is abnormally large, bowel may leave the abdomen, pass through the inguinal canal and protrude through the scrotal wound. Some vets, therefore, employ a closed technique for castration which seals off this opening. For such a technique to be employed successfully, general anaesthesia, clean surgical conditions and a ligature are obligatory.

Complications of Castration

HAEMORRHAGE

Dripping of blood after castration is common and of no significance, provided the drips are not running into one another and the rate of drip is slowing down. Applying cold water to the scrotum, either from a bucket or a hose pipe is often apparently effective, although there is a danger that the bleeding vessels may retract further into the wound and the bleeding continue internally. Lay persons should not therefore interfere.

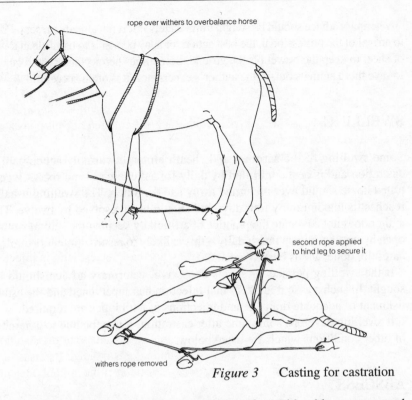

rope over withers to overbalance horse

second rope applied
to hind leg to secure it

withers rope removed

Figure 3   Casting for castration

Streaming of blood, however, is a matter of considerable concern and veterinary advice should be sought. Some advocate packing the wound and waiting, but the author's preference is to anaesthetise the animal again, find the bleeding point and ligate it. Haemorrhage can be prevented by the use of an adequate, well-maintained emasculator.

Haemophilia is very rare in horses, but the author has seen two horses bleeding profusely after castration, both of which had unidentified clotting defects.

A rare complication of profuse haemorrhage is irreversible blindness due to damage to the retina.

PROLAPSE OF THE BOWEL

Passage of a loop of bowel down the inguinal canal and through the castration wound can occur while the castration is being performed, as the horse stands up (or attempts to) after a general anaesthetic, or up to forty-eight hours after castration. This is the complication of castration most likely to be fatal because the bowel becomes dry and dirty or may get torn or damaged by the horse's feet. Moreover, the bowel gets trapped in the canal, its blood supply is severely reduced (strangulation) and this causes colic.

Veterinary advice should be sought immediately if it is not already present. Prior to arrival of the professional, the best action for a lay person is to use a clean towel or sheet to keep the bowel off the ground. Sometimes heroic surgery is required to save these animals but, in the author's experience, it is often successful.

SWELLING

Some swelling of the scrotum and sheath almost invariably accompanies castration and is best controlled by daily forced exercise – no recently cas-trated horse should ever be turned away and forgotten. The swelling usually reaches its maximum by four days and should have resolved by twelve. The author does not advocate the practice of artificially keeping the scrotal wound open by putting fingers into it daily – this is likely to result in infection, unless carefully done, and is best avoided.

If the swelling persists or seems excessive, veterinary advice should be sought. In such a case it is likely that infection has supervened and the estab-lishment of adequate drainage and injections of antibiotics are required.

If swelling develops some time after castration, it may be due to a number of other conditions which are listed below.

ABSCESS

A scrotal abscess is characterised by a spherical, fluctuating, painful swelling, and the horse can sometimes be quite ill from poisons produced by pus in the abscess. Abscesses usually develop within a few weeks of castration. The abscess should be opened by a veterinarian and drained, and the cavity kept open until healing has advanced. Occasionally an infected ligature will be at the root of an abscess and resolution will only occur if the whole abscess is surgically removed.

CHAMPIGNON

This condition derives its name from the French word for 'mushroom' and is characterised by a mushroom-like growth of proud flesh from the scrotal wound. It develops a few weeks after castration and must be cut out under gen-eral anaesthetic. Fortunately, it is quite rare today.

LIGATURE SINUS

This condition is characterised by the development of a small opening in the scrotum which discharges pus and of a hard lump in the groin. It usually takes several years to develop and the animal may present as lame on that side before the discharge is noted. The cause is an abscess developing round a ligature used for castration. The abscess and the sinus tract leading from it to the outside must be excised.

SCIRRHOUS CORD

Like ligature sinus, this condition develops years after castration and is characterized by a large hard lump in the groin, sometimes with multiple openings discharging pus. It is caused by chronic infection with a staphyloccocal organism and is extremely difficult to treat. Occasionally it can have spread into the abdomen before it is recognised; the prognosis is then hopeless. Surgical excision should be attempted, perhaps after a long course of suitable antibiotic treatment has reduced its size.

CYSTIC ENDS

Soft, fluctuating swellings can develop in the scrotum of castrated horses, months or years after castration. They are very soft, fluid-filled cysts and can appear and disappear, sometimes quickly, sometimes slowly. They cause the horse no trouble, but can be surgically removed if they are considered a blemish.

CRYPTORCHIDISM (RIG, RIDGELING)

Cryptorchids are animals with improper testicular descent and the condition may be bilateral or unilateral (see p. 361). The retained testicle may lie high up within the inguinal canal but external to the body wall, or it may lie within the abdomen internal to the inguinal ring. General anaesthesia is essential when castrating to allow exposure of and exploration for such hidden testicles.

OTHER TECHNIQUES

Cryosurgery

Cryosurgery is the technique of destroying tissues by the local application of intense cold. The tissue is rapidly frozen to a temperature of -20°C (-4°F) or lower, then slowly thawed and subsequently refrozen. The number of freeze–thaw cycles used depends on the type of tissue under treatment, the depth of penetration required and overall area to be destroyed.

Tissues contain large amounts of water, both extra- and intracellular, and thus ice formation within the tissues can readily be induced. Freezing causes the cells to swell, followed by death and rupture of the cell membranes. The frozen tissues die and gradually slough off to leave a well-demarcated, healthy, granulating wound.

Cryotherapy is most frequently utilised for the removal of skin tumours (see chapter 42), especially squamous cell carcinoma, sarcoids, cutaneous granuloma and exuberant granulation tissue. It has been found that the technique, used alone or in combination with prior surgical excision, has improved the overall success rate by decreasing the number of treatments per case and reducing the incidence of recurrence at the original site.

Cryosurgery is also used in ophthalmic surgery for cataract extraction. Latterly it has also been developed as a technique for neurectomy of the lower limb; it is said to reduce the risk of secondary neuroma formation.

Lasers

Lasers are a relatively recent addition to the surgeon's armamentarium. At the present time there are two main types of laser: the high-energy ('hot') laser and the low-energy ('cold') laser.

The former produces a high energy 'lightbeam', capable of both cutting and burning tissues, which is used to treat the base of a wound after surgical excision of a tumour or tissue mass. Hot lasers are most frequently used in the removal of skin tumours, epithelial carcinomas, sarcoids and to treat beds of granulation tissue. They are also used in the more refined techniques of ophthalmic surgery for treating retinal detachment.

Cold lasers are a more recent innovation and have been used mainly in the fringe areas of physiotherapy, cosmetic surgery and acupuncture. At the present time there has been little published scientific data to substantiate the claims made for the therapeutic benefits of this tool.

Currently in the veterinary field these lasers are being used for management of specific soft-tissue injuries, such as sprained tendons, ligaments, tendon sheath injury, haematomas and open wounds. It is not known how the laser beam affects tissue response or assists the rate of healing of different tissue types, which is said to follow treatment.

It is claimed that this class of laser can significantly reduce the healing time for open wounds of soft tissue. Practical experience has shown that recent tendon injuries may be cosmetically improved, but that the underlying structural damage remains materially unaffected. This may lead to a horse being returned prematurely to work, only to break down.

Different types of lameness have been treated with the cold laser both locally and at sites distant from the injury, the laser being applied over the nerves supplying the injured area. Benefits from this technique may be related to a desensitising or local anaesthetic effect, as can be seen with acupuncture.

Note: Lasers produce a concentrated beam of light which can be reflected from glass or metal surfaces and the operator should be aware of this risk. The laser should never be pointed at the eye, either directly or indirectly.

Electromagnetic stimulation
The application of an electrical current across the fracture site of a bone injury stimulates bone repair under certain circumstances. Under normal conditions unstressed bone has a static surface electrical potential, which alters in response to mechanical stress (i.e. loading). If the bone is fractured, the inherent electrical charge of the bone becomes rearranged, with a negative polarity induced at the fracture site. It has been found in cases of non-union of fractures and pseudoarthrosis that application of an electrical charge across the fracture site stimulates repair.

Direct current may be applied via implated electrodes (an invasive technique which has inherent problems with electrolysis). Another method is by electro-magnetic induction of current in the tissues under treatment. Pulsing electromag-netic fields (PEMFs) are produced by passing pulsed electrical current through special circular coils placed on either side of the bone under treatment. The tissue between the coils is thereby exposed to an electromagnetic field which induces changes in the electrical potential of that tissue and modifies cellular activity. By varying the electrical pulse in size, shape and rate, it is possible to produce the ideal electrical conditions for the particular tissue type under treatment.

PEMFs are commonly used for treatment of stress fractures of the anterior cortex of the cannon bone, bucked shins, sesamoid bone fractures and as an adjunct to standard orthopaedic surgical procedures. Both sesamoid fractures and cortical fractures of the cannon bone have a tendency to heal slowly, frequently with nonunion; it is thought that PEMF therapy can significantly reduce the healing time and improve the final union.

At present there are several systems on the market. The Blue Boot, which is designed to be strapped to the leg, is completely portable and contains a rechargeable energy pack. There are other rechargeable portable systems and also larger, mains-operated systems which give the operator a choice of pulses.

Slinging as an aid to surgery
A sling is employed as a means of support to an injured horse when it is essen-tial that it be kept in the standing position, as, for example, in cases of pelvic fracture, which may become displaced with serious complications under the strain of the animal lying down or getting up. The apparatus may also be used for lifting recumbent animals.

A patent sling consists of a middle piece or suspender which supports the body and is attached on each side by a metal ring to a bow (a metal tree), which is in turn attached to a strong overhead support by an endless-chain pulley.

Breast straps at the front of the bodybelt prevent the horse from falling forwards, and breechings at the rear afford support if the horse sits back.

The sling should be adjusted to a height at which the horse may stand unsupported of its volition. It should also be able to lean backwards against the breechings and thereby derive postural support. On no account should the horse be suspended without its feet touching the ground, unless it is being raised from a recumbent position.

A horse in a sling should be checked regularly to make sure that the apparatus is properly adjusted and that pressure sores do not develop. Extra padding may be needed at potential pressure points. A laxative diet is essential.

Some horses, by their very nature, are unsuitable candidates for slinging. To prevent recumbency, such cases should be tied up by the head collar with a loop of string connecting the stable chain to the ring of the head collar.

Firing

Firing is the application of hot irons to the area of a damaged tendon, bone or joint with the purpose of inducing a severe inflammation (a counter-irritation) in an attempt to effect a cure. It is a procedure virtually confined to the horse and has been handed down over centuries.

In the present day it has been superseded as a means of therapy by the introduction of more refined treatments developed from a newer understanding of pathology and carried out with equipment developed as a result of technological advance.

Recent scientific research has been unable to demonstrate any benefit from firing damaged tendons and, despite some dissenting views, veterinary opinion is against its use.

Blistering

This is the term for the application of a chemical irritant to produce vesication (blisters) and counter-irritation, in other words, to induce an inflammatory response as a therapeutic measure.

The use of vesicants (blistering agents) is a contentious subject and is not advocated by the veterinary profession. The efficacy of blistering is likely to remain based on subjective opinion rather than on scientific fact.

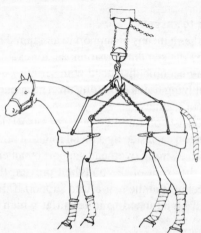

Figure 4
A sling

41
WOUNDS:
THE FIRST-AID KIT

Wounds are commonly seen in horses as a result of falls, being kicked or bitten by other horses, colliding with or getting entangled in fencing, hitting jumps, etc. A wound is defined as 'an injury to the body caused by physical means with disruption of normal continuity of body structures which is followed by healing.'* A wound may be closed, that is, the skin remains intact as in bruising, sprains and ruptures, or open with various degrees of skin damage.

OPEN WOUNDS

Open wounds can be grouped according to the nature of the damage.

Incised wounds   These wounds have clean straight edges and often bleed quite freely. There is usually very little associated bruising and they normally heal quickly and simply. Examples are surgical incisions using a scalpel and cuts caused by sharp pieces of metal or glass.

Lacerations and tears   These wounds have torn rather than cut edges and may be irregular in shape. There is usually some associated bruising and the amount of bleeding is variable. These wounds often result in tags or flaps of skin, the blood supply of which is compromised, resulting in death of the skin (necrosis) at a later stage. Lacerated wounds are the result of getting caught on protruding nails or posts and sometimes wire.

Puncture wounds   These can be more serious than they appear and are characterised by a small skin opening with soft-tissue penetration to a variable depth. They are caused by bites, being staked on fences or jumps, treading on nails, pieces of wire, pitchforks, and so on.

* *Dorlands Medical Dictionary*, 26th ed.

The object causing the puncture wound can carry with it, to the depth of the injury, either foreign material (for example, a splinter) or bacteria, which can become established and cause deep infection. The skin wound may be so small as to not be seen.

Puncture wounds should not be probed or explored excessively because such action may disrupt blood clots or force any foreign body deeper. This type of wound always requires the administration of tentanus vaccination and antitoxin. Drainage must be established and encouraged so the wound can heal from the inside out. A poultice (e.g. Animalintex) can be applied to try to draw out any contaminating material and help keep the wound open.

Penetrating wounds   These are wounds which penetrate into one of the body cavities, such as the thorax or abdomen, and are very serious. There may or may not be injury to internal organs.

Emergency first aid in these cases involves covering the wound with sterile gauze or bandage to prevent further contamination and/or the escape of organs or tissues, and to reduce the amount of air sucked into the body cavity and hence prevent infection.

Abrasions   These are very superficial skin wounds, resulting from rubbing or scraping against an irritant surface. Examples are saddle chaffs and shoulder rubs from ill-fitting saddles and rugs respectively. Abrasions may also result from falling on the road, but, although the skin injury may seem superficial in these instances, the bones of the limbs which have poor protection may be damaged even if not exposed through the wound.

These wounds should be gently but thoroughly cleansed and if possible lightly bandaged.

Treatment
Open wounds involve damage to some of or all the following: skin, muscles, nerves, blood vessels, tendons, bones, internal organs. All wounds, unless incurred during asceptic surgery, are contaminated by bacteria, which may become established and result in an infected wound.

The main aims in wound treatment are: to control haemorrhage; to turn the contaminated wound into a clean one; and to promote rapid healing.

Haemorrhage to a limited degree helps to flush a wound free of contaminating material, and it may be difficult to decide whether it is more important to try to control the haemorrhage or cleanse the wound. This depends on the degree of haemorrrhage and the degree of contamination. If bleeding is minor, cleanse the wound and apply a dressing, preferably sterile, which will help to control the bleeding. If bleeding is more extensive, there are several methods available to reduce or stop it completely.

Control of bleeding

Ligature   If a large vessel is severed, it must be ligated before excessive blood loss occurs. If an artery is involved, bright red blood will be escaping in spurts. If it is a vein, the blood is darker and flows continuously. The damaged ends of the vessel should be grasped in a forceps and a ligature of sterile catgut or other sterile absorbable material placed around them and tied tightly so that it does not slip. If the vessel cannot be clamped, firm direct pressure should be applied with a finger onto both cut ends until help arrives.

Clamping with and without torsion   Small vessels, especially arteries, will seal if clamped for several minutes with an artery clamp or forceps. Twisting the clamp or forceps (torsion) until the vessel stretches and breaks causes elastic recoil and can be used to seal many smaller arteries and veins, although veins lack the full elasticity of arteries and may not seal without being ligated.

Pressure   This may be applied directly by placing a clean dressing to the wound and holding it firmly in place until bleeding stops. On the limbs a pressure bandage with several layers of absorbent material or a wad of material underneath can be applied over the wound. This must be left in place until bleeding has stopped.

The pressure bandage must be applied tightly but should be removed once haemorrhage has ceased to avoid interfering with the circulation. Tourniquets should not be used unless haemorrhage is severe, as they can, if incorrectly applied, exacerbate the bleeding by interfering with venous drainage from the area.

Topically applied substances   Some chemicals can be applied to the bleeding surfaces to control haemorrhage. They include silver nitrate, ferric chloride, ferric sulphate, alum and tannin. These substances work by precipitating proteins in the damaged vessel to block it and allow clotting to occur. Pressure should be used to reduce haemorrhage and the wound should be cleansed before the substance is applied, as excessive amounts of blood or a blood clot will interfere with the effectiveness of the chemical.

Locally applied materials   These are used surgically to encourage clotting and include oxidized cellulose, calcium alginate and absorbable gelatin sponges. They act as a framework on which a clot can develop. They can be left in a clean wound as they are absorbable.

Electrocautery, diathermy, electrocoagulation   These methods use heat or electric current to seal vessels or coagulate tissues to stop haemorrhage.

Cleansing and débridement

Simple hosing is the best way initially to cleanse many wounds, especially if they are large or heavily contaminated (dirty), because it produces a constant flow of water in large volumes and under variable pressure. Excessive pressure should be avoided as it may force foreign material deeper into the wound or open up new tissue planes, allowing spread of infection. The skin surrounding the wound should also be hosed clean of mud and debris.

Smaller wounds, and larger ones after initial hosing (performed for up to fifteen or twenty minutes), should be gently cleansed with a *dilute* solution of a mild skin antiseptic in *warm* water using either a syringe or a hand pump and pieces of clean cottonwool or Gamgee. Suitable solutions can be made up using iodine-based washes such as povidone iodine, chlorophene, cetrimide and chlorhexidine. If possible, the surrounding area should be clipped or shaved before cleansing, care being taken that hair does not enter the wound by packing it with clean gauze.

After a wound has been cleansed the remaining, often embedded, foreign material and dead or damaged tissues may need removing (débridement). Physical or chemical restraint (tranquillisation or general anaesthesia), with or without the use of local anaesthesia, may be needed, depending on the nature of the wound, the amount of contamination, the facilities available and the temperament of the patient. A pair of tissue forceps, a sharp pair of scissors and a scalpel are essential instruments for débridement. If the wound is extensive, this procedure may have to be repeated at a later date as some tissue will die despite correct treatment. During débridement all care must be taken to preserve tendons, nerves and blood vessels, but tags of skin or other damaged or dead tissue should be removed.

Drainage

Some wounds, especially puncture wounds or wounds in which there is a large gap left due to loss of normal tissue, will require drainage which must be maintained for a variable period of time to allow healing. This may be achieved either by leaving the wound open, with or without enlarging the skin opening, or by creating a second skin opening and establishing drainage with or without the use of drains.

These drains are pieces of latex or plastic which are sutured into the wound with one or both ends communicating with the outside. They allow the passage of fluid and debris from the depth of the wound. Care should be taken, however, over placement and protection to prevent drains being torn or acting as routes for infection to enter the wound. They should not exit through the wound itself as this will interfere with healing.

Healing

A clean wound will begin the process of healing immediately after the injury. Wounds heal in several ways depending on the nature and site of the injury. Healing by first or primary intention can only occur in non-contaminated incised wounds where the edges are or can be brought together. For this type of healing to occur, the wound must also be fresh and sutured to bring the skin edges into direct contact with each other.

The wound should be stitched as soon as possible after the injury has occurred. If the skin edges are not under tension, a simple pattern of interrupted sutures or a continuous suture may be used. The former permits better apposition of skin edges than the continuous pattern; also, if a knot comes untied, only one suture is lost. The continuous suture can be inserted more quickly.

Subcutaneous and deeper tissues may be brought together using a absorbable suture material before the skin is closed. However, if structures such as tendons and ligaments need to be sutured, stainless steel should be used for its strength and durability as these tissues need a long time to heal. If the edges of a wound can only be brought together under tension or if extensive swelling is likely, tension sutures, using either buttons or tubing to spread the tension over a larger area, or a vertical mattress suture pattern may be used. Sutures should remain in place for at least ten days, and longer if necessary.

If the wound cannot heal by primary intention, it must undergo the processes of granulation, contraction and epithelial cell multiplication and migration. This is called healing by second intention.

Large skin and tissue defects on the body tend to heal with relatively little scarring because the skin is loose and wound contraction can occur readily. On the limbs, however, there is little or no loose skin and wound contraction is limited. The formation of excessive granulation tissue (proud flesh) in wounds to the limbs also interferes with healing, as the epithelial cells cannot migrate over the proud flesh to create a new skin covering. Little can be done to facilitate wound contraction on horses' limbs and skin grafting may be necessary to complete healing. The forces of wound contraction are so great that, if scarring occurs over or near a joint, the skin may be pulled so tight as to prevent proper joint movement.

Proud flesh can be kept to a minimum by the use of pressure bandaging and immobilisation. However, once present, it must be removed either surgically or by the use of caustic powders or solutions. These substances include copper sulphate (bluestone) and silver nitrate. Care should be taken when using these to ensure that the delicate band of advancing epithelial cells around the edges of the wound is not damaged. Formalin may also be used to reduce excessive proud flesh, but, again, this must not come into contact with healthy tissue.

Dressings

Bandaging wounds serves many purposes. One is the immobilisation of the region to aid healing. Another is to keep the wound clean and protect it from infection and to prevent further trauma. Pressure, as applied through a bandage, can aid in reducing swelling and oedema and in controlling haemorrhage. Not all wounds require or are suitable for bandaging. Some are best left open, kept clean and free from debris, and treated with either a wound powder or spray and allowed to granulate. Wounds on many parts of the body and upper limbs must be treated in this way. On the other hand, where rigid immobilisation is necessary, for example, with leg wounds where a tendon is exposed or damaged, or with some wounds around the joints, the limb should be placed in a cast to allow tissues to heal.

All dressing should be non-adhesive and may be impregnated with sterile petroleum jelly (Vaseline) or antibiotics. They should preferably be sterile but at the very least clean. Padding, such as cottonwool, combine or Gamgee should be used to help distribute the pressure of the bandage and absorb any discharge, from the wound. There are many types of bandages available, from light stretch crepe through stable bandages to adhesive elastic bandages. Care must be taken with the stretch bandages not to apply them too tightly as this may interfere with the blood circulation to the area and below.

Drugs

Systemic antibiotic treatment may be necessary in serious or heavily contaminated wounds. Penicillins, sulphonamides and trimetho-prinsulphonamide combinations are most frequently used. Anti-inflammatory drugs are also occasionally indicated as they help to reduce pain, inflammation and swelling.

Factors affecting healing

There are not many ways to stimulate healing to progress faster than it does in a clean, 'healthy' wound, and the rate of healing is the same in a large as in a small wound. However, many factors interfere with and delay healing. The most important of these is infection, which results in further tissue damage, discharge and inflammation. An infected wound must be thoroughly cleaned, drainage established and antibiotics administered. Topically applied antibiotics are often unable to reach the bacteria in infected wounds because of the barrier produced by dead tissue and discharges, and systemic antibiotics must be used instead.

Other local factors which may affect healing include blood supply to the wound, associated soft-tissue damage, such as bruising and haematomas (blood sacs), skin temperature, and the availability of loose connective tissue to allow wound closure. Many systemic disorders may also interfere with wound healing: these include protein or vitamin A or C deficiency, zinc deficiency, age and some hormonal, cardiac, liver and kidney abnormalities.

CLOSED WOUNDS

Closed wounds include bruises, contusions, sprains, and muscle and tendon rupture. Contusions result from a blunt force causing haemorrhage, bruising and oedema without breaking the skin. Signs of contusion include swelling, heat and pain at the site of injury, and discolouration of the overlying skin if it is pink (or depigmented). Kicks from other horses often result in contusions with the formation of haematomas under the skin due to leakage of blood from damaged vessels. Treatment of contusions involves initial immobilisation of the region and cold hosing or the application of ice packs to reduce heat and swelling. Subsequently applying heat to the area encourages the absorption of excessive fluid.

Large haematomas often require draining, but this is best left for two or three days to allow haemorrhage to cease. The drainage hole should be made in the most dependent (lower) point of the haematoma and should be kept open by vigorous cleaning until there is no more discharge from it. If allowed to close early, the haematoma sac may refill with blood or fluid and require redraining.

Other closed wounds include sprains, ligament tears and ruptures, and muscle tears and ruptures (see Chapters 14 and 15)

BURNS

Burns may be caused by excessive heat – for example, flame, hot solids, steam or water or other hot liquids; excessive cold or freezing, such as frost bite; electric current; substances such as acids and alkalis; or radiation. They are classified as follows:

First-degree burns   These involve only the very superficial epithelial layers of the skin and result in temporary reddening and loss (sloughing) of these layers, which are rapidly replaced from deeper layers. Mild to moderate sunburn is a first-degree burn.

Second-degree burns   These involve almost the full thickness of the epidermis and damage some of the accessory skin structures such as sweat glands and hair follicles. They heal by the multiplication of surrounding cells, which migrate into the tissue defect, usually under a scab.

Third-degree burns   These cause damage to the full thickness of the skin and some of the subcutaneous tissues, and result in ulceration and sloughing of the full thickness of the skin. They often require skin grafts to complete healing.

Very deep burns may also affect the muscles and tissues underneath. The hair coat of mammals protects them, to a small extent, from burns by flames or hot objects, but may also act to mask the full extent of an injury. The reddening of skin in a first-degree burn may go unnoticed, especially where the skin is pigmented.

In second-degree burns there is damage to the dermis and loss of the epidermal layers, resulting in leakage of serum from blood vessels the development of oedema in surrounding tissues and a crust on the surface. Third-degree burns result in the coagulation of the skin, thrombosis (blocking) of vessels and subsequent obstruction to the nutrient supply to the upper tissue layers, resulting in the formation of a black, leathery scar (an eschar). Damage to nerve endings results in loss of sensation. These burns, if large in area, often require skin grafting.

Electric burns appear as cold, pale yellow, bloodless, painless lesions. These are worse if the hair is wet because wet tissue conducts electricity more efficiently. There may only be a small skin lesion, but a much larger area of damage may have occurred under the skin. These wounds generally heal slowly and there may be some tissue sloughing.

Although the wounds themselves can appear dramatic, burns can have more serious effects on the whole body. In burns due to fire or steam, swelling and oedema of the nasal passages and pharynx may result in death from asphyxiation. Shock may develop immediately or as a result of the loss of large amounts of fluid from the damaged area. This can be fatal.

Another long-term effect of severe burns is the development of anaemia due to depression of red blood cell formation in the bone marrow. Infection is common after serious burns, and toxaemia may develop and result in the death of the animal within a few days or sometime later.

Treatment
Treatment of burn victims must take into account both the local and the systemic consequences of the injuries. Burns are extremely painful and the affected animals should be handled quietly and gently at all times. If the burns are extensive or severe, your veterinarian should be called immediately. Fluid replacement and maintenance therapy is most important. Fluids may need to be administered intravenously at first, although, once the animal has stabilised, giving water by stomach tube and encouraging the horse to drink may be adequate. Painkillers may also be necessary to reduce the chance of shock and make the animal more comfortable. Useful painkillers are the narcotics (e.g. pethidine) and certain anti-inflammatory drugs. The horse should be kept quiet, warm and comfortable.

Local treatment of the burned or scalded area involves *gently* washing the area with a very dilute antibacterial solution or wash (e.g povidone iodine). Avoid the use of oily or greasy ointments, tannic acid, silver nitrate, iodine, methylated spirits or other household remedies. Wet dressings consisting of sterile gauze soaked in warm isotonic saline or surgical chlorinated soda solution should be applied to the area. Water-based creams with antibiotics may be applied to the wounds and covered with a sterile dressing. Silver sulphadiazine (flamazine) is specifically used for burns.

Treatment of burns due to chemicals
The most important initial step is to rinse the area free from any remaining chemical. If the burn is caused by an acid, bath the area with an alkaline solution such as baking soda in warm water. If the burn is caused by an alkali, e.g. quicklime, bathe the area with a fifty-fifty vinegar and water mixture. In either case, or if the causative chemical is unknown, the area should be rinsed freely with clear water and then treated as any other burn.

Burns due to cold
Fortunately burns due to excessive cold are uncommon although freeze branding is becoming increasingly popular as an aid to identification of horses in some countries. In temperate climates frostbite may occur if a horse is allowed to stand in mud and water during very cold weather. This results in damage to the superficial skin layers, leakage of serum from the capillaries and oedema of the affected areas, which become swollen and painful. The skin may appear cracked and the condition is often called cracked heels or mud fever in its milder form (see p. 306).

Treatment consists of keeping the affected areas clean and dry and applying a soothing, non-greasy cream to soften the scabs. The cream may contain an antibacterial substance such as a sulphonamide to prevent infection. It is better to try to prevent cracked heels either by not washing a horse's legs in winter or by thoroughly drying them immediately if washing is necessary or if the animal has been standing in cold water or mud. Do not allow horses to stand for any period in mud or water in cold weather and ensure they are kept in good health and condition throughout the year.

LIGHTNING STRIKE AND ELECTRIC SHOCK

Both these events usually result in death with little external evidence of injury apart from a line of singed hair or burned skin along the course of the current. Occasionally, more obvious evidence of lightning strike is present, such as a struck tree nearby or a branching pattern on the hair from the point of strike. Rigor mortis is usually present for a very short period only and the carcase decomposes rapidly. Post mortem reveals widespread petechial (pinpoint) haemorrhages throughout the intestine, endocardium (lining of the heart), meninges, central nervous system and viscera (internal organs). It may be difficult to differentiate between septicaemia, anthrax, lightning strike and other causes of sudden death unless further tests are performed.

Surviving animals appear dazed or unconscious, with severe depression of both cardiac and respiratory functions. Respiration is slow, laboured or gasping. The pulse is weak and slow. The pupils may be dilated or constricted, and convulsions are common. A varying degree of paralysis is also common; its disappearance is a good sign of recovery. Recovery may take hours or days, but in some cases permanent paralysis or blindness follows.

Electric shock arises from contact with overhead cables, wire fencing or other sources of electric current, particularly if the immediate area is wet. At post mortem the heart appears flabby and there is marked congestion of the lungs, heart and other organs.

Treatment for a surviving victim of electric shock or lightning strike is largely a matter of good nursing. Plenty of bedding, food and water should be available and the animal's condition constantly monitored. Support bandages on all limbs may be useful if the animal is weak or is paralysed in one leg.

The First-Aid Kit

Every responsible horse or pony owner should have a basic first-aid kit in the tack room. It is best kept in a small, clean, preferably waterproof box. This ensures that the kit remains clean and dry, and can be taken with the horse whenever it travels away from home.

The contents of the box are for dealing with any minor injuries which may occur either in the stable or paddock or while out riding. These are usually superficial cuts and grazes, such as those resulting from kicks, wire cuts, overreaching, thorns, etc.

If the injury is severe, first aid should only be temporary procedure and a veterinarian contacted as soon as possible.

The contents of a basic first-aid kit are as follows:

Antiseptics
An antiseptic cleansing agent, such as povidone iodine or chlorhexidine (diluted for use), is essential for cleaning wounds. Hosing is generally a very good way of flushing out debris from the wound area (see p. 640) and then the antiseptic solution can be applied at the final stage. If a hose is not available, the antiseptic should be added to a bucket of clean, preferably warm, water. The wound should be cleaned thoroughly, staring at its centre and working outwards.

Wound powders and sprays

After cleaning a wound which is not going to be bandaged (either because it is in an area which is impossible to bandage or because it is very superficial), a dressing of either powder, spray or gel/cream should be applied to help prevent infection and aid in the drying of the wound.

Powders such as acrimide are antibacterial and those such as aureomycin contain antibiotics. During the summer fly-repellent powder containing coumaphos should be used. This is to prevent fly strike (flys laying eggs in the open wound).

Some horses object violently to sprays. If this is the case the spray should be squirted onto cottonwool at some distance from the horse and then dabbed on the wound. Some antibiotic sprays contain gentian violet (purple spay), which is an effective antifungal agent. These sprays are particularly useful when treating areas on and around the feet.

Never use powders or sprays on or around the eyes of a horse.

Creams and ointments

An antiseptic ointment such as Betadine or Savlon is useful for applying to mild skin problems such as cracked heels and mud fever, and a light healing cream such as Dermisol can be used on dry non-adherent dressings before bandaging.

Bandages

It is useful to have a good selection of open-weave, adhesive and crepe bandages. These can be obtained from most chemists or from a veterinarian.

Dressings are employed after the injured area has been cleansed to control haemorrhage, to keep an open wound clean, and also for support and protection. Most wounds which involve the full thickness of the skin should be bandaged if possible because this prevents dirt from entering and helps to hold the edges of the wound together.

Crepe bandages give support and slight pressure without restricting movement. Adhesive bandage helps to hold a bandage onto a difficult area such as the knee or hock and should be applied directly to the skin above the bandage and over the material dressing.

All bandages must be applied with care. It is important that there is adequate padding (such as Gamgee) underneath and that they are kept flat and not wrinkled. Except in cases of severe haemorrhage, when they may be used tightly for short periods (not more that fifteen minutes at a time), bandages should be applied with a light, even pressure. Overtight bandaging can cause disruption to the blood circulation of the skin and underlying tissues and result in necrosis and sloughing.

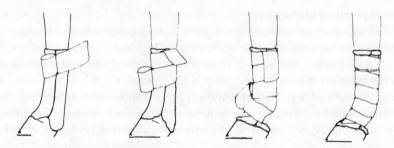

Figure 1   Stable bandage

Sterile, non-adherent dressings

These are applied where the surface of the skin is broken and are placed over the wound before bandaging. Some of these dressings are impregnated with antibiotic and are either greasy or have a non-adherent surface. The greasy form should only be used when the wound is fresh, as it will keep it moist and encourage excessive granulation tissue if used over an extended period of time. When the wound has nearly healed it should not be bandaged but treated with wound spray or powder (see above) to encourage it to dry and scab over.

Cottonwool and Gamgee

Cottonwool is useful for cleaning wounds, but should not be applied directly as it will stick to an open wound. A non-adherent dressing should be applied first and covered with a layer of Gamgee or cottonwool before bandaging. This will absorb any discharge and protect the wound from trauma.

Scissors

Curved, blunt-ended scissors will be needed for cutting hair away from a wound and straight ones for cutting tape and bandages.

Poultices

Poultices may be hot or cold. Hot ones are used either to increase the blood supply to an area, to draw out infection, as with pus in the foot, or to encourage an abscess to burst. Hot poultices should never be hotter than you can tolerate yourself. Never warm a poultice in the microwave as it continues to heat up after removal from the appliance. Cold poultices are used to decreased inflammation associated with the swelling and bruising caused by blows or kicks.

Several proprietaries of gauze and wool impregnated with boracic powder are widely used for hot poultices. Kaolin is excellent for foot problems as it has good heat-retaining properties and an antiseptic action. If nothing else is available, bran may be used mixed with an antiseptic and hot water. However, this is not really recommended as the wet bran is a good culture medium for moulds and bacteria.

There are several types of cold poultice on the market which are cooled in the fridge before use, but the best way to reduce inflammation is by cold hosing or by applying ice cubes between layers of Gamgee.

Thermometer

A clinical thermometer should be used to take a horse's temperature if it is showing symptoms of any illness. The mercury is shaken down and the bulb end of the thermometer placed in the horse's rectum for at least one minute. The normal temperature variation for the horse is 38-38.2°C (100.4-100.8°F). A rise in temperature of 0.7-1°C (2°F) or more above normal should be considered cause for concern and a vet should be consulted.

Figure 2   Exercise bandage

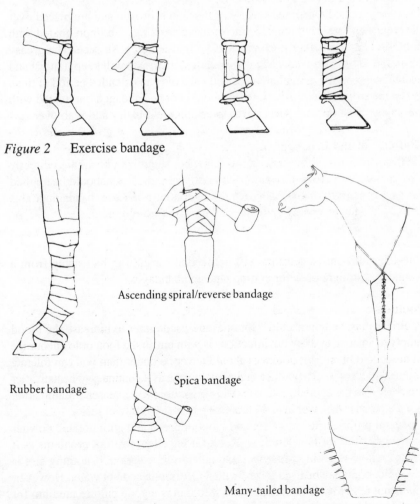

Ascending spiral/reverse bandage

Rubber bandage

Spica bandage

Many-tailed bandage

Figure 3   Bandage techniques

42
CANCER AND OTHER EQUINE LUMPS AND SWELLINGS

Abnormal lumps or swellings may appear externally or internally on horses and ponies, as they may on all animals, for a variety of reasons. They may appear suddenly or gradually over time, most commonly as a result of injury, infection or a mal-development (cysts) or chaotic transformation of otherwise normal body tissue (cancer). Of greatest importance to the horse and its owner is an early accurate diagnosis of the nature of the lump or swelling, the application of appropriate treatment and the monitoring of healing. The owner will wish to know the prognosis, i.e. the likely outcome, for recovery.

Cancer is understandably an emotive word. In most cancers, the reasons why the normal and orderly turnover (cell death and replacement) of body tissues in a specific area suddenly fails and abnormal chaotic cell growth occurs, remains unknown. The terms 'tumour' and 'neoplasm' may also be used to describe the swelling and new growth of an abnormal tissue type. It is important to understand that most swellings and lumps are not cancerous and of those that are, many can be cured by appropriate treatment. Some non-cancerous swellings and lumps, following serious injury and/or infection, can in fact be more difficult to resolve.

Diagnosis
As in all aspects of human and veterinary medicine, an early accurate diagnosis is the most important first step towards effective treatment and management. Veterinary advice should be sought at an early stage to make an accurate diagnosis. An experienced visual inspection of the lump's site and appearance will often give useful clues, and digital palpation for pain, heat and consistency will help differentiate haematomas, abscesses, cysts and tumours.

If necessary, and in addition to visual inspection and digital palpation, veterinary surgeons can use ultrasound scan technology to look at the internal structure of lumps to see if they are full of clear fluid (seromas) or turbid fluid (blood or pus). Ultrasound scan can also be used to locate lumps in internal organs, e.g. abscesses or tumours in lungs, liver, spleen and intestines. Modern X-ray (radiography) and nuclear scan (scintigraphy) technology can sometimes reveal the site and consistency of internal lumps. If fluid-filled, some may be withdrawn for visual and laboratory inspection. The fluid can be examined under the microscope (cytological examinations) to confirm the presence of pus or tumour cells and cultured in an incubator on special growth medium (agar) to identify the cause of the infection and to establish its anti-biotic sensitivity pattern to guide effective antibiotic treatment.

In most cases, in order to make a definitive diagnosis, especially at an early stage, microscopic (histopathological) examinations must be undertaken. Where the lump is single and discrete, especially involving the skin, this is best achieved by complete surgical removal of the lump with a rim of normal surrounding tissue, so that the pathologist can clearly sample and examine representative pathology, confirm adequate removal and look for signs of invasion of surrounding tissues, blood and lymphatic vessels to help deter-mine prognosis. If complete removal is not possible, e.g. where local vital tissues have been invaded, or for internal lumps, a biopsy (a piece taken by incision or needle penetration) can sometimes provide adequate tissue for a pathological diagnosis to be made. The problem with small, especially needle biopsy samples, is that they sometimes provide insufficiently representative samples upon which to make a confident diagnosis or may miss the primary pathology entirely.

TREATMENT

This entirely depends upon the diagnosis and the site or organ involved.

TYPES OF SWELLINGS OR LUMPS

Traumatic injury with a breach in the skin surface may result in externally visible **haemorrhage**. If contained within the skin or subcutaneous (under the skin) tissues and the haemorrhage is very mild, it causes discoloration of pale coloured skin forming a **bruise**. If more significant, a swelling or lump full of blood develops, called an **haematoma** ('blood blister'). Bruises, haematomas or haemorrhages caused by traumatic injury are usually best treated immedi-ately with the application of cold (cold hosing and/or ice packs) to aid the clotting process thereby minimising blood loss, the size of the resultant swelling and time to recovery. If they are large, as they can be following a kick injury to the brisket or hind quarters, they may need cold hosing and time (5-7 days) to form a **seroma** where the bleeding vessel has sealed and the blood has clotted and separated into serum. The serum is drained by surgical lancing and the wound and swelling heal in time.

If not associated with traumatic injury, haemorrhage may be a secondary complication of another medical condition, e.g. warfarin poisoning, some liver diseases and rare conditions such as haemophilia. These need urgent veterinary attention.

Infection following the introduction of pathogenic micro-organisms (bacteria or fungi) through the skin or their settling in an area of tissue after being transported via the blood stream may cause the sudden development of a hot painful **abscess**. Examples are subcutaneous abscesses caused following skin penetration injuries, most commonly associated with the ubiquitous equine skin cotaminating bacterium *Streptococcus zooepidemicus*, throat gland (sub-mandibular and parotid lymph nodes) abscesses caused following respiratory tract inhalation of the highly contagious strangles bacterium *Streptococcus equi* and bone and joint abscesses in foals caused following the flow of *Escherichia coli* bacteria around the bloodstream from the healing navel.

Abscesses are most commonly discretely hot and painful, from local tissue stretching and the production of toxins by the multiplying bacteria. The body's natural defence mechanisms include increasing blood supply to the area, bringing in white blood cells (leucocytes) whose task it is to kill and eat (phagocytose) the invading bacteria. The ensuing battle between the defending and invading 'armies' causes destruction of local tissue and pus (dead tissue, leucocytes and bacteria) forms. The initially hard abscess 'ripens', as pus forms, and 'points' as the skin and subcutaneous tissues over the abscess are progressively destroyed until they burst and pus discharges, eliminating the infection. The wound and swelling heals with time.

Abscesses are usually best treated with the application of heat (hot water bathing and/or hot poulticing), to aid natural defence mechanisms by increasing blood supply and speeding the formation of pus and the ripening process. When adequately 'ripe', the abscess can be surgically lanced and drained, to make sure that drainage occurs at the best place (not into adjacent vital organs or structures), speeding recovery. In general terms, although caused by infection, abscesses are best not treated with antibiotics because this often delays the healing process, by inhibiting pus formation and therefore ripening and discharging, and sometimes encouraging the dissemination of invading micro-organisms via the bloodstream encouraging the formation of infection elsewhere in the body. The best example of this is with strangles infection. Although *Strep. equi* is usually highly sensitive to treatment with penicillin, by the time an abscess forms and the diagnosis can be made, factors such as the developing fibrous wall and the central dying tissue inhibit penetration of the antibiotics into the area of infection. Partial cure delays the resolution of the abscesses and encourages release of infection into the blood stream causing abscesses in the chest and abdomen, resulting in chronic ill-thrift, i.e. the so-called 'bastard strangles'. A practical compromise is to wait for the abscess/abscesses to ripen, burst/be lanced and then use a full therapeutic course of appropriate antibiotics.

Some infections do not progress to form abscesses, but produce dense masses of cells including lymphocytes (another type of white blood cell involved in immune responses) and fibrous (scar) tissue which form long-lasting hard lumps which are called **granulomas**. Examples are **tubercles**, which can occur in the skin, lungs, intestines and other internal organs, caused most commonly in horses by the avian (bird) strain of the bacterium *Mycobacterium tuberculosis*. Long term treatment with specific anti-tubercular antibiotics is required. Some fungal skin infections and some chronic bacterial infections caused by *Staphylococcus aureus* (**botryomycosis**) cause granuloma formation. Their cores (centres) can become very hard when calcium, the hard mineral in bone, is formed. Blood supply into them is poor and so conventional antibiotic treatment is seldom successful and some are best treated by surgical removal. Treatment with sodium iodide by very careful intravenous injection (the drug is very damaging if released outside the vein) is sometimes helpful. Another example is the so called **'nodular skin disease'**, which forms granulomas which contain eosinophils (another white blood cell), believed to be in response to the death in-tissue of intestinal parasitic larvae (probably small strongyles) migrating in the horse's skin. They can be single or multiple and can disfigure the neck, brisket and shoulder area.

Not all granulomas are caused primarily by infection. Equine wounds, especially when they involve areas which are constantly mobile, i.e. on the legs, often produce **exuberant granulation tissue**, consisting of actively growing and multiplying blood vessels and fibrous tissue, which becomes ulcerated, bleeds and secondarily infected, and prevents the wound edges from closing. This is often called **'proud flesh'**. Depending on size and position, it is sometimes best treated by surgical 'de-bulking', followed by careful applications of copper sulphate crystals onto the bed of granulation tissue only, to gradually reduce it and allow wound healing to complete. When anticipated in a healing wound, it may be prevented by the judicious use of steroid creams. However, if over-used, these creams can delay the normal processes of wound healing. Proud flesh may be confused with sarcoids (see Figure 1) and may require removal/biopsy for laboratory differentiation. Proud flesh can sometimes transform into a sarcoid.

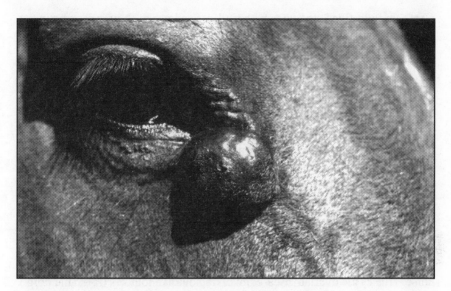

Figure 1   A sarcoid tumour on a horse's eyelid

Calculi (hard mineral 'stones') are the most common cause of lumps in the bladder of horses, and less commonly occur in the kidneys. They form from the mineral constituents of urine which, in the horse, is most commonly calcium carbonate. They cause haematuria (blood in the urine) and secondary cystitis (bladder infection). Kidney stones may cause pain and weight loss. If stones pass down and block the ureters (the tubes taking urine from the kidneys to the bladder) or urethra (the tube taking urine from the bladder to the vagina or penis), this can cause pain and, in the case of the urethra, urine blockage. In the bladder they can be palpated and examined by ultrasound scan per rectum and viewed by endoscopic examination (cystoscopy). In the kidneys stones can be seen on ultrasound scan. If producing problems, they require removal, either surgically or, in the case of small bladder stones in co-operative mares, by careful digital manipulation. Technology available in human medicine has been used to 'explode' the stones into smaller particles, sometimes with success. Attempts to disperse or dissolve the stones by dietary adjustments (altering the acidity/alkalinity of the urine) are seldom success-ful but may help to prevent re-formation in horses prone to stone formation.

Choleliths are lumps which uncommonly form in the bile duct, within the liver, of some horses. They are concretions of bile constituents and can cause abdominal discomfort, weight loss, jaundice and other signs of liver disease. Their presence can be confirmed by trans-abdominal ultrasound scan. If the common bile duct is occluded, they require attempts to remove or disperse them via abdominal surgery.

Cysts are fluid-filled structures with well-defined walls. They may occur in the skin or internal organs (e.g. kidneys) as a result of a local developmental error. In such cases they may be present and obvious from birth or may be present from birth but only apparent later when they grow to a size which causes an externally-recognisable lump or, when internal, signs of organic disease. Skin cysts, such as **epidermal and dermoid cysts** are best treated by surgical removal which, assuming normal wound healing, usually results in a complete cure. **Dentigerous cysts** cause painful hard lumps at the base of an ear in young horses. X-ray examinations confirm the aberrant growth of a tooth structure and this needs skilful surgical removal. **Polycystic kidneys** are rare in horses but if extensive enough are life-threatening in that they can cause progressive incurable renal failure. **Hydatid cysts** are not uncommonly found in the livers of horses who are in contact with dogs, typically hounds, who are infected with the parasite *Echinococcus granulosus* and who pass infective parasites in their faeces. Unless they are very large, extensive and embarrassing important blood vessels or the bile duct, these cysts seldom cause signs of clinical disease in the horse. True cystic ovarian disease, involving ovarian follicles (follicular cysts) or the corpora lutea (yellow bodies) (luteal cysts) is rare in mares. **Bone cysts** are believed to be a form of osteochondrosis (OCD), now a well-recognised problem of the joints of many types of young, growing race and other performance horses throughout the world. OCD remains an incompletely understood condition but it involves focal errors of bone development from cartilage (endochondral ossification) and can result in ulceration of joint surfaces or the formation of cystic spaces adjacent to growing joints. Cysts can occur in most bones but the bones of the stifle joint, especially the tibia, are most commonly affected. Bone cysts cause varying degrees of lameness and joint distension. Some heal or become symptomless naturally with prolonged rest and others require surgical intervention where the cyst is identified, its lining scraped (curetted) and packed with bone chips removed from the horse's hip.

New bone formation causes lumps and swellings following injury, infection or degeneration of bones and joints. It is not cancerous but can become disfiguring and painful, especially when it inhibits the mobility of a joint. It can progress to form, or be part of the development of degenerative joint disease, which is a form of arthritis. Diagnosis is confirmed with x-ray examinations. Treatment is with careful management in relation to exercise and body weight and the judicious use of non-steroidal anti-inflammatory medication, e.g. phenylbutazone.

Tumours are swelling or lumps and the term is now most commonly used for those that are cancerous, i.e. they result from abnormal chaotic cell growth in single or multiple sites. **Neoplasm** is another synonymous term used. They are defined as being **benign**, when they are usually solitary, do not invade other local tissues and do not recur following surgical removal, or **malignant**, when they invade local tissues, especially blood and lymphatic vessels and either recur locally, in regional draining lymph nodes or at remote sites in other organs, i.e. **metastasise**, following surgical removal. The prognosis for benign tumours following timely surgical removal is therefore good, whereas that for malignant tumours is not so good and, in some cases, is poor.

With the exception of warts (papillomas) on the lips of young horses, which sometimes occur in epidemic form and are believed to be primarily incited by a papilloma virus infection, the reason why horses develop cancers remains as unknown as it is for other animals. As cancer is by definition a state of cellular chaos it can develop in any tissue in any organ of the body but an interesting feature is that different animal species suffer more commonly from particular types of cancer, e.g. the common equine skin sarcoid in contrast to the rarity of mammary, uterine and cervical cancer in mares. Also, patterns of equine cancer vary geographically, e.g. the lymphosarcoma is the most common equine intestinal tumour in the UK whereas in the USA it is the gastric squamous cell carcinoma.

It is important for horse owners to remember that not all tumours are bad news and many, if diagnosed and treated early, can be successfully cured.

Equine Cancers

SKIN

The surface layer (epithelium)

Papillomas (warts) are not uncommonly found around the lips of foals and yearlings, appearing in epidemics, i.e. several individuals are affected at the same time or within a short space of time. They are small, usually multiple, raised, non-painful, cauliflower-like benign tumours. They are believed to be caused by a papilloma virus and disappear naturally when specific immunity is developed. If persistent it sometimes helps to remove some in a manner which encourages release of viral particles into the blood stream to stimulate immunity by 'vaccinating' the horse. Rarely, it may help to submit tumour tissue to a laboratory who are able to produce an autogenous vaccine for injection. A number of 'wart creams' have been commercially available but are usually very irritant or caustic and must be used with great care if the treatment is not to cause more damage than the disease will.

Squamous cell carcinomas are important potentially-malignant tumours of the eyelids, particularly the third eyelid (nictitating membrane), the skin of the penis, particularly at its tip, i.e. the urethral process, and less commonly of the vulva, particularly on or around the clitoris in horses. They can form large cauliflower-like masses which commonly become secondarily infected and very unpleasant. They require early diagnosis and radical surgical removal before they grow too large, invade local tissues and spread to local lymph nodes. If removed early, there is often a complete cure, but if not they frequently recur. Complete amputation of an affected third eyelid or clitoris is recommended, earlier rather than later, and is usually very effective. Penile amputation is usually a last resort and amputees thereafter require careful sheath management. It is reported that radioactive gold implantation may help in cases where complete surgical removal is impossible because of invasion of surrounding tissues, e.g. around the eye.

Basal cell carcinomas occur uncommonly in horses at a variety of skin sites. They are solid, raised, discrete tumours involving the surface layer of the skin only, which are usually benign and respond well to complete surgical removal.

Melanomas are tumours of the pigment-producing cells of the surface layer of the skin and can be easily recognised by their solid, raised black appearance. They are very common in grey horses to the extent that it has been said that all grey horses will eventually develop them if they live long enough. They occur most commonly around the anus, tail, vulva, sheath and abdomen, although they can occur anywhere in the skin. They are usually benign but multiply locally and elsewhere to the extent that surgical removal is seldom a practical undertaking and many grey horses live out their lives with them. Occasionally, they may ulcerate, bleed and become secondarily infected and then removal is sometimes attempted, but when they invade around the anus, as is common, this is seldom possible. It has been reported that long-term treatment with an anti-gastric ulcer drug (cimetidine) has helped some cases but more experience with this form of therapy needs to be gained before reliable claims can be made. Malignant melanomas are rare in the horse but unfortunately metastasise aggressively throughout internal organs. They are untreatable and affected horses require euthanasia on humane grounds.

The skin glands

Sebaceous and sweat gland carcinomas occur rarely in horses at a variety of skin sites. They are solid, raised, discrete tumours involving the surface layer of the skin only, which are usually benign and respond well to complete surgical removal.

The dermis (main layer of skin)

Fibromas are tumours of the fibrous architecture of the skin and are the most common skin tumour of horses. They occur most frequently on the head, limbs and groin. They are non-painful, solitary, hard, pale in colour and can be easily moved over the subcutaneous tissues. The skin surface may thin and the tumour can sometimes easily 'shell out' (like shelling a pea) cleanly with digital manipulation. They are benign but can recur locally. If this is not possible they should be removed surgically because of their potential to transform into sarcoids.

Sarcoids, sometimes called 'angleberries', are also very common skin tumours in horses. They are sometimes classified as low-grade fibrosarcomas. They also occur most frequently on the head, especially around the eyes (Figure 1) and ears, limbs, groin and abdomen. They are often raised and discrete, sometimes multiple, and less commonly flat and more diffuse. Many ulcerate, bleed and become secondarily infected. They are often multiple and are said to be of low-grade malignancy in that they frequently spread locally and recur after conventional surgical removal. They sometimes appear along the line of wound healing after an injury and sometimes transform from 'proud flesh' exuberant granulation tissue (see above) or a previously benign fibroma. Laboratory differentiation of surgically-removed tissue is essential to confirm the diagnosis.

Many and varied treatments, including combinations of conventional, cryo (freezing) and laser surgical removal have been used for sarcoids over many years with variable success. Repeated fortnightly injections with anti-tubercular (BCG) vaccine or implantation with radioactive gold seeds or iridium wires has been successful for some, especially those around the eyes. Currently, good results are often obtained with the application of a specially-formulated 'sarcoid cream', available from the University of Liverpool Veterinary School, sometimes following surgical 'de-bulking' of the tumour. Where the tumours are extensive and involving many skin sites, such treatments may be impractical and some success has occasionally been achieved by repeated periodic vaccination with an autogenous vaccine, i.e. one specifically prepared from tumour tissue from the horse involved. It has to be said that some cases defeat all attempts at treatment, but this is less common now than it used to be, with earlier diagnosis and treatment, using combination therapy.

Fibrosarcomas are much less commonly seen in the skin of horses and usually involve the lower limbs. They are seldom malignant in terms of metastasis but can become very extensive and invasive to the extent that they are sometimes uncontrollable and then require euthanasia on humane grounds.

Haemangiomas and haemangioendotheliomas are rare tumours of the walls of the blood vessels in the skin. They have been seen primarily on the shoulders and neck. Haemangiomas are benign and form cavernous blood-filled spaces like varicose veins, which are prone to injury and haemorrhage. They can sometimes be surgically removed with careful attention to closure of the large blood vessels supplying the tumour and seldom recur. Haemangioendotheliomas are aggressively locally-invasive, malignant and very difficult to remove and affected horses require euthanasia on humane grounds.

Lipomas are tumours of the fat deposits and are rarely seen in or under the skin of horses. Benign tumours are easily and usually successfully removed by surgical excision. A rare case of aggressively malignant mixed myxoliposarcoma has been seen, initially involving a hind leg, which required euthanasia on humane grounds.

Mastocytomas, involving the mast cells, are uncommon in the skin of horses, but can occur at any site. They are usually single, raised and often ulcerated. In the horse they are usually benign and respond well to early complete surgical removal.

Histiocytomas and lymphosarcomas are tumours of the lymphatic (immune) cells, which can occur anywhere in the skin. Histiocytomas are rare in horses and are usually single, raised and non-ulcerated, and they respond well to complete surgical removal if performed early. Lymphosarcomas are the most commonly seen tumours of the intestines of horses in the UK (see below), but the generalised (lymphoma) and skin forms are much less common. Skin lymphosarcomas are often part of the generalised condition and produce widespread thickenings of the skin, which do not ulcerate. They are usually a sign that metastasis to internal organs has already occurred and affected horses require euthanasia on humane grounds.

GASTROINTESTINAL SYSTEM

The mouth

Fibromas and **fibrosarcomas** of the gums and **osteogenic fibromas** of the jaws are uncommonly seen in horses. They are usually benign but there can be difficulties in removing them when, like osteomas (see below) they invade the bone around the teeth.

The stomach

Squamous cell carcinomas are the most commonly reported gastric tumour in the horse. They appear much more common in some countries, e.g. USA, than in others, e.g. UK, for reasons which are unknown, but may reflect differences in diet. They are invasive, often malignant tumours of the squamous (part closest to the oesophagus) portion of the stomach, can erode through its wall, causing peritonitis, and can metastasise to adjacent organs, e.g. the diaphragm and liver and throughout the peritoneal cavity (the large cavity that contains the abdominal organs) and less commonly the thoracic cavity (the cavity in the chest which contains the lungs and heart). The condition is untreatable and affected horses require euthanasia on humane grounds.

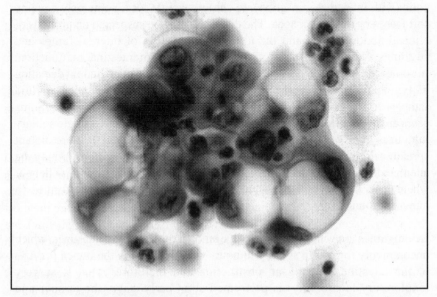

Figure 2   Microscopic picture of cancer cells in a horse's peritoneal (abdominal) fluid

Adenocarcinomas of the glandular (part furthest from the oesophagus) portion of the stomach are much less common. They are malignant tumours which aggressively metastasise throughout the abdominal and thoracic organs.

For both types of tumour, affected horses loose their appetite and weight and show varying degree of colic. The diagnoses can be made by gastroscopic examinations of the stomach, during which biopsy samples may be obtained. Microscopic (cytological) examinations of peritoneal fluid samples may also be a helpful diagnostic aid. The condition is untreatable and affected horses require euthanasia on humane grounds.

The intestines

Lymphosarcomas are the most commonly seen tumours of the intestines of the horse in the UK. The tumours develop either primarily in the lymphatic tissue of the walls of any areas of the intestines or may spread metastatically to the intestines from the lymphatic tissue in other organs, e.g. the spleen. They are either round firm solitary tumours which can block the lumen (cavity) of the intestine, causing an obstruction, or may diffuse throughout the wall of the intestine, causing intestinal malfunction in terms of motility and absorptive capability. Intestinal lymphosarcoma may be part of a generalised lymphoma, where tumours develop throughout the body, bloodstream and skin.

Affected horses show a wide variety of clinical abnormalities from acute colic (with intestinal impaction), to chronic weight loss. Some may develop soft faeces or frank diarrhoea. The diagnosis may be suspected on grounds of clinical abnormalities and the ultrasonic detection of internal lumps and swellings. Oral glucose absorption tests may confirm intestinal malfunction. In some cases, the diagnosis may be confirmed by the microscopic detection of lymphatic tumour cells in blood samples, peritoneal or pleural fluid samples or in organ biopsy samples, e.g. the rectum, intestines or spleen. Some cases are not confirmable until examined postmortem. Where a single solitary tumour is involved and there are no obvious signs of local or more distant spread, surgical removal of the affected bowel (enterectomy) may be attempted. Where the tumour has spread locally or has metastasised widely or where generalised lymphoma is involved, euthanasia should be performed on humane grounds.

Leiomyomas are benign tumours of the smooth muscle of the intestines, which uncommonly form firm solitary tumours which can block the lumen (cavity) of the intestine, causing an obstruction and therefore colic. If surgery (exploratory laparotomy) is performed at an early stage, the tumour and surrounding intestine can sometimes (depending on site and accessibility) be removed (enterectomy) with successful results.

The rectum

Adenomas and **adenocarcinomas**, i.e. the benign and malignant forms of glandular tumours of the rectal wall are very rare in horses.

The peritoneal surfaces

Lipomas are benign tumours which form in the fat deposits around the intestines and elsewhere in the peritoneal cavity. They are benign tumours which are seldom of consequence themselves, unless they transform into the malignant form, called the **liposarcoma**. In older horses and ponies, as the tumours become older, they loose their blood supply and form a stalk, which lengthens and can loop around a section of intestine, strangulating its blood supply. This results in acute colic and the death of the length of strangulated intestine. Affected horses require urgent abdominal surgery (laparotomy) to confirm the diagnosis, to remove the fatty tumour and to release the strangulated intestine. In many cases, the affected intestine is non-viable and must then be removed (enterectomy). If surgery is delayed, the strangulated intestine leaks, causes peritonitis and the horse may require euthanasia on humane grounds.

Mesotheliomas are uncommon tumours of the lining cells of the peritoneal (abdominal) cavity and less commonly the pleural (thoracic). They are invasive, malignant tumours which metastasise across the surfaces of either cavity and cause massive fluid swelling of the abdomen, with acute colic, or of the chest, with respiratory difficulties. The diagnosis can be made by microscopic examination of peritoneal (Figure 2) or pleural fluid. The condition is untreatable and affected horses require euthanasia on humane grounds.

LIVER, PANCREAS AND SPLEEN

Hepatomas are rare tumours of the liver in horses. They can cause fatal internal abdominal haemorrhage.

Bile duct carcinomas are occasionally seen in the liver of horses. They form in the walls of the bile ducts and cause blockage to bile flow, resulting in jaundice and progressive liver failure. The diagnosis can be suspected following abnormal blood test results for liver disease with ultrasound scan examinations of the liver and can be confirmed by liver biopsy. The condition is untreatable and affected horses require euthanasia on humane grounds.

Pancreatic tumours have not been reported in horses.

Splenic tumours in horses are most commonly lymphosarcomas (see above), and much less commonly haemangiomas and haemangioendotheliomas (see above).

RESPIRATORY SYSTEM

Nasal passages and sinuses

Atheromas and nasal polyps are benign fibrous tumours which are usually solitary and, if large enough, may cause obstruction to the affected nasal passage, when they can be removed surgically, with a good prognosis for complete recovery. Atheromas grow in the nostrils and cause a visible swelling. Nasal polyps may only be found during endoscopic investigations of noisy respiration.

Squamous cell and adenocarcinomas are highly invasive and sometimes malignant tumours which can occur in the nasal chamber, sinus and guttural pouch linings. They can cause a 'snoring' respiratory noise and the horse to be depressed, loose appetite and weight. They may cause distortion of the facial bones, over the tumour. X-ray examinations reveal a space-occupying mass where an air-filled chamber should be and the diagnosis can be confirmed by biopsy examination. Some cases have responded very successfully to radiation therapy, but most affected horses require euthanasia on humane grounds.

Progressive ethmoid haematomas are unusual benign tumours of the upper respiratory tract surfaces which only occur in horses. They cause nasal haemorrhage and abnormal respiratory noise from obstruction. They are diagnosed on endoscopic examination and often respond well to skilled surgical removal, which involves an approach through the nasal sinus and a great deal of haemorrhage. Some recur at the same site, especially if it was not possible to remove all the tumour tissue at the first attempt.

Lungs

Adenomas and adenocarcinomas are very rare benign and malignant forms of tumours of the lung of horses.

Secondary tumour metastases sometimes occur in the lungs of horses after metastatic spread from a variety of malignant tumours elsewhere in the body.

GENITAL ORGANS

Penis

Squamous cell carcinoma of the penis has been discussed under skin tumours (see above).

Testicles

Seminomas are uncommon benign tumours of the old stallion, who gradually develop one large usually non-painful testicle. Digital palpation and ultrasound examination reveals a solid, homogenous testicle with no fluid or cystic spaces. Treatment is to remove the abnormal testicle by unilateral castration. The other testicle is usually unaffected and fertility is maintained unless its temperature is increased by the adjacent enlarged testicle, causing thermal damage to sperm production.

Teratomas appear to be less common now than they were reported to have been in the older veterinary literature, when heavy working horses were common. They affect young horses and usually involve one testicle. They grow and develop abnormal non-ovarian tissues such as hair and teeth. The latter can be seen during ultrasound scan examination. Treatment is by surgical removal, as for seminomas. They are usually benign but it is reported that in rare cases one of the non-testicular tissue components may metastasise.

Leydig and Sertoli cell tumours are exceedingly rare in horses.

Prostate gland tumours have not been recorded in horses.

Vulva and vagina

Squamous cell carcinoma of the clitoris or vulva has been discussed under skin tumours (see above).

Fibromas may unusually occur in the vaginal wall of mares, producing a hard 'polyp'. They are benign and may be relatively easily removed by surgical excision through a large duck-billed speculum, under local anaesthesia, with the mare standing in stocks.

Cervix and uterus

Leiomyomas and fibroleiomyomas are hard benign tumours of the smooth muscle in the wall of the cervix or uterus. They are usually small, discrete and innocuous, but can ulcerate and bleed if they grow large. Such cases will require surgical removal either through a large duck-billed speculum, under local anaesthesia, with the mare standing in stocks or by major abdominal operation (hysterotomy) under general anaesthesia or sometimes standing under local flank anaesthesia, as appropriate to the mare and the site of the tumour.

Adenomas and adenocarcinomas are exceedingly rare malignant tumours of the uterus in mares. One case reported in the veterinary literature metastasised to the lungs and required euthanasia on humane grounds.

Ovaries

Granulosa cell tumours are the most common tumour of the mare. They are benign, affect both young and old mares and have only very rarely been reported to involve both ovaries. The typical finding is of one large (sometimes very large) and hard ovary, whilst the other is very small and inactive. The mare does not show normal oestrous cycles, but may behave unusually, depending upon the abnormal hormones that the tumourous ovary produces. Some mares become virile and aggressive (excessive testosterone production), whilst others become nymphomaniacal (excessive oestrogen production) and others become highly maternal (excessive progesterone production). Other mares show no signs of abnormal behaviour.

Ultrasound scan examinations confirm one large polycystic ovary, whilst the other is very small, solid and inactive. The diagnosis is not always straight forward in the early stages, but if repeated examinations performed over time confirm the large ovary to be growing and the small ovary to be shrinking, the diagnosis can be accurately made. Abnormally high hormone levels can occasionally be measured in blood samples taken from affected mares, most commonly those who are aggressive and virile (high testosterone and/or oestrone sulphate levels). The diagnosis cannot be ruled out by normal hormone levels in blood samples.

The treatment is to remove the one large ovary surgically, either by a major abdominal operation (laparotomy) under general anaesthesia or by 'keyhole surgery' (laparoscopy) with the mare standing under local flank anaesthesia. The ovary must be fully removed and its large blood vessels safely ligated (tied off) to prevent haemorrhage. The ovary can then be submitted for laboratory examinations and the diagnosis can be confirmed. Following removal of its hormonal inhibition, the other (small) ovary will, over time, grow and regain its function and the mare resumes her oestrous cycles and her fertility.

Teratomas appear to be less common now than they were reported to have been in the older veterinary literature, when heavy working horses were common. They are benign and usually involve one ovary. They grow and develop abnormal non-ovarian tissues such as hair and teeth. The latter can be seen during ultrasound scan examination. Treatment is by surgical removal, as for granulosa cell tumours.

Adenocarcinomas are malignant tumours of the ovary which are rarely seen in mares. They cause colic, abdominal fluid distension (ascites) and ill-thrift when they metastasise throughout the peritoneal cavity, growing on and in the abdominal organs, e.g. kidneys, intestines and liver. Affected mares require euthanasia on humane grounds.

Cystic ovaries are not commonly seen in mares. Occasionally, a persistently large ovary may develop while the mare continues to enjoy apparently normal oestrous cycles with the other ovary remaining of normal size and cyclic activity. The large ovary does not usually have the typical polycystic ultrasound appearance of a granulosa cell tumour. These mares can conceive from the normal ovary and undergo an apparently normal pregnancy to produce a healthy foal. The large ovary sometimes resolves back to normality during the pregnancy and must be assumed to have been 'cystic'. Others persist as being enlarged, sometimes containing a large semi-turbid fluid containing cyst. When removed surgically, some have been confirmed as follicular cysts (originating from an ovarian follicle) and other as luteal cysts (originating from a corpus luteum). Occasionally mares bleed excessively into their ovaries after ovulation, forming a haematoma. Some haematomas can become very large and even painful and if they do not resolve may require surgical removal.

Providing the mare is not adversely affected by the abnormal ('cystic') ovary, time should be given to allow opportunity for natural resolution before surgical removal is considered. It has often been suggested that behavioural changes or uncooperative behaviour in mares is caused by 'cystic' ovaries. Some such cases have had their ovaries removed only to find that they appear normal on laboratory examination and the mare continues to behave badly. It may be wise to consider test therapy with progesterone and to show beneficial behavioural effects before making a decision for ovariectomy in such mares.

Mammary glands

Adenomas and **adenocarcinomas** are very rare in mares, but are malignant and affected horses require mastectomy or euthanasia on humane grounds. Lumps or swellings in the udder are more likely to be inflammatory in origin, i.e. abscesses or granulomas. Lumps or swellings on the udder are more likely to be skin tumours, e.g. fibromas or sarcoids (see above).

KIDNEYS AND BLADDER

Transitional cell papillomas and carcinomas have only very rarely been reported in the bladder of horses. They cause haematuria and secondary cystitis. Bladder carcinomas are invasive and potentially malignant. Renal (kidney) carcinomas are rare but are aggressively malignant in the peritoneal cavity. Bladder and renal carcinomas are untreatable and affected horses require euthanasia on humane grounds.

Polyps are benign fibrous lumps which have rarely been recorded in the bladder of horses, causing haematuria and secondary cystitis. They can be removed surgically via cystotomy.

The most common cause of haematuria and secondary cystitis in horses is bladder calculi (stones) (see above).

MUSCULOSKELETAL SYSTEM

Muscles

Rhabdomyomas and **rhabdomyosarcomas** are benign and malignant forms of tumours of the muscles, most commonly forming in the limbs and heart muscles. They are extremely rare in horses.

Bones

Osteomas are benign but disfiguring tumours of the bones, most commonly seen in the head, especially the jaw of younger horses, even foals, where they can disrupt tooth growth. Diagnosis is made on the basis of x-ray and biopsy examination results. They can sometimes be removed surgically with good results.

Osteosarcomas are the malignant form, which are rare in horses, where again they occur most commonly in the bones of the head. They grow rapidly, are painful, locally invasive and can metastasise widely. Diagnosis is made on the basis of X-ray and biopsy examination results. The condition is untreatable and affected horses require euthanasia on humane grounds.

Chondromas and chondrosarcomas, involving the cartilage component of bone, are very rare in horses.

Keratomas are unusual but well-recognised benign tumours of the horse's hoof. Lameness and disfigured hoof growth, particularly at the front of the hoof, is often the first sign. X-ray examinations reveal an apparently circular 'hole' in the hoof wall, which is in fact filled by developing tumour tissue rather than hoof. If diagnosed before major hoof deformity and secondary complications develop, these tumours respond well to surgical removal of the abnormal hoof wall and careful protective bandaging until new replacement hoof grows down.

Joints and tendon sheaths

Synoviomas and **synoviocytomas** are benign and malignant forms of tumours of the lining membranes of joints and tendon sheaths. They are extremely rare in horses.

ENDOCRINE GLANDS

Thyroid glands

Adenomas are relatively common in horses, causing a non-painful swelling of one side of the thyroid gland in the throat, like a goitre. They are benign and only require surgical removal if they are causing obstruction in the throat or appear to be adversely affecting the horse's behaviour, either hyperexcitability or persistent lethargy. **Adenocarcinomas** are the uncommon malignant form, which grow rapidly and are difficult to remove surgically as they invade adjacent vital structures in the throat, i.e. trachea, carotid artery, jugular vein and nerves.

Pituitary gland

Adenomas are slow-growing and benign and not uncommonly seen in usually old horses. The pituitary gland is located inside the base of the skull, immediately beneath the brain and attached to it by a stalk. The gland is responsible for regulating a number of other hormone-producing glands, e.g. the testicles, ovaries and the adrenal glands. Disruption of the adrenal gland's ability to control blood cortisol levels can lead to an interesting condition known as Cushing's syndrome in affected horses, where they become unable to shed their hair coat and become characteristically long and curly coated, they sweat in patches, drink and urinate excessively and their abdomen becomes 'pear shaped'. They are susceptible to complicating liver failure and recurrent laminitis. The diagnosis of Cushing's disease is made on the basis of these typical clinical signs, and by showing high blood and urine glucose levels, high blood insulin levels and abnormal blood cortisol regulation. Typical cases are straightforward to diagnose but early cases in younger horses may present quite a challenge, with often conflicting hormone test results.

Treatment with daily anti-cancer medication by mouth has been successful in some younger cases who have not developed serious secondary complications.

Adrenal glands

Adenomas may occur in the cortex (outer layer) of the adrenal glands, next to the kidneys, of older horses who show no obvious signs of clinical abnormality. **Adenocarcinomas** are the malignant form, which is rare, but can cause colic, weight loss and abdominal fluid distension as the tumour metastasises aggressively throughout the peritoneal cavity. **Phaeochromocytomas** rarely occur in the medulla (inner structure) of the adrenal gland and disrupt the horse's ability to regulate fluid and electrolyte balance. Euthanasia is required on humane grounds.

BLOOD VASCULAR SYSTEM

Lymphomas and lymphosarcomas can occur in any blood or lymphatic vessels anywhere in the body. They are the most common intestinal tumours of horses in the UK (see above).

Lymphoma is the generalised form of the disease where the cancer of the lymphocytes (immune cells of the blood and tissues) spreads throughout the body. The horse is depressed, looses appetite and weight and shows a variety of symptoms depending upon which internal organs are most affected. Laboratory examinations of blood samples reveal very high white cell counts and microscopic examinations confirm large numbers of circulating cancerous lymphocytes. The skin may be 'lumpy' with tumour tissue and cancerous lymphocytes can be found in peritoneal and pleural fluids and in biopsy samples taken from a variety of organs. The condition is untreatable and affected horses require euthanasia on humane grounds.

Haemangiomas and haemangioendotheliomas are unusual benign and malignant tumours of the blood vessel walls. In horses they are most commonly seen in the skin (see above) and spleen.

Plasma cell myelomas are rare malignant tumours of antibody-producing cells in the bone marrow, which may form in the spinal column or limb bones. They, and sometimes lymphosarcomas, produce large quantities of abnormal antibodies which can be demonstrated in the blood of affected horses by special tests (protein electrophoresis). The condition is untreatable and affected horses require euthanasia on humane grounds.

CENTRAL NERVOUS SYSTEM

Astrocytomas have rarely been reported to occur in the cerebrum and cerebellum of the brain of older horses, **papillomas and carcinomas** in the choroid plexus and **meningiomas** in various parts of the brain, causing major neurological abnormality. These conditions are untreatable and affected horses require euthanasia on humane grounds. Brain tumours are, in general, extremely rare in horses and neurological abnormality is much more likely to be caused by injury, infection or toxicosis.

It can therefore be seen that equine lumps and swellings can be caused by a variety of conditions, the least common of which are serious cancers. The most important action is to achieve an early accurate diagnosis so that appropriate treatment can be applied while treatment can be successful and before secondary complications occur. Your veterinary surgeon will be able to help you with this or, if appropriate, he or she may wish to find expert help.

Management
and Husbandry

How we manage, feed and maintain our horses is one of the most important subjects for the lay reader. It is very much a part of the responsibility of owners, managers, trainers and lay personnel associated with horses. Chapters in this section cover the following subjects:

* Behavioural problems in horses frequently encountered by owners.

* Diets and feeding of horses for various purposes. Energy to support performance and work is necessary if we are to achieve the objectives for which we keep our horses; and the inclusion in the diet of basic substances required for growth is essential, especially for young horses. At the end of the chapter is a table of causes and symptoms of malnutrition.

* The chapter with the description of the relationship between soundness and conformation has been retained from the previous edition of this book. The assessment of conformation is a subjective matter and the older veterinary practitioners probably had greater insight into the subject than their present-day counterparts.

* *Equus caballus*, the modern horse, has been bred by man into types as different as the Falabella and the Shetland, the

Clydesdale, the Shire and the racehorse. These differences have been produced by selection based on the genetic composition of what we now describe as breeds. Successive chapters in this section deal with genetics of the horse, and the importance of selective breeding.

* Finally in this section an equestrian has a number of
practical comments to make about the care and management of the hunter.

43
BEHAVIOURAL PROBLEMS

There are a number of problems encountered in the day-to-day management of horses which can be grouped together loosely as behavioural problems. These include weaving, windsucking, crib-biting, excessively mareish behaviour, unusual aggression, rearing, bucking, nappiness, extreme coldback behaviour, unwillingness to work on the bit, headshaking, unwillingness to load into a trailer or horsebox, and travelling badly. This is by no means a complete list but it encompasses the most common problems. Some of these problems may have a primary veterinary cause, for example, back pain causing nappiness or a nutritional deficiency predisposing to woodchewing. However, many of the problems are true behavioural problems, perhaps related to previous or current management practices, or are of unknown cause.

It is important to recognise that horses and ponies vary considerably in their temperaments, their willingness to oblige and to submit to handling and working. Although not exceptionally intelligent animals, they are strong, much stronger than any person, and readily recognise a handler who is apprehensive or not a strict disciplinarian, and many will be inclined to try to take advantage of such a situation. Once a horse has got away with unruly behaviour it will often try to do so again. What starts as a very minor problem can become a major problem which may make, for example, the horse unsuitable to be ridden by that particular rider or somebody of similar experience and ability. That is not to say that the problem is incurable – given the right handling the horse may become extremely amenable – but generally a difficult horse will always need skilful (not necessarily forceful) handling. Some problems may be persistent despite expert handling: for example, there have been a number of top-class international showjumpers which have been extremely difficult to mount.

One particular horse-rider combination may be totally unsuited. A rider must be prepared to recognise this and at times be ready to admit defeat and sell the horse to a more suitable rider. Another problem can arise if a relatively inexperienced rider is receiving advice from an expert in whom he or she understandably has faith. Occasionally this so-called expert is not such an expert (he or she may be very competent to handle easy horses, but may have limited experience with a large variety of difficult horses). It can be very difficult for an independent adviser to convey this diplomatically to the rider and to advise that the rider seeks the help of a different expert.

It is also important to realise that sometimes it is necessary to be quite aggressively firm in order to get a horse to submit to discipline. Quiet kindness certainly has a role in horse management and must not be undervalued, but this is not always the most appropriate method.

An objective assessment of some behavioural problems is not easy. Ideally it requires a thorough understanding of horses' temperaments and psychology, a knowledge of veterinary medicine and an ability to recognise good and bad handling and riding of horses, and to identify when there is a mismatch between horse and rider. The aims of investigation of a behavioural problem include identifying whether the problem has a painful or other medical cause, or is purely behavioural or related to the relationship between the horse and its rider or manager.

REARING, BUCKING, NAPPINESS

A horse which repeatedly bucks, rears or naps may become a potential danger to the rider, particularly if the behaviour is unpredictable and may occur on a road. A similar approach is adopted to the investigation of all these problems. First, it must be established how long the horse has been in the owner's possession. Does it have a history of awkward behaviour? How soon after purchase did the problem arise? Could the onset be related to any specific incident – a fall, for example? Does the horse act similarly on the lunge or only when ridden? Does it behave the same with different riders? It is also important to learn whether the behaviour occurs only under certain circumstances – for example, only at a competition; if this is the case, it is unlikely to be related to a medical problem. Then the temperament of the horse and of the rider is assessed and the ability of the rider and or manager. Does, for example, the rider sit straight or put weight heavily on one side, predisposing to the development of back muscle soreness? The fitting of the saddle and bridle and the suitability of the bit are assessed. It is also useful to review the feeding of the horse – it may be receiving too much food and may be much more manageable when receiving considerably less.

A complete physical examination of the horse is performed to try to identify any medical problems. Special attention is paid to the mouth – the presence of sores in the corners, sharp edges on the teeth, an oddly positioned tooth, especially if it is slightly movable and the bit is likely to come in contact with it. Wolf teeth rarely cause a problem unless they are movable or positioned abnormally far forward. Other areas meriting particularly careful attention are the back, sternum and ribs, and, of course, the limbs. A horse with a low-grade bilateral lameness may be unwilling to go forward and may nap.

It is important to evaluate the horse not only at rest and in hand, but also ridden, both by the regular rider and by a genuine expert – a horseman rather than somebody who may have official qualifications but may lack widespread experience of problem horses. In some cases it may be necessary for that person to ride the horse for several days in succession before an answer can be reached.

Based upon the results of all these investigations, additional diagnostic tests may be indicated, for example, radiography, assessment of concentrations of serum muscle enzymes in the blood before and after exercise. Nuclear scintigraphy (bone scanning) can be useful in cases with multiple sites of pain or when symptoms are subtle. Soft tissue scintigraphy can also be performed to look for some injuries to soft tissues (muscle, ligament etc.). In some cases it can be very useful to treat the horse with a painkiller such as phenylbutazone to assess whether the problem is pain-related. The horse must be treated at a sufficiently high dose for its bodyweight, and for long enough in order to make a proper judgement of the drug's efficacy. The horse must also be maintained in work. The author usually recommends that a horse of 500 kg bodyweight should be treated with 2-3 g phenylbutazone daily for at least four weeks.

Possible causes

Underlying medical problems which may cause this type of behaviour include back pain, neck pain or a mouth or tooth problem. The reader is advised to refer to the relevant chapters in this book for further information. Other causes include poorly fitting tack, a rider problem, overfeeding and a genuinely difficult horse. The question 'Is the horse suitable for the rider?' must be asked.

Treatment

If a medical cause is found this can be treated accordingly. If no underlying cause is identified, then it is usually worthwhile seeking the help of a genuinely expert horseman. This may simply be with a view to improving the horse so that it is suitable to be sold to a more experienced rider. If the horse is nappy it may benefit from a complete change of job for a while; for example, a horse that has become nappy in the show ring may benefit tremendously from spending a season hunting or being turned out for several months.

THE HORSE THAT WILL NOT WORK ON THE BIT

The horse is said to be working 'on the bit' if it is pushing evenly with its hind limbs, with impulsion, is reasonably relaxed in the back, and is accepting the bit so that the head is positioned slightly in front of a vertical line. The conformation of the horse may limit its ability to do this properly and to maintain it throughout all movements. Many inexperienced riders do not appreciate the importance of the horse pushing properly from behind: unless the horse is moving freely forward with adequate hind-limb impulsion it cannot be said to be on the bit. In order to achieve this the horse must be pushed forwards – it is not achieved by pulling the horse's head into the appropriate position and restricting its forward movement. This tends to create stiffness and possibly an irregular hind-limb rhythm. There is a certain knack in encouraging horses to work on the bit and this is probably one of the most elusive skills for inexperienced or uneducated riders, or for those who lack real feel for the way the horse is responding to the aids. There are medical causes for a horse's reluctance to work on the bit, many of which are shared with the horse that naps, so the reader is advised to refer to the preceding discussion.

Treatment
If a medical cause is identified it must be treated appropriately if possible. Conformational abnormalities which make it mechanically and physically difficult for the horse to work on the bit must be recognized and the shortcomings of the horse appreciated. It may be suitable for many purposes other than dressage. A change of rider may provide the key to success: a horse which is difficult to get on the bit may be improved dramatically by an experienced, skilled rider, and when worked in this way for several weeks may begin to find it easier. It will develop strength in the appropriate muscles and may become appreciably easier for the regular rider to cope with. Work on the lunge with the horse in a Chambon or running (draw) reins may serve the same purpose provided the horse is encouraged to work sufficiently hard from behind. If done carefully, it may also be helpful to ride the horse in draw reins. It must always be remembered that the engine is in the rear of the horse and that the horse must be pushing properly from behind if it is to be on the bit.

EXCESSIVELY COLD-BACK BEHAVIOUR

Cold-back behaviour refers to the horse which tenses abnormally or sinks (lowers) the back either when tacked up, when the girth is tightened or when the rider mounts. Some horses arch the back and buck repeatedly. A few horses throw themselves to the ground, which can be very alarming and is potentially dangerous.

Causes
In many horses there is no underlying cause. The horse performs quite normally in all other respects so it may seem illogical to presume that some-

thing hurts only when the saddle is placed on the horse's back or when the rider mounts. Nevertheless this is not true of all cases. Causes of cold back behaviour include poorly fitting tack resulting in a sore back (for example, a saddle with too narrow a tree causing undue pressure on the areas on either side of the withers), an overtight girth (especially if the girth has an elastic insert), other causes of back pain, a previous fracture of a rib or the sternum, and girth galls.

Investigation
Investigation of this problem follows much the same pattern as that for napping. Particular attention is paid to the back and chest, the fitting of the tack, the way the horse reacts when the saddle is lowered into place, when the girth is tightened and when the horse first moves forward, the way in which the rider mounts (whether he or she pulls excessively on the saddle, sticks a toe into the horse's side, sits down heavily onto the horse) and whether or not the rider sits straight. The reaction to a roller being placed on the back is compared.

Treatment
If an underlying cause can be identified appropriate action can be taken. If no cause can be identified there are several approaches which may help. The saddle can be placed on the horse several minutes before the girth is fastened. A clean, thick, well-fitting numnah may be used beneath the saddle. The girth is done up loosely at first, the horse is walked forwards and the girth is then tightened slowly. Although superficially it would seem that a girth with an elastic insert would allow more give, and would thus be better tolerated by the horse, such a girth tends to be done up more tightly than non-elasticated girths; some horses may resent this but behave normally if a non-elasticated girth is used. Some horses benefit from being lunged for a while, with the saddle on, before the rider mounts. The rider may either be given a leg up or use a mounting block so that the girth need not be excessively tight and the saddle is not unduly pulled as the rider mounts. Initially it may be necessary for the horse to be led. Some horses remain very difficult, and although this may be acceptable in a competition horse, managed by a professional, such a horse is generally unsuitable for an amateur who rides for pleasure.

HEADSHAKING

Headshaking is a poorly understood syndrome in the horse which occurs most frequently during the summer months and is often worst when the weather is sunny, rather than overcast, and warm. Headshaking behaviour varies from a slight twitch of the head from side to side, or a slight nod, to vigorous up-and-down movements of the head. The horse may repeatedly try to rub its nose against one of the forelimbs, or may strike out repeatedly with its forelimbs. In the majority of affected horses the behaviour occurs only when the horse is ridden, but a few horses demonstrate headshaking at rest or when worked on the lunge. The problem may be sudden in onset and disappear just as suddenly, or it may be persistent or intermittent, occurring only during the summer. Some horses may be severely affected if worked outside but much better if worked indoors, suggesting that exposure to high concentrations of ultraviolet light may be an inciting factor.

Causes
In the majority of horses it is not possible to identify a cause despite an intensive investigation. Possible causes include poorly fitting tack, lameness, a tumour or other type of growth in the head, the presence of mites in the ears, vision difficulties, infection of a tooth root and an allergic type of reaction or undue sensitivity to something in the environment. In some horses headshaking seems to be triggered by bright sunlight.

Investigation
A complete physical examination must be performed, paying especial attention to the head, neck and back. The eyes are examined carefully (see chapter 9) and an endoscopic examination of the upper respiratory tract is performed. Radiographs of the head are obtained. It is worthwhile treating the ears with a drug that kills mites (an acaricide). It is sometimes helpful to see if the behaviour is altered by painkilling or tranquillising drugs.

Treatment
If an underlying cause is identified this can be treated appropriately, but in the vast majority of cases the cause remains obscure. Some horses improve if a stocking is placed over their nose when ridden. Others are helped by a change of occupation. Many horses show total remission of clinical signs during the winter, only for the problem to recur the following summer. It has been suggested that neuralgia of the facial nerve (pain associated with the facial nerve) might be a cause, and cutting the nerve has been performed with generally poor results. More recently a combination of drugs (carbamazepine plus cyproheptadine) used to treat trigeminal nerve neuralgia in humans has been tried with headshakers with some success. In a few of those cases where bright light is a triggering factor coloured contact lenses have resulted in complete remission of the signs. This is an extremely frustrating condition to deal with because so little is known about why it happens, so there is no logical method of approach to treatment.

EXCESSIVELY MAREISH BEHAVIOUR

Some mares are very unpredictable in their performance especially when in season. They may show reluctance to go forward freely, swish the tail excessively, repeatedly pass small volumes of urine or wink the vulva, or uncharacteristically refuse to jump. The exact underlying cause remains uncertain but presumably it is the result of variations in the concentrations of certain hormones at different stages of the oestrous cycle. In many mares the problem is controlled by suppression of oestrus, which can be achieved by the administration of a prostagen drug, allyl trenbolone. This drug is administered in the feed, and while the mare is being treated the oestrous cycle will be suppressed. After cessation of treatment the mare will return to oestrus in approximately eight days. In some mares, however, the 'mareish' behaviour persists even during treatment. In these mares the cause of behaviour is most likely to be temperamental rather than hormonal.

AGGRESSION

Abnormally aggressive behaviour may be seen in mares, entire males and castrated males. Aggression may be directed towards other horses or towards handlers. In some instances this type of behaviour may reflect poor handling or be a response to fear. In other circumstances the horse may be trying to establish its dominance in the social hierarchy in which it is placed. In a mare the underlying cause may be hormonally related: a mare with a granulosa cell tumour of an ovary usually has abnormally high levels of the hormone testosterone in the blood. If the ovary is removed, testosterone levels decline and the aggressive behaviour disappears. Entire males may show aggression and following castration often become easier to handle. Some rigs show aggressive behaviour, but a recent study comparing behaviour before and after castration showed that there was only limited improvement in aggressive behaviour postoperatively.

THE HORSE THAT IS DIFFICULT TO CLIP

Some horses will not tolerate part or all of their body being clipped. This may be manifest as an unwillingness to stand still, shaking or twitching the skin and kicking with both the fore- and hind limbs. The problem may arise because the horse has been badly handled in the past, or is unduly sensitive to the noise of the clippers, or the clipper blades have been blunt and pulled the skin, or the clippers have become excessively hot.

Some horses can be satisfactorily controlled by the use of a nose twitch, an ear twitch and/or a lip shank, provided they are skilfully handled. It is important that sharp clipper blades are used, that the clippers are not allowed to overheat, and that the job is performed as quickly as possible. In the past tranquillisers were of little use: acepromazine produced minimal sedation and the horse was more likely to kick unpredictably; xylazine was more potent but horses could still kick unexpectedly, and often tended to sweat, which made clipping difficult. The introduction of detomidine and romifidine represents a considerable advance. These have a very powerful effect, last for up to an hour (depending on the initial dose) and do not encourage the horse to sweat. However, difficult horses may still kick. Either drug can be used in combination with butorphanol, an opiate-like drug, and this combination produces excellent results – the horse stands immobile with the limbs planted on the ground and seems unaware of what is going on.

TRANSPORTATION PROBLEMS

Transportation problems include the horse that will not load into or, less commonly, walk out of a trailer or horsebox, the horse that 'scrambles' when the trailer is in motion, and the horse that worries excessively and develops loose faeces, sweats a lot or goes off feed.

UNWILLINGNESS TO LOAD

Unwillingness to load may reflect stubbornness or be the result of previous bad experiences (travelling too fast, especially around corners, poor balance between the trailer and towing vehicle so that the trailer shunts the towing vehicle, falling off the ramp during loading or unloading) or be genuine apprehension. It is usually not related to a pathological problem.

The problem must be approached thoughtfully. The trailer or horsebox should be positioned so that the slope of the ramp is as slight as possible, either with the ramp resting on a slope or on a loading bay. If possible the sides of the ramp should be enclosed so that the horse is unable to swing from one side to the other. The ceiling of the trailer should be as high as possible and the interior as light as possible. The walls should be a pale colour and if possible the front doors should be open. The horse should be allowed as much room as possible in the trailer, so the partition should either be removed or tied back. The horse must be held by a strong, experienced handler and be adequately restrained using a chain shank over the nose, or applied as a lip chain, or as a bit, or using a bridle or Chiffney. Whichever method is adopted, it is useful to have a lunge rein or a long lead rope so that if the horse does pull back the handler will not lose hold. The handler should wear gloves to protect his hands.

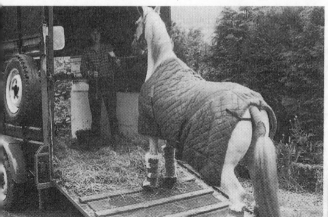

Figure 1
Enticing with food often succeeds in getting the pony on the ramp but no further. The open jockey door gives a sense of space and light

Figure 2
A helper stands to the side and behind the pony, carrying a lungeing whip but not actually using it. The pony capitulates

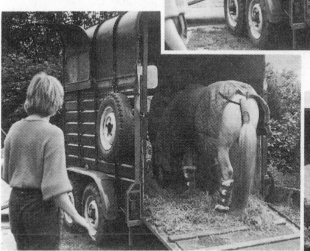

Figure 3   Reward

Figure 4
The partition is in place and the breeching strap is in position to prevent a hasty backward exit

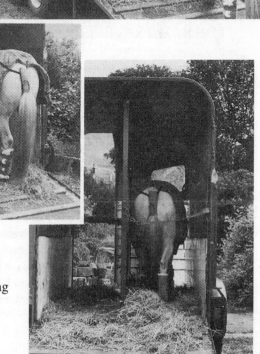

The limbs of the horse should be protected with boots or bandages because serious injuries can result from a horse scraping a leg against the ramp of a trailer or horsebox. The handler should offer the horse a bowl of feed as a reward. At least two extra people are usually necessary. In some cases it is useful to put a rope around the hindquarters and pull the horse forwards. Sometimes the horse can be encouraged forward with the bristles of a broom prodded into the hindquarters but great care must be taken in case the horse kicks back. Restrained force may include cracking a lunge whip behind the horse or hitting it on the hindquarters with a broom, but it is important to remain calm and disciplined.

Whatever method of approach is adopted, it is important to have plenty of time available and to remain as calm as possible. With a difficult loader the calm, quiet, enticement approach is sometimes successful. This requires a great deal of time and patience but is definitely the way to start with a horse which has not travelled previously. The horse is enticed with food and rewarded when it makes progress. However, this approach often succeeds in getting the horse onto the ramp with its head just over the threshold, but no further. More often restrained force is necessary, the horse only being rewarded once it is safely locked inside. It is useful to repeat the loading procedure on several occasions, to feed the horse in the trailer, and not to travel anywhere. In some cases it is helpful to load another horse first or to load the horse from the front of the trailer if that is possible. Occasionally sedation of the horse is beneficial.

THE BAD TRAVELLER

If the horse is going to maintain its balance when travelling it must straddle all four limbs. If apprehensive or claustrophobic it may not do this. If the limbs are not straddled the horse will tend to fall either to the left or to the right, especially when going around corners, and may lean against the side or the partition of the trailer and kick. This behaviour may persist even when the vehicle has come to a stop. Apprehension must be overcome and feeding the horse in the trailer a number of times without travelling anywhere can be helpful. Some horses travel badly on their way to competitions but are much better on the home journey. With such horses it can be helpful to break the routine and travel to a place and just go for a hack. It is vitally important that the trailer does not shunt the towing vehicle and that the horsebox or trailer is driven slowly, especially around corners. Some horses will travel perfectly calmly if they are allowed more room, for example, if the partition of a double trailer is removed. Other horses travel better facing backwards rather than forwards (this can be done in a trailer); in a horsebox, they can stand cross-wise (diagonally).

STABLE VICES

The most common stable vices are crib-biting (wood-chewing), windsucking and weaving. Windsucking is the aspiration of air, done by the horse arching its neck and sucking in air. Some horses do this while holding onto something with their teeth; others do it unaided. It results in a grunting type of noise. Weaving is swinging the head and neck from side to side, rocking on the front feet. These vices can also be called stereotypies – repetitive behaviours, constant in form, that serve no real purpose. Most arise from boredom and are probably the result of horses being maintained in an unnatural environment.

CRIB-BITING

Crib-biting or wood-chewing occurs in both stable-kept and grass-kept horses. It tends to be an infectious habit, copied by other horses. Although a nutritional deficiency may be an underlying cause, if the horse is being fed a balanced diet and has free access to a mineralised salt block this should not be the case. A chronic crib-biter will develop abnormal wear of the incisor teeth.

The problem can be controlled by minimising the number of surfaces which the horse has available to chew: for example, removing the manger, placing a strip of metal over the top of the door or placing a grille on the door. Any surfaces which remain should be painted or covered in a noxious substance such as creosote. Some horses are helped if they have a companion – a small pony, a sheep or a goat. Others are improved if a solid object, such as a rubber ball, is hung from the ceiling.

WINDSUCKING

Traditionally windsucking has been described as a cause of recurrent colic or of failure 'to do well', but the vast majority of horses that windsuck suffer no adverse effects at all. If the habit is severe the muscles on the underside of the neck, which the horse contracts when it arches its neck to suck in air, may hypertrophy (get bigger) and this might be regarded as unsightly. In the majority of horses the habit can be effectively controlled by placing a tight leather strap around the top of the neck; this seems to prevent the horse from arching its neck. Various surgical procedures have been tried, the most successful of which involves removing a piece from several of the muscles on the top of the underside of the neck (the omohyoideus and sternothyrohyoideus muscles) and cutting their nerve supply (the accessory nerve). Although this operation is successful in some horses, others subsequently relapse and some are not improved at all. It also results in a slight cosmetic defect where the muscles have been removed. The author would not recommend the procedure if the habit can be controlled by a leather strap, and would also not be averse to buying a horse with this problem although it is a habit which should be declared at the time of sale.

WEAVING

Weaving is usually a sign of boredom or anxiety – some horses will only do it when they are about to be fed – and it may result in excessive wear of the front shoes. In a few cases the horse rocks from side to side to relieve the weight on painful feet. It is a problem rarely seen in a horse kept at grass. It is usually controlled by placing a V-shaped grille on the stable door.

44
THE NUTRITION AND FEEDING OF HORSES

Basics of horse nutrition

The following chapter is divided into five sections. The first deals with basic information. The second section deals with the digestive system. Nutrient requirements are discussed in the third section. The characteristics of various feeds are given in the fourth and feeding programmes are discussed in the fifth.

Horses must be fed a diet which supplies the essential ingredients – energy, protein, vitamins and minerals – in order to perform at their best. There is no one best diet. Many different rations can be used to supply the necessary nutrients. The ingredients of a diet depend on many factors, such as availability of feedstuffs, economics, palatability and, of course, tradition.

For many horses, feeding does not need to be complicated. Dr. Dean Scoggins of the University of Illinois suggested that horse feeding can and should be simple. Certainly for the maintenance horse this is true. He suggested that horses should have fresh air, high quality forage, trace mineral salt, fresh clean water and grain as needed, with a footnote that many horses only need what grain it takes to catch them. I would add that the horse must be free of dental and parasite problems for the diet to be effective. Of course, the nutrition of the lactating broodmare, foal and performance horse is much more complicated.

Today, feeding mismanagement probably causes more problems than improper dietary formulation. Many horses are overfed, fed too much at one time, or have their feed changed abruptly. In many parts of the world the use of commercial rations fortified with vitamins and minerals has significantly increased over the last few decades and has greatly decreased the incidence of simple nutrient deficiencies that were once common. However in those countries that do not have ready access to balanced diets, deficiencies are likely to occur.

Dr. Pat Harris wrote, 'One of the biggest changes in the last part of this century has been the increased use of manufactured commercial feeds for horses.' The impetus for such feeds came initially in the 19th century from the military and those involved with using horses for transportation. At the start of the tewntieth century 'compressed food cakes consisting of a mix of oats, beans, corn, bran and sometimes chaff' were mentioned as possible feeds but it was recommended that they be broken up before being fed damp. The few manufactured feeds available tended to be expensive and contained poor quality ingredients such as ground corn stalks and sawdust. By the late 1920s, for convenience, 'prepared chop' could be purchased which was reported to contain mainly cereal straw, bruised oats (of indeterminate quality), broken maize, kibbled locust beans, and other beans, but it was recommended that 'horse owners should buy and mix the food for the horses themselves, then they know exactly what their animals are getting and that the food is of good quality.' Pelleted feeds were being fed as early as 1917 but their popularity did not increase dramatically until the 1960s. Increased competition and improved knowledge, as well as more ethical companies and government regulations have resulted in a large industry producing mainly high quality pelleted and coarse mix feeds (sweet feeds) often tailored for the different types or uses of the horse.'

Figure 1 Digestive system of the cow

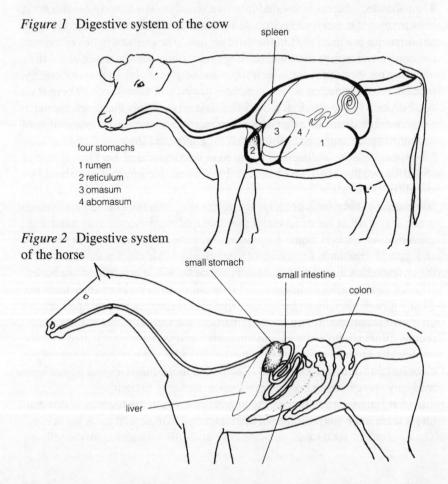

four stomachs

1 rumen
2 reticulum
3 omasum
4 abomasum

spleen

Figure 2 Digestive system of the horse

small stomach

small intestine

colon

liver

Although I have attempted to base all recommendations on scientific studies, there remains a great deal of art to feeding horses. The following words, written by Professor William Henry in 1901, are still true: 'The skill of the artist horse feeder enters into the very life of the creature he manages along with the food he supplies.'

DIGESTIVE PHYSIOLOGY

Understanding the digestive system of the horse is essential for proper feeding and management. The horse and its relatives have a unique system among domestic animals (Figure 2). Cattle, sheep and goats have a large rumen (or specialized 'first' stomach) in which bacteria digest fibre. The horse also has bacteria which digest fibre, but they are located in the large intestine (colon and caecum). Pigs, dogs and cats have much simpler digestive tracts and therefore do not digest fibre as efficiently as the horse.

Some of the differences between the horse and the ruminant are advantageous to the horse and some are disadvantageous. For example, the ruminant can utilize the products of bacterial metabolism, such as vitamins and amino acids, more efficiently than the horse because the bacterial products of the rumen can pass into the small intestine, where digestive efficiency is high. In the horse the bacteria are in the large intestine, which is beyond the primary site of digestion and absorption. The horse has a much higher incidence of colic than other domestic animals because of the complicated structure of the intestine. The horse is more susceptible than a ruminant to mould and many other toxins because the bacteria in the rumen can detoxify some compounds before they are absorbed. Of course, if a horse had a large rumen, it would be more difficult to ride.

The rate of passage of digesta is faster for horses than for cattle. Thus horses do not digest fibre as efficiently as do ruminants because the intestinal bacteria do not have as much time to act on the fibre. On the other hand, the faster rate of digesta passage allows the horse to eat larger amounts of poor-quality feed than the ruminant, and thus the horse is more likely to survive when fed poor-quality roughage than the ruminant. For example, studies in Africa with zebra and antelope indicate that zebra do better than antelope when only poor-quality roughage is available because the rumen of the antelope becomes filled with poorly digested material. The zebra does not digest fibre as efficiently but because more food passes through, more energy is obtained. Of course, this does not mean it is a good idea to feed poor-quality roughage containing low concentrations of nutrients to horses. Poor-quality roughage is more likely to lead to impactive colic than good-quality roughage and most owners want more for their horses than mere survival.

The digestive tract
The digestive tract extends from the mouth to the anus and can be divided into different components:

Mouth Correct dental care is essential for good nutrition. If the horse cannot chew properly, food intake and efficiency of food utilization may decrease. Poor teeth are a major cause of thin horses. Improperly chewed food can also lead to choke or impactive colic. For information on dental care, see Chapter 54.

Oesophagus This tube is 120-150 cm long. Choke (see p. 45) is the most common nutritionally related problem. It is most often seen in animals which do not moisten feed adequately when chewing. Thus greedy eaters are prone to choke. Preventive measures (in such cases) can include moistening the feed, feeding small amounts several times a day or the age-old trick of putting smooth, large stones in the manger to decrease the rate of intake.

Stomach The horse's stomach is relatively small and the horse seldom vomits. Thus overfeeding may cause gastric distension and even rupture of the stomach. Horses fed significant amounts of grain should be fed two or more times daily. No more than 2 kg of grain should be fed at one time.
  Food normally does not remain in the stomach for a prolonged period but passes into the small intestine. However, the digestive process starts in the stomach. Some fermentation and digestive action occurs.

Small intestine This is the primary site of digestion and absorption of soluble carbohydrates (such as starch), protein, lipids, vitamins and many minerals. However, the site of starch digestion can be influenced by many factors such as type of starch granule and processing. Barley starch has a lower rate of digestion in the small intestine than oat starch. It is usually best if the starch is digested in the small intestine. If the starch reaches the lower intestine it is fermented by bacteria and the end products are volatile fatty acids. The fermentation of starch decreases the pH in the large intestine which can lead to colic and/or founder. Control of parasites is essential for the health of the small intestine. Heavily infested animals have greatly reduced capacity to utilise nutrients.

Large intestine This is a very large organ consisting of the caecum and colon. The colon has several sections. Bacteria similar to those found in the rumen of cattle live in the large intestine. Bacteria produce enzymes which digest fibre, the end products being volatile fatty acids (acetate, propionate and butyrate), which are absorbed and used by the horse as energy sources. Horses fed high-fibre diets may obtain one third or more of their energy from volatile fatty acids. Some of the bacterial protein can be used to supply amino acids, but the efficiency of utilisation is low.

The bacteria also supply some water-soluble vitamins but, as with the protein, utilisation is not great. Therefore the diet of a horse with great demands, such as rapid growth, must contain the essential amino acids and water-soluble vitamins. The ruminant, however, can survive without either if nitrogen and carbohydrates are supplied for the rumen bacteria.

NUTRIENT REQUIREMENTS

Water   This is the nutrient required in the largest amount. It comprises about 70% of the body. It has many necessary functions, since it is being involved in digestion, body-temperature regulation, lubrication and metabolism. Water, however, is often neglected. Automatic water bowls may become fouled and horses will not drink. The incidence of impactive colic increases during winter because owners neglect to provide water for their horses or because the horses may be reluctant to drink extremely cold water. Waterers with heating elements may increase intake but cases of electric shock to horses have been reported when the heaters are not properly maintained.

The requirement for water depends on many factors: environmental temperature, amount of work performed (i.e. sweat production), level of milk production, rate of bodyweight (bwt) gain, and faecal and urinary loss. The estimates vary from 20 to 60 litres per day, depending on conditions. If possible, the best policy is to allow the individual to drink all it wants. If the horse has reasonable and consistent access to water, it can regulate its own intake. As Dr. Hinton writes: 'The simplest and most obvious way to prevent dehydration is to allow horses to drink whenever they wish.' Hinton suggests that 'working horses be given the opportunity to drink every hour or so. They should be allowed sufficient time to take what they require and it must be remembered that they may pause and lift their heads during the course of a drink.' Of course, if a horse is very hot and thirsty, it may need to have its water intake limited to a series of small drinks because a single large intake is thought to cause laminitis and colic.

Energy   A deficiency of energy can diminish growth rate, reproductive performance, athletic performance, resistance to disease, parasites or other stress and can affect the appearance of the horse. Excess energy causes obesity, lamintis, colic, reduced resistance to some diseases, and perhaps skeletal problems. It also causes the owner unnecessary expense.

The energy content of feeds can be expressed in many different ways. The net energy system developed in France is used in many European countries. The digestible energy system, expressed in megajoules (MJ), used in this chapter. Digestible energy is determined by measuring the gross energy in feed and faeces with a special device know as a bomb calorimeter. Intake minus faecal loss equals digestible energy.

Estimates of energy requirements are provided in Tables 1 and 2. The figures show how work and lactation can greatly increase the requirement. For example, let us assume that a horse weighing 500 kg is worked 60 minutes at a fast walk, 60 minutes at a medium trot and 15 minutes at a gallop and that the weight of tack and rider is 70 kg. The maintenance requirement would be 69 MJ (Table 1).

The energy above maintenance for the work would be (570 kg x 1 hr x 10.5 KJ/kg/hr) + (570 kg x 1 hr x 39.7 KJ/kg/hr) + (570 kg x 0.25 hr x 96.1 KJ/kg/hr) or 5985 + 22,630 + 13,694 = 42,309 KJ or 42.3 MJ. The total requirement would be 69 + 42.3 or 11 1.3 MJ daily.

Of course the energy requirement depends on the desired body condition. The values in Tables 1 and 2 are only guidelines. If the horse is too lean, provide more energy; if it is too fat, decrease energy intake.

Body condition can be evaluated by visual appraisal, by weighing the horse or by more sophisticated methods such as ultrasound. Routine evaluation is helpful in the assessment of management practices, feeding and health programmes. It is recommended that horses be visually evaluated according to body scores such as those listed in Table 3 and also weighed monthly. If scales are not available, tapes which are placed around the heart girth can be used to estimate weight. Properly formulated tapes are reasonably accurate for most types of animal. Mares in middle to late pregnancy are obvious exceptions.

Protein   Proteins are chains of amino acids. Amino acids which cannot be synthesized by the body and must be supplied in the diet are called essential amino acids. The requirements for essential amino acids have been studied extensively in many species, but knowledge is limited concerning the requirements of the horse.

It is known that the weanling requires 0.7% dietary lysine for a reasonable rate of growth, but there are no recommendations for the other amino acids. A deficiency of protein causes a decrease in food intake and rate of gain in foals and it affects the quality of the coat, making it rough. Protein intake above the requirement is utilised for energy but with less efficiency than carbohydrates or fats. Nitrogen is excreted in the urine. Thus overfeeding of protein increases urinary excretion and water intake. Because protein sources are usually more expensive than energy sources, overfeeding of protein is uneconomical and increases pollution of the environment. Estimates of protein requirements are shown in Tables 1 and 2.

Minerals   The horse requires at least twenty-one different minerals. Calcium, phosphorus, magnesium, sodium, chloride and potassium are called major minerals because they are required in large amounts. The other minerals are called trace minerals because they are required in smaller amounts, not because they are less important.

Calcium is required for muscle function, blood clotting and bone development.

A deficiency of calcium in a young animal causes rickets, a condition in which the bone is not fully hardened. The bones become weak and the long bones may bow.

Bone is a dynamic tissue. It is constantly being remodelled, calcium removed and replaced. The condition known as **nutritional secondary hyperparathyroidism** (NSH) causes more calcium to be removed than is deposited, weakening the bones. In some bones, particularly those of the skull, connective tissue invades the affected bone, which actually increases in size. Hence a common name for the condition is big-head disease.

NSH usually results when a diet containing low levels of calcium and high levels of phosphorus is fed. The high level of phosphorus impairs the utilisation of calcium, the blood level of calcium drops, stimulating the parathyroid gland to release a hormone which increases the rate at which calcium is removed from bone. The condition is often caused by feeding high levels of wheat bran, which has a calcium to phosphorus ratio of 1:12. Hence NSH is also called bran disease.

The role of bran in the aetiology of the disease was first described in the scientific literature by Dr. Varnell, an English veterinarian, in 1860. In spite of the fact that the dangers of feeding high levels of wheat bran without calcium supplementation have been known for many years, the condition is still occasionally reported by veterinarians.

Calcium requirements are listed in Table 4. The amount of calcium needed in the diet depends on its availability. As mentioned, high levels of phosphorus decrease the utilisation of calcium. Studies in Australia demonstrated that many tropical forages contain oxalate, an organic compound, which can bind calcium and decrease utilisation.

Legumes such as lucerne are excellent sources of calcium. Grains have very low levels of calcium. Inorganic materials, such as those listed in Table 5, are excellent sources of calcium.

Phosphorus is also involved in bone formation. About 80 per cent of the body's phosphorus is in bone and a phosphorus deficiency can result in improper mineralisation of bone. A deficiency of phosphorus also causes the blood level of phosphorus to decrease but, unlike the case of calcium, the decrease does not stimulate the parathyroid hormone to release phosphorus from the bone.

Phosphorus requirements are shown in Table 4. The phosphorus content of forage depends on the soil. The phosphorus content of grains is much higher than that of hay. Grains, however, have a significant percentage of phosphorus in the phytic form, which is not utilised efficiently by horses. Several inorganic sources (Table 5) are effectively utilised by horses.

Magnesium is required for bone formation and for many enzymes. If the blood level of magnesium greatly decreases, the animal develops **tetany** (muscle spasm). The condition is usually associated with stress, such as being transported.

Electrolytes (potassium, sodium and chloride) are important in osmotic pressure regulation and acid-base balance. Forages usually contain high levels of potassium. Potassium nutrition can be of concern, however, especially when horses sweat profusely because sweat contains a high concentration of potassium. Sodium is lacking in most conventional feeds. Thus, free choice intake of salt is recommended in all cases and electrolytes are often needed by working horses.

The function and deficiency signs of trace minerals are summarized in Table 6. The trace mineral content of foodstuffs depends on several factors such as the mineral content and pH of the soil where the crops were grown.

Vitamins   Vitamins are divided into two categories: fat-soluble and water-soluble. Vitamins A, E, D and K belong to the former. Fat-soluble vitamins (with the exception of vitamin E) are more likely to be stored in large amounts in the body and are more likely to be toxic than water-soluble vitamins when fed in excessive amounts. The functions, requirements and signs of deficiency and toxicity are listed in Table 7.

Green, leafy plants and high-quality hay are excellent sources of many vitamins. Vitamin supplements are more likely to be needed when large amounts of grain and poor-quality hay which has been stored for longer than a year are fed. Biotin is not included in Table 7 but it has been found that 10-15 mg supplemental biotin daily may help repair cracked and/or poor-quality hooves.

Nutrient requirements can be expressed in two ways, units per day or percentage of the ration. Many horse owners prefer the latter system. The requirements for several nutrients expressed as percentages of the ration are shown in Table 8.

FEED

Grains, succulents (such as pasture) and roughages (such as hay) are the most commonly used sources of energy. Grains (also called concentrates) usually contain 85-95% dry matter. They contain high levels of digestible starch, thus providing a high level of digestible energy (Table 10). Any of the common grains can be fed if their characteristics are taken into account. Owners usually prefer oats to the other grains because they are safer due to the higher fibre content and because the horse finds them palatable. Maize is a very good energy source and is widely used in many parts of the world but requires more careful management than does oats because of its high energy concentration. Barley has a digestible energy content somewhat between that of maize and oats.

Pasture and other succulent foods contain high concentrations of water. Thus the energy content is usually expressed on a dry-matter basis, that is, MJ per kilogram dry-matter. The desired types of pasture plants depends on many factors such as soil, climate, drainage and traffic patterns. Therefore it is impossible to make specific recommendations without knowledge of local conditions. A general recommendation is that the mixture be about one third legume, if possible.

Good quality pasture is still an excellent basis for a feeding programme. The old saying that 'Dr. Green is an excellent veterinarian' is still true. Proper use of pasture provides a much higher level of antioxidants than present in hay, such as vitamin E and carotene. Dr. David Pugh of Auburn University stated in a presentation at the North American Veterinary Conferences in 2000 that 'grass is magic but hay is dead.' Certainly much of the antioxidant content is lost during drying and storage. Pasture can reduce the incidence of colic, ulcers, equine motor disease, signs of respiratory diseases and abnormal behaviours.

Of course pasture is not a perfect diet. Excessive intake of lush pasture can cause founder and colic. Pasture may be lacking in certain minerals depending on the content of the soil. Toxic plants or harmful products such as endophytes may be present in the grass.

Pasture can also be a source of parasite infestation. Prompt removal of faeces will greatly reduce the parasite load and improve pasture utilisation. Horses will not normally graze on pasture near faecal piles. However, they will graze near piles if the pasture is in short supply.

Hays have a much higher fibre content than do grains. Fibre is not digested as efficiently as starch. Thus the digestible energy concentration in hay is not as great as that in grains (Table 10). The energy concentration in hay depends on several factors, but the most important is the stage of maturity at harvesting. The fibre content increases as the plant matures, thus older plants contain lower concentrations of digestible energy.

Legume or grass hays can be fed to horses. Legumes such as lucerne usually provide more protein than is needed by mature horses, causing them to urinate more in order to excrete the unneeded nitrogen. The greater excretion, however, does not cause kidney damage as is frequently suggested. Legume hays usually provide more energy and vitamins than grass hays. As mentioned earlier, legumes contain much more calcium than grasses.

Many of the protein supplements used in livestock feeds are by-products of vegetable oil production. The composition of several oil meals is listed in Table 10.

As mentioned earlier, some classes of horse require specific amino acids in the diet. The level of lysine is of particular concern. Of the commonly used meals, soybean meal has the greatest lysine content at 2.3%, compared with 1.7, 1.6, 1.2 and 1% for cotton seed, groundnut, linseed and sunflower meals, respectively. Dried peas can also be an effective protein source. They contain less protein (26%) but have 1.8% lysine. Thus the protein-lysine ratio is better than for many of the other vegetable proteins. Any legume seeds such as soyabeans and peas must be heat-treated to destroy components which inhibit utilisation. Over-long heating can also decrease protein utilisation.

Animal products such as dried skimmed milk and fish meal are excellent sources of amino acids and can be fed to horses (see, p. 601). However, they are much more expensive than plant sources. Locust beans are not high in protein but are considered to be very palatable.

FEEDING PROGRAMMES

Mature horses at maintenance This class of horse is usually the least demanding. Average- to good-quality hay consumed at a rate of 1.5-1.75 kg per 100 kg bwt, water and trace mineralised salt fed but free choice should supply all the necessary nutrients. If the soil is lacking in trace minerals, additional minerals may be needed. During cold weather the energy requirement will be increased and some grain may be helpful.

Working horses A primary concern for working horses is energy intake (Table 2). Horses at the racetrack may need 1.5 kg hay and 1.5 kg grain per 100 kg bwt or more. The source of energy can be important. If the hay is of very poor quality, intake may be limited. Maize, oats and barley can all be used as energy sources. The advantages and disadvantages are discussed above.

The addition of fat increases the energy density of the ration. Several studies indicate that the addition of 6-10% fat such as vegetable oil or animal fat may have some benefits for working horses.

The protein requirement is not greatly increased by work. It is true that some nitrogen is lost in sweat, but as the general intake is greatly increased to meet the energy needs, so protein intake is also increased. Thus there is no need to increase the protein concentration of the diet. In fact, excess protein can decrease performance.

Work increases the mineral requirements because of the loss in sweat, but, as with protein, if the diet contains a percentage of minerals adequate for maintenance, the horse will, in most cases, obtain additional minerals when eating to meet energy needs. There are exceptions, however. Electrolyte losses may be of particular concern in horses which sweat profusely, such as endurance horses or three-day-event horses. **Synchronous diaphragmatic flutter (thumps)** has been related to low serum calcium and potassium levels in endurance horses. Several commercially packaged electrolyte supplements are available.

Selenium might also be of concern because selenium is required for muscle function. The diet should contain about 0.1-0.2 parts per million (ppm) selenium. Excess selenium can be toxic (see p. 597), thus supplementation by addition to feed or by injection should be done very carefully.

As energy intake increases, the requirement for B vitamins increases because the B vitamins are cofactors necessary for energy utilisation. Reports have suggested that some racehorses have marginal intakes of thiamin, one of the first signs of which is anorexia. If a supplement is desired, it should provide about 25 mg thiamin daily.

Stabled racehorses may require a folic acid supplement, but horses on pasture apparently do not. Stabled horses utilise folic acid more effectively if large doses are given weekly than when smaller doses are given daily. If poor-quality hay is fed, a vitamin A supplement may be needed. A supplement of 13,000 IU vitamin A in such cases would not be unreasonable. Horses may perform poorly with lower than normal levels of vitamin A in the blood.

Broodmares Energy is also of great concern when feeding mares. Underfeeding of fillies can delay the onset of first heat. Severe underfeeding of pregnant females can cause embryonic death.

The pregnant mare, early in gestation, does not have nutrient requirements greatly different from those of the non-pregnant mare. During the last ninety days of gestation the foetus is developing rapidly and the mare's needs are increased.

The energy needs of the lactating mare are a function of the level of milk production. The amount of milk produced varies greatly among mares, but some mares will produce amounts of milk equivalent to 3 and 2% of their bodyweight during early lactation (one to twelve weeks) and late lactation (thirteen to twenty-four weeks) respectively. A 450-kg mare producing milk at these levels would require about 70% more energy during early lactation and about 48% more energy during late lactation than needed or required for maintenance.

The pregnant mare's protein needs for energy is increased significantly over that for maintenance only during the last ninety days of gestation. Mares fed legume hays such as lucerne or clover (usually 11-15% protein) and grain such as oats (12% protein) or maize (9% protein) would not need a protein supplement. When a grass hay such as late-cut timothy hay is fed, a protein supplement may be needed. For example, if a grass hay contains only 8% protein, and if 5.5 kg hay and 1.5 kg grain are fed, the grain mixture should contain about 16% protein. The lactating mare needs about 12.5% protein in her ration. As with the pregnant mare, the need for a protein supplement depends on which hays and grains are used.

The calcium and phosphorus requirements, when expressed as percentages of the diet, are similar for pregnant and lactating mares. Of course, total intake of minerals is much greater for the lactating mare because she eats more food. Adequate intakes of trace minerals, particularly copper and zinc, are essential for the pregnant mare to prevent skeletal problems in the foal.

Orphan foals   An adequate intake of colostrum or another source of antibodies is essential for survival of the foal, but good nutrition is also important. A foster mare can be a very effective source of nutrients. The least troublesome type of mare is probably an older, cold-blooded one, and the worst type is a young, flighty Thoroughbred. A foster mare should be checked for disease; milk samples should be taken following examination of the udder, and her tail should be thoroughly washed and disinfected. She should be brought to the stable and hooded so that she cannot see, and a strong-smelling substance placed on her muzzle. The same substance can be used on the foal's head, neck and tail. A simple but sturdily constructed fostering gate will allow the foal to suck without danger of being kicked.

Nanny goats can also be very effective nurses, particularly during the first few days. Foals at the Critical Care Center at the University of Florida are routinely fed goat's milk. Mare's milk in early lactation usually contains 10.5-11 per cent total solids, 1.4-1.8% fat, 2-2.3% protein and 6.5-7% lactose. Goat's milk usually contains 14% total solids, 4% fat, 3.6% protein and 5% lactose and therefore is slightly richer than mare's milk.

Mare's milk replacers are now available, and very effective. When milk replacer is fed in a bottle, the foal should be fed near another horse, which acts as a decoy, and never at the doorway of the stable. If fed at the doorway, the bottle-fed foal will spend all its time inside the door waiting for the human voice and the next feeding. Foals can quickly learn to drink from a bucket.

It is important to monitor carefully the weight changes of the foal in order to evaluate the feeding programme.

Weanlings   Weanlings are much more susceptible to nutritional problems than older horses. For example, the protein requirement, expressed as a percentage of the diet, is almost twice that of the mature horse at maintenance. Of course, the requirements are dependent upon the desired rate of growth. More attention must be given to balancing the ration when a rapid rate of gain is desired. Rapid growth and overfeeding can cause severe skeletal problems. Osteochondrosis (see p. 224), flexural deformities (see chapter 19) and physitis (see p. 214) are often claimed to be induced by overfeeding. Genetic factors are also probably involved in the incidence of the disease.

The optimal growth rate is not known, but the results of several surveys suggest that the average light horse might be expected to obtain about 47, 67 and 80% mature weight and about 83, 91 and 95% mature height at the withers by six, twelve and eighteen months respectively. Estimates of body-weight at various ages in relation to mature bodyweight are shown in Table 9.

Nutrition is more than just balancing the nutrients in the diet. There are many aspects involved. Proper selection of feeds that are palatable is important and parasite control is essential as the benefits of a balanced diet are greatly reduced by a heavy infestation of parasites. Horses should be fed at regular times - they are creatures of habit and regular feeding times helps to reduce stress and digestive problems.

Horses are susceptible to poisoning by mouldy feed (see p. 603). Although moulds cannot always be detected by eye, tests are available for the detection of many mycotoxins. Mangers, buckets and feed tubs should be kept clean, not only to deter the spread of disease, but also to decrease waste, improve feed intake and prevent the formation of mould.

Feed by weight not by volume. There are considerable differences in density among horse feeds. Wheat bran weighs about 225 g per quart whereas maize weighs 775 g per quart.

Abrupt changes in the type of feed should be avoided. Colic, inappetence or diarrhoea may result when horses are changed abruptly from a low- energy to a high-energy feed. Reasonable levels of fibre should be provided. There is no established requirement for fibre, but a level equivalent to at least 0.22 kg hay per 100 kg bwt seems to be adequate.

In conclusion, the eye of the master remains still an important part in the feeding of the horse. Fortunately, the master also has more scientific help at his disposal than ever before.

Table 1 Daily Energy and Protein Requirements of Various Classes of Horse*

| | Expected mature weight (kg) | | | | | |
| | 400 | | 500 | | 600 | |
	DE (MJ)	Protein (kg)	DE (MJ)	Protein (Kg)	DE (MJ)	Protein (kg)
Maintenance, mature	56	0.54	69	0.66	81	0.78
Mares, last 90 days of gestation	68	0.67	79	0.82	94	0.97
Lactating mare, first 3 months	96	1.14	118	1.42	140	1.71
Lactating mare, 3 months to weaning	84	0.84	102	1.05	118	1.26
Weanling	54	0.68	63	0.75	71	0.86
Yearling	65	0.70	82	0.85	84	1.02
Two-year-old	64	0.65	79	0.80	87	1.00

*From the National Research Council, *Nutrient Requirements of the Horse*, National Academy of Science - National Research Council publication, Washington, DC. 1989.

Table 2 Digestible Energy Requirements above Maintenance for Horses at Various Activities*

Gait	DE (KJ) hour Per kg bwt+
Slow walk	7.1
Fast walk	10.5
Slow trot	27.1
Medium trot	39.7
Fast trot/slow canter	57.3
Medium canter	81.5
Gallop	96.1
Strenuous effort	163.0

*Adapted from J. D. Pagan and H. F. Hintz, 'Equine Energetic II. Energy expenditure in horses during submaximal exercise', *Journal of Animal Science*, vol 63 (1986), pp.822-30.

+Weight of horse plus rider and tack.

Table 3   Condition Score for Horses*

Score

1   *Poor.* Animal extremely emaciated. Spinous processes, ribs, tailhead and hooks and pins projecting prominently. Bone structure of withers, shoulders and neck easily noticeable. No fatty tissues can be felt.

2   *Very thin.* Animal emaciated. Slight fat covering over base of spinous processes; transverse processes of lumbar vertebrae feel rounder. Spinous processes, ribs, tailhead and hooks and pins prominent. Withers, shoulders and neck structures faintly discernible.

3   *Thin.* Fat build-up about halfway on spinous processes; transverse processes cannot be felt. Slight fat cover over ribs. Spinous processes and ribs easily discernible. Tailhead prominent, but individual vertebrae cannot be visually identified. Hook bones appear rounded, but easily discernible. Pin bones not distinguishable. Withers, shoulders and neck accentuated.

4   *Moderately thin.* Negative crease along back. Faint outline of ribs discernible. Tailhead prominence depends on conformation, fat can be felt around it. Hook bones not discernible. Withers, shoulders and neck not obviously thin.

5   *Moderate.* Back level. Ribs cannot be visually distinguished but can be easily felt. Fat around tailhead beginning to feel spongy. Withers appear rounded over spinous processes. Shoulders and neck blend smoothly into body.

6   *Moderate to fleshy.* Slight crease down back. Fat over ribs feels spongy. Fat around tailhead feels soft. Fat beginning to be deposited along the sides of the withers, behind the shoulders and along the sides of the neck.

7   *Fleshy.* Crease down back. Individual ribs can be felt, but noticeable filling between ribs with fat. Fat around tailhead is soft. Fat deposited along withers, behind shoulders and along the neck.

8   *Fat.* Prominent crease down back. Difficult to feel ribs. Fat around tailhead very soft. Area along withers filled with fat. Area behind shoulder filled in flush. Noticeable thickening of neck. Fat deposited along inner buttocks.

9   *Extremely fat.* Extremely obvious crease down back. Patchy fat appearing over ribs. Bulging fat around tailhead, along withers, behind shoulders and along neck. Fat along inner buttocks may rub together. Flank filled in flush.

*D.R. Hennecke, G.D. Potter, J.R. Kreider, 'A condition score relationship to body fat content of mares, during gestation and lactation,' *Proceedings of the 7th Equine Nutrition Phsyiology and Symposium,* 1981, p. 105.

Table 4 Daily Calcium (Ca) and Phosphorus (P)
Requirements for Various Classes of Horse

	Expected mature weight (kg)					
	400		500		600	
	Ca(g)	P(g)	Ca(g)	P(g)	Ca(g)	P(g)
Maintenance, mature	16	11	20	14	24	17
Mares, last 90 days of gestation	29	22	35	26	41	31
Lactating mare, first 3 months	45	29	56	36	67	43
Lactating mare, 3 months to weaning	29	18	36	22	43	27
Weanling	33	18	34	19	40	22
Yearling	23	13	29	16	36	20
Two-year-old	19	11	24	13	31	17

*National Research Council, op. cit.

Table 5 Calcium (Ca) and Phosphorus (P) Content of Some
Mineral Supplements

	Percentage		Amount contained in 1 tablespoon (g)	
	Ca	P	Ca	P
Calcium carbonate	34	0	10	0
Defluorinated phosphate	32	15	10	5
Bone meal	30	14	9	4
Dicalcium phosphate	27	21	8	6
Monocalcium phosphate	17	21	5	6
Monosodium phosphate	0	22	0	7

Table 6 Summary of Trace Mineral Functions, Deficiency Signs and Requirements.

Mineral	Some functions	Some deficiency signs	Requirement*
Iron (Fe)	Part of the haemoglobin molecule and therefore involved in oxygen transport; part of some enzymes which speed up important bodily chemical processes	Anaemia: lack of stamina, poor growth	40 mg/kg feed for maintenance; 50 mg/kg for growth
Copper (Cu)	Iron absorption, haemoglobin synthesis, skin pigments, collagen metabolism	Anaemia, hair pigment loss; bone disease, swollen joints, deformed thin bones	10 mg/kg feed
Zinc (Zn)	Activator of many enzymes	Skin problems: hair loss, scaly skin, poor wound healing; reproductive, behavioural and skeletal abnormalities	40 mg/kg feed
Iodine (I)	Thyroid function	Goitre, poor growth, low body temperature, impaired development of hair and skin, foals weak at birth	0.1 mg/kg feed
Manganese (Mg)	Synthesis of bone and cartilage components, cholesterol metabolism	Reproductive problems: delayed oestrus, reduced fertility, spontaneous abortion, skeletal deformities in the newborn	40 mg/kg feed
Potassium (K)	Maintenance of acid-base balance	Decreased rate of growth, reduced appetite and hypokalemia (decreased serum level of potassium)	
Selenium (Se)	Removal of peroxides from tissues	White muscle disease, low serum selenium and serum glutathione peroxidase concentration	0.1 mg/kg feed

*Based on National Research Council recommendations. Dry matter basis.

Table 7   Summary of Vitamin Functions, Deficiency Signs and Requirements

Vitamins	*Some functions*	*Some deficiency signs*	*Requirements**
Vitamin A	Growth and development of bone and epithelial cells, night vision	Night blindness, corneal cloudiness; impaired growth; reproductive problems: poor conception rate, abortion, loss of libido, testicular degeneration; convulsions, elevated cerebrospinal fluid pressure; decreased vitamin A in tissues and serum	2000 IU/kg feed for maintenance and working horse; for 2000 growing horses; 3000 for reproducing or lactating mares
Vitamin D	Absorption of dietary calcium and phosphorus	Skeletal disease: poor mineralization of bone, bone deformities; impaired growth; low blood calcium and phosphorus	300 IU/kg feed
Vitamin E	Antioxidant in tissues	Decreased serum tocopherol, increased red blood cell fragility, elevated serum glutamic-oxalic transaminase (SGOT); muscular dystrophy	50 IU/kg feed for maintenance 80 IU for growing, working or pregnant or lactating mares
Vitamin K	Blood clotting	Haemorrhagic disease in species that require the vitamin	Unknown
Thiamin	Co-enzyme in energy metabolism	Accumulation of acids in tissues; loss of appetite and weight, impaired growth; incoordination, muscular weakness and twitching; hypoglycemia	3 mg/kg feed
Riboflavin	Co-enzyme in many enzyme systems	Impaired growth and feed efficiency; eye problems: conjunctivitis, lacrimation, aversion to bright light	2 mg/kg feed
B12	Co-enzyme in several systems	Deficiency signs have not been described in horses	Probably synthesized in the intestine

IU = international unit

*Based on National Research Council recommendations

Table 8 Minimum Nutrients Concentration in Diets for Horses and Ponies Expressed on 90% Dry-Matter Basis*

	Digestible energy (MJ/kg)	Crude protein (%)	Ca (%)	P (%)
Mature horses and ponies at maintenance	7.5	7.2	0.21	0.15
Mares, last 90 days of gestation	8.4	9.0	0.39	0.30
Lactating mare, first 3 months	9.8	12.0	0.47	0.30
Lactating mare, 3 months to weanling	9.2	10.0	0.33	0.20
Weanling (6 months of age)	10.9	13.0	0.50	0.28
Yearling (12 months of age)	10.5	11.3	0.39	0.21
Long yearling (18 months of age)	9.6	10.0	0.31	0.17
Two-year-old (light training)	9.4	9.4	0.28	0.15

Ca = calcium, P = phosphorus
*Adapted from National Research Council, op. cit.

Table 9 Estimates of bodyweight at various ages in relation to mature bodyweight.

	Mature weight (kg)					
Age (months)	200	400	500	600	800	1000
2	60	105	130	155	180	210
4	85	150	180	220	250	315
6	110	185	230	275	340	420
8	125	220	275	320	400	500
10	140	245	301	360	450	565
12	150	270	335	400	500	630
14	160	290	360	435	540	670
16	165	305	380	460	580	730
18	170	320	400	480	620	780

Table 10   Estimates of Composition of Foodstuffs for Horses (Dry-Matter Basis)*

	Dry matter (%)	DE (MJ/kg)	Crude Protein (%)	Ca (%)	P (%)	Mg (%)	K (%)	Cu (mg/kg)	Zn (mg/kg)
Cereals									
Barley	86	15.0	10.8	0.08	0.40	0.13	0.45	9	17
Maize	86	16.1	9.8	0.05	0.26	0.12	0.35	4	20
Oats	86	13.5	11.0	0.09	0.37	0.17	0.44	6	36
Rye	86	14.7	13.3	0.07	0.36	0.12	0.42	8	36
Sorghum	86	15.5	10.8	0.04	0.33	0.20	0.39	12	12
By-products									
Brewer's grains dried	90	11.3	22.4	0.30	0.60	0.17	0.09	24	30
Distiller's grains, dried	90	12.1	30.1	0.11	0.44	0.10	0.20	48	35
Sugar-beet pulp	90	12.2	9.0	0.75	0.10	0.30	0.20	14	10
Sugar-beet molasses	75	12.9	7.4	0.12	0.03	0.30	6.20	22	18
Sugar-cane molasses	75	12.9	4.1	1.05	0.15	0.47	3.80	80	30
Wheat feed, middlings	88	11.9	17.6	0.10	0.90	0.60	1.40	10	106
Wheat feed, bran	88	11.1	17.0	0.12	1.45	0.60	1.60	14	120
Miscellaneous									
Locust bean plus pods	86	13.0	6.9	--	--	--	--	--	--
Peas, dried	89	13.8	26.5	0.13	0.47	--	1.14	--	--
Oil cakes									
Cotton-seed meal	90	13.3	45.7	0.20	1.20	0.50	1.40	20	70
Groundnut meal	90	14.0	48.1	0.29	0.68	0.17	1.25	17	22
Linseed meal	90	12.5	40.4	0.40	0.89	0.66	1.53	29	36
Soyabean meal	90	14.0	50.3	0.31	0.70	0.30	2.20	30	50
Sunflower cake (no hulls)	90	12.9	48.3	0.41	1.10	0.81	1.10	4	--

				Ca	P	Mg	K	Cu	Zn
Roots									
Carrots	13	12.8	9.3	0.40	0.35	0.20	2.80	10	–
Turnip	9	11.2	12.2	0.60	0.26	0.14	2.90	21	–
Grasses									
Cocksfoot, young	23	8.6	18.4	0.55	0.29	0.30	2.50	12	–
Cocksfoot, mature	27	8.2	10.0	0.35	0.23	0.20	2.00	10	–
Rye-grass, perennial, mature	25	8.4	10.5	0.50	0.25	0.20	1.65	10	–
Timothy, in flower	25	8.5	9.6	0.45	0.25	0.14	1.65	5	17
Green legumes									
Clover, early flower	19	8.6	18.0	1.90	0.30	0.40	2.20	9	17
Lucerne, early flower	23	8.8	19.0	2.0	0.30	0.50	2.25	9	18
Hays									
Clover, good	86	8.4	16.1	1.50	0.25	0.40	1.70	11	18
Clover, poor	86	8.0	12.0	1.00	0.21	0.30	1.50	7	14
Grass, early cut	86	8.5	13.0	0.55	0.25	0.20	1.35	7	18
Grass, late cut	86	8.0	8.5	0.30	0.19	0.15	1.00	5	14
Lucerne, half flower	86	9.0	18.0	1.60	0.25	0.29	1.90	9	16
Lucerne, full flower	86	8.3	15.5	1.20	0.21	0.28	1.75	8	14
Oats, milk stage	86	8.3	9.0	0.30	0.24	0.60	1.20	4	–
Straws									
Barley	87	5.8	3.4	0.27	0.07	0.19	2.0	5	7
Oat	87	6.2	3.4	0.25	0.09	0.17	2.3	9	6
Rye	87	5.8	3.7	0.25	0.09	0.07	1.0	5	6
Wheat	87	5.8	3.7	0.21	0.08	0.12	1.4	4	6

Ca = calcium, P = phosphorus, Mg = manganese, K = potassium, Cu = copper, Zn = zinc
*The values are from several sources. The dashes indicate that no values were found. The values are expressed on a dry-matter basis in order to compare feeds that contain different amounts of water. As mentioned earlier, the energy and protein content of forages depends greatly on the stage of maturity and times of harvesting. The mineral content of plants depend on several factors such as the genus, species and variety, the type of soil on which the plant was grown, the weather during the growing season and the stage of the maturity of the plant at harvest. The values in the table should be considered as guides or general indicators. If possible, the balancing of rations should be based on analysis of your foodstuffs.

Table 11 Malnutrition

Malnutrition is defined as an abnormal intake of nutrients. Although we usually think of this term in relation to starvation and underfeeding, it applies equally well to excessive intake of nutrients, which, in many cases can be just as harmful.

Below are outlined the most common states of malnutrition seen in practice. Deficiencies of minerals and vitamins are dealt with in chapter 44 and poisoning by excess of the same in chapter 38.

Nutrient	Shortage		Excess	
	Condition	Symptoms	Condition	Symptoms
Carbo-hydrate	Weight loss	Poor covering of bones, prominent ribs and pelvis, hollow neck	Obesity	Ribs not palpable. Development of crest in all sexes. Sluggish exercise tolerance
	Milk shortage in lactating mares	Foal sucks for longer than usual. Does not sleep after feeds. Poor growth	Obesity with laminitis	Bilateral lameness. Stiff gait in front. Stands rocked back from front feet. Hot feet (feel near coronet). Lameness worse on gravel or stones
	Poor fertility	Repeated return to stud (other factors often involved)	Azoturia	Severe cramping of muscles after short bursts of exercise. Hind limbs very stiff. Severe pain, swearing, etc. Overfeeding while in irregular work
	Stunted growth	Underweight, small yearlings		Overfeeding while in irregular work
			Flexural limb deformities in foals	Club feet, upright pasterns in rapidly growing foals (other factors also involved)
Protein	Protein starvation	Muscle wasting associated with fat belly. Often linked to poor worming programme in face of apparently adequate feeding programme. Neck	Poor performance	Overzealous use of protein supplements can occasionally lead to poor athletic performance

Nutrient	Problem	Signs	Problem	Signs
		hollow at sides, quarters sunken behind bony pelvis	Diarrhea	Loose, often dark-coloured, foul-smelling faeces. May follow sudden introduction or overuse of high-protein supplements such as soyabean meal and milk powder
	Milk shortage in lactating mares	See above	Flexural limb deformities in foals	See above
	Poor fertility	See above		
	Susceptibility to disease	Low protein levels in blood may reduce immune system's ability to fight infection		
Roughage or fibre	Spasmodic colic (caused by poor gut movement associated with low-fibre diet)	Pain, sweating, rolling, looking at flank	Impaction colic (often linked with sudden fall in regular exercise)	Small, hard or absent droppings. Low-grade, dull pain. Horse lies down a lot. May roll onto back and lie still. Can progress to severe pain. Often linked to horse eating bedding or straw being used as feed
	Laminitis (caused by overeating cereal to satisfy bulk intake)	See above	Nutritional secondary hyperparathyroidism ('bran disease' - see p. 691)	Swelling of joints and bones of head. Shifting lameness. Brittle bones, leading to pathological fracture

45
THE RELATIONSHIP BETWEEN SOUNDNESS AND CONFORMATION

The examination of horses as to soundness and their selection as to suitability are part of the work of veterinarians which requires sound judgement and the employment of knowledge tempered with experience. The relationship between soundness and conformation has long been recognised.

> A horse is sound when he is free from hereditary disease, is in the possession of his natural and constitutional health and has as much bodily perfection as is consistent with his natural formation.
> The rule as to unsoundness is, if at the time of sale or examination, the horse has any disease, which either actually does diminish the natural usefulness of the animal, so as to make him less capable of work of any description, or which in its ordinary progress will diminish its natural usefulness; or if that horse has, either from disease (whether such disease be congenital, or arising subsequently to birth) or from accident has undergone any alteration of structure that either does at the time or in its ordinary course will diminish the natural usefulness of the horse, such horse is unsound.

Conformation is the manner in which the horse is formed or put together. Bad conformation may not be unsoundness in itself, but it may often lead to unsoundness. The study of conformation should consist of the appraisement of points of structure and the estimation of their significance in the horse as a whole. Let us now consider what we require as broad principles of conformation.

In the first place the horse, whatever its breed or job, should convey to the eye suitability in make and shape, with no obvious fault which would upset the whole make-up. In short, the horse must have presence – that undefinable something which, at first impact to the eye, impresses one with the suitability of the horse for its particular work. If the horse meets you well and, on a cursory inspection, shows no outstanding faults of conformation, it is more than likely that on further examination it will be found to be more or less sound. It is presence, allied with good movement, which enables one to pick out the first half dozen in a strong class in the show ring, or rapidly to select a few animals of the right type in the busy atmosphere of a crowded sale yard and then proceed to a more detailed examination.

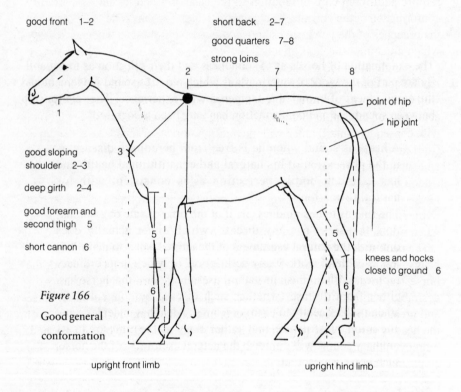

good front   1–2

short back   2–7

good quarters   7–8

strong loins

point of hip

hip joint

good sloping shoulder   2–3

deep girth   2–4

good forearm and second thigh   5

short cannon   6

knees and hocks close to ground   6

Figure 166

Good general conformation

upright front limb

upright hind limb

Figure 1   Good general conformation

Head and neck

The head should be of a size proportionate to the size of the horse itself, with a straight face line and well-defined features. The forehead should be broad, full and flat, and the ears of medium size, finely pointed and carried alertly. The eyes should be prominent, clear and large, with eyelids of uniform curvature. The muzzle should not be too fine, the nostrils large but not dilated, with thin lips and the incisor teeth sound and regular. The lower jaw should be well defined, clear at its angle, and the space between the two branches of the lower jaw should be wide in order that the larynx may be fully accommodated, with room for large muscular attachments. Any deformity of the jaw, such as a parrot mouth or an undershot jaw, is an unsoundness depending entirely on a fault of conformation. Such horses are bad doers as a rule, and require additional care in feeding. In the case of breeding animals a faulty conformation of the jaw may be passed on to their progeny. The width between the branches of the jaw is an established feature of the Arab horse and one to which great importance is attached.

The angle at which the head meets the neck is one of the most important features of conformation. If this angle is too acute, the head and neck are not well set on; in the extreme, a 'cock-throttled' appearance is shown. By the acuteness of this angle there is the possibility of compression of the larynx, with consequent interference with respiration. When, in such a case, the depth from ear to throat is also marked, it is suggestive of commonness or jowliness and such a horse is not likely to bridle well or to carry its head kindly when ridden or driven. An overlarge head places a strain upon the forehead, and means that more muscular power from the great muscles of the neck is required to maintain it in position. Such horses often tire easily and die on the hand when ridden or driven.

The neck should be of proportionate length, reasonably crested but not too heavy, and its muscular development should be in proportion to the work the horse has to do. A long, lean neck on a Thoroughbred or riding horse is desirable; a shorter, well-muscled neck is an essential part of a draught horse and prepares the collar area for the reception of the draught. The carriage of the head is very largely determined by the shape and nature of the neck and, moreover, the junction of the neck with the body determines, very largely, the slope and carriage of the shoulder. Actually, the neck of the draught horse is rarely very short, but the muscular development of the neck and crest may make it appear to be somewhat shorter in proportion, for example, to that of the riding horse. The jugular groove should be easily determined, and in the well-bred horse the trachea should be well marked out.

The withers should be of good height and well defined. Withers which are too high are undesirable and are sometimes associated with deficient spring of the chest, while low, thick, heavy withers are undesirable in the light horse and interfere with the free mobility of the shoulder. In the Hackney, low, thick withers

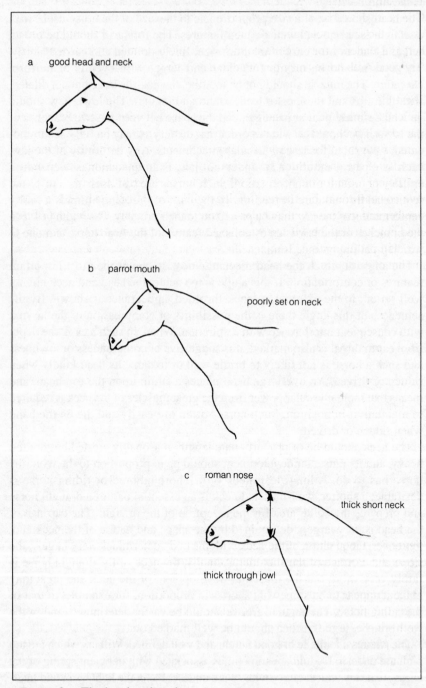

a   good head and neck

b   parrot mouth

poorly set on neck

c   roman nose

thick short neck

thick through jowl

Figure 2   The head and neck

are usually associated with deficient action and a bad shoulder, and while strong withers are desirable in the draught horse, withers which are too low and fleshy result in the saddle not maintaining its correct position and, in the draught-horse, there is a tendency for the collar to rock. It should be noted, however, that some very good Arab horses may be found to have rather low withers.

Chest

The chest should be deep and full, the ribs should be long, well sprung and spaced well back, so that the edge of the last rib is not too far away from the point of the hip. Flat, narrow ribs are undesirable and tend to reduce the capacity of the chest. Such horses are often poor doers, due to there being insufficient room for the heart and lungs. If too narrow, not only will the horse have no heart room, but the two forelegs will emerge from the body too close together and give rise to the dealer's expression 'both legs coming out of the same hole'. If the chest is too wide, the horse will be found to have a rolling gait, will paddle with its forelegs, and will be found to waste a considerable amount of muscular action when endeavouring to walk freely.

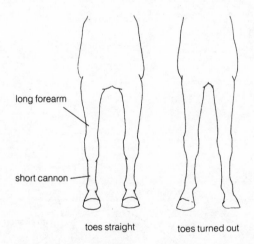

long forearm

short cannon

toes straight   toes turned out

Figure 3   Good chest, straight front legs
Figure 4   Poor chest, legs 'from the same hole'

Measurement of girth is of the greatest importance, and in a horse of 16 hands the girth measurement should be at least 6 feet. At one time, when purchasing a large number of horses for travelling long distances daily in double harness, I was instructed by the director of the firm that I must never purchase a horse that did not have 6 feet of girth. It was maintained, quite rightly, that this was the minimum measurement that gave the heart and lungs room to function adequately when the horse was in hard work.

A prominent sternum is sometimes encountered. This is a conformation which I dislike intensely: it gives the horse a pigeon-breasted appearance and is often seen in ill-balanced horses whose forefeet are too much under them. It is often associated with a flat chest and insufficient heart room, and such horses are often bad doers when put into hard work.

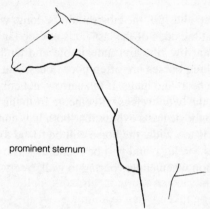

prominent sternum

Figure 5   Pigeon breast

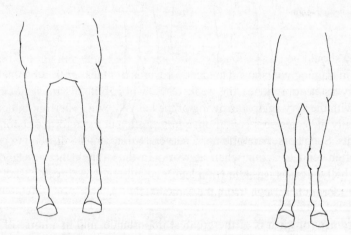

Figure 6   Wide chest, bench knees and pigeon toes
Figure 7   Narrow chest, small knees and feet turned out

Back

The back should be short and strong, but it must be remembered that the relative shortness of the back must be governed by the work the horse has to do. The Thoroughbred and the riding horse must have some length of back if they are to travel quickly, while the draught horse must be short of back and closely coupled. The term 'long back' is often used loosely. A horse for fast work must have some length of back and the confusion arises when the length of the back and the length of the loin are not defined. It is the loin which must be as short as possible in all circumstances; the loin is the least supported portion of the back and it is the horse with the length of loin which particularly gives the impression of slackness and too much length behind the saddle.

In the conformation of the back one may have a hollow back, in which the back is unduly dipped (and which must not be confused with the hollowing of the back with old age); and the roach back, in which there is an upward curve of the back and loin. Both are undesirable, and in my time I have noted a number of roach-backed horses which have eventually turned out to be shiverers. Horses with odd conformation of the back very often do not lie down regularly when in the stable and so shorten their working life.

Particular care should be taken when examining so-called 'cold-backed' horses (those that dip their back as the saddle is put on - see p. 676). Some of these horses may have an abnormality of the withers and saddle-bearing area and only very careful examination will reveal this. Often such an abnormality may not be noted on palpation of the withers and saddle area, but only be discovered by standing behind the horse and viewing along the back to the base of the neck. Any alteration in the shape of the withers or saddle-bearing area is then more easily detected.

The belly should be proportionate to the size of the horse, but not too big. The horse in training will show a tendency towards lightness of the abdomen, particularly as it approaches the peak of its work, but this must not be confused with the very sharp narrowing of the belly known as herring-gutted, which usually indicates poor condition, with insufficient room for the abdominal contents. Such horses are often of a nervous temperament, difficult to get fat, and often tend to scour when at work. In the draught horse a good capacious belly – or, as it is sometimes termed colloquially, bread-basket – indicates a good constitution and a good feeder; when needed for long hours of work such a conformation is essential.

In all geldings of any breed, always look for a well-developed sheath. It is a practical point that lack of development of this appendage usually indicates a weak constitution and, again, such animals are often bad doers.

The croup is an area of great importance in conformation. It comprises that part of the body between the loins and the setting of the tail. The pelvis and sacrum are involved in its formation and so effect a compact connection between the hind leg and the trunk. In most cases a nearly horizontal croup is

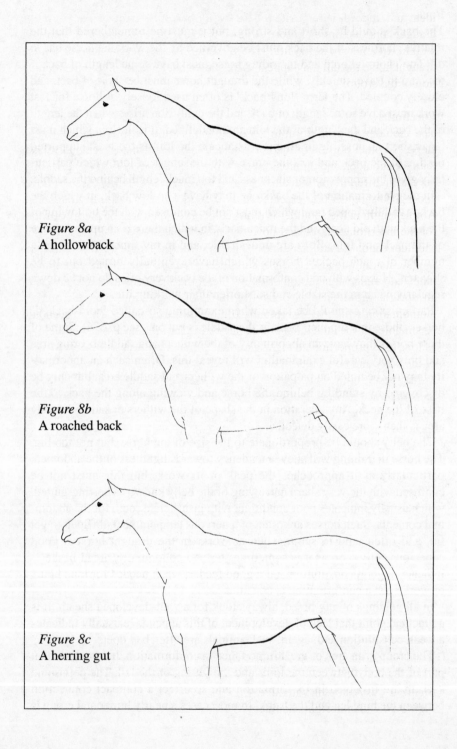

Figure 8a
A hollowback

Figure 8b
A roached back

Figure 8c
A herring gut

ideal and, indeed, is requisite for the development of great speed; but in the draught horse a more inclined croup will fill the requirements of ability to shift weight. In a nearly horizontal croup, the tail is well set on, whereas in the draught horse the tail may appear to be somewhat lower owing to the inclination of the croup.

Forelimbs
The shoulder, in proportion to good withers, should be of ample length and slope. No other portion of the horse's anatomy comes under greater criticism than the shoulder, and opinions on the type and suitability of the shoulder may vary with different individuals. Ample slope is essential in any breed of horse and a good shoulder is as essential in the draught horse as in the Thoroughbred. Ample length in the shoulder is required in order that there be plenty of room for the insertion of large and powerful muscles. Moreover, full action of the shoulder cannot be attained unless there is sufficient length of back to accommodate its obliqueness. Upright shoulders give rise to a shortened gait and, indeed, to undue concussion of the whole of the foreleg, while in many cases an upright shoulder is associated with a horse standing over in front – a combination which will eventually diminish its usefulness. The arm should be suitable for the attachment of its large muscles and, in all cases, should be as long as is proportionate to the shoulder, while the elbow should stand clear of the body and be well defined. Elbows that are turned in are objectionable, as they result in the feet being turned out, and, in the opposite tendency, the feet are turned in. In both cases undue strain is directed to the fetlock and feet; both conditions tend to produce lameness in the lower part of the leg and speedy-cutting and interference are common faults.

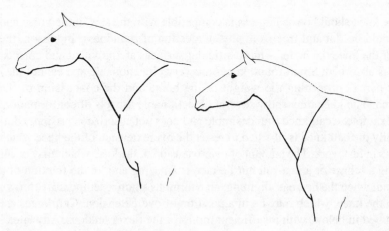

Figure 9   A sloping shoulder
Figure 10   An upright shoulder

The forearm should be long, wide, thick and well developed. From the point of view of speed, the conformation should be such as to present a long forearm and a comparatively short cannon. In the Hackney with high knee action, the forearm will be found to be comparatively short, but it should be remembered that if the forearm is too short, the action will be of a choppy nature and will not produce sufficient freedom to allow the horse to move with pace and action and to reproduce that impressive one, two, three, four, which is so desirable and essential.

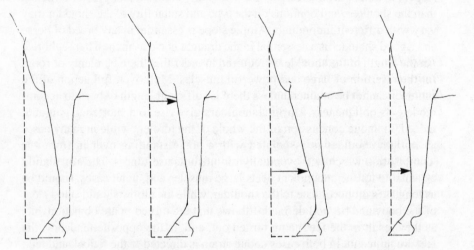

Figure 11   From left to right: correct forelimb conformation, forelimb set too far back, forelimb sloping back from the vertical, forelimb set too far forward

The knee should be as large as is compatible with the size of the horse and it should be flat and free from any suggestion of roundness. In reason, the larger the knee the better – more articular surfaces are provided and concussion is absorbed. Small round knees are very objectionable and cannot play their part in absorbing the weight of the horse and the concussion of the ground. The knee may show several objectionable aspects of conformation. For example, a calf knee is undesirable and does not absorb concussion; additionally the calf knee is ill-fitted to resist the overextension of the knee which occurs in fast work. The amount of overextension of the knee which may occur during a 'chase or a fast-run hurdle race is amazing and, in the fraction of a second, when the horse is alighting, an enormous strain is temporarily thrown upon the knee, which may be in a position of overextension. Calf knees are often tied in below, with insufficient room for the flexor tendons. Any lateral deviation of the knee is a serious breach of conformation. Such conditions give rise to unequal distribution of the bodyweight and tend to produce injuries to the supporting and connecting ligaments as a whole.

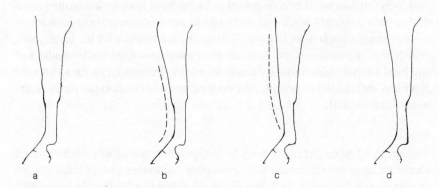

Figure 12a   Straight limb, but open knees
Figure 12b   Back at the knee
Figure 12c   Over at the knee
Figure 12d   Tied in below the knee

A markedly forward direction of the knee is known as 'over at the knee' or 'kneesprung' and it may be congenital or acquired. Many young horses with slightly forward knees are very sure-footed and have great freedom of movement. When acquired, this conformation is usually the result of excessive work combined with contraction of the tendons, and such horses will frequently stumble and be unsafe to ride.

The cannon should be short and strong with width from front to back, and this gives a good measurement of bone below the knee. Nevertheless, it should be remembered that in the long run it is not the amount of bone, but the quality of it which really counts. The cannon of the draught horse is shorter than that of the Thoroughbred, and in all well-formed animals the metatarsus is always longer than the metacarpus. The tendons must be clearly defined, with no suggestion of gumminess, and, when viewed from the front, cannon, fetlock and pastern must be in a straight line. No conformation is more likely to lead to unsoundness than a round cannon bone with fleshy tendons; such legs will not stand up to hard work.

The fetlock should be wide, thick and free from blemishes. When the fetlock is narrow in the antero-posterior direction, the tendons are always closer to the cannon bone and become more subject to strain at work.

The pastern should be of medium length and slope and both extremes have their drawbacks. The excessively long pastern, which is often lowjointed, is weak, and not only does it throw great strain on the tendons but it is an important factor in the production of sesamoiditis. The short, upright pastern is very strong, but it absorbs concussion to a greater extent and may result in the early formation of ringbone *if* associated with an indifferent foot. There is no doubt that the worst combination met with in the pastern is that of excessive length

and lowjointedness. This conformation in the hind limb is sometimes associated with a straight hock and stifle and is one of the worst conformations
of the draught horse that I know of. It leads to trouble with the hock joint,
which is subjected to excessive strain above and below. while the tendons of
the hind limb rapidly show evidence of strain. In such a conformation the
hind leg, throughout its length, has no mechanism for relieving the concussion of the ground.

Feet

Perhaps in no other part of the body is conformation related to soundness more
closely than in respect of the feet. Xenophon, centuries ago, pointed out the
importance of the foot in the horse and insisted that in all cases of examination
of the legs, one should look first at each foot. With defective feet the usefulness
of the horse is diminished, and whatever the job it does its working life is
limited, and eventually disease or inability will make its appearance. Feet must
be of a similar size and odd feet must arouse suspicion at once. Occasionally a
horse may be found which has had odd feet since birth, but for all practical
purposes the odd-footed horse is an unsound horse. A good foot must be well
shaped, not too large or too small, with a strong, deep, wide heel and a well-
developed frog, and the colour of the horn should be dark or blue. Seen from the
front, a well-developed foot should present a level surface, free from rings or
grooves, and showing no tendency to contraction at the quarters. Any form of
contraction is an unsoundness. When lifted, the foot should present a deep, wide
heel with a good frog having a shallow, medium lacuna. Any difference of the
angle of the slope in the wall of either foot should be regarded with suspicion.

McCunn has drawn attention to the important significance of any 'waisting'
of the hoof, accompanied by a lateral groove in the wall on either side. Such
a foot is almost invariably unsound and a horse with such a foot usually
develops some form of pedal osteitis.

I dislike a frog with a deep, split-up cleft, particularly in the draught horse;
such feet, in my opinion, frequently develop thrust or canker.

*Of all faults in conformation of the feet, a weak heel is the worst, because
without sufficient depth and width of heel, no horse will remain sound for long.*
Such a conformation exposes the navicular area to injury and particularly
encourages injury to the wings of the pedal bone, resulting in osteitis.

The foot may appear to be an excellent one when viewed from the front, but
the real test of its value is to see whether it possesses sufficient depth of heel.
A narrow hoof head should be avoided and in this connection it is always
essential, in heavy horses, to raise the hair at the coronet in order to examine
the top of the hoof. A horse with a narrow hoof head, with a tendency to bulge
slightly on its anterior aspect, is likely to develop pyramidal disease or low
ringbone when put to hard work. Flat feet are weak feet, and horses with such
rarely remain sound for any length of time.

It should always be remembered that on the foundation of the horse's feet rests its upper structure. In many cases the horse with indifferent feet will begin to prefer the centre of the road and will avoid the extreme camber of the near side.

Hind limbs
The hind limbs are the essential elements of propulsion in the horse and are associated with groups of muscles larger and more powerful than those of the forelimb. It has been pointed out that the greater obliquity of the shoulder and the more horizontal position of the croup in horses of speed tend to diminish the scapulo-humeral and coxofemoral angle, and so facilitate the forward and backward movement of the limbs. The thigh should be long, well-muscled, deep and well let down. Looked at from behind, it should be thick, with ample muscular development; above all, it must not show any signs of a split-up appearance. In this respect one should remember the old axiom of 'a head like a duchess and a bottom like a cook'. The second thigh should be well developed, and the stifle should be well forward in position.

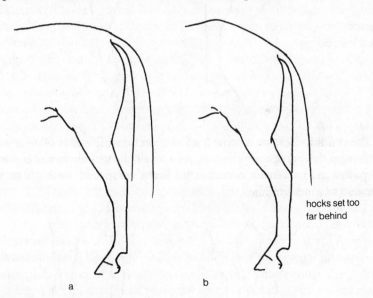

Figure 13a   Horizontal croup
Figure 13b   Goose or apple rump

Hocks
The hock constitutes the most important joint in the process of propulsion, and a good, well-developed, well-positioned hock is essential for soundness. The hock should be big in proportion to the size of the horse, wide and deep, with a well-marked point and, above all, well supported beneath and with no tie-in

immediately below. Above all, the hocks must be a pair and remember that the strong hock found in the young horse may fine down with increasing age. A slender, narrow hock is bad, just as a full, round, fleshy hock must be disliked.

The true value of the hock, apart from its size, depends upon the greater or less inclination of the tibia above and the cannon below. The so-called sickle hock results in the cannon bone taking an inclination forward so that the hind leg is brought under the body. Such a conformation is most undesirable. It leads to excessive strain of the hock joint above and of the tendons below, and usually results in unsoundness. In all cases, however, it must be remembered that for draught horses the hock may have a little forward inclination compared with that of the riding horse. This sickle-hock conformation is sometimes found in a big horse which stands over in front. Such a horse will usually be a source of trouble, either from overreaching or pulling off his foreshoes when galloped.

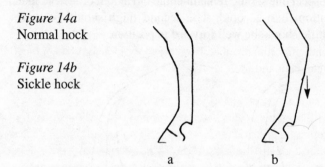

Figure 14a
Normal hock

Figure 14b
Sickle hock

a			b

The condition known as cow hock is objectionable and is often associated with other defects of conformation. As a result, the toes are turned out and loss of power and movement occurs as the limbs are moved outwards instead of forward in a straight line.

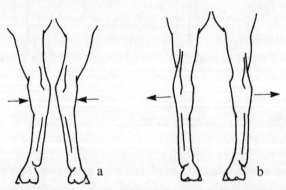

a			b

Figure 15a	Cow hocks
Figure 15b	Overwide hocks

Bowed hocks are equally objectionable, the hocks being set wide apart and the toes turned in. In this conformation the animal will be noted to twist the hock out as the foot comes to the ground and the foot develops a screwing movement as it touches the ground. In such animals the hocks tend to develop thoroughpin and bog spavin, while the coronet and feet become upright. Such animals are very hard wearers on their shoes and the toe is invariably knocked out too soon. The screwing action of the foot on reaching the ground is particularly likely to produce lameness. A good hock should be large and well directed and in its relation from the point through the back of the cannon to the ground should be vertical.

With regard to the limbs as a whole, in the forelimb, looked at from the front, a perpendicular line dropped from the point of the shoulder should divide the leg and feet into two lateral halves. Viewed from the side, a perpendicular line dropped from the tuberosity of the scapular spine should pass through the centre of the elbow joint and meet the ground at the centre of the foot. In the hind limb, viewed from the rear, a perpendicular line dropped from the point of the buttock should divide the leg and foot into two lateral halves. Viewed from the side, a perpendicular line dropped from the hip joint should meet the ground midway between heel and toe.

The horse's action
Good conformation is associated with correct movement. A horse must walk well, and if this movement is carried out correctly the horse will usually be satisfactory in his other paces. Action should be straight and true, with no dishing, brushing or interfering, and the toe should be well extended, especially in the riding horse. In the active draught horse and the Hackney, the knees and hocks should be well flexed and carried from the forearm and thigh in a straight and forward direction. In these breeds the horse must move over the ground and not pick the feet up and put them down in the same place again.

The action of the Thoroughbred and riding horse should be low and sweeping, with extension of the toe and a good carry forward of the hind leg. Avoid a horse that goes on its heels - this is bad movement and will usually be found to be associated, sooner or later, with unsoundness.

Wind
Lastly, soundness of wind and conformation. That conformation may influence soundness of wind is, to my mind, undeniable. From the point of view of size and height alone, it is well known that a big horse, e.g. a heavyweight hunter with height, is more likely to be unsound in his wind than a horse of moderate size. How many times do we examine a big, goodlooking hunter and immediately in our mind wonder if he will prove to be a roarer or a whistler? The relative immunity of the pony breeds from roaring and

whistling and the marked tendency of the fat, short-backed, wide-barrelled pony to become broken-winded is, indeed, well known.

As already noted, the set of the head upon the neck also has some influence. Not every whistler or roarer will have paralysis of the recurrent nerve, and conformation may, and in my opinion does, play a part in the production of such unsoundness.

Finally, 'a good horse is one with many good, few indifferent and no bad points'.

Never hesitate to buy a sound, well-made horse because it is in poor condition. Such horses, under good management and feeding, grow just as you would wish them to; and remember that fat or gross condition may hide a multitude of faults.

Without an understanding of conformation no one can develop that knowledge of soundness and unsoundness which is desirable in those who undertake examinations of the horse. It must never be forgotten that within the framework of its conformation lies the horse's essential soundness.

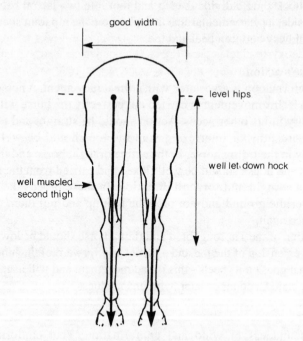

Figure 16   Good hindquarters and straight limbs

46
GENETICS OF THE HORSE

Genetics is the science of heredity; the study of how characteristics or traits are transmitted from parents to offspring. Animals and man inherit their characteristics via genes. Genes control characteristics by governing the changes which take place in development and are specifically ordered arrays of the four different chemical groups (called bases) which, in linear arrangement, make up the deoxyribonucleic acid (DNA) chains which form the backbone of the chromosomes. Chromosomes are found in the nucleus of every cell. Every species has a specific number of chromosomes. The horse has 64 chromosomes with 62 being autosomes and two sex-chromosomes. There are two of each autosome in every cell so that all cells of all horses have 31 different autosomes each present twice. The sex chromosomes are of two sorts, a large X chromosome and a small Y chromosome. In females there are two X

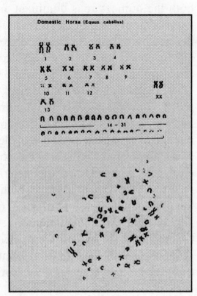

Figure 1
Karyotype and chromosome spread from mare: $2n = XX$

chromosomes and no Y but in males there is only one X and one Y. An individual receives one copy of each autosomal type and an X from its mother and a single copy of each autosomal type and either an X or a Y from its male parent. The fertilisations involving a Y chromosome develop as males as the Y carries the major gene for maleness.

Each gene has its own position on a specific chromosome; this is called the gene locus. Since each chromosome type, except the X and Y in males, is present twice, each individual has two copies of each gene except that males have only one copy of those genes which are on the X or the Y. Genes can occur in different forms called alleles. Different alleles of the same gene affect the same characteristic by all acting at the same point in development but produce slightly different end-expressions. Because each gene is present twice, it follows, that if a gene has more than one form (allele), it can be represented in an individual as two identical alleles or two different alleles. Some genes can have a large number of alleles but, because only two copies of the gene are present in any individual, any animal can only have two copies of the same allele or one copy of two alleles. Individuals in which the two alleles are the same are said to be homozygous while those which have two different alleles are heterozygous. Because each individual passes only one copy of each chromosome type to any one of its offspring, an homozygote can only pass to all its offspring the allele for which it is homozygous, while an heterozygote will pass a copy of one allele to half its offspring and a copy of the other to the rest.

The two alleles present in an individual can react in development in different ways. In some cases an allele can cover the presence of another. Such an allele is said to be dominant and the allele which is covered up is recessive. In animals which have a trait controlled by the expression of a dominant allele both the homozygous dominant and the heterozygote will have the same expression of the trait and the allelic constitution of the individual cannot be defined by its appearance or behaviour. This can be seen in the gene which allows coat colour to be either black or chestnut. Chestnut horses have two copies of the chestnut allele while blacks can have either two copies of the black allele or one copy of the black and one of the chestnut. The homozygote will however pass only the dominant allele to all its offspring while the heterozygote will pass that allele to only half with the rest having the chestnut allele. No matter what is the allelic constitution of mates all the offspring of the homozygote will show the expression of the dominant allele. If the heterozygote is mated to another heterozygote some of the offspring (25%) will receive a recessive allele from both parents and will show the expression of the recessive allele. The types of offspring left by homozygotes and heterozygotes will be different.

Sometimes the two different alleles present can both show their presence. In these cases the heterozygote is intermediate in expression between the two different homozygotes as in leopard spotting where one homozygote has no spots, the other has spots in a restricted area and the heterozygote is spotted all over. In other cases the alleles both show their effect without any interaction. This is the case with many alleles governing blood types. The homozygotes score only as the blood type of that allele while the heterozygotes score as both blood types.

It is frequently necessary to know how common alleles are in a population. If there is no dominance this is easy as we can simply count them; each animal which shows only the expression of one allele and is therefore homozygous carries two copies of that allele while the animals with intermediate expression or with both expressions are heterozygotes with one copy of each allele. The alleles cannot however be counted directly from the phenotypes when dominant/recessive relationships are present. Some of the recessive alleles will be hidden in heterozygotes. In this case we can estimate the frequency of the recessive allele as the square root of the frequency of the expression of the recessive trait. This arises because where two alleles **A** and *a* are present in a population at frequencies of p and q respectively the allelic combination **AA** will occur at p^2, **Aa** will occur at 2pq and **aa** will occur at q^2. The consequence of this is that recessive traits are shown at frequencies much lower than the frequencies of the allele itself but many recessives remain concealed in heterozygotes. If the recessive trait is undesired or even disease associated it is therefore important to be aware that there will be many more carriers of the unwanted allele than animals actually showing the trait. If the trait shows in 10% of foals there will be 42% heterozygotes (carriers), if it shows in 1% there will be 18% heterozygotes.

Sometimes the expression of one gene may be affected by the allelic constitution of another. A well-known example of this is the expression of Bay pattern. The allele governing this pattern can only be expressed if the animal is capable of making black pigment. To be Bay, a horse must therefore have at least one black allele of the black/chestnut gene. If the animal is homozygous chestnut the presence of a bay allele at the bay/non-bay gene cannot show as the animal cannot make the black pigment necessary for the lower legs, mane, etc. In this case the chestnut allele of the black/chestnut gene is epistatic to the bay pattern allele of the bay gene.

Another set of allele expressions which can be modified by other genes are all those controlling characteristics associated with one sex only. These are called sex-limited expressions. They arise because the expressions of the genes controlling them depend on the hormonal background in which they are working. The alleles give one set of characters in males because of the presence of male hormones and another in females where their action is altered because of the presence of female hormones. The most spectacular of these are those associated with milk production. The male has exactly the same genetic constitution as the female but the presence of male hormone and the absence of female hormone prevents the development of the necessary glands and udders.

Many traits, especially perhaps those associated with growth, or behaviour, or performance, are the combined expressions of many different genes with the ultimate expression being the sum of the effects of the expression of lots of genes. Such quantitative traits are said to be additive in their genetic control.

The X and Y chromosomes, as well as being markedly different in size, are very different in the number of genes which they carry. The Y can be regarded as carrying only the gene which ultimately causes the embryo to be male rather than female, while the X has lots of genes which act in the same sorts of ways as genes on the autosomes. Genes which are present on the X chromosomes are called sex-linked genes and their alleles frequently have different frequencies of expression in the sexes. This is because in the male where there can only be one copy of the gene present there can be only one allele and therefore no heterozygosity can exist. The allele cannot be covered by dominance. If it is present it must show itself. In the female it can be hidden by dominance and will only show itself, if it is a recessive, when it is present as an homozygote. Sex linked recessives show their expressions in males at the frequency of the allele in the breed and in females at the square of this frequency. Sex linked dominants show more frequently in females than males.

The genetic make-up of an animal is all the alleles which it carries and is called the genotype. The total of all the characteristics of the animal which can be scored is the phenotype. The phenotype is always known but it cannot always, because of dominance, epistasis and interaction with environmental pressures, be used to define the genotype. The only situation where the genotype of an animal can be defined is where the individual shows the expression of homozygosity for a recessive allele and no epistasis is involved.

In general, as animals become inbred, they lose heterozygosity and become more homozygous. This means that the frequency of recessive alleles being hidden by dominance decreases and it becomes easier to define the genotype from the phenotype. Inbreeding is the mating together of animals which share ancestors and line breeding is a form of this. The degree of inbreeding can be calculated from a pedigree and is called the coefficient of inbreeding (table 1). This coefficient is the probability that two alleles of any gene are copies of one which was present in an ancestor occurring on both sides of the pedigree (the genotype is said to be homozygous by descent for these alleles). All pure breeds are, by definition, inbred as they are homozygous for those alleles the expression of which define the characteristics of the breed. This homozygosity has been achieved by breeding together animals which are all descended from the original ancestors showing these characters. Inbreeding is therefore not always bad and is a necessary technique for the production of pure-breeding populations. The homozygosity which accumulates as inbreeding is practiced is however random, and is as likely to affect recessive as dominant alleles. Many deleterious alleles are recessive so that inbreeding can lead to an increase in the frequency of their expression and thus to a decrease in the usefulness of the animal. On the other hand the demonstration of the presence of unwanted recessives in a population allows the formulation of breeding plans to remove them. A much more difficult result of the random accumulation of homozygosity by inbreeding can be the appearance of inbreeding depression. This is a general drop in fitness, fertility and productivity which can, in some cases, be correlated with increasing inbreeding coefficients. It is associated, not with homozygosity for any specific alleles, but with a general increase in homozygosity. Inbreeding depression is not an inevitable result of inbreeding but only a possible consequence. It is best to attempt in most breeding programmes to keep the inbreeding coefficients below 0.06. The levels of inbreeding in breeds can be minimised if the breeds are maintained as separate lines for a number of generations. This may allow the increase of inbreeding coefficients within the lines but that can be easily reversed by crossing the lines and beginning again to set up a new set of lines from the crossed offspring. The breed can only be kept pure if the lines are of the same breed. Crossing between breeds will also eliminate inbreeding depression by getting rid of homozygosity but will result in hybrid offspring which cannot breed true as they will segregate to offspring with a mixture of characteristics from the breeds involved in the crosses.

The opposite of inbreeding depression is hybrid vigour where crossed animals show greater performance than their parents. This is relatively rare in crosses between lines but some crosses between specific breeds can show it e.g. the performance of some warm blood crosses with other types have outstanding performances far beyond those of either their sire or dam. These cannot however be produced other than from their respective pure bred parents as only that cross gives the correct mixture of alleles to show the effect. The animals themselves, because they are hybrids, cannot breed true.

Table 1 Coefficient of Inbreeding

$F_x = (1/2)^{n_1+n_2+1} (1 + F_a)$

where F_x = coefficient of inbreeding of individual x.

n_1 = the number of generations between one parent and a common ancestor.

n_2 = the number of generations between the other parent and the same common ancestor.

F_a = coefficient of inbreeding of the common ancestor. (When this is not known F_a is given an arbitrary value of 0.)

The genetics of coat colour
The coat colour of the horse is under the control of a number of genes which have a number of alleles and between which there are a number of epistatic reactions. All horses have all of these genes and the colour differences between individuals arise only because of the different alleles of the genes present in the different animals.

It is well known that matings between bay horses can produce bay, black or chestnut animals, matings between black parents can produce either black or chestnut foals but matings between chestnut horses can only produce chestnut offspring. This series of colours and patterns arises because a bay horse is genetically a black horse in which the development of the black pigment is restricted to the extremities by the action of the dominant allele of the bay gene the other allele of which allows the development of black all over the body. The dominant allele causing the development of the bay pattern is designated **A** and the non-bay is **a**. Bay horses must then be either **AA** or **Aa**. The production of the black pigment is governed by another gene which has two alleles. These are the dominant **E** allowing black pigment to be formed and the recessive **e** which does not permit the formation of black but allows only the production of chestnut pigment. Because **E** is dominant over **e** both **EE** and **Ee** horses form black pigment and are black but **ee** animals are chestnut. Because bay horses form black pigment, even though this is restricted to the extremities by the action of the **A** allele of the bay gene, all bay horses must have both a dominant **E** and a dominant **A**. If an animal with a **A** lacks **E**, i.e. it is **AAee** or **Aaee**, it will be chestnut as it cannot form black and **A** cannot show its effect. The genotypes possible in bay, black and chestnut horses are given in the table below.

Colour	Possible genotypes
Chestnut	**eeAA, eeAa, eeaa**
Black	**EEaa, Eeaa,**
Bay	**EEAA, EEAa, EeAA, EeAa**

It should be clear from this that all gametes produced by chestnut horses must carry **e** and thus matings between chestnuts can only produce chestnuts as the status of the **A** gene does not matter as it cannot work on chestnuts. Matings between blacks can produce either blacks or chestnuts because it is possible, if both parents are **Eeaa**, for both to produce either **Ea** or **ea** gametes. If an **Ea** gamete is involved in fertilisation the foal will be black because it will have **E** but if both gametes are **ea** the foal will be **eeaa** and thus be chestnut. Matings between blacks and chestnuts with **A** can produce bay foals because an **E** comes from one parent and an **A** from the other. Matings between **EeAa** bays can produce bay, black or chestnut foals because the gametes are **EA**, **Ea**, **eA** or **ea** and the random fusion of these can produce any of the genotypes in the table.

Grey horses are born any colour but become grey as they mature. This is governed by the grey gene for which the **G** dominant allele causes greyness to develop while the **g** recessive allele allows persistence of the birth colour. Because **G** is dominant, grey horses must have either one or two **G** alleles, and all grey animals must have at least one grey parent because they must have had **G** from a parent and that allele, because of its dominance, must have shown in the parent. Matings between **Gg** greys will produce some offspring which are **gg** and thus will not become grey but remain some other colour/pattern determined by the allelic constitution of the other colour/pattern genes.

There is a rare dominant allele **W** of the white gene which produces all-white animals. Coloured horses are all **ww** so that colour can develop but **WW** conceptuses die so that all white horses of this type are **Ww**. They cannot therefore breed true as matings between them will produce some **ww**, and thus coloured, foals.

Another colour gene with an allele which in its homozygous state caused death of the conceptuses is roan. All roan horses are **Rr** and all non-roans are **rr**.

There are a number of inherited white-mark patterns commonly found in horses. These are:
1. the variously sized and variously distributed white areas on the feet and the face;
2. the large white areas found on piebalds and skewbalds;
3. the similar but sometimes more diffuse pattern found in paints;
4. the extensive whitening found on apaloosian or leopard-spotted horses.

The inheritance of 1 is complex and may be governed by a number of genes with a number of alleles. The exact positioning of the white appears to involve a random element dependent on the migration of colour cells from their site of production in the body to the site of their expression in the coat.

The expression of piebald and skewbald is controlled by the Tobiano gene in which the **TO** dominant allele gives the white marks and the recessive **to** allele gives no such marks. If **TO** acts on a genetically black animal the offspring is piebald while if it is present in an otherwise chestnut animal the animal is skewbald. All piebald or skewbald animals must therefore have at least one **TO** allele.

Paint horses are heterozygous or homozygous for the dominant allele **O** of the overo gene. Animals not showing this pattern are therefore **oo** while those with it are **OO** or **Oo**.

Appaloosa animals show the pattern of leopard spots on a white background because of the action of the **LP** allele of the appaloosa gene. In the heterozygous state (**LPlp**) this allele produces an animal with spots distributed all over its body but when homozygous (**LPLP**) the spots are restricted to areas of the body with the rest being non-spotted. Horses with no leopard spotting are **lplp** homozygotes. The colour of the spots is dependent on the other colour genes being expressed in the animal.

Blood typing

A good example of normal genetic variation (or genetic polymorphism) is the series of genes which control the red blood cell antigens and the different serum proteins. Depending upon their different cell surface antigens, red cells can be divided into groups and this is what is meant by the term 'blood group' (Table 2). In addition, present in serum and within red cells, there are a number of different proteins and enzymes which are polymorphic and therefore can be used to identify individual horses (Table 3). The protein complement plus the red cell antigens make up the blood type of the horse.

Table 2 Blood Group Systems in the Horse

Antigen type	Alleles
A	A^a, A^b, A^c, A^{bc}, A^-
C	C^a, C^-
D	D^{bc}, D^c, D^{ce}, D^{cef}, D^d, D^{ad}, D^{de}, D^{df}
K	K^a, K^-
P	P^a, P^b, P^-
Q	Q^a, Q^R, Q^{RS}
U	U^a

Table 3 Protein Polymorphism Used in Blood Typing in the Horse

Protein/Enzyme	No. of alleles
Albumin	3
Transferrin	10
Prealbumin (Pr)	9
Prealbumin (XK)	3
Esterase	7
6 Phosphogluconate dehydrogenase (PGD)	3
Phosphoglucomutase (PGM)	3
Phosphohexose isomerase (PHI)	3

The efficiency with which blood typing can be used to categorize an individual depends upon the number and frequency of alleles for each system. Different breeds have different alleles or a different frequency of alleles in the population. For example, the red cell factors D & and K' have not been found in Arabs but are present in Thoroughbreds, while the enzymes PGM and PHI are found in Arabs but not Thoroughbreds. The greater the number of characteristics tested, the larger the number of alleles at each locus, and the broader the spread of frequency of each allele within a population, the less likely it is that any two individuals will be found to have exactly the same genotype. This is important because blood typing is mainly used as an individual's 'fingerprint' and hence utilised in questions of doubtful parentage. Whereas an animal can be excluded as a parent by means of blood typing, it can never be proved to be the parent.

Variation in DNA which does not code for genes
Only a small portion of the DNA in the strands forming the backbone of the chromosomes actually acts as genes. Most of the DNA present is of unknown function and in this DNA there is a great deal of variation. Much of this variation consists of repeated sequences of the bases from which DNA is formed. The blocks of bases are the same in the same positions on pairs of chromosomes but they can be represented by different numbers of copies of the repeated bases. One chromosome of a pair can have x repeats while its partner can have y repeats. These different repeat numbers are transmitted via gametes to offspring in the same way as alleles of genes and can be treated as alleles of non-coding DNA. As they always occupy the same positions on a chromosome they can, if found closely associated with a gene, be used as flags for alleles of that gene. Allele 1, on one chromosome of a pair, will be next to repeat number x, and allele 2, on the other chromosome of the pair, next to repeat number y. An individual homozygous for allele 1 will then have two copies of repeat number x, a homozygote for allele 2 will have two copies of repeat number y, and an heterozygote will have one copy of x repeats and one of y repeats. Via special techniques called the Polymerase Chain Reaction and Electrophoresis, the sections of repeats with a small part of the adjoining DNA which may include part of a gene can be copied many times in vitro and can then be spread on a slab of special medium. In electrophoresis, in response to an electric current, the pieces of DNA move along the medium and the distance they move is inversely proportional to their size. Small pieces move further than large pieces so that low number repeats move further than high number repeats. An homozygote for a low number repeat will then show a band quite far up the slab of medium and an homozygote for a high number repeat a band lower down the slab. An heterozygote will show two bands one in the high number position and one in the low number. If the repeat blocks are associated with specific alleles of a functional gene homozygosity or

heterozygosity at that gene can be recognised from the position and number of the bands on the gel. This technique is very useful in screening possible parents to see if they carry unwanted alleles of particular genes especially those recessives which, in the homozygous state, cause disease. Such a test is available for Severe Combined Immunodeficiency Disease (SCIDS) which is found in Arabian horses and is inherited as an autosomal recessive (a recessive allele of a gene on an autosome). In the homozygous state this allele kills the foal and is thus a recessive lethal allele. The application of this test allows the identification of animals carrying one copy of the recessive lethal allele and thus allows them to be removed from the breeding population, thus preventing the transmission of the unwanted allele to the next generation. Clearly, if all the carriers of the allele can be identified and, in one generation, all such carriers removed from the breeding group, the allele can be totally removed from the breed. If, however, carriers of unwanted alleles are common in a breed their total removal from the breed in one generation may cause an unacceptable reduction in the numbers of breeders. The production of foals, free from the symptoms of the disease, can however be achieved by never mating together parents both of which are carriers.

DNA variants of the sort described above can also be used in parentage testing as they are transmitted to offspring in the same way as alleles of any other gene. They may have advantages over conventional blood type based parentage testing as there are many of them in all species and many have a large number of alleles. The allelic constitution of an animal for these variants can be generated from any tissue sample and, for parentage testing, the favoured tissue is hair follicle. These are collected by plucking hair samples from the tail or mane (making sure that there are obvious follicles attached to the hairs) and this process can be done by an owner without veterinary intervention. The samples can be sent dry to the testing laboratory in a sealed envelope.

Developmental abnormalities
When abnormalities are present at birth, these are said to be congenital. Such abnormalities may be caused by deleterious genes and therefore are heritable. However, they could also be caused by other agents during pregnancy, such as virus infections, drug administrations, extremes of temperature and exogenous chemicals. Such abnormalities would not be passed on to the next generation, but they might look exactly like those anomalies which are genetic in origin. It is therefore often not easy to determine whether or not a specific abnormality is caused by deleterious genes. Even when a genetic cause is strongly suspected, it may not be possible to define the mode of action and inheritance of the gene or genes involved. For this reason definitive advice on development anomalies is often not possible.

A number of congenital abnormalities are recognized in the horse but only a very few have been proved to be genetic in origin.

Reproductive System

Developmental abnormalities of the reproductive tract occur due to single gene anomalies and also to whole chromosome abnormalities.

TESTICULAR FEMINIZATION

This condition is due to an X-linked gene, the testicular feminizing gene (tfm), which renders the target organs incapable of responding to testosterone. The result is that, during embryogenesis in a genetic male, the gonads differentiate to form testes but the testosterone-dependent male duct system falls to develop. The female duct system is inhibited in the normal way and the uro-genital sinus, being unable to respond to testosterone, develops as a blind-ending vagina. Externally the animal is a phenotypic female, while internally there are abdominal testes and little or no tubular genitalia.

Inheritance and recommendation
Females carry the tfm gene in the heterozygous state and 50% of their offspring will receive the tfm gene. All male offspring receiving the gene will be affected and will present as infertile 'females'. Female offspring receiving the gene will be reproductively normal but may pass the gene to their offspring. If an affected animal is diagnosed, the dam should not be used for rebreeding. The sire will not have contributed to the condition and can safely be re-used.

XY GONADAL DYSGENESIS

This condition is superficially similar to testicular feminization. The animal is a genetic male but presents as an infertile 'female'. Internally there is normally some development of the Mullerian duct system with a cervix and a uterus. However, there is always a complete absence of normal gonadal tissue.

Inheritance and recommendation
Gonadal dysgenesis is thought to be due to an autosomal gene, but the mode of inheritance is not known. It may be that both parents have contributed to the condition (autosomal recessive) or that it is passed on only through the dam (malelimited autosomal dominant). In either case it is advisable not to repeat the mating.

XY SEX REVERSAL

This is a condition seen in Arabs, Quarter horses, Thoroughbreds and Paso Fino breeds. The animals again present as infertile 'females' although genotypically they are male. Phenotypically they can range from 'mares' showing oestrous cycles and sporadic follicle production to 'mares' that are overtly masculinized.

Inheritance
This varies. In most cases it appears as an X-linked or autosomal sex-limited dominant trait. In one case there was inheritance through the male either as an autosomal sex-limited dominant trait or as a Y chromosomal mutation with the carrier having some germ cells with the normal gene and other germ cells with the mutant gene.

XO SYNDROME AND XO/XX MARES

Some mares have only sixty-three chromosomes because one X chromosome is missing. These are described as 63 XO mares.

Pure XO mares tend to be small in stature with an infantile uterus and small, underdeveloped, fibrous gonads. They present as animals which fail to cycle. Clinical symptoms in cases of mares which have both abnormal (X0) and normal (XX) cells are more varied. There is often some development of the ovaries with irregular signs of oestrous behaviour, while others show no signs of oestrus at all.

Inheritance and recommendation
It is not known whether it is the maternal or paternal X that is missing in these cases, which are rare. There is no record of any mating having produced more than one normal offspring, therefore no particular breeding policy is necessary.

INTERSEXES

Intersexuality (part male, part female) in the horse can be due to an autosomal gene. In these cases the animal is a genotypic female but externally there is an enlarged clitoris which may be rather penis-like. There is often an increase in the distance between the anus and vulva. Internally the gonads are testicular and may lie anywhere along the line between the normal ovarian position and the inguinal ring.

Other intersex types have had abnormal chromosome complements (e.g. 63X0/64XX/65XXY, 63X0/64XY, 64XX/65XXY) but their phenotype is very similar to the 64XX intersexes.

Treatment

The problems associated with these animals are behavioural. Most have some male characteristics and may try to mount other females. Removal of the gonads solves this problem but requires major surgery. Secondly, because of the position of the penis-like organ, the animal will urinate backwards in an arc, even although it will squat like a female. This may create problems for the unwary.

CRYPTORCHIDISM

Cryptorchidism (see p. 361) is hereditary but the mode of inheritance is not always clear. In the Welsh Mountain pony it is thought to be due to an autosomal recessive. Unilateral cryptorchids should not be used for breeding, and mares producing a cryptorchid foal should be eliminated from the breeding stock.

Haematopoietic and Lymphatic Systems

HAEMOLYTIC DISEASE
(NEONATAL ISOERYTHROLYSIS)(see also p. 453)

This is a condition seen in young foals of any breed after they have suckled the dam's colostrum. It is characterized by an acute jaundice and may result in death if not treated.

The condition is caused by the production by the mare of antibodies to the foal's red blood cells. These antibodies pass into the foal via the colostrum. The mare only produces antibodies if her blood group and that of the foal are incompatible and she has been previously sensitized. Hence it is usually only seen in mares which have already produced a number of normal foals.

Treatment

This consists of replacement blood transfusions to the foal with blood from a compatible donor. It is advisable to remove some of the foal's blood to limit damage to the kidneys due to haemolysis.

Preventive measures

Before mating takes place the mare and stallion should be checked for blood group compatibility. Serum from the mare is mixed with erythrocytes from the stallion and if these haemolysize any offspring may develop haemolytic disease if it inherits an incompatible blood group from the sire. The mating may be abandoned at this stage.

Alternatively the mating can proceed and the foal's blood checked at birth before it suckles the colostrum. If the foal's blood is compatible with the mare's, suckling can take place as normal. However, if the foal's blood is incompatible with that of the mare, colostrum from a compatible nurse mare should be given for forty-eight hours and the foal prevented from suckling its own dam. After this period antibodies are not absorbed from the digestive tract, so suckling can be permitted.

HAEMOPHILIA

This is a rare condition in which the normal clotting mechanism is impaired. In the horse it is due to a deficiency of Factor VIII. Only male foals are affected. They appear normal at birth but within a few days develop haematomas.

Inheritance and recommendation
The inheritance is a sex-linked recessive gene.

The condition is passed on by the mare since females are heterozygous carriers, and males are affected hemizygotes. Thus the dam of an affected animal and any of her daughters should not be used for breeding.

STRUCTURAL ABNORMALITIES OF THE HEART

A number of congenital abnormalities of the heart are thought to be genetic in origin but the mode of action and inheritance are not known. These include interventricular septal defect, patent ductus arteriosus, patent foramen ovale, persistent right aortic arch, and the tetralogy of Fallot.

Immunodeficiency

There are three similar conditions which are due to a failure of the normal immunological defence systems of the horse.

COMBINED IMMUNODEFICIENCY (CID)

This is a condition seen in Arabian-bred foals and which is due to a simple autosomal recessive gene. There is a combined B- and T-lymphocyte deficiency, and affected foals are markedly lymphopaenic (that is, there is a marked decrease in the proportion of lympocytes in the blood), with less than 1000 peripheral blood lymphocytes/mm blood. The foals are incapable of responding to immunization and produce no immunoglobulins of their own.

Affected foals develop clinical infections, usually a pneumonia, due to adenoviruses with secondary bacterial invasion, which are always fatal. The life expectancy depends upon the amount of passive protection the foal receives from the dam's colostrum, but to date all foals have died within five months of birth.

Recommendation

Because both the mare and the stallion are carriers of the recessive gene, they should not be used for breeding.

PRIMARY AGAMMAGLOBULINAEMIA

This condition was seen in a male Thoroughbred foal. The T-lymphocyte levels and functions were normal but there was a complete absence of functional B-lymphocytes. The animal eventually died at the age of seventeen months after repeated infections causing pneumonia and arthritis. It is suggested that the condition is similar to the sex-linked disorder in humans.

SELECTIVE IGM DEFICIENCY

Low or complete absence of serum IgM has been seen in foals of Arabian and Quarter horse breeding. The T- and B-Iymphocyte counts were normal as were the levels of other immunoglobulins. It is not known whether this is a primary, genetic-based condition.

Eye

ANIRIDIA

Aniridia is an absence of the iris and is usually associated with cataract.

Inheritance and recommendation

The condition is due to an autosomal dominant gene. Since the gene is dominant, discarding all affected animals will eliminate the condition.

OTHER ABNORMALITIES

A number of other congenital abnormalities occur, though rarely (see Table 4). Many are thought to have a genetic component in their aetiology but the modes of inheritance are not known.

Table 4 Congenital Eye Abnormalities in the Horse

Aniridia (known to be due to an autosomal dominant gene)

Anophthalmia (complete absence of an eye)

Atresia of the naso-lacrimal duct (blockage of the tear duct)

Cataract (see p. 181)

Coloboma iridis (abnormal development of the iris resulting in part of it missing)

Congenital keratopathy (developmental abnormalities of the cornea usually resulting in loss of opacity)

Corneal dermoids (opaque, skinlike growth on the normally opaque cornea)

Detached retina (detachment of the retina from the back of the eyeball resulting in blindness)

Ectropion (eversion of the eyelids exposing the mucous membranes)

Entropion (see p. 179)

Glaucoma (swelling of the eye due to increased fluid pressure)

Melanosis of the cornea (black pigmentation on the cornea)

Microcornea (abnormally small cornea)

Night blindness (Inability to see in weak light because of a defect in the retina)

Optic nerve hypoplasia (incomplete development on the optic nerve resulting in blindness)

Recommendation

When inheritance is suspected but not proven, the safest procedure is to refrain from breeding from stock that have produced an affected foal.

Nervous and Musculoskeletal Systems

CEREBELLAR HYPOPLASIA
(CEREBELLAR DEGENERATION)

A hereditary form of cerebellar hypoplasia is seen in Arabians. In this condition the animal is unable to control the extent or degree of muscular action, which results in overreaching (hypermetria), paddling and head tremors. Signs usually appear at four to six months of age.

Inheritance and recommendations
The condition is thought to be genetic in origin, although possible viral causes have not been excluded. It is advisable not to rebreed from parents of an affected foal.

HEREDITARY ATAXIA

A form of ataxia (Incoordination) seen in the German Oldenberg breed is genetic in origin. Symptoms appear from three weeks onwards, when the foal shows loss of muscular coordination. The animal is liable to fall and is unable to rise. Death usually occurs within two weeks of symptoms first appearing.

Inheritance and recommendation
The ataxia is due to a single autosomal recessive gene. Both parents of an affected animal are carriers and should not be used for breeding.

WOBBLER SYNDROME (see also p. 326)

Wobblers are young horses, more commonly males, between the ages of six and twenty-four months, which show signs of ataxia, weakness and spasticity of the pelvic limbs. It is a complex syndrome with more than one aetiology. In one form the symptoms are due to a compression of the spinal cord due to cervical vertebral malformation. There is thought to be a genetic component to the syndrome in that there is a predisposition to a narrow vertebral canal and susceptibility to bone and cartilage disease.

OCCIPITO-ATLANTO-AXIAL MALFORMATION (OAAM)

A familial abnormality of the atlas, with fusion to the occiput, is seen in Arabians. Foals may be born dead because of medulla oblongata compression. Alternatively, the less severe cases range from tetraplegia to abnormal head and neck carriage.

Inheritance and recommendation
It is suggested that in Arabs this is due to a simple autosomal recessive. Parents of an affected foal should not be used for breeding.

TORTICOLLIS (WRYNECK)
Affected animals have a twisted neck due to involuntary contraction of the cervical muscles. In the congenital form the condition is due to an autosomal recessive, and thus both parents are carriers and should not be rebred.

OTHER ABNORMALITIES
Other congenital abnormalities of the musculoskeletal system are listed in Table 5. Evidence of any genetic component and mode of inheritance for these conditions is weak.

Table 5   Congenital Abnormalities of the Musculoskeletal System

Arthrogryposis (literally 'crooked joint'; abnormal
        contraction of the muscles causing crooked,
        fixed joints)
Contracted flexor tendons (see p. 330)
Multiple exostosis (see p. 221)
Patella luxation and fixation (see p. 255)
Polydactyly (see p. 221)

Digestive System

ATRESIA COLI

This is a closure or lack of development of the ascending colon in the region of the pelvic flexure. Death will occur due to an inability to defecate unless the condition is corrected surgically.

The condition is due to a simple, autosomal recessive gene, so neither parents should be used for breeding.

PARROT MOUTH AND SOW MOUTH

Parrot mouth is when the lower jaw is shorter than the upper, while sow mouth is when the lower jaw is longer than the upper. Both conditions are considered an unsoundness.

Both conditions are believed to be genetic but the mode of inheritance is not known.

WHITE FOAL SYNDROME

There are a number of different genes which produce the white coat colour. One, which produces a white foal with blue eyes, is recessive. The foals are born alive but die within a few days because of a large constriction of the large intestine.

Neither parent of affected foals should be used for breeding.

MISCELLANEOUS

EPITHELIOGENESIS IMPERFECTA (HAIRLESSNESS)

Affected foals have patches of skin which lack hair and in these areas the skin is leathery. Sometimes one or more hooves are missing. Most foals die within a few days of birth.

The condition is due to an autosomal recessive gene, so neither parent should be rebred.

UMBILICAL AND INGUINAL HERNIAS

Males tend to have inguinal hernias more commonly than umbilical, while in females it is vice versa. Quarter horses seem more prone to umbilical hernias than other breeds.

The mode of inheritance is not known but affected animals should not be used for breeding.

LETHAL DOMINANT WHITE

As the name suggests, this is a dominant gene that produces a white foal with blue or hazel eyes. Homozygous foals die in utero and all white horses with the dominant white gene are heterozygotes. When such horses are mated, 25% of the embryos will be homozygous for the white gene and will therefore die in utero. The cause of death is not known.

47

SELECTIVE BREEDING
– ESSENTIAL TO COMPETITIVENESS!

Which stallion should I choose for my mare? This is the most common question breeders put up, usually in good advance of the breeding season. I have experienced it for a long time, both as a geneticist and adviser on breeding issues, as well as when being responsible for the activities of a breed society. And as a practical breeder I certainly do it myself. Many thoughts are given to this subject by the breeders, and very rightly so. An old saying is: 'Select the best to be mated to the best, and then hope for the best!' The answer may not be as easy as that, but it certainly expresses the idea of strong selection, while there are no guarantees in what you get. Let's clarify the issue a little.

Which stallion should I use – what about the mare?
Firstly, the question on which stallion to use needs to be returned to the breeder with a whole range of questions. Which mare is it? What are her qualifications to be or become a broodmare? What is her pedigree? If bred before, what is her fertility record, and what kind of progeny has she produced before? How have they been tested or shown? We need to clarify the quality of the mare before any choice of stallion can be discussed. And not only that. We need to make sure that the mare has such qualities that there is a good opportunity that she can be pregnant without too much trouble, and that she can transmit good genes to her progeny. All mares are not worth breeding. Some selection must take place if we are going to be able to produce competitive horses for the market. And the market for sport horses has become more demanding by time. The riders and trainers do not worry too much from where or which country the horses come, only that they have the right qualities for their purposes.

What are your breeding goals?
The facts needed about the mare only explain part of the story that needs to be clarified. Another question to be settled concerns you as a breeder and the

objectives you have with this breeding activity. What sport discipline do you aim to produce a horse for? For what market? Maybe, for your own purpose, or for supplying the children with a horse? Or maybe for the export market? The demands may be quite different, and as a consequence also the choice of both mares and stallions to use.

Objective information about available stallions needed

Depending on the answers to all these questions the response to the initial question will vary a lot. To what extent they will vary depends, however, in the end on which stallions are available, the conditions for their use, and the kind of information that is available about the stallions. How have they been tested? What kind of breeding values have they got based on the performance of their progeny? Again, as many questions as for the mares need to be answered about the stallions. As stallions quite often are followed by rumours about their inherited qualities, it is extremely important to find real facts as a basis for any decisions.

It is obvious from the above that a whole series of questions need to be attended in a systematic manner if we are going to be successful as breeders. Some of the issues depend largely on the individual breeder, his or her knowledge and ability to evaluate horses, but a lot is dependent of the joint efforts of the breeders within the framework of their breed societies. The breeding programme and testing and selection methods applied, giving rise to the objective information needed, are usually the responsibilities of breed societies. In order to cast some light more systematically on these issues we need to clarify some principles of horse breeding that at the end of the road will help us to make the right choices of stallions for our mares. We will limit ourselves to the breeding of sport horses and have an international look at the situation, as much research has taken place in the past decades in this field in Europe.

SOME BASIC GENETIC PRINCIPLES

Mares and stallions provide half of the genes each, but ...

The relative merits of the mare and the stallion is often discussed among breeders. Let us make this part short and conclude that each foal gets half of its genes from each one of the parents. We shall not mix this up with the fact that the mare also influences the foal with the environment that she provides, from the time the fetus is placed in the uterus to the later mental development of the foal as a result of the temperament of the dam while rearing the foal. Thus, the choice of mares for breeding is very important, but not just for the genes they transmit.

Stallions give many more foals

The opportunity of the individual mare to contribute to the improvement of the breed, compared to the individual stallion, is severely limited by the fact that the reproductive capacity of the mare is much less than that of the stallion. While mares may on average give birth to ten foals, a stallion may produce 50-100 times more foals, especially in larger populations where artificial insemination is practised.

Broodmares should always be among the better half...
In order to maintain the number of mares in a population one must select about 40% of the fillies born to replace their mothers and contribute to optimum genetic progress. This assumes that these new broodmares are selected at the age of five or earlier and stay in breeding until better mares are found. If selected at later ages, many more of the remaining mares must be used to maintain the population size, a practice that would lead to very weak selection and progress despite the fact that you may know more about the individual horse, the good ones as well as the bad ones. A regular practice to select mares for breeding after a sports career is therefore not a viable strategy, although it occasionally may be practised.

...while stallions should be much more strongly selected
Stallions on the other hand can be selected at a much higher intensity. One percent of the colts born will in most cases be enough. However, the rate is dependent on a number of facts such as the population size, testing procedures and use of artificial insemination. This is why testing methods applied for evaluating the characteristics of stallions need to be much more accurate than those for selection of mares. Altogether this means that in an optimum breeding programme of a breed, testing and selection of stallions account for 70-80% of the overall progress achieved in the breed. Nevertheless, as an individual breeder you must look into your opportunities to select good mares for the breeding objectives you have set for your own operation.

Inbreeding and linebreeding belong to history
In early days most breeds were formed by practising some form of inbreeding, of which linebreeding is a mild variant. These breeding practices were applied in order to get more uniform animals within a population and to get rid of some weak animals or defects that may have occurred in the population. Linebreeding was practised by accumulating genes from some previous individuals known to transmit superior genes. Through in- and linebreeding more gene pairs are becoming homozygous, i.e. alike in the chromosomes from both sire and dam. A weak point of in- and linebreeding is that defective genes are also accumulated in such a way that they may become lethal or sublethal in its homozygous forms. Such genes are otherwise kept hidden and will not cause any problems, provided the gene frequency is kept not too high. An easy principle to follow in order to avoid inbreeding, and thereby some weaknesses, is to check that the same ancestor is not appearing more than once in the first three generations of the foal pedigree.

A second reason to leave these breeding practices to history is that they were applied during times before modern methods for estimation of breeding values were known or available. Today the situation is completely different. We now have a much better understanding of the principles of inheritance and how to make use of that in designing testing schemes to offer rapid genetic progress in the various horse populations, i.e. to find the best breeding stock for efficient use.

Traits are more or less heritable

Determining the breeding objective means that you have decided which trait you will put most emphasis on in order to meet the requirements of the market you look for. It is then important that you choose to select for traits that show a reasonably high *heritability*. This value, ranging from 0-100%, expresses the accuracy of selection for the trait you have chosen, or the likelihood of similarity between parents and their offspring.

In producing *dressage* horses, apparently good basic gaits are a prerequisite as well as a good rideability and temperament for the sport. All these traits show reasonably good heritabilities, of the order 30-50%, especially if the horses have been doing a performance test of some length. Evaluations based on one-day tests yield less accurate information, somewhat lower heritabilities, 20-30%, but are quite sufficient for mare testing as many mares can be tested and a good basis for selection is provided. *Conformation* is usually positively correlated to results from performance tests for gaits and dressage, but can never replace these tests. Still a good-looking horse of sufficient size for the rider, with a good neck and shoulder, and correct set legs, is desirable. Subjectively scored conformation traits show heritabilities of the order 10-30%, whereas measured wither height shows a heritability of 40-60%.

Freejumping offers good opportunities for selection

For *showjumping* purposes the conformation plays less of a role, although the horse must have a sound constitution and a good rideability and balance through a long and well set neck. More important though, is that the horse must show natural talents for jumping. For selection purposes it is therefore critical that both stallions and mares, as prospects for breeding, are tested for their jumping ability. Such tests are usually done in combination with the gaits evaluations in performance tests of various kinds. Studies show that freejumping tests show higher heritabilities, often about 50%, than tests under rider, and therefore provide very good information to be used for selection purposes. As an example it could be mentioned that the Holsteiners, which no doubt have been very successful in international showjumping, have mainly been selected for jumping ability based on freejumping of 2 1/2-year old colts.

Select among young horses and use highly qualified judges

Of course, as in the case for dressage, these early tests of sport performance may be considered less accurate for prediction of sport results at the most advanced levels. However, such results are not available in the young horse when the selection has to take place, and furthermore the influence of the rider has become very large. Competition results therefore usually show lower heritabilities, 20% or less, than well conducted performance tests of younger horses. There is one important reservation though. As we deal with subjectively scored traits, the accuracy, or heritability we find is very much dependent on the quality and experiences of the judges used for the performance tests.

In summary it could be concluded that selection of stallions for both dressage and showjumping should be based on well designed performance tests. These could vary in length from one week to several months, but should provide the most important information about stallions to allow good decisions to be made by the breeders in their choice of males for best matings of their mares. In the selection of broodmares it is equally important that they are performance tested as 3-5 year olds, but one-day tests in combination with a pedigree evaluation and the knowledge of the breeder about the characteristics of the mare, is sufficient.

Don't look too far back in the pedigrees!
As regards the pedigree evaluation, horse breeders seem by tradition to put too much emphasis on generations far back. If the breeding values of both the sire and dam are well known, very little, if anything, will be gained by considering generations beyond the grandparents on the sire side and the third generation on the dam's side. The difference between the sire and dam depends on the more accurate information usually available on the sires through their many progeny.

Breeding values based on progeny information
– an important tool for selective mating
Progeny evaluations based on performance tests as 3-5 year olds are very important as a second step for selection, mainly to cull stallions whose progeny do not meet expectations. Results from such tests or competitions form the basis for genetic evaluations of stallions, and sometimes also mares, in several European countries today, e.g. in Denmark, France, Germany, Ireland, the Netherlands and Sweden. The horses get breeding values, so-called BLUP-indexes, for different traits, and they account for the heritability of the traits and include information on the individual itself as well as on all tested relatives. The method, named after its properties for selection (Best Linear Unbiased Prediction), provides the best information for selection and culling of breeding stock. It has been the task of the breed societies in each country to cooperate with scientists to develop the most appropriate testing and evaluation scheme, and thereby provide the breeders with as accurate information as possible about the breeding stock available. In Sweden, for instance, such testing systems started in the early 1970s and nowadays provide breeders with

objective and genetically correct information on both sexes for a number of traits regarding dressage, jumping and conformation. In that way the breeders can more easily make the 'right' choices of stallions to fit a given mare.

SOME GUIDELINES IN SUMMARY

Let us return to the initial question about which stallion to use and summarise the steps to be taken, realising that the information on the breeding stock may not always be optimal. Here are some guidelines:

1. Be precise on your breeding objective and the market needs you want to meet.

2. Make sure that your mare is a suitable broodmare with good test results and pedigree for the sport in question. If test or competition results are lacking, have an established trainer to evaluate the horse for you if you feel uncertain. Lay out both strengths and weaknesses of the mare. Try to be objective, although you may be attached to the horse! Any broodmare should always belong to the better half of the population.

3. Screen among the stallions available which ones best fit your primary breeding goal. If you have high ambitions with your breeding you should be aware of the opportunities of utilising artificial insemination and that many stallions from different countries may be available through transported chilled semen. Use the internet to find information from breed societies and stallion owners, domestically and abroad. Look at performance test or competition results to evaluate young stallions and estimated breeding indexes, if available, for the older ones. Distinguish between fact and advertisements!

4. Find out which of the stallions have strengths where your mare needs to be compensated. Don't consider stallions with the same weaknesses as the mare. Consider the size and type of horse desired, e.g. lighter, with more substance, etc. For production of eventing horses the use of a thoroughbred stallion may be desirable.

5. Check the pedigrees of the potential stallions selected this far, firstly to avoid undesirable inbreeding, and secondly to verify that the pedigree supports the breeding objective set.

6. Check the conditions for use and see which conditions best meet your requirements or wishes.

7. Now pick the two to three stallions that you find suit best and try to inspect them before the final decision – and that decision will be yours and depend on sense and taste!

Remember, in following a procedure such as this one, you have a good opportunity to succeed, but due to chance in the combination of genes from the stallion and mare, there are no guarantees of the product! We only know that a consistent selection according to the principles given here, in combination with a good eye for what type of horses you want, gives a high probability of success.

Good luck! Take care of the foal, and enjoy the enlightening time of having a new foal, even though it may happen not to be a star. All foals should be given their best opportunities to develop.

48
THE HUNTER

Finding the right horse

Buying a horse can involve a great deal of money nowadays, but selling horses is a very old business with its own set of customs and its own particular traps for the unwary. Basically there are three different ways of buying a horse: by private treaty, at public auction or through a dealer.

A great many riding horses are bought privately and this method has certain advantages for both parties. The seller can be more certain of finding a good home for his or her horse and has a chance to assess the suitability of the prospective rider. The buyer can ascertain details of the horse's history and often have the animal for a trial period. However, it is wise not to become too friendly with the vendor – it is surprising how easily ethical considerations are abandoned when there is a need to be rid of a troublesome beast.

Public auction is the method of sale most popularly associated with horses. Auctions have a vivid atmosphere and are frequented by characters as entertaining and as various as those in a Dickens novel.

For the vendor the auction has the advantage of widening the field of purchasers; more people will attend an auction than will reply to an advertisement. In addition they are collected together in a specific place for a specific length of time, with no opportunity to go away and think about whether or not to buy. However, because there are a number of horses to choose from, presentation is all-important.

For a buyer, however, an auction is a difficult path to tread, where his or her judgement is put to the test in the instant. On no account should an inexperienced person buy a horse at an auction without help. The overriding rule of all auctions, however reputable they might be, is *caveat emptor*, apart from some basic conditions. These vary from place to place, but they usually exclude from the sale ring, unless declared, whistlers or roarers and horses prone to such vices as crib-biting. Some auctions may give a guarantee that a horse is a good hunter, but such conditions offer but a meagre safety net.

Most hunters are in an auction for a good reason, which the purchaser must endeavour to find out. By no means all horses are bad ones, however. A master of hounds may be selling up or perhaps an owner simply cannot get on with his or her mount and wishes to be rid of it quickly. A good judge of a horse and, sometimes more importantly, of the person selling it can often pick up a bargain. In addition, there is a variety of horses to choose from. In essence an auction presents the biggest risks and potentially the biggest gains.

A middle course is the dealer. By going to a dealer a purchaser can see a number of horses at leisure and also has some of the advantages of buying privately, such as a trial day's hunting. The key lies in choosing the dealer: a good dealer will have reliable sources of horses and, with an eye to his reputation and perhaps a second sale, will do his best to match rider and horse.

A bad dealer will be professional at lying and cheating, and can survive for many years doing so. There is no federation or association of dealers to protect a purchaser, but reputation is a good yardstick, and it is always worth asking knowledgeable friends whom they would recommend. The dealer's attitude is all-important; if he is willing to allow a prospective purchaser to ride the horse thoroughly, then he is probably quite reputable. However, he cannot be expected to run down his own horse.

For the buyer a policy of reticence without being rude is wise. A stream of trumpeted assertions and stipulations will not only annoy a vendor who may otherwise be helpful, but it will also allow him or her to say less. An experienced dealer in particular will soon stress the horse's good points which match the purchaser's opinions. Reticence, on the other hand, will often draw the truth and give you a chance to learn more and make a better assessment.

There are many points to bear in mind when buying a horse, some of which should not be compromised while others are more flexible. The most important point, which must never be compromised, is to insist on a horse that is quiet in traffic. Modern roads make a badly behaved horse a constant danger. Many are a little nervous of large lorries and may shy slightly when one goes by, which is just about tolerable with an experienced rider, but it is a vital principle to have a horse that is quiet in traffic.

Beyond this, good manners are important, but they are more a matter of personal taste than absolutes. By manners I mean that the horse should stand still when required, that it should be able to go away from other horses, that it should be kind in the box, and so on. Many experienced riders will put up with a fidget, but will get very annoyed if a horse will only follow other horses, whereas other riders are happy to go in a crowd but, as they like to chat, would get cross if their mounts were to keep going round in circles.

Soundness is also a prerequisite in a good hunter. It is surprising how some purchasers will be carried away by ability – or talk of it – and will overlook even glaring unsoundness. They may think they are buying a horse on the cheap, but it is a false economy for there is nothing more expensive or frustrating than a lame horse.

Hunting puts great stress on a horse, particularly on its legs. Not only is it asked to carry large weights over jumps at speed – a job for which it is in no way designed – but it has to cross plough, grass and metalled road in quick succession, standing one moment, going flat out the next.

A hunter which has done some work will not be without blemish. Knocks, scars and cold lumps on knees are rarely of consequence; nor are windgalls, though they are a sign of wear. The foot, the seat of 90% of lameness, is most vulnerable in a hunter, and any wear such as ringbone (see pp. 233) or sidebone (see p. 304) – any bony growth in fact – should rule out a horse.

The thickening of a tendon (see pp. 264 ff.) should also be viewed with great suspicion. This is usually the result of either having been ridden over plough for a period, or having tripped in a hole, or poor conformation. Tendons can recover and may never give trouble again, but it is worth getting professional advice.

This brings me on to my next point: the importance of having a horse vetted (see chapter 51). The veterinarian is not responsible for selecting a good horse, but he or she can save you from buying a wreck. It is advisable to consult a veterinarian experienced in purchase examinations because such a person will be able to spot quickly the most important points.

There is disagreement as to the value of radiography when having a horse vetted, but if you are spending several thousand pounds on a horse, a radiographic view of the foot may save you from wasting your money by revealing the start of osteitis or navicular disease.

As to ability, a horse must suit the rider and the country in which he or she hunts. Someone who is seventy and hunts over Lincolnshire plough hardly wants to buy a Thoroughbred that is excellent over fly fences and gallops on. He or she would be better advised to buy a steady half-bred which can jump safely and find its own way out of trouble, and which probably costs far less.

Basically the horse should be able to jump the local obstacles. An inability to do so will soon leave you far behind and miserable. The need for speed varies, from the shires – Leicestershire and the like – where quick runs over hedges and ditches make a good galloper desirable, to plough country, where a broad, sure foot rather than speed is the order of the day.

Horses which follow a shire pack will tend to be Thoroughbreds and quality half-or threequarter-breds. The Irish Draught is marvellous for producing good sense and an instinct for self-preservation, which compensates for the lack of speed and better action of the pure-bred horse.

In plough country you will find many different types of horse, Irish Draught, cobs and native crosses, all of which are excellent in tricky situations. A touch of Thoroughbred is desirable in such horses, as the breed imparts an ability to last and try when tired.

As for other countries, a half-bred horse is generally considered best for hilly country, while the followers of the moorland hunts often use native ponies or crosses.

In the foregoing discussion I do not mean to define types absolutely because some Thoroughbreds are marvellously clever across ditches, for example, and, just as importantly, some riders get on better with one type rather than another. Also the amount of time available to devote to the horse must be taken into account: a half-bred or a cob can take much rougher treatment and be hunted from less exercise than a Thoroughbred.

A rider should buy a horse of appropriate size for his or her needs. There is a growing preference for big horses, perhaps to make the fences look smaller. However, the bigger the horse the greater the likelihood of problems in wind and limb.

Training a hunter
It is impossible to describe in full detail how to get a hunter fit, but, although you should bear in mind that every horse is different, starting right is half the battle won.

After a season's work hunters are turned out to grass to rest and put on condition, and also to rest their legs, but they should not be allowed to get fat, because this may strain the heart and legs on restarting work. Cubhunting starts after harvest, so every horse should be in work by August at the latest.

There is no harm bringing a horse in from the field, riding it and turning it out in July up to the time when it is in serious work and the nights are drawing in. The object of exercise is to build up muscle. If a horse starts to lose condition without gaining muscle, it should be brought in whatever the weather.

Others can stay out for some of the day, coming in at night. Some indeed are better out for an hour, under rugs, each day well into the winter to keep them keen and fresh.

It is tempting for a rider who likes leaping over fences at the gallop to hurry a horse, but every hunter should be walked for at least two weeks, starting with half an hour and working up to an hour or so. Jogging can then be introduced, initially with little bursts, using gentle hills, building up to two hours or so.

After about another two weeks a hunter will usually be ready for cubbing. At this stage you can canter a little, so that by six weeks of work your horse will be nearly fit to hunt. Again it must be stressed that the time taken to reach fitness will vary according to the individual.

There are three main dangers to look out for when getting a horse fit: coughs, back soreness and leg trouble. A cough in a horse which has just come up from grass is often due to dust in straw and hay, which should be damped; a good airflow without a draught will help. This can be achieved by leaving open the top door of the stable.

Back sores are caused by rubbing tack, particularly the saddle. Leather linings, as opposed to old-fashioned serge, and girths are the usual culprits, so the best solution is to use a numnah under the saddle and candlewick or webbing girths (girths should always be used in pairs, because they can occasionally break).

Many an old groom would be horrified at the use of numnahs, but they save wear on back and saddle, and even the best saddle will not fit a fat horse well. The back can be hardened with lead lotion, salt water or rubbing alcohol. If a sore develops, it should be protected by felt with a hole cut out over the area of the sore to prevent further rubbing.

Swelling in the legs which is not painful, hot or bowed (a sign of tendon trouble) is usually due to the effect of corn on the blood and is common. Such swelling can be walked off by and large, but it is best to reduce the grain ration until the legs are normal and the horse doing work.

Once a horse is being hunted regularly it will need relatively little work, unless it has a tendency to stiffen up. If a horse is hunted on Mondays and Fridays, it should be walked out on the following days. On Thursdays it should again be walked out with perhaps one half-speed canter. You should aim to be out for between one and two hours – the more walking the better. This is as much to keep the horse interested as anything else.

Feeding

The theory of feeding is discussed at length in chapter 44, but it is worth looking at how feeding works in practice in relation to a specific example, namely, the hunter.

First, it has to be remembered that every horse is different and, given the endless variety of feeds available, feeding an individual animal is a matter of skill, sensitivity and experience, a matter of art, in fact, as much as science. It is an irony that the rise in research into and knowledge of nutrition has been matched by a decline in the quality of feed for horses, mainly due to the emphasis on quantity in farming.

Feed is divided into two sorts: hard (concentrates) – oats, bran and so on – and soft – hay and grass. As a horse becomes fitter, you should feed more of the former and less of the latter.

Oats are the main source of protein and they should be plump, heavy – a 55kg bushel is ideal – hard and sweet-smelling. To help digestion they should be bruised or rolled – not more – if possible on the day of use, though this is not vital.

Of the alternative grains, the best is barley, which is used in many parts of the world and was often the basic diet of army horses. Barley is a harder grain than oats, and should be well rolled or boiled whole as a substitute for part of the oat ration. It is better at keeping on flesh than oats, but horses unused to it can often show adverse reactions, such as swollen legs.

Wheat used to be fed a good deal to carthorses and, being high in vitamin E, is thought by some to be good for young showjumpers. However, it is not a good feed for horses. Maize, which is fed flaked to keep on flesh, is more likely to produce an empty saddle than anything else as it is high in energy but relatively low in proteins and vitamins.

The pure digestible protein level for a hunter should be 12-14%, and oats and barley often contain only 8 or 9% nowadays, so you may also have to give a higher-protein food. Beans used to be fed in small quantities, and they are indeed very high in protein, but they are also full of carbohydrates, producing energy and fat.

Far more worthwhile (but expensive) is linseed, with 35% pure protein, or soyabean meal, with 45%. Linseed should be soaked overnight, and then boiled to a jelly or heated with more water to produce a nutritious tea. This is not a tidy process, but the result is very popular with the horse.

Soyabean meal is easier to use because it needs no cooking, but it is less palatable and needs mixing well, up to about one part soyabean meal to twelve parts oats (the ratio should be slightly higher for linseed).

The other main constituent of a feed is wheat bran. Bran should generally be fed damped (it can be fed dry, especially after a physic, but can cause choking). Broad bran should have large flakes, be full of flour and perfectly dry, not musty. Nowadays so-called broad bran has lost all its flour and is steamed and rolled heavily to reconstitute the broad flakes; it will provide bulk but not much else.

Such a diet would, of course, be very boring and there are several other food-stuffs that add interest, the most common of which is sugar-beet pulp or nuts, the residue of processed farming beet. It should be soaked for twenty-four hours before feeding and has an appetising sweetness. Like all foods rich in carbohydrates, it is good at keeping flesh on a horse. Although it is not too heating, it does little to promote fitness and should be used in smallish quantities. Another appetiser is palm kernel, which is high in oil and good for the coat and digestion.

Carrots, which are easily digestible, are good for cooling the blood and a help with poor-winded horses. Other roots such as swedes and turnips are also palatable sources of vitamins and bulk, but need to be introduced gradually because horses can be put off them if overfaced.

Extreme luxuries are eggs, which can be fed six at a time for four days and no more to a horse in strong work, and beer at the rate of two bottles a day for, say, seven days when leading up to a competition. However, this should be stopped three to four days before competing.

Of course, the fun of creating concoctions is lost if you feed nuts (cubes), but they have their advantages, as do all convenience foods. They are easy to feed and there is no waste; the mix is likely to be consistent, though some of the constituents are not ideal – wheat and fish meal, for example, which is excellent protein but indigestible. You should only use reliable manufacturers who have a proven reputation, because they can be relied on to use good-quality foodstuffs.

Some horses, including top-class racehorses and yearlings, do very well on nuts, but they can become boring and, as they have less bulk, can be less filling. Horses, like any other animal, prefer to feel full, whatever their requirements.

So much for the concentrates; the rest of the feed for hunters is grass and its derivative, hay.

The two main classes of hay are seed hay and meadow hay, the former grown as a crop in rotation over three years or so, the latter cut from permanent pasture. Seed hay is more controlled and contains desirable grasses such as timothy, which is high in fibre and carbohydrates but low in digestible protein and minerals, clover, which is rather the opposite and a laxative, and the staple rye-grass. The best seed hay is generally second-year lay, as it will contain a wider variety of herbs.

Meadow hay, consisting of older grasses, will be far more variable in every way and its quality will depend on the grassland management of the farmer. It is likely to be lower in protein but may contain a variety of herbs which are both nutritious and highly palatable.

For a hunter, good meadow hay is the most desirable. Good hay should smell sweet and be free from dust. The most common fault with meadow hay is that it hangs onto flowers, especially clover. It should be crisp to touch and a soft green, neither yellow, which is a sign of dampness, nor bottle green, which indicates excessive nitrogen and overproduction of grass. The latter is not so serious, but such hay is less digestible and less palatable.

Lucerne hay (alfalfa) can be fed, but with caution as it can be very high in protein, but its role is limited in England, which is not its natural environment.

A new sort of forage feed has come onto the market under various brand names. Basically it is vacuum-packed hay or silage, often enriched by molasses, and is known as haylage. Depending on the type of grass from which it is made, it can be high or low in protein; the former is claimed to be virtually a complete food. Time will tell if this is true for a hunter in full work, though it might well be the case. Variable quality and unpalatability to a horse unaccustomed to such feed can be problems. It is free from dust but expensive compared with hay and prone to mould if not stored carefully.

With the advent of research and the decline in the quality of foodstuffs, mineral and vitamin supplements have become very popular. If high-quality foodstuffs are available such expensive additives are unnecessary, but they can be useful and harmless if given as the manufacturers direct.

Cod-liver oil is also a useful supplement, enabling a horse to convert vitamins and giving it a shiny coat. Salt is also important and can be added to the feed, but a permanently available salt lick is preferable.

The following is an example of a diet for a stabled middleweight hunter, 163 cm (16.1 hh). This is only a guide. One should look carefully at the individual horse and the work it is doing, and vary the feed accordingly. Feeding, in the end, is an art.

> Early morning (an hour and a half before exercise)
> 2 lb oats
> 1/2 lb soaked sugar-beet pulp
>
> Midday
> 3 lb oats
> 1/2 lb bran
> 1/2 lb soaked sugar-beet pulp
> 1 lb barley
> 1/4 lb soyabean meal
>
> Night
> 6 lb oats
> 1/2 lb bran
> 1/2 lb soaked sugar-beet pulp
> 1/2 lb soyabean meal or cooked linseed

Hay (up to 18 lb per day) should be fed throughout the day and water should be freely available.

On a hunting day the early-morning feed should be replaced by the following, fed at 7-8 a.m.:

> 3 lb oats
> 3 lb bran
> 1/2 lb soyabean meal (this should be quite wet and warm)
> 1/2 lb soaked sugar-beet pulp

The evening ration of sugar beet can be increased to 2/3 lb if the feed is regularly eaten up.

The diet should also contain mineral supplements, salt, cod-liver oil and carrots. In addition, three times a week 2 x 15ml of the following mixture may be mixed into the feed:

> 7 oz saltpetre
> 7 lb Epsom salts
> 7 lb bicarbonate of soda

Horses generally do better if fed at night but as their stomach is small they should be fed little and often. It is important to keep to a routine both in feeding and exercising, as horses have a very well-adjusted clock in their head.

Harness

A great many people, perhaps impressed by the magnificent sight of a saddler's shop, keep far too much equipment for a hunter. The most basic needs are, of course, a saddle and a bridle.

The important aspects of fitting the saddle are that the shoulders should be free to move without hindrance and the spine and withers untouched. The weight of the saddle should be borne by the ribcage and not by the loins, which are prone to soreness and least able to bear weight.

The best way to buy a saddle is to take several and try them on the horse. Failing this, one can simulate the withers and ribcage with a stout but pliable cable moulded to the horse's shape. This can then be taken to the saddlers.

These days the great majority of saddles are lined with leather. Leather linings are longer lasting and easier to use than linen or serge linings, but are much harder on the horse's back, necessitating the use of numnahs. However, a leather lining is easier to clean.

Numnahs are saddle-shaped pads made of sheepskin, felt or synthetic fibre. They fit underneath the saddle to which they are attached by straps. They should be kept clean and uncreased, otherwise they will cause soreness rather than prevent it. They are particularly useful on thin-skinned horses.

There are various types of girths. Leather girths have the same benefits and drawbacks as leather linings, whereas webbing girths are serviceable but encourage sweating. My own favourite is candlewick, which has to be scrubbed clean and changed if fraying occurs, but which is tough, kind to the horse and smart.

The bridle, like the saddle, should be fitted carefully, but is easier to adjust. The most important element is the bit, which lies between the canine and molar teeth and acts on the lips, the bars of the mouth, the tongue and the jaw to help stop and balance the horse. If it is sitting right, a bit should cause, at most, one wrinkle in the side of the horse's mouth, while the ends of the bar of the bit should be about 1 cm free of the mouth at each side - not more and not less, otherwise it will pinch the mouth.

There are innumerable types of bits. Some horses pull and need a strong bit. However, a horse often pulls because the rider uses the bit too much. In addition, a more severe bit will work only for a short time, until the nerves in the mouth deaden further and leave the rider with a worse problem. Ironically, stronger bits, such as gags and curbs, need much more careful handling and far more skill, especially when jumping, because being caught in the mouth will cause a horse to rush its jumps. It also has to be remembered that excitement can cause a horse to pull, a problem no bit will solve, but a good seat and quiet voice might.

I believe a snaffle is usually best, but if a severe bit is required, the double bridle, with two bits, is the most satisfactory because the horse can be ridden on the snaffle bit most of the time and on the curb when necessary. Both horse and rider need to practise its use, especially as there are four reins, but it is an art well worth learning.

There are also several types of noseband available. Again, the noseband should be chosen with thought and, with the majority, fitted high enough so that pressure is applied to the bone of the nose and not to the air passages.

The other method of constraint is the martingale, the running version of which is often part of the hunter's kit, even if it is not tight enough to do its job. However, the neck strap in dire circumstances may be useful.

Clipping

In cold weather any horse in hard work should be clipped, because the long hair will make a horse sweat and then take chill. There are three main types of clip: a full, which leaves only a saddle patch and legs; a trace, which takes off below where traces would come: the belly, lower neck and jaw but excluding the legs, and a blanket, which takes in the neck, head and shoulders as well, leaving a blanket shape.

The first is the one for a stabled hunter in hard work, but a trace clip is useful, especially if one wants to turn a horse out during the day under a rug.

Some people clip all over the first time (a horse will need clipping at least twice in a season), but this is unnecessary and robs the horse of valuable protection, as does clipping the inside of the ears.

Clipping is an art gained by practice. You should start with a clean, dry horse and clip against the coat in as broad a sweep as possible, without forcing. It helps to tense the skin lightly and to keep the clipper blades sharp and well oiled. Some horses dislike being clipped so it is advisable to let them hear the clipper beforehand so they become accustomed to the noise, and to do the sensitive areas last. In extreme cases it is best to ask your veterinarian to administer a tranquillising drug (see p. 679). When clipping or pulling manes (which are never cut) it is better to resort to a twitch or a tranquillising drug rather than engage in a brawl.

Clothing

Clothing is a major item of expense with a hunter. There are many kinds of rugs to choose from, but the jute night rug is still the most useful. This is a top rug, under which one can put any number of blankets, either purpose bought or made from old bed blankets. Underblankets should be folded back over the jute rug at the withers to prevent chafing and to keep them in position. All of these should be surrounded by a webbed surcingle with a pad to protect the horse's withers. This strap should be done up snugly, but not too tightly, as it will be there for long periods. There should also be a strap and buckle at the front to prevent the rug slipping.

hunter

blanket

trace high

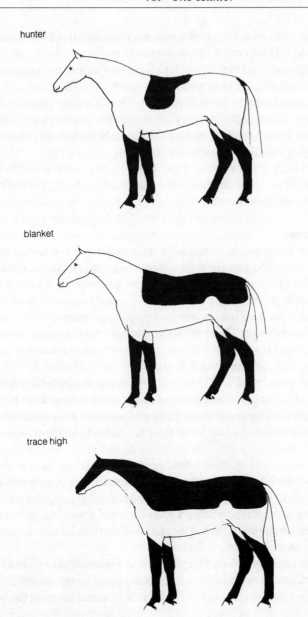

Figure 1 Types of clip

Some rugs have one or two straps instead of a surcingle. If this is the case they should be wide, so that the rug is not pulled down on the withers, which would cause pinching.

The jute rug is also perfectly adequate as a day rug; light day rugs are an unnecessary luxury.

If a horse is turned out with a rug or if it is being roughed off, a New Zealand rug is generally used. This is made of tough canvas with a soft lining, and has a surcingle and leg straps to keep it in place. These are necessary because the horse may roll and move around its paddock at speed.

Synthetic rugs have come to the fore recently. They are easy to look after, to dry and to clean, and are light, but they are not cheap, can rip easily and do not breathe as well as rugs made from natural fibres. However, they are very handy in a variety of situations, especially outdoors.

The other rug which is indispensable is the sweat rug. Basically this is a string vest for use, as its name implies, immediately after a horse has worked, to let him dry without chilling.

Boots and bandages

The extremities of the horse have attracted all sorts of garments. The most important extremity is the leg, for which, without trying, I can think of 15 types of boots and five types of bandage. Most of these are designed in response to particular problems.

Some owners take out their horses wrapped up like mummies, with enough boots to equip a football team. The two basic bandages necessary for a hunter are the stable bandage, which is used on the legs for warmth and to foster good circulation, and the tail bandage, which is used for protection when travelling.

The stable bandage is broad and long, and covers the leg from the knee to the coronet. The leg should be wrapped in Gamgee and the bandage bound evenly (most important) and not too tight. Most bandages have tapes which should be tied at the side of the leg, not at the front or back, in a bow, with the ends tucked in.

Nowadays there are soft synthetic bandages which can be used without Gamgee and which have Velcro fastenings. The latter are very convenient, but tend to wear out.

Bandaging every night is not necessary with a normal horse, but it is useful for tired limbs after hunting, both for support and warmth as legs lose heat rapidly after the pores have opened during work.

The tail bandage is used not only to protect the tail when travelling, but also to shape it. It is made of stretch fabric, three inches or so wide, and should be applied to a lightly damped tail – never the other way round because the bandage will shrink.

The procedure is: place the left hand under the tail, holding the end of the bandage, and wrap the bandage round with the right. Keep the left hand in place until the end is secured, and then wrap several turns at the top to catch the top hairs and give the bandage an anchor.

You should bandage to the end of the dock bone and then back up, tying the tapes about a third of the way down, again in a bow.

Figure 2a
Protective or brushing boots – these boots do not prevent a horse from striking into itself, but do minimise the damage incurred

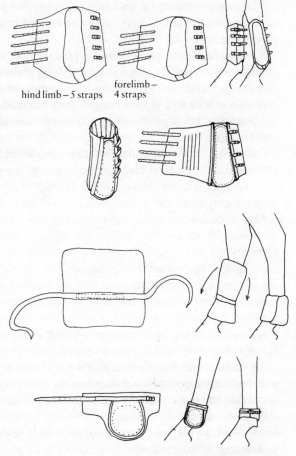

hind limb – 5 straps

forelimb – 4 straps

Figure 2b Tendon boots are fitted to the forelimb with the straps in front. They provide support to the tendons when jumping

Figure 2c
A felt Yorkshire boot, tied around the hind fetlock protects the fetlock and upper pastern region of a horse which moves closely behind. It is an alternative to a fetlock boot

Figure 2d
A hind fetlock boot protects the fetlock and part of the pastern region of a horse which moves closely behind

Figure 2e
A sausage boot, placed around the pastern of a forelimb, prevents the heel of the foot coming in contact with the elbow when the horse lies down. It may help to prevent a capped elbow developing

Figure 2f
A rubber ring. The ring is placed around one or both hind pasterns to protect the insides of the pasterns

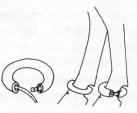

Figure 2g (below)
An overreach boot, which protects the pastern and heel regions provided that the boot fits correctly. If the boot is too big, it may be easier to put on but will sit too low and not completely protect the pastern

To remove the bandage, undo the ties, grasp the top in both hands and slide it down. When applied every day for several hours, it will give the tail a pleasing shape.

Exercise bandages are designed to give support to tendons and protect legs from knocks. They are unnecessary, indeed undesirable, for normal horses, whose legs should be strong enough without support. Indeed, they are only of limited use with bad-legged horses. They are made from stretch fabric, like tail bandages, but shorter, and should be put over Gamgee, between the knee and the fetlock joint.

Unroll 6-8 inches and, having taken one wrap round, hold the bandage obliquely. Then, letting the spare hang down, wrap the bandage around the legs, keeping it fairly firm but even. Having reached the fetlock, work back up the leg, tying as for stable bandages. The ends may be secured by sewing if hard work is envisaged.

Grooming

Grooming is performed mainly for our benefit, although it may improve the horse's circulation. For the most part we like to see clean horses, but horses themselves like to roll in the mud, acquiring an effective duvet against the weather.

A basic grooming kit consists of a dandy brush to remove the mud, a body brush, which is used in circular sweeps to remove dust and to brush the tail, a curry comb, which is pulled across the body brush to clean it every few sweeps, a rubber curry comb, which is excellent for removing tough mud, a water brush for laying the mane and tail, a mane comb, used when pulling a mane, two sponges for cleaning the nose and the dock, a stable rubber – a cloth – for the final polish, a hoofpick, to clean out the foot (away from the frog), and oil for moistening the foot and sole.

This is not the place for a detailed discussion of grooming, but one should be wary of washing large areas of the horse without the facility to dry it in the warm. Surplus water should be removed with a scraper and the horse rubbed and walked under a light rug until dry.

In addition to a grooming kit, you will also need a first-aid kit (see chapter 41).

Injuries

A horse is a highly complex animal and prone to injury when asked to do things not suited to its frame, such as carry weight at speed over fences. It is remarkable indeed that horses do so much with injuries similar to those we experience when playing a contact sport. For the most part these will be knocks, bangs or cuts, with only the occasional disaster, but a lot depends on the horseman.

'Horseman' is a word I use with care: many good riders never make successful followers of hounds because they fail to be observant stablemen, judging a horse's health, or prudent pilots, spotting wire on a hedge or a hole in the ground. It is surprising how some people always seem to be in the front rank but rarely lame a horse, while others are frequently on their feet at the meet, their horses at home.

Every owner should be aware of his or her horse's character and appearance when it is healthy; it should be keen in its work, eating well, bright-eyed and with a shiny coat and loose skin. The most obvious sign that a horse is unwell is deviation from the norm – failure to eat, listlessness or a dull coat.

The most common illnesses with hunters – generally pretty tough characters are colds, which they can catch when meeting so many other horses, and colic (see p. 46), rarely seen in the wild but common enough when a horse is receiving relatively little natural roughage and large amounts of concentrates. An owner should be alert to a persistent cough, listlessness, a runny nose or, worse, fever, and should keep an eye on the horse's droppings, which should be distinct but not too firm.

The most common injuries to a hunter are cuts on the legs. With luck these will be superficial, in which case treatment with antiseptic powder or spray will be sufficient. Alternatively the wound can be wrapped with a bandage soaked in salt water (one teaspoon salt to one pint water). This dressing should be renewed every twenty-four hours until the wound is healed.

Some horses have actions that make them liable to injury. An extravagant hind action may cause a horse to overreach; some horses move close in front and will brush (hit their fetlocks). Overreaching can also come about by accident, particularly on heavy ground, if a front foot is held by the mud.

Such accidents have to be solved mechanically. All hunters should have their hind shoes set so that the toe of the hoof is slightly prominent, as it is the metal shoe that does the most damage. Also overreach and brushing boots will afford good protection.

With an overreach the bulb of the heel is usually cut and may only require treating with sulphanilamide powder to prevent excess scar tissue forming. More care should be taken with a deeper cut. The hole should be washed and filled with a poultice of brewer's yeast until it has nearly healed. This should take a week or so, although complete healing will take a week longer.

An overreach higher up on the fetlock joint is more serious because the tendons may be affected even if the cut is small. Any swelling indicates bruising and fluid escaping from the sheath. Poultices may be applied to draw any moisture and keep the wound clean, but in case of doubt about the seriousness of the injury, you should call your vet. When the swelling has subsided you can start walking the horse if it is not lame.

Another wound which may appear small but which sometimes can be more serious results from a kick. The underlying bone may be affected, especially in the thigh. Rest, and advice from the veterinarian, are recommended in these circumstances.

Puncture wounds are common, especially in the foot. With any puncture wound there has to be free passage for the serum to drain, and this can be done by either a blacksmith or a vet. For details of treatment, see p. 638.

Wounds in the leg caused by thorns and the like should be treated with poultices, either Animalintex or one made from Epsom salts and glycerine on lint and covered by greaseproof paper to hold in the heat. Success in treatment is indicated by a clean area, with several small points of blood, denoting a good supply.

In all cases of wounding vaccinations should be taken against tetanus (see p. 475). Indeed, all hunters should be vaccinated annually; a small cut, which may easily be missed, may otherwise prove fatal.

There is another type of injury found in older hunters, the result of wear and tear over the years. It includes chronic osteitis, sidebone, ringbone, navicular disease and pedal osteitis. These manifest themselves in various forms of lameness and hard, bony swellings. All will require diagnosis by a veterinarian and are described in detail in the section on the musculoskeletal system.

Preparing for a hunter's day
The etiquette of hunting has been dealt with at length in other books, but enjoying the day and surviving intact to enjoy another are the most important points of all. Several days before going hunting the horse's shoes should be checked. On the day, the heels should be greased to keep the wet out of sensitive areas, especially if the horse is prone to cracked heels.

A hunter should travel in a tail bandage and whatever rugs are necessary to keep him warm without sweating. Night rugs should not be used if possible, as they may get wet or dirty in the general scramble.

It is best to put the tack on before going, with the girth done up loosely, because it is awkward to fiddle with an excited horse in the confined space of a horsebox or trailer.

Unbox a mile or two away from the meet, walk a little way and then trot on gently to loosen horse and rider. So often horses get out at the meet, stand, getting cool, while their owners chatter, and then are asked to set off at speed.

During the day the rider should observe the hounds and the going, and take care of the horse. These can be done at one and the same time. This does not mean you have to display excessive caution, just alertness and common sense. For example, it is pointless to clatter down a road when hounds are not running or when there is a decent verge, yet so many do just that.

Seeing what others do is helpful but it is far more satisfying to take your own line, watching the direction of the hounds not the field. This may be possible even in small ways: a long queue may form to jump and leave other parts of a hedge clear simply through lack of confidence.

The next problem is when to go home. It is far better to do two half days than one full day in a week. The important point is not to exhaust the horse; it is for an owner to know his or her horse well enough to judge when to go home. A horse may stop pulling or fidgeting, or it may slow down markedly or start hitting fences.

The horse should be walked to the box and cooled off as much as possible, then untacked, rugged up to keep warm without sweating, and then taken home.

Most people wash off their horses vigorously when they return home, but this is unnecessary. Brush out saddle sweatmarks and feel down the legs carefully for thorns, chips of wood or stone flakes. A tired horse likes to be warm and dry and prefers to eat in peace rather than be clean.

This does not imply leaving it unobserved. The horse should have a good deep bed, be bandaged and have its rugs changed; this latter point may need fine judgement. Frequent observation is necessary, especially if a horse is trace-clipped, in case it gets cold under the lighter rugs or gets too hot and breaks out in a sweat again under heavier rugs. Some horses are prone to sweating, but generally a dry horse is fit to be rugged up.

If you have many horses to do, then some will have to be cleaned that night. If possible this should be done with a brush and cool water; hot water opens the pores and increases the chance of a cold. A sponge is preferable to a hose, because the water will not then penetrate the coat and chill the horse so much, but the latter is commonly used in livery yards.

After a day's hunting I like to use a mixture of methylated spirit, vinegar and water in equal quantities to wipe on the legs at night – in fact a daily application will do no harm. The mixture is a good cooling agent and astringent. A stronger version, for a horse with windgalls or slight heat in the legs, is fuller's earth soaked with vinegar as a mudpack, under Gamgee and bandage or a flannel soaked in Epsom salts. This should be changed every few hours.

It is also a good time to check again for thorns and so on. By the next day most of the mud will have dropped off, but the remainder should be brushed off and the tail washed if necessary. The horse should then be checked for soundness and allowed to pick grass and relax.

Miscellaneous

This final section of the book contains chapters on the following subjects:-

- Exercise physiology and performance analysis – relatively new developments in the field of veterinary studies

- Two chapters relating to the purchase of horses; the first discusses the examination of horses for veterinary certification, and the second looks into the legal implications of buying and selling horses

- A key aspect of veterinary service – the training of the veterinary nurse;

- Determining the age of a horse by examination of the mouth. Although little has been added to the subject in recent years, it is still important, especially for non-Thoroughbred breeds of horses

- Finally, a chapter on colours and markings, based on the latest system from the Royal College of Veterinary Surgeons

49
EQUINE EXERCISE PHYSIOLOGY

Although it is true that investigations of energy metabolism in working horses had been conducted in the late 19th and early 20th centuries, modern day equine exercise physiology can reasonably be considered to have begun in earnest in the 1980s, with the seeds being sown by a relatively limited number of interested scientists and veterinary surgeons in the preceding 20-30 years. In the 1980s a great deal of research concerning equine exercise physiology was aimed at describing and defining the 'normal' responses to exercise and training. Whilst a considerable amount of basic research is still undertaken, a great deal more applied research and studies relating to disease or dysfunction are now a major part of equine exercise physiology. For example, the knowledge base relating to normal responses to exercise has meant that investigations of loss of performance syndrome (where a horse has performed well or as expected in the past but is now performing below a previous level) or poor performance syndrome (where a horse has never performed to the expected level – probably based on breeding) are carried out routinely at many centres around the world. Furthermore, whilst much of the initial work in equine exercise physiology was funded by racing and the findings applied to the racehorse, today equine exercise physiology crosses all equestrian sports and the pleasure horse, and has even seen application in working equids.

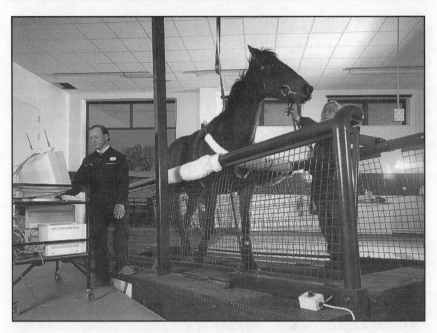

Figure 1   A horse working on the treadmill at the Animal Health Trust in Newmarket in an environmentally controlled laboratory

Treadmills

In 1986, around the time when Dr David Snow contributed the first chapter on exercise physiology to the 17th edition of Veterinary Notes for Horse Owners, the first high-speed treadmill for research use in Britain was installed at the Animal Health Trust's Balaton Lodge site in Newmarket. This was followed by the installation of a treadmill at Bristol University Veterinary Schools' Langford site. Today there are treadmills for research and clinical use installed at the Animal Health Trust, the veterinary schools at Edinburgh, Liverpool, Bristol and London and at a number of colleges or universities running equine courses, including Hartpury College, De Montfort University and Warwickshire College. The first treadmills at Newmarket and Bristol were able to reach speeds of 12 metres per second (m/s), or 27 mph, on a level surface or on inclines up to 7° (~12% or 1 in 8). Today, many of the high-speed treadmills can reach speeds of upwards of 16 m/s. To put this in context of flat racing for example, a horse in a 5 furlong (1000 metres) race would achieve an average speed of around 17-18 m/s, whilst a horse racing over 12 furlongs (1 1/2 miles or 2400 metres) would have an average speed of around 15-16 m/s (in each case the average speed would of course vary with factors such as the class of race, the individual course and the going). When the maximum speed is only 12 m/s, the workload can be increased by inclining the treadmill. So for example, to achieve the workload experienced by a horse in a 1 1/2 mile flat race on a treadmill limited to 12 m/s, the treadmill would probably be inclined to around 5°, which would allow for the fact that the horse was not carrying a jockey and running at sub-maximal speed. With the newer tread-mills, which can actually reach the speeds encountered in racing, it is therfore only necessary to elevate the treadmill to account for the absence of a rider. It is now known that an incline of ~3° is sufficient to account for the work that would have been done if the horse carried a rider.

There is no doubt that a very large part of our increase in knowledge of the response of the horse to exercise that has occurred in the last 15 years has been due to studies carried out on treadmills. This is because in the field the researcher is limited as to what equipment can be used, either by the size of the equipment, the need for mains power or sensitivity to movement. However, after such an intense period of 'laboratory' based study of equine exercise physiology, many researchers believe that studies in the field still have an important role to play. The treadmill has the advantage that the same exercise (speed and duration) can be reproduced almost infinitely and on constant going, with controlled environmental conditions (temperature, humidity and air move-ment over the horse; the latter usually achieved by large industrial fans placed in front of the horse). These aspects make treadmill exercise ideal for the stringent requirements of scientific study, in which we often wish to only vary one factor between two separate exercise sessions; for example exercise with and without a nutritional supplement.

However, there are disadvantages to studying horses during treadmill exercise. For example, the horse is forced to exercise at the exact speeds set by the scientist. These may be near to the point in which the horse may naturally change from trot to canter or canter to gallop and the horse may switch between the two and therefore not be settled. In the field, when a horse changes legs, it may slow down fractionally, whereas on the treadmill it is forced to continue running at the set speed whilst accomplishing this. It is also difficult to run time trials of maximum effort on a treadmill.

The treadmill surface (nearly always a rubber belt running over a large metal plate) is generally harder than most surfaces the horse would encounter during canter and gallop in the field. On early treadmills the force transmitted to the legs during trotting was found to be around to be around three to four times that for trotting on sand or wood chip tracks but around a third of that for trotting on asphalt. On modern treadmills the steel plates have improved suspension reducing the impact of the legs on the surface. Whilst most treadmills must be considered to equate to firm going, the surface is uniform, flat and non-slip. Whilst long-term, intense exercise at fast canter and gallop is best avoided for horses with poor conformation (e.g. horses very upright in front), the risk of injury appears to be no different to that when training normally on grass or all-weather surfaces.

Treadmill *versus* **Track**

Prior to the widespread use of treadmills, the little equine exercise physiology that took place was undertaken in the field. With treadmills becoming easily obtainable and the increased interest in equine exercise physiology, there was an inevitable move to primarily laboratory based studies. Researchers had many questions which could not be answered in the field due to problems with variation in going or climate, inability to control speed and equipment limitations. These problems were largely overcome by using treadmills. However, horses do not compete on treadmills and so there is always a place for studies in the 'real world' under true competition conditions. At the 5th International Conference on Equine Exercise Physiology held in Japan in 1999, a workshop session was devoted to the issue of treadmill *versus* field comparisons. Certainly for those involved in trying to solve the heat and humidity issue for the Atlanta Olympic Games, studies of horses competing in actual competition were essential to construct treadmill exercise protocols that would reproduce the effort and pattern of competition. The results of the laboratory studies were then used to make modifications to the speed and endurance test which were actually investigated back in simulated competition conditions in the field. Thus, both field and laboratory (treadmill) based studies of exercise physiology have a place.

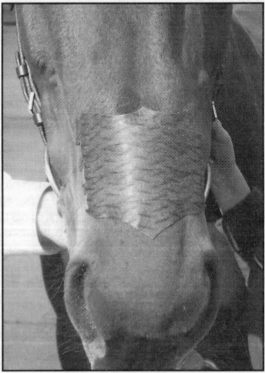

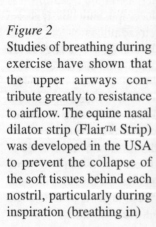

Figure 2
Studies of breathing during exercise have shown that the upper airways contribute greatly to resistance to airflow. The equine nasal dilator strip (Flair™ Strip) was developed in the USA to prevent the collapse of the soft tissues behind each nostril, particularly during inspiration (breathing in)

Respiratory System

The size of the horse and its ability to move air in and out of the lungs at air-flow rates 10-15 times higher than those seen in man has meant that measurements of ventilation during exercise have always been technically challenging. Simple scaling up of devices used for measuring airflow (pneumotachometers) at rest or during exercise in man were disappointing as these devices generally posed a significant resistance to the movement of air at the high flow rates achieved by the horse during exercise, with the result that either horses did not breathe 'normally' or that the flows measured were below the true maximum. However, in the mid to late 1980s, a new design of flowmeter or pneumotachometer using ultrasound and with very low resistance was developed. This system enabled measurements of airflow up to maximal exercise with virtually no resistance. This technology has enabled researchers to describe in great detail the normal responses of the respiratory system in exercise and training, and in disease.

One important outcome of research in this area has been the finding by a number of different groups, working independently, that the equine respiratory system does not respond to training. This is quite fortuitous for those involved in clinical evaluation of poor or loss of performance syndrome, which frequently involves the respiratory tract, as the training status of the horse is relatively unimportant in making the assessment. This is in marked contrast to assessment of the cardiovascular or muscular responses to exercise which will vary greatly with training status. A further important implication of the lack of any response to training is that if the lung is damaged, for example by disease (e.g. pneumonia, or COPD – 'broken wind'), then it is not possible to make up for any deficiencies in lung capacity or function with training. However, the fact that the respiratory system of the horse does not respond to training, may partly explain why there is now increasing evidence to suggest that this system may be a major factor limiting performance, even in the fit and healthy horse.

The horse is an obligate nasal breather (i.e. it can only breathe through its nose, unlike humans) and a consequence of this is that the upper airway (from the nostril to the larynx) has been shown to be responsible for the majority of the resistance to the movement of air, both during inspiration and expiration at rest and during exercise. A form of nasal dilator strip, similar to those designed for human athletes, has recently been developed for horses. These strips are designed to prevent the collapse inwards of the skin that covers the nasomaxillary notch above each nostril. Research on these strips is still in progress and whilst there is some evidence that they may be effective in some horses, scientific opinion is still divided.

A further peculiarity of equine respiratory function during exercise is that at canter and gallop the horse is obliged to take one breath with each stride. This is termed 1:1 respiratory-locomotory coupling. Whilst human cyclists or runners may choose to entrain their pedalling frequency or stride with their breathing, unlike the horse, they are not obliged to do so. During exercise, the harder an animal works, the harder it must breathe in order to move more oxygen from the atmosphere into the lungs. The oxygen is then transported in the blood to the working muscles. Thus, whilst the human athlete could increase the amount of air, and therefore oxygen, moved in and out of the lungs each minute during exercise (the respiratory minute ventilation) by increasing either the rate of breathing (respiratory frequency), the depth of breathing or both, the horse primarily increases its level of ventilation during canter and gallop by taking bigger breaths (increasing the tidal volume – the volume of air moved in and out per stride) as it goes faster, whilst the respiratory frequency (and therefore stride frequency) increase much less.

There are a number of exceptions when the one to one relationship between breathing and stride is not maintained. Firstly, if the horse has to swallow, which usually occurs around 1-2 times a minute during canter and gallop in a healthy horse. Secondly, at slow canter a horse may choose to take one breath over two strides. As the horse moves into a faster canter, he may alternate between periods of 1:1 and 1:2 breathing. However, with increasing speed the horse should switch to predominantly 1:1 breathing and by around 500-600 m/min, the horse should have around 98% of breaths coupled 1:1 with stride.

Perhaps one of the disappointing areas in respiratory research is that there is still no universally agreed explanation for the condition known as exercise-induced pulmonary haemorrhage (EIPH). EIPH refers to bleeding (haemorrhage) from blood vessels within the lung (pulmonary) which occurs during strenuous exercise (exercise-induced). Whilst it has been documented for over 300 years that a small percentage of racehorses show blood at the nostrils after racing (e.g. Bleeding Childers, Herod), it was not until the introduction of fibreoptic endoscopes that it became clear that blood observed at the nostrils during or following strenuous exercise nearly always originated from the lung.

With the more widespread use of endoscopy in veterinary practice and veterinary research, it is now clear that 40-75% of Thoroughbred horses will have some blood in their trachea (windpipe) after racing. The degree of bleeding varies considerably between individual horses, with horses showing visible blood at the nostrils often being referred to as 'bleeders'. Whilst originally thought to be a Thoroughbred 'problem', it is now clear that any breed or type of horse undertaking strenuous exercise may experience some degree of EIPH. The condition has been observed in Thoroughbreds following flat racing and steeplechasing, Standardbred racing (trotting or pacing), polo, show jumping, cross-country and barrel racing. EIPH has also been shown to occur in racing greyhounds, camels and humans after intense exercise.

The bleeding that occurs as a result of intense exercise in horses is not randomly or uniformly distributed throughout the whole lung, but affects the dorso-caudal (uppermost and rearmost) part of the lung; effectively in the area of lung under the back of the saddle. In a young two-year-old horse in training or young riding horse (around 4-5 years old), with strenuous work (fast canter and gallop and possibly jumping), the very tips of the lung will tend to be affected. As the horse ages and works more, a larger amount of lung is affected and the bleeding tends to become worse. It may be that continual bouts of EIPH cause structural changes in the lung as a result of the repair process and this may explain the trend for more frequent and severe bleeding with age.

As the amount of blood in the trachea after intense exercise can vary greatly between horses and even in the same horse over a period of time, various grading systems have been developed to describe the amount of blood seen endoscopically after exercise. Despite the fact that it is now 25 years since it was generally accepted that horses bleed in their lungs after intense exercise, the cause is still not known. The most popular theory is that the bleeding occurs because of very high stresses (known as transmural pressures) acting across the walls of the tiny capillaries (small blood vessels) in the horses's lung during exercise leading to stress failure. The blood is only separated from the air spaces within the lung by a very thin membrane, which facilitates uptake of oxygen by the blood. During exercise, horses develop tremendously high pressures in the pulmonary blood vessels and it is hypothesised that this could be sufficient to rupture the vessel walls. This is the basis behind the use of the drug *Lasix* (frusemide) in North America. *Lasix* is a diuretic, a drug which causes increased urine production and hence loss of water from the blood circulation. This causes the blood pressure both at rest and during exercise to be lower. However, the scientific evidence that bleeding is due to high pressure is poor and as yet there are no scientific studies that prove that *Lasix* either reduces or prevents EIPH, indeed in some surveys of the condition in the USA in the 1980s, horses racing on *Lasix* were no less likely to bleed than untreated animals. In addition, high blood pressure theories of EIPH cannot immediately explain why the bleeding occurs in the upper and rear part of the lung. Perhaps one reason for the popularity of *Lasix* is that it has been shown to improve performance, because a treated horse will be carrying around 20-30 kg less weight.

A theory has recently proposed that EIPH results from the high impact of the front legs on the ground during fast cantering, galloping and jumping. When the front legs hit the ground during galloping, the shoulder is pushed hard onto the rib cage. When the foot is planted on the ground, the force is transmitted to the lung and a shock-like 'wave' passes through it. Because of the shape of the lung this 'wave' becomes amplified and most intense in the rear and upper part of the lung. The damage is similar to that experienced in the lungs of people in car accidents where they are hit hard in the front of the chest by the steering wheel. In this situation, the damage and bleeding that occurs in the lung is not usually at the front of the lung where the chest has been hit, but at the back. A similar situation could exist between the back and top part of the lung and the chest wall.

In a survey, 26% of flat trainers and 54% of National Hunt trainers thought that bleeding affects racing performance. In a survey carried out in the UK, it was found that the incidence of EIPH following racing was not different between a random sample of horses and poorly performing animals. In a study under laboratory conditions performed at the University of Sydney, with horses exercising on a treadmill, it was shown that placing 200ml of blood in the left and right lungs significantly reduced performance. This amount of blood was thought to be equivalent to Grade 3 (the middle grade of bleeding) on our scale of 0 to 5.

There is evidence that EIPH may cause permanent alterations in the blood supply to the affected parts of the lungs. Fortunately, EIPH only affects a relatively small amount of the total lung. However, the presence of blood in the airways may of itself also lead to inflammation. Inflammation is the process that occurs when body tissues are damaged. For example, in the case of a cut in the skin, the inflammatory response results in increased blood flow to the area, with redness, swelling, heat and pain. Some studies have suggested that inflammation may occur in the lung as a result of EIPH.

At present, without knowing the true cause of EIPH it is extremely difficult to make recommendations on management to prevent, reduce or treat the condition. Many suspect that airway inflammation, following infection or as a result of poor stable hygiene (allowing contamination with moulds, dust and ammonia), may accentuate EIPH. Others believe that upper airway conditions such as laryngeal hemiplegia ('roaring') may worsen bleeding. Only once we have a clear understanding of the causes of EIPH and access to techniques to accurately quantify the bleeding within the lung will it be possible to improve our management of this condition.

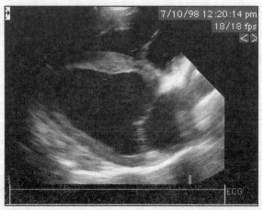

Figure 3   Two ultrasound images of horses with different size hearts. The left ventricle (LV) is the main chamber pumping arterial blood (containing oxygen)

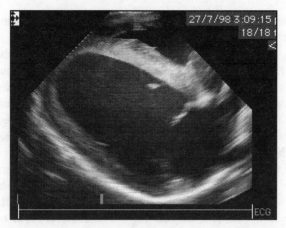

around the body. In theory, horses with large hearts should have an advantage in races over longer distances (such as flat racing over 1 1/2 miles, National Hunt (jump) Racing or in endurance). The first heart has a smaller pumping chamber (ventricle) and is from a moderate flat racehorse whilst the secound heart is from a Group I winner that raced over 1 1/2 miles.
(Pictures courtesy of Dr L.Young.)

Cardiovascular System
The heart is a muscle and it is now clear that it responds to training in a similar way to the locomotory muscles (muscles used for movement). Studies using ultrasound to image the heart before and after training have shown that far from being an organ that simply varies in overall size between horses, there are also differences between horses in the thickness of the walls of the heart. Many of these studies have been carried out in Thoroughbred racehorses with the aim of identifying elite horses, or eliminating poor horses, before training starts. Not all the studies carried out have come to the same conclusions. Some have found a relationship between heart size and performance whilst others have found no difference in heart size between good and bad performers. Horses with large hearts, in which the wall of the left ventricle (the chamber that pumps oxygenated blood out of the heart into the arterial system) is relatively thin, show a trend to be better than average over the longer flat race distances (+10 furlongs). This should not be surprising as it is clear that delivery of oxygen to the muscles determines how hard and for how long they can work. The delivery of oxygen to the muscles is dependent on the volume of blood in the circulation, the number of red blood cells and the speed at which the blood can be pumped around the body. The latter is known as the cardiac output (in litres per minute) and is heart rate (in beats per minute or b.p.m.) multiplied by the volume of blood pumped out of the heart with each beat, referred to as the stroke volume (in litres). Thus, at the same heart rate, the

horse with the bigger heart will usually have a larger stroke volume and there-fore be able to deliver more oxygen to the muscles.

In general, most training programmes for horses can be considered to be aerobic programmes, that is they increase the capacity of the muscles to use oxygen. This would include training of racehorses, endurance horses and eventers. In these types of training programmes, the heart would generally be expected to show some increase in size. The exceptions are in training programmes for short duration, explosive sports such as Quarterhorse racing or possibly showjumping.

Heart rate monitors designed for human use have been commercially available for around 30 years and are widely used by keen joggers and professional athletes alike, as well as in research. In the 1980s the heart rate monitors used by researchers or horse owners were most frequently modified versions of the human monitors or rather crude and cumbersome equine models. Today, companies such as POLAR produce heart rate monitoring systems specifically for use with horses. These systems are much easier to use and more robust than the early systems, and the ability to record a whole exercise session and download the information into a computer for further examination and analysis means they are more widely used in training, research and competition. More detailed information about heart function during exercise can be obtained from an electrocardiogram (ECG). The ECG is the characteristic electrical activity of the heart that occurs with each beat. Advances in technology have meant that recording the ECG during exercise is now a procedure that can be easily carried out by many veterinary practices in the field.

Muscle
During the 1980s there was a tremendous increase in knowledge concerning the composition, function and response to training of equine locomotory muscles, mainly due to the application of the muscle needle biopsy technique. This involved collecting small samples of muscle under local anaesthesia from large muscle groups such as the those of the hindquarters. Much of the pioneering work was carried out by Dr David Snow, initially at Glasgow University and later at the Animal Health Trust. At that time there was great interest in the possibility of using the muscle biopsy to predict performance in advance of training and racing or other competition.

It is now clear that there is great variation in muscle composition between breeds, and even between Thoroughbred horses who have often been thought to be relatively homogenous, in terms of variables such as the numbers of the different types of individual muscle fibres (classified as type I or slow twitch; type IIA or fast twitch high oxidative (aerobic or 'staying' fibres) and type IIB or fast twitch high glycolytic (anaerobic or 'sprinting' or 'speed' fibres)), sizes of fibres and numbers of the small blood vessels (capillaries) surrounding each muscle fibre. However, a number of studies have been unable to show any definite relationship between muscle composition assessed by muscle biopsy and subsequent performance, at least in racing. Part of the problem may be that the numbers of different muscle fibres within a muscle do not simply vary between individuals but also as a function of different parts of the same muscle. Effectively a single muscle group such as those of the hindquarters may have a number of different compartments which are not easy to identify when looking at the outside. It is also now clear that the muscle fibre proportions also vary with the depth at which the muscle biopsy sample is taken. Most samples in earlier studies were taken at a depth of 6 cm. However, studies have now shown that the proportion of slow twitch fibres is lowest at the surface of the muscle but increases with depth. Thus, a muscle sample taken at 6 cm depth in a horse with a muscle only 8 cm deep will naturally contain more slow twitch fibres than a sample taken at 6 cm from a horse with a 12 cm deep muscle.

In general terms, we now know that most training programmes for horses result in the muscles becoming better at using oxygen, that is they increase the aerobic capacity of the muscles. In the previously untrained, young horse, the individual muscle fibres are relatively large, with few capillaries and there are big differences between fibres in their capacity to use oxygen. Thus the young horse is a born sprinter. With predominantly aerobic training, the muscle fibres decrease in size, the number of capillaries around each fibre increase and all fibres show an increase in their ability to use oxygen. This is generally the response for horses trained for medium distances flat races and longer, jump racing and for the endurance and event horse.

Although the advances in knowledge of how muscle functions during exercise have shown that it is not possible to predict performance using muscle biopsy, this has contributed greatly to the understanding of 'tying-up' or exertional rhabdomyolysis. Work by Dr Pat Harris in the UK showed that many cases of severe muscle damage during exercise were related to dietary imbalances in electrolytes such as sodium, potassium, chloride, calcium, magnesium and phosphate. In addition, Dr Stephanie Valberg in the USA has demonstrated that in some horses there is a genetic component to 'tying-up' described as polysaccharide storage myopathy (PSSM). This is a condition connected to the metabolism of glycogen within the muscle. Glycogen is essentially a string of glucose molecules linked together and is the equivalent of starch in plants.

Nutrition
The last 15 years has seen great progress in the field of nutrition of the exercising horse. Dr David Snow noted in the 17th edition that at the time of writing (~1986), little was know about the requirements of the exercising horse. Major topics of research and advance within the last 15 years have been in the areas of: 1) the effect of time of feeding in advance of exercise or

competition; 2) what should be fed prior to and during exercise or competition; 3) the use of high fat diets; 4) the interaction of diet with water balance; 5) the use of dietary ergogenic (performance enhancing) aids and nutraceuticals (food or food ingredients considered to provide medical or health benefits, including the prevention and treatment of disease; 6) optimal nutrition to ensure maximal performance, as opposed to adequate nutrition; 7) the development and use of haylage products to minimise exposure of stabled animals to moulds; 8) new fibre sources; 9) micronisation in feed production. Many of these topics are covered in the chapter on nutrition.

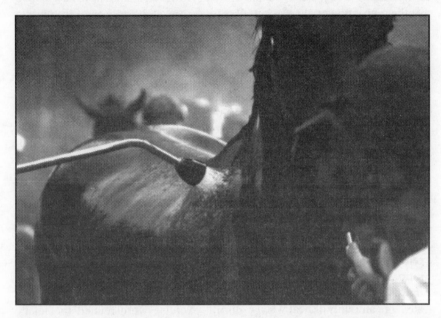

Figure 4   A major advance in the management and welfare of horses during competition, especially in thermally stressful environmental conditions, has been research which has led to acceptance of the need to cool horses effectively during or following competition.

Thermoregulation

Prior to the 1990 Olympics in Barcelona, very little was known about how the horse controlled its body temperature (thermoregulation), especially in conditions of high thermal stress. The environmental conditions in Barcelona were hot and dry, with little wind and strong sunlight (solar radiation). In the three-day event speed and endurance test, the combination of conditions was such that many horses either became fatigued and could not complete the cross-country or finished exhausted and with very high body (rectal) temperatures. Following Barcelona therefore, the governing body of international equestrian sport, the Federation Equestre Internationale (FEI), launched an initiative to stimulate research in the area of equine thermoregulation in heat, or heat and humidity. This was particularly warranted as the next Olympics would be held in the even more thermally stressful climate of Atlanta in the southern USA.

Prior to 1990 there was somewhere in the region of ten published papers on equine thermoregulation in the heat and 15 in the cold. Between 1990 and 2000, there were a further 14 papers published in relation to cold conditions, but 81 papers related to heat. The enormous increase in knowledge between 1990 and 1996 was applied successfully in the preparation for and management of horses at the 1996 Atlanta Olympic Games with the result that there were no heat related problems in any of the horses competing.

The main findings can be summarised as follows:
Transport - horses should be allowed one day recovery for every two hours of flying.

Acclimatisation – nearly all horses can adapt to cope better with dry heat or humid heat by a period of at least 14 days acclimatisation.

Environmental thermal load – accurate assessment of environmental thermal stress is essential to planning and management. An index used by the American military, known as the Wet Bulb Globe Temperature (WBGT) index was adapted and validated for use with equestrian sports and used during both the build up and the Games themselves. This index takes into account heat, humidity, cooling effects, of wind and heating effects of solar radiation.

Dry heat versus humid heat – for the same air temperature, the higher the humidity, the greater thermal stress imposed

Cooling – Horses are large animals with a low surface area to bodyweight ratio (~1m^2 per 100kg). This allows them to keep warm in cold climates, but makes it difficult for them to get rid of heat in hot conditions. Horses generate large amounts of heat when exercising and may be unable to dissipate this effectively in thermally stressful conditions. Effective cooling, without any adverse effects, was shown to be best achieved using large volumes of ice-cold water (0-4°C) over the whole body

Heat tolerance – horses are able to tolerate much higher body temperatures than people. Horses can tolerate rectal temperatures of 42°C for short periods during or after exercise without adverse effects, whereas a temperature of 40°C (104°F) in a person would be a cause for serious concern.

Phase A (First phase of Roads and Tracks) – Phase A in a Three-Day Event Speed and Endurance Test is designed to be a warm-up phase. In very hot or hot and humid conditions, undesirable increases in body temperature above that needed for warming-up and unnecessary fluid loss through sweating may be induced even prior to the steeplechase. Therefore, in thermally stressful conditions Phase A should be shortened.

Phase C (Second phase of Roads and Tracks) – Phase C is designed to allow recovery of horses from the steeplechase prior to undertaking the cross-country phase. In hot or hot and humid conditions, horses are unable to recover on Phase C and actually become hotter and more dehydrated with increasing time or distance. Mandatory 10 minute cooling stops on Phase C were shown to allow effective recovery by reducing temperature and thus reducing sweat loss and dehydration.

'10 min box' – the time in the '10 min box' should be increased to 15 or even 20 min to allow more time for recovery and more frequent veterinary monitoring of horses to determine fitness to start the cross-country.

Cross-Country – the number of fences, total distance and height or difficulty of fences may need to be altered in thermally stressful conditions.

General management – if it is not possible to move the location of a competition or the time of year, then it may be possible to avoid the most thermally stressful times of the day by an early morning start. The risk of heat related injury will increase with the level of thermal stress and objective criteria based on the WBGT index should be used to determine the level at which modifications to the competition should be made and when a competition should be halted or abandoned.

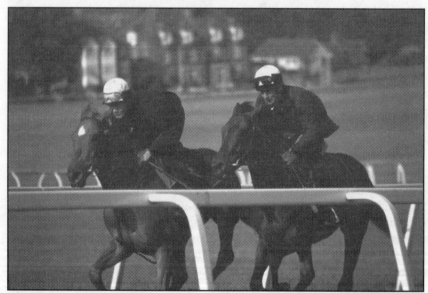

Figure 5   There are unfortunately still relatively few scientific studies of training programmes due to the cost of undertaking such investigations. However, in order to reduce training and competition related injuries, studies of different training programmes to identify those which minimise damage to the musculo-skeletal system whilst still achieving the required levels of fitness are required.

Training

The aim of training is twofold: firstly, to improve performance and secondly, to minimise the risk of injury or illness as a result of exercise. Unfortunately, scientific studies of training are expensive to undertake due to the cost of buying and keeping horses, the training time itself and the fact that minor injuries frequently occur, even in normal training, and disrupt studies. Thus, there are relatively few good studies of training and even fewer comparing different training methods such as conventional *versus* interval training methods. However, we do now know that the response to initial long, slow type training in terms of increases in fitness and adaptation of the muscles and cardiovascular system reaches a plateau by around 3-4 weeks from starting a training programme. The implication is that continuing long, slow work beyond 3-4 weeks has little benefit in terms of increasing fitness, which can only be brought about by increasing the intensity of the work but which may be detrimental to other body systems, for example, the skeleton.

Overtraining syndrome has been clearly identified in human athletes and is characterised by a gradual reduction in performance in highly fit athletes at National level or higher, usually undertaking a large volume of training close to peak fitness. There is no obvious cause, such as an injury or viral infection, and reduction in intensity or volume (amount) of training is usually recommended. Many racehorse trainers believe that a similar syndrome occurs in horses in training, particularly once horses are at racing fitness. However, analysis of blood samples and other tests have generally failed to identify any marker of overtraining in the horse. A recent treadmill study of overtraining on Standardbred racehorses in Australia at the University of Sydney found that a decrease in performance was only associated with changes in behaviour and weight loss.

If a period of training is followed by a period of reduced training or complete inactivity, a detraining or deconditioning response usually occurs. This is generally associated with decreased fitness and performance. In man the detraining response is usually rapid, with marked losses in fitness and performance in a matter of weeks. However, loss of fitness with detraining in the horse from a high level of fitness appears to be both small and slow. In fact, in one study, race fit Thoroughbred horses galloping twice a week were 'detrained' by being restricted to box rest and 20 min walking a day. After 15 weeks, there was no detectable change in cardiovascular or respiratory function or aerobic capacity. The only change was that during exercise after detraining the horses produced more lactic acid (lactate) than when fit. The implication is that when a horse is fit, a short period of missed work, for example due to a minor injury, will have little impact on fitness.

Biomechanics

Biomechanics is the study of biological systems (bio) and the way in which movement occurs and the associated changes in pressures and forces (mechanics) at rest and during exercise. There are essentially three branches of biomechanics. The first, kinematics, describes movement but does not deal with the forces involved. For example, video of a horse during exercise or over a jump can be used to obtain kinematic data but will provide no information on forces, for example on joints or between the feet and the ground. Kinematic measurements would include variables such as stride length, stride frequency and joint angles. Kinetics is the study of the forces (such as pressure and acceleration) involved in movement, but without information on movement itself, i.e. where the limb is or the angles of the joints. For example, force plates which horses are trotted over provide detailed kinetic information on the contact between the limb and the plate surface, but don't provide any information on the movement of the foot and limb. The third area of biomechanics deals with the structural properties of bone, cartilage, tendons, ligaments and muscles. Studies may be carried out in the laboratory on limbs taken from horses that have been destroyed. For example, measurements of bone strength can be obtained by placing a leg in a press that places increasing load on the bone until it fails (fractures). The load the bone can stand until it fractures is a direct measurement of strength. Investigation of structural properties in the live animal can be undertaken using non-invasive techniques such as radiography, ultrasound or single photon-absorptimetry or invasive techniques such as bone biopsy to obtain a small sample for further analysis. This approach to biomechanics can be used in assessing the impact of factors such as diet and training on structural properties and in understanding the mechanisms of injury and repair of supporting structures such as bone and cartilage.

In many scientific studies, kinetic and kinematic data are obtained at the same time allowing complete biomechanical analysis of movement. Advances in computational power and technology have been admirably exploited by those in the field of equine biomechanics, which is now a science with its own specialised nomenclature and a highly specialised area of exercise physiology. Some of the techniques currently used in biomechanics include video and optoelectronics (with markers placed on defined anatomical points), electromyography (analysis of the electrical signals from muscles as they are used), measurements of limb acceleration using accelerometers attached to the limbs and measurements of forces between the foot and the ground (ground reaction forces) using force plates and force shoes.

There can probably be considered to be three main themes in equine biomechanics: 1) basic studies to understand movement; 2) the application of biomechanics to disease and injury; 3) application of biomechanics to select horses that have characteristics that make them elite in running or jumping.

Lameness and orthopaedic conditions are the most common cause of wastage in the racing industry. The underlying reasons and the approaches to prevention are still not clear. Orthopaedic problems may be the result of many factors including age at the onset of training, training methods, discipline, training surfaces, nutrition and conformation. Diagnosis of lameness and evaluation of responses to treatment can readily be undertaken by application of a variety of biomechanical techniques. The critical issue is whether these approaches are more sensitive or provide additional information to the veterinary surgeon. At present it is not clear if this is the case and requirements for sophisticated and expensive equipment, a considerable understanding of biomechanics and complex analysis procedures required to analyse kinetic or kinematic data, mean that such approaches to lameness are restricted to specialised biomechanics groups.

An important contribution of biomechanics has been in optimising track design to limit orthopaedic injuries. The modifications to tracks were made on the basis of kinematic studies undertaken on racing Standardbred horses. Biomechanical techniques have also been applied to analysis of shoeing. For example, one kinematic study demonstrated that reducing the hoof angle by 10° resulted in the toe hitting the ground first. Not only would this movement probably affect performance it was also considered to predispose to injury.

The relationship between movement (locomotion) and performance has been studied the most in trotting races, galloping races, show jumping and dressage. In trotting races, the best performers have been shown to have a high maximal stride frequency and long stride length. In galloping horses, the maximum speed that can be reached is mainly determined by the stride length rather than the stride frequency. In three-day event horses analysed during the steeplechase phase at the Seoul Olympics, successfully performing horses were found to have stride lengths between 1.85 and 2.05m. For showjumpers at the highest level of competition, a number of biomechanical factors have been identified as being associated with good performance, including low take-off speed, close placement of the hind-limbs to the jump, a long stride, a takeoff angle of around 15° to the ground and low level of braking with the forelimbs. In Dressage, it has been shown that a low stride frequency has been identified as necessary for a good quality of trot and that the horse should place its hindlimbs as far as possible underneath itself. Horses achieving the highest scores at Olympic level have been shown to extend their gallop stride by increasing stride length without changing their stride frequency (i.e. lengthening).

Dr Eric Barrey, at the French based INRA research station, concluded in a recent review of biomechanics that 'the number of concrete applications [of biomechanics] available for trainers, riders, breeders and veterinary practitioners is too limited compared to the amount of work that has been done' and acknowledged that the advances in equine biomechanics must be used to develop applications that can be used under field conditions rather than in the highly specialised laboratory setting with complex and expensive equipment.

Summary
Exercise physiology has matured and established itself as an important discipline dealing with the issues of performance and injury or disease in the competing or working horse. As new technological developments in equipment, imaging and molecular biology based techniques, including genetics, continue to evolve, it is likely that greater and more rapid advances will take place. Whilst there will continue to be great emphasis on the health and welfare of the competition or working horse, it is inevitable that there will continue to be a strong interest in performance related factors.

50

INVESTIGATION OF POOR PERFORMANCE AND LOSS OF PERFORMANCE

Equine clinicians are frequently presented with horses in whom the major or sole presenting sign is poor performance, loss of performance or reduced exercise tolerance. Investigation of poor performance or loss of performance can present the clinician with a considerable diagnostic challenge. Diagnosis of medical causes of impaired performance are important, not merely from the point of view of the disappointed owner or trainer, but also because appropriate reduction of exercise whilst suffering from disease is of welfare importance for the horse. This chapter aims to discuss the various causes of impaired performance and how they are investigated clinically.

The terms 'poor performance' and 'loss of performance' are sometimes used as though they were interchangeable, but it is best to use them correctly and to categorise individual cases accordingly. 'Poor performance' implies a low level of performance in an animal or group of animals that have not previously shown a higher level of achievement. 'Loss of performance', on the other hand, implies a low level of performance in an animal that has shown a higher level of achievement in the past. It can be important to distinguish the two conditions, since the loss of performance case is the more likely to stem from a medical problem.

The causes of impaired performance (i.e. both loss of performance and poor performance) can be categorised as follows:

1. A low level of inherent ability
2. Inadequate or inappropriate training
3. Participation in inappropriate competition
4. Dysfunction of one or more physiological system(s)
5. Lack of motivation

It is without doubt that the most frequent cause of poor performance is a lack of talent, yet this diagnosis can be a difficult one for the clinician to arrive at with certainty, as well as for the owner to accept, and requires a thorough investigation in which all other possible causes of impaired performance are eliminated as far as possible. Inadequate or inappropriate training may also result in an animal that shows poor performance in the absence of any medical disorder. Lack of motivation is difficult to quantify in the equine athlete and may in itself result from the effects of work in the presence of disease or injury.

The clinician's main task in the investigation of poor performance is to determine whether there is dysfunction in one or more of the physiological systems necessary for optimum athletic performance, i.e. whether disease or injury is present. Overt disease is generally easy to detect, but low-grade disorders, insufficient to cause clinical signs at rest, yet sufficient to limit performance when the demands of exercise force utilisation of the body's physiological reserve capacity, are more difficult to diagnose but are frequently a cause of impaired performance.

For example, the resting Thoroughbred racehorse breathes around eight to ten times per minute with a tidal volume (volume of air inhaled per breath) of around four to five litres, giving a minute ventilation (volume of air breathed per minute) of around fifty litres. During strenuous exercise the minute ventilation can increase to more than 2000 litres per minute. Given such a huge reserve capacity it is unsurprising that mild respiratory disease may escape detection when the horse is examined at rest. Low grade disease without overt clinical signs but sufficient to affect physiological function is termed sub-clinical and diagnosis of such conditions can present the equine clinician with a severe diagnostic challenge. The techniques used for the investigation of poor performance/loss of performance will vary from case to case.

Various methods for the objective assessment of racing ability and training state have been used in the horse. Resting haematological variables are not good indicators of fitness, but various parameters of exercising heart rate and blood lactate such as V_{200} (the speed at which heart rate is 200 bpm) and V_{LA4} (the speed at which blood lactate concentration is 4mmol.L^{-1}), have been used in exercise tests. It has been suggested for example, that V_{LA4} is higher (meaning that blood lactate starts to accumulate at a higher speed) in Standardbreds that perform well compared to poor performers. With increasing fitness, heart rate at submaximal speeds decreases and blood lactate accumulation is delayed so that V_{200} and V_{LA4} both show an increase with training. There are drawbacks, however, to the use of such parameters for fitness testing or comparison of ability between individuals. Firstly, there is the need to standardise testing procedures and conditions, which can be very difficult in the field. In addition, since both the heart rate and the blood lactate responses to exercise are affected by other factors such as disease, age and excitement, it is difficult to interpret their relevance to fitness in isolation. Finally, the relevance of these variables depends on the horse's use, and in sprinting animals high concentrations of blood lactate may represent a desirable high anaerobic potential rather than lack of fitness.

The term 'overtraining' is frequently used to describe the syndrome in which horses lose performance after a prolonged period of time in training. A similar condition has been described in human athletes, but usually only at high levels of training and when associated with other psychological stresses. It has been difficult to reproduce overtraining in experimental studies in horses and when it has been seen, after very high levels of training, no consistent haematological or physiological markers of overtraining have been demonstrated. The signs associated with overtraining appear to involve reduced performance and behavioural changes and in human athletes it has been suggested that subjective ratings of fatigue, stress, muscle soreness and sleep are more accurate predictors of the onset of overtraining than are physiological variables. Whilst there are reports that overtraining in Swedish Standardbred racehorses is associated with an increase in red blood cell volume, other workers have generally been unable to demonstrate this.

Poor performance and loss of performance investigation may be divided into those involving individual animals and those in which a whole stable or part of a stable are affected. In the latter case, the search for a common factor affecting the group of animals, such as infectious disease, a nutritional deficiency, inappropriate training or an adverse environmental factor is important. In either situation a detailed and precise clinical history is vital and this is most easily obtained from owners and trainers who keep good medical, feeding and training records. In the investigation of a whole stable problem it may be necessary to obtain appropriate diagnostic samples from all of the whole group or a representative sub-group. Animals showing signs of frank disease should be sampled and techniques such as routine haematology, virus serology, nasopharyngeal swabbing and collection of lower airway secretions (using tracheal wash or bronchoalveolar lavage) sampling may be of value.

It is frequently the case that investigation of the poorly performing equine athlete reveals the presence of more than one abnormality, the proportion of such cases having been estimated in one study to be over 80%. In such cases it is important to determine which of the abnormalities are clinically significant and which are incidental findings.

In investigating the nutritional status of the stable, nutrient analysis of feeds and accurate measurement of amounts fed will provide information as to the adequacy of the diet. It can be necessary to follow feeding practices through by direct observation to ensure that the theoretical feeding practice actually translates into the practical situation, e.g. do the amounts that are thought to be fed tally with the amounts measured using the utensils used daily for dispensing? Similarly, when obtaining feed samples for analysis these should be taken under the normal circumstances of feeding rather than being measured out especially for the analysis.

Various studies have identified orthopaedic disorders and respiratory diseases as the two major causes of lost training time and wastage in racehorses in training and these also represent the most frequent causes of loss of performance in these animals and other types of performance horses. The prevalence of orthopaedic abnormalities in racehorses in training is high and they can contribute significantly to impaired performance, yet their importance is often underestimated by trainers. On occasion it may be useful to resort to exercise testing with and without analgesia to demonstrate the effects of orthopaedic conditions on exercise tolerance.

Both upper and lower respiratory tract disorders can impair performance. The accurate diagnosis of dynamic upper airway obstructions may necessitate treadmill examination and is detailed below.

Lower respiratory tract disease occurs frequently due to both infectious and non-infectious causes. Traditionally, lower respiratory tract disease in racehorses in training has been attributed to 'the virus', but it is now clear that there is no single viral entity that causes respiratory disease in the horse, but rather several different agents including equine influenza, equine herpesviruses and rhinoviruses. Respiratory disease caused by these different agents cannot be reliably differentiated on clinical grounds alone and requires specific diagnostic tests such as nasopharyngeal swabbing for (isolation of virus from throat swabs) and viral serology (for identification of an increase in circulating antibody levels to specific viruses in response to an infection). Moreover, it has become clear in the last decade that bacterial infections are a more frequent cause of airway inflammation in horses in training than viral ones. A study of racehorses in the United Kingdom has reported a prevalence of 13.8% for lower airway disease and in the majority of cases in this study bacterial infections were involved. Other studies involving both racehorses and mixed groups of horses have demonstrated a strong association between lower airway inflammation and bacterial infection with agents such as *Streptococcus zooepidemicus*, *Actinobacillus/Pasteurella* spp. and *Streptococcus pneumoniae*.

Environmental factors may also frequently be involved in respiratory problems in racehorses and other performance horses. It has been reported that horses bedded on straw in looseboxes are twice as likely to suffer from lower airway disease as animals bedded on shavings in barns and a recent study showed that stabling was associated with airway inflammation in a group of young Arabian horses.

The most frequently occurring medical condition of adult horses in the United Kingdom is probably recurrent airway obstruction (RAO – previously known as chronic obstructive pulmonary disease), a respiratory hypersensitivity or allergy with some similarities to asthma in man. In the majority of cases the agents responsible are mould spores found in the stable environment. RAO can cause significant reduction in lung function and yet it is often overlooked in the evaluation of respiratory disease in racehorses.

The prevalence of sub-clinical respiratory disease in all types of competition horses is high and its detection is complicated by the poor sensitivity of coughing as a marker of the presence of respiratory disease in the horse. A recent study reported that in a group of racehorses monitored routinely by endoscopic examination for the detection of lower airway disease, only 38% of the animals with lower airway inflammatory disease were reported to be coughing. The use of endoscopic examination of the respiratory tract and the evaluation of respiratory secretions obtained by tracheal wash or bronchoalveolar lavage is a powerful tool for the detection of such sub-clinical disease (Figure 1)

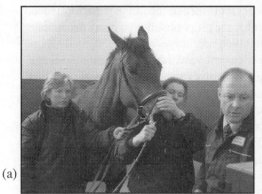

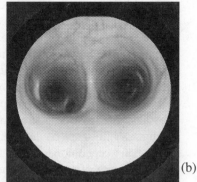

(a)   (b)

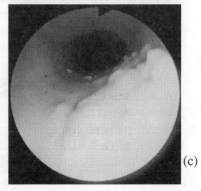

(c)

Figure 1 (a) Endoscopy of the respiratory tract can usually be carried out in the unsedated horse, permitting observation of the upper airways, trachea and large bronchi (airways). *(b)* In this normal horse, the trachea can be seen bifurcating into the main bronchus of each lung. *(c)* A horse with a large amount of mucopus in the trachea due to marked lower airway inflammation, (photographed at the lowest point of the trachea a few inches further forward than Figure 1b).

Bleeding into the airways associated with strenuous exercise has been recognised in the horse for centuries, although it is only relatively recently that it has become apparent that the source of the haemorrhage is the lungs. This condition is known as exercise-induced pulmonary haemorrhage (EIPH) and it occurs frequently in horses performing strenuous exercise. For example, in one study of British Flatracehorses the prevalence of the condition was found to be 40% in two-year-olds, 65% in three-year-olds and 82% in horses aged four years and older. It appears likely that virtually all racehorses in full training experience some degree of EIPH and its effect on performance in uncertain. Only one survey has found a relationship between EIPH and finishing position and in view of the frequency with which the condition occurs, the presence of EIPH on endoscopic observation of the trachea shortly after a race should be interpreted with care. In a group of horses subjected to post-racing endoscopic examination following poor racecourse performance, the prevalence of EIPH has been found to be no greater than that of a random sample of racehorses. The presence of a small amount of blood in the trachea after racing or the detection of EIPH by laboratory examination of a tracheal wash or bronchoalveolar lavage sample should not therefore prevent a comprehensive investigation of a poorly performing equine athlete as other factors may be implicated as a cause of impaired performance.

Cardiological abnormalities occur frequently in the horse but are often not of clinical consequence. In a recent survey a prevalence of heart murmurs of over 80% was reported in Thoroughbred racehorses and another study found that murmurs due to mitral and tricuspid valvular regurgitation (leakage) increased in two-year-old Thoroughbred horses after nine months of race training. Whilst in a small number of animals leakage of blood through a heart valve is sufficiently severe to impair exercise tolerance, in the majority of cases they have no discernible effect on performance. Similarly, abnormalities of cardiac rhythm may be detected in many animals at rest, and whilst atrial fibrillation (a condition in which the atria of the heart do not contract normally) can be a cause of reduced exercise tolerance, many arrhythmias are not of clinical consequence. The use of colour flow Doppler echocardiography, which permits imaging of blood flow through the heart, combined with exercise testing to assess the cardiac response to exercise, are powerful aids to determine in which cases cardiac function is limiting to performance (Figure 2).

Figure 2   Colour flow Doppler echocardiagram showing blood flow through the heart (picture courtesy of Dr Lesley Young)

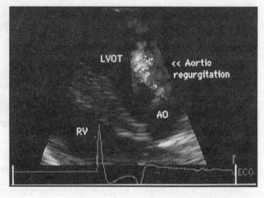

A not uncommon presentation is the horse in which a history of reduced exercise tolerance and/or lethargy is reported. Affected animals may have no other signs of ill-health, but in some periodic inappetence or muscle stiffness are reported. Blood samples obtained from infected animals sometimes show alterations in the numbers of white blood cells, with low total white blood cell count and/or reductions in the number of neutrophils (a type of white blood cell) being the most frequently reported changes.

A definitive diagnosis in these cases is not always possible and when signs are very vague it may be difficult to determine whether the patient is really ill.

It must be remembered that a small number of individuals will normally have white blood cell values that lie outside the reference range.

A wide range of possible causes of this syndrome have been suggested and it has been compared to the chronic fatigue syndrome of man, which is also believed to be multifactorial in origin. A common term used for the condition is 'post-viral fatigue', although few cases have detectable evidence of an initial viral infection. Some workers have reported evidence of enterovirus infection in a number of affected horses, whilst others have suggested that a bacterial infection may be involved in some patients.

In mild cases in which a full investigation fails to reveal a definitive cause, some patients respond to the implementation of a carefully graded exercise plan bringing the horse into full work over an extended period.

The use of exercise testing for the investigation of exercise-related disorders has increased with the advent of the high-speed treadmill. Observation of field exercise has been used by the clinician for centuries to examine animals with reduced athletic capacity but the use of standardised exercise testing is a more modern practice.

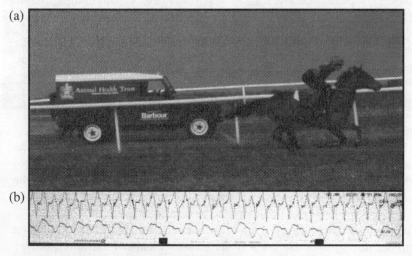

Figure 3 *(a)* Field exercise testing: Electrocardiogram, respiratory rate and pattern of breathing are measured telemetrically in the pace car, which indicates to the jockey the correct running speed . *(b)* A typical exercising electrocardiogram (upper trace) and impedance plethysmograph showing the pattern of breathing (lower trace).

Field exercise testing may be useful in some cases and both cardiac and respiratory rate and rhythm can be recorded in the field by electrocardiography and impedance plethysmography respectively during exercise (Figure 3). The drawbacks to field testing are the limited degree to which conditions can be standardised and the limited range of measurements that can be made. The advent of the high speed treadmill has permitted far greater standardisation of conditions such as running speed, track surface, incline, temperature, humidity, etc., as well as allowing measurements to be made which are difficult or impossible to perform at high speed in the field.

Treadmill exercise can be used to measure exercise tolerance in terms of run time to fatigue, providing a measure of exercise capacity, as well as facilitating measurement of physiological function during exercise. One study suggested that there is likely to be a relationship between treadmill run time and racing performance, noting that the best racehorses generally had the longest run time to fatigue on the treadmill. A similar relationship has been evident in patients tested at our Centre.

(a)
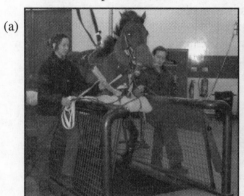
(b)
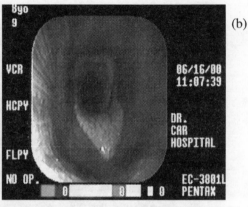

Figure 4
(a) Horse galloping on a high-speed treadmill. Note the facemask and flow meters that permit measurement of airflow without impairing respiration. *(b)* Endoscopic image of the upper airways of a normal horse galloping on the treadmill.

Treadmill exercise testing (Figure 4) facilitates both arterial and venous blood sampling during exercise, as well as measurements of cardiorespiratory function such as heart rate, electrocardiogram, respiratory rate, respiratory airflow rate, expired gas compositions, stride rage and length and total red blood cell volume. Measurement of maximum oxygen uptake (V_{O2max}) is an extremely useful measurement that can be made during treadmill exercise and this assessment of aerobic capacity is a valuable indicator of athletic potential. Measurement of physiological responses to a standardised treadmill exercise test can be used to detect body systems in which there is abnormal function during exercise and also to assess the effects on exercise tolerance of abnormalities detected during a resting examination.

Possibly the most useful single clinical diagnostic test facilitated by treadmill exercise is, however, exercise videoendoscopy. The prevalence of upper airway obstructive disorders in racehorses is relatively high and in many cases these disorders are dynamic, that is, they are only apparent during exercise. Conditions such as severe recurrent laryngeal neuropathy ('roaring') and permanent epiglottic entrapment can be diagnosed during a resting endoscopic examination. On the other hand, disorders such as dorsal displacement of the soft palate (DDSP – often referred to as 'soft palate disease' or erroneously called 'tongue swallowing') and dynamic laryngeal collapse, only occur during exercise when the tremendously high respiratory airflow rates cause dramatic changes in upper airway pressures and fatigue occurs in respiratory as well as locomotor muscles. Exercise endoscopy is indicated for horses in which an abnormal respiratory noise, that cannot be diagnosed using resting endoscopy is heard during exercise, as well as in cases in which endoscopic findings are equivocal. Additionally, since some horses with dynamic upper airway collapse present with no history of abnormal noise, it is also indicated in the investigation of the poor performance/loss of performance horse. The importance of exercise endoscopy can be gauged from the findings of clinicians at the University of Sydney, who reported that a complete and correct endoscopic diagnosis was made at rest in only 25% of a group of horses referred to them for treadmill investigation.

In our Centre, exercise testing begins with a routine orthopaedic evaluation to determine whether there are any musculoskeletal conditions present that might 1) be limiting performance and 2) be likely to be worsened by treadmill exercise. Following this examination a short period of treadmill acclimation follows, consisting for around 90% of horses of two or three practice runs. A small percentage of horses require a longer period of acclimation, but only about 2% are unresponsive to treadmill training.

The protocol used for physiological exercise testing varies with the type of horse being tested. For racehorses and higher level eventers the following exercise protocol is used for physiological testing:

Speed (metres/second)*	Gait	Duration (minutes)	Incline (%)
1.7	Walk	5	0
4.0	Trot	3	8
7.0	Canter	2	8
8.0	Canter	1	8
10.0§	Canter	1	8
11.0§	Gallop	1	8
12.0§	Gallop	1	8
13.0§	Gallop	1	8
1.7	Walk	10	0

* One metre/second is equivalent to 2.25 miles per hour (3.6 kilometres per hour)

§Test concluded when the patient has difficulty maintaining treadmill speed.

Such an incremental test permits exercise capacity to be investigated and if oxygen consumption at the end of each step is plotted, V_{O2max} may be calculated. In an average Thoroughbred horse in full training V_{O2max} is around 150-160 ml.kg^{-1}.min^{-1}, whilst elite animals of championship status have been found to have values for V_{O2max} in excess of 200 ml.kg^{-1}.min^{-1}. For less athletic animals or horses involved in less strenuous activities, protocols involving a lower workload, produced by exercise at a lower speed and/or incline, are used.

For exercise endoscopy, incremental exercise test protocols are also used, with the starting point, duration and rate of increase of steps again depending on the type of animal being tested. Since conditions such as DDSP frequently only occur towards the end of a race or event when fatigue is occurring, when racehorses and eventers in full training are investigated, it is important that the exercise test continues until either a diagnosis of upper airway obstruction is made or the horse shows signs of fatigue. Table 1 shows a summary of the relative incidence of dynamic upper airway disorders in horses presented for exercise endoscopy at our Centre over a two-year period. In suitable cases, the diagnostic value of treadmill exercise testing is high and the safety record of such tests is excellent.

In summary, whilst this has of necessity been only a brief introduction to the subject, it will be apparent that accurate diagnosis of the poor performance or loss of performance case can be challenging to the equine clinician. It requires detailed attention to the patient's clinical history, thorough clinical examination and, frequently, recourse to advanced diagnostic methods.

Table 1   Prevalence of dynamic upper airway obstructive disorders in 152 horses referred for treadmill videoendoscopy.

	%
Dorsal displacement of the soft palate	37.5
Soft palatal instability	20.4
Dynamic laryngeal collapse	10.6
Axial deviation/vibration of the aryepiglottic folds	10.5
Pharyngeal collapse	9.9
Epiglottal entrapment	0.7
Epiglottal retroversion	0.7

51
THE PURCHASE OF HORSES AND VETERINARY CERTIFICATION

It cannot be emphasised too strongly that would-be purchasers of a horse should, whenever possible, have it examined by a veterinarian, and should not complete the purchase until they have in their possession the certificate indicating the result of this examination.

A buyer may not consider this necessary when the seller can produce a recent certificate of such an examination, but nevertheless the wisest plan is to obtain an independent opinion, because the animal may not have shown symptoms of a serious defect previously.

Should the buyer wish to have the animal on trial, he must remember that nothing must be done to it, such as removing a mane or replacing the shoes (even if those the animal is wearing require removal) until he has made up his mind whether to retain or return, because should he do so, it constitutes 'purchase' and legally the seller is entitled to refuse return.

The buyer must understand that, from the standpoint of the veterinarian, the animal can only be classified as suitable or unsuitable for purchase. The veterinary certificate will list the defects detected in the horse and offer an opinion on the significance of the fault in relation to the purpose for which the animal is being purchased – for example, racing, dressage or breeding.

Very often a prospective buyer may have noticed a particular vice, and he should always mention this to the veterinarian because some vices or bad habits are not always found at the time of an examination for purchase. He should also remember that a veterinary certificate does not indicate freedom from vice. Nevertheless, the seller is under an obligation to disclose to the buyer any vice or bad habit that is within his knowledge as failure to do so can nullify the transaction and the animal can be returned.

Traditionally the maxim *caveat emptor* has been the rule of the law, and a party who has bought a defective horse has no remedy, unless there is evidence either of express warranty or of fraud. In the general sale of a horse the seller only warrants it to be an animal of the description it appears to be and nothing more; if the purchaser makes no inquiries as to its qualities and it turns out to be unfit for use, he cannot recover against the seller.

Recently consumer legislation has altered this situation and sales have been nullified on the basis of manifest or 'hidden' defects being shown to have been present before or at the time of sale. The current situation, including the professional liability of a veterinarian who undertakes an examination for purchase, is discussed in Chapter 52.

Common conditions rendering a horse unfit for purchase
It is impossible to lay down rules for conditions that render horses fit or unfit for purchase. All decisions must take account of the future use for which the horse is required and, to a certain extent, the value placed on the individual. For example, a horse with partial vision may be suitable for purchase for breeding while being unsuitable for all athletic duties. Similarly, a horse with total laryngeal hemiplegia (paralysis) will usually be considered unfit for purchase for racing or breeding, but will be capable of use as a hack or even as a hunter.

However, it is helpful to consider the most common defects of the organ systems which are likely to appear on veterinary certificates.

Defects of eyes   Absence of an eye, collapse of an eye, any form or size of corneal opacity, lenticular or capsular cataract, paralysis of the iris, or blindness from any cause constitute serious defects. Inflammation or injury of the iris and pupil (iridocyclitis) and loss of orbital pressure may be an indication of periodic ophthalmia and should be considered a serious defect. Photophobia and conjunctivitis may be temporary or indicative of a more serious problem. Other more subtle abnormalities detected with an ophthalmoscope are rare but usually serious – for example, retinal atrophy.

Defects of wind (the respiratory system)   The chief abnormalities of wind are laryngeal hemiplegia (whistling or roaring), chronic obstructive pulmonary disease (COPD, broken wind), coughing and bleeding.

The main respiratory disorders are discussed in detail in chapter 2. However, in relation to purchase, the condition of laryngeal hemiplegia, frequently demonstrated clinically as an abnormal inspiratory noise described as a 'whistle' or a 'roar', has been the cause of great controversy in recent years. Examination of the upper airway of horses has been greatly facilitated by the introduction of flexible fibreoptic endoscopes which allow visual examination of the larynx before and after exercise. Thus, the examination of wind of highly priced horses will often involve exercise and endoscopic tests. The results of such examinations have not always been simple to interpret. The laryngeal paralysis (usually left-sided) may be partial or complete. Cases of partial paralysis may or may not produce abnormal inspiratory noises and detectability of the noise may be altered by the fitness of the horse or concurrent respiratory infection.

There is little doubt that many horses with partial paralysis perform satisfactorily. However, the progressive nature and probable heritability of the defect make unreserved recommendation of affected horses impossible. Soft palate paresis causing 'gurgling' and 'choking' also causes respiratory embarrassment. It is generally manifested under severe stress and so is not generally recognised during the extent of the normal prior to purchase examination. It is also normally unrecognisable by endoscopy at rest but any suspicion of this condition would be grounds for the rejection of the horse.

Other respiratory sounds are emitted under exertion by some horses, but unless they are connected with disease, injury, operation or acquired alteration of structure, they should not be regarded as unsoundness of wind. High-blowing may be due to excitement (showing condition or freshness). It should, and often does, disappear with exercise or as the horse settles down to steady work.

The term 'bleeding' is more correctly called exercise-induced pulmonary haemorrhage (EIPH – see p. 86; see also epistaxis - p. 66). As this name suggests, affected horses bleed into the substance of the lung during strenuous exercise and this may adversely affect their performance. After exercise blood passes into the respiratory tract and may appear at the nostrils, particularly as the horse lowers its head. Endoscopic examination of horses worldwide shows that a high percentage of horses have blood in their trachea (windpipe) after exercise. A smaller number show bleeding at the nostrils. Nevertheless, clinical evidence or a history of bleeding constitutes a serious abnormality sufficient to advise against purchase for strenuous athletic duties.

Persistent purulent nasal discharges may be bilateral, related to infectious bacterial or viral diseases, or unilateral in cases of sinusitis or guttural pouch disease. Coughing is a common sign of respiratory disease and may be related to infection or allergy and may be temporary or persistent. Purchase should be delayed until coughing has ceased or the condition investigated to the purchaser's satisfaction.

Defective limb or action   Lameness, if present in any degree is a serious abnormality. The cause is immaterial. The action may be peculiar or objectionable, such as dishing, but when due to conformation it does not amount to lameness. Stringhalt is a definite defect and shivering a serious one, which is often rapidly progressive.

Thickening or inflammation of tendons, especially the flexor tendons of the forelimbs, must always be considered a serious defect when purchasing a horse for athletic duties. Such tendon strains are frequently recurrent despite treatment. Osteoarthrosis of joints is of great significance when related to lameness or pain, but many mature horses may be unaffected by old injuries and even fractures. In these cases the examining vet's opinion is all-important.

Incoordination of the hindlimbs or all four limbs must always be regarded as a serious defect. The most common cause in young horses is pressure on the spinal cord in the neck region (the wobbler syndrome - see p. 326). Other causes are traumatic injuries to the head and neck and certain infections such as the neurological form of rhinopneumonitis and protozoal encephalomyelitis (seen in horses imported from the USA).

Existing disease or effects of disease or accident   Diseases of the heart, respiratory and digestive systems, urinary and genital organs, skin, feet and eyes all constitute serious abnormalities. Dribbling of the urine may be due to a calculus or sabulous (gritty) accumulation in the bladder or congenital malformation. If diarrhoea is present, it must be noted; it may be temporary but the purchaser should await its disappearance. Sometimes profuse staling occurs when the animal is being ridden: this may be only a peculiarity of temper, but must be mentioned. For disorders of these systems, see the relevant chapters.

Blemishes   Any blemish, such as scars or firing marks, devalue a horse but may be of no consequence if the animal is not lame. Broken knees may indicate a tendency to fall in some cases, the significance of which will depend upon the work the horse may have to perform. All blemishes must be mentioned. Capped hocks and elbows do not interfere with work but some people object to them as an eyesore. Firing marks, either from thermo-cautery or crio-cautery (freeze firing), should be noted but their significance is overshadowed by the condition which necessitated this form of therapy. In the case of splints and curbs, the condition itself may have become of little consequence but most will remain a cause for concern.

Vices and bad habits   When these impair the natural usefulness of the animal, they will render it unfit for purchase. Several may pass unnoticed at the time of the examination, for example, windsucking. A horse that is a crib-biter or a windsucker must be rejected. A windsucking horse is said to 'crib in the air', that is, without seizing any object or supporting the chin, and the habit produces no abnormal wear of the teeth as in crib-biting. Crib-biting can cause damage to the object which is grasped, particularly in the instance of paddock rails. Box walking and weaving may cause horses to lose body condition rapidly and can upset other horses within sight or hearing. These vices may be temporary, associated with a change of environment or separation from companions. A distinction must be drawn between vice and mere force of habit. It is sometimes the case that a horse may prove unsuitable to the new owner and may develop bad habits as a result of this (see chapter 43).

Defective conformation   This is largely a matter of taste or opinion: a horse should not be rejected because of 'bad shape'. Only when the conformational defect can be accurately described as a deformity should it be declared. Naturally there is a great difference of opinion among veterinarians, judges and owners, and reference should be made to Chapter 45.

Responsibility of the examiner for purchase

The responsibility is to the one who pays the fee and the opinion given after the examination may be oral or written. The latter is preferable.

The veterinary profession has received very clear instructions on both the method of examination and the type of certificate to be used. The procedure is laid down in the Royal College of Veterinary Surgeons/British Veterinary Association Joint Memorandum, *The Examination of Horses on Behalf of a Purchaser* (revised edition), BVA Publications, London, 1974. All veterinary certificates should be issued on these forms; where insufficient space is available on the sheet, additional sheets may be attached to the official form. The format of the certificate is shown on p. 807.

Procedure to be adopted when examining a horse for purchase

Before the animal is brought out of the loosebox or stable, it should be observed, undisturbed, by the examiner. Very often a vice such as crib-biting or wind-sucking will be spotted which might escape notice later on. Its attitude while resting should receive particular attention. Standing with one forefoot in advance of the other or frequent shifting of the weight from one forefoot to the other is suggestive of foot lameness or disease. Having watched the animal for a few minutes, the examiner should enter the box or stall, approaching the animal on its left (near) side and making it move over to its right (off) side, paying particular attention to the movement of the tail and hind limbs for signs of stringhalt, shivering and incoordination.

The teeth can now be examined for age, the pulse taken and the heart auscultated (this must be done again later after testing for wind), and a preliminary examination of the eyes can be made (this again to be repeated after testing for wind when the pupils will be well dilated). The horse is then led out quietly with a bridle or halter and stood in a convenient spot to enable the examiner to walk around it. During this preliminary inspection the colour, markings (natural and any acquired such as firing marks) and sex can be written down. In addition the following defects may be seen: nasal discharge, deformity of the face, lips or nostrils, corneal opacities, scars, skin eruptions, bursal distensions, marks of brushing, speedy-cuts, capped elbows and hocks, bowed or thickened tendons, odd feet, sandcracks, asymmetry of the pelvis, muscle wasting, thoroughpin, spavin, curb, windgalls and so on.

The person in charge of the horse should now be asked to walk it away from the examiner, giving it full use of its head, i.e. *not* holding the bridle or halter close to the head, for a distance of not less than 30 metres, and then back. It should be trotted over the same distance. It is a rather common fallacy that any lameness will become more apparent the faster the animal moves. The horse should be turned in a tight circle around the handler and backed, which will demonstrate stringhalt and shivering.

Each veterinary examiner has his or her own method for the next procedure. Some prefer to examine both fore and hind limbs, for example, in sequence, but personally I prefer to start on the horses left (near side) and, having finished here, proceed to the right (off side), working backwards from the hind limb to the front leg, the same examination being identical on both sides.

Starting at the head, I examine the eyes, teeth (the tongue is grasped and the condition of the cheek teeth noted on both sides), nostril, the submaxillary space, parotid gland, poll, throat, larynx, trachea (at this stage it is convenient to make the animal cough by squeezing the trachea and note the tone of the cough). I note if there is any sign of a jugular pulse, then raise the jugular. Then I examine the withers, shoulder point, forearm, knee, cannon, flexor tendons, fetlock, pastern and coronet; next, the elbow, back of forearm, knee, cannon, fetlock, and suspensory and sesamoid region, pastern and foot, testing the lateral cartilages for their elasticity. Holding the foot in the left hand, I press with the fingers of the right into the hollow of the heel, and flex the foot, noting any evidence of pain such as flinching. The foot is then examined for any signs of corns, thrush, seedy toe or canker. Whenever possible, the shoes should be removed if a really satisfactory examination is to be made; if the seller objects, this cannot be insisted upon, but a note should always be made to this effect.

Having finished here, I proceed to the chest, back, loins and croup, crural (leg) region, stifle, front of leg, hock, cannon, fetlock, pastern and coronet; next the quarter, buttock, thigh, back of leg, point and sides of hock, flexor tendons, suspensory, fetlock, heels and hind foot, which is to be raised, the hock flexed and the limb abducted. Next I raise the tail and inspect the anus, vulva, perineum and dock. While the fore and hind limbs are being examined, the inner side of the opposite limb should be carefully inspected, paying special attention to the groin, sheath, scrotum and testicles if entire and in the mare the udder. The inside of the groin is frequently a site of sarcoids (warts or fibrous tumours) which can cause trouble (see p. 659).

The wind should now be tested, and this is guided, to a certain extent, by the breed and condition of the animal. For example, if the animal is a mare advanced in pregnancy, this may be neither practicable nor advisable. In the case of the lighter breeds it is customary for the animal to be ridden, starting off with a slow canter round the examiner and then, at a signal from him or her, the animal is put into a gallop, to be finally pulled up (preferably after coming up an incline) beside the examiner when he or she so indicates. Alternatively, and this is usually employed with all stallions and yearlings, the animal should be lunged until sweating occurs.

After testing for wind, the heart should be re-examined. It should not be forgotten that an unfit horse, in some instances being fed for sale, may take as long as half an hour after a wind test before his breathing and heart settle down.

**CERTIFICATE OF VETERINARY EXAMINATION
OF A HORSE ON BEHALF OF A PROSPECTIVE PURCHASER**

CERTIFICATE No:
V 19672

This is to certify that, at the request of (Name & Address) _____

_____

I have examined the horse described below, the property of (Name & Address) _____

_____

at (Place of Examination) _____ on (Time & Date) _____

NAME of horse (or breeding)	**INSTRUCTIONS** 1) WRITTEN DESCRIPTION SHOULD BE TYPED OR WRITTEN IN BLOCK CAPITALS 2) WRITTEN DESCRIPTION AND DIAGRAM SHOULD AGREE 3) ALL WHITE MARKINGS SHOULD BE HATCHED IN RED 4) WHORLS MUST BE SHOWN THUS "X" AND DESCRIBED IN DETAIL
BREED OR TYPE	
COLOUR	LEFT SIDE / RIGHT SIDE
SEX	
AGE by documentation	FORE REAR VIEW / HIND REAR VIEW
APPROX. AGE by dentition (See Note 1 - overleaf)	
	HEAD AND NECK VENTRAL VIEW / MUZZLE / LEFT RIGHT / LEFT RIGHT

IDENTIFICATION

Head: _____

Neck: _____

Limbs: LF _____
RF _____
LH _____
RH _____

Body: _____

Acquired marks/brands/microchip: _____

REPORT OF EXAMINATION (See Note 2): I find no clinically discoverable signs of disease, injury or physical abnormality other than those here recorded (or recorded on the attached sheet)

_____
_____
_____
_____
_____ **Cont'd on attached sheet Yes/No**

Radiological or specialised techniques included in addition to the standard procedure _____

Report appended YES/NO   Blood taken and stored for testing for NSAIDs and other substances YES/NO   **WARRANTY (see Note3)**

THE OPINION (See Note 4): <u>On the balance of probabilities the conditions set out above</u> | ARE | ARE NOT | Delete clearly as appropriate

<u>likely to prejudice this animal's use for</u> _____

Owing to _____ stages _____ of the standard procedure were omitted **(See Note 5)**

Veterinary Surgeon's Signature _____ Date of Signature _____

Veterinary Surgeon's Name (in block capitals) _____

Address _____

NOTES - See overleaf

A normal heart should settle in about six to eight minutes after any but the most excessive exercise. Also the respiratory system cannot function efficiently in the presence of a diseased or disordered heart, and a careful examination of the respiratory movements should enable the examiner to detect a defective heart. When carrying out an examination for wind, if it happens to be a windy day, proximity to trees should be avoided and the examiner should stand with his back to the wind. Every precaution must be taken to avoid extraneous noises.

The eyes should be examined directly after the test for wind and while the pupils are dilated. This examination must be carried out in an enclosed area with diminished lighting. The nearer to darkness, the more satisfactory will be the examination. In the event of the examination being made inside, be careful to avoid white-washed walls behind the animal. These may cause a reflection in the eyes, giving the external appearance of cataract. The examination of the eyes should be made with an ophthalmoscope.

The height is taken at the highest point of the withers, ensuring that the animal is standing on level ground and with all four feet in alignment. The shoes, where practicable, can now be removed, the feet examined, and the soles pressed with the pincers to detect any sensitivity. Thin soles increase an animal's susceptibility to bruising. The animal should now be rested for half an hour and then led out and trotted away from and back to the examiner.

In the case of a harness horse it is important that the purchase is not completed until the animal has been driven for a few miles; the journey should include an ascent and a descent of a hill. This may identify any faults which would render it useless for the purposes for which it is being bought and which would not be detected in the customary examination for purchase. If possible, the person who is going to drive it later on should do so now.

The following recommendations are taken from an unpublished paper prepared by Major A. C. Fraser, BVSc, PhD, MRCVS, on the subject of examination of wind. He emphasises that, when examining a horse for wind, the object is to exert him, not to exhaust him.

1. With Thoroughbred horses in training the pace given should be a halfspeed canter over 3-4 furlongs, followed by a faster gallop over a distance agreed upon with the trainer.
2. Hacks, hunters and polo ponies should be tried more slowly over a longer distance.
3. Draught animals should be harnessed and driven uphill with a wheel locked.
4. Untrained animals or those too young or too small to be ridden may be lunged at this stage.

In summary, the animal should be given sufficient exercise to achieve the following objects: to make him breathe deeply and rapidly so that any abnormal breathing sounds may be heard; to cause his heart to beat strongly so that any abnormalities may be detected; and to tire him somewhat so that any strains or injuries may be revealed by stiffness or lameness after a period of rest.

The use of special techniques
Advances in veterinary science have led to the use of various techniques to extend the scope of the standard examination for purchase. Particularly,

radiographic examination of the lower limbs, fibre-optic endoscopic examination of the upper respiratory tract and blood sampling have become popular in cases of expensive racehorses, eventers and showjumpers. Rectal palpation and vaginal examination of the internal genital organs of fillies going to stud and bacterial cultures of the external genital organs of mares and stallions prior to purchase have become commonplace. Collection of semen samples for quality evaluation from stallions and colts out of training is sometimes required.

These techniques may be useful when correctly applied by a veterinarian and used in conjunction with his clinical examination. The danger of all such tests is that they become fashionable and may be requested by the purchaser without full appreciation of the limitations of the particular test. This can lead to problems of interpretation. Such extra tests should be performed whenever the examining veterinarian feels that they would be helpful, and the implications of the results of such tests should be discussed in advance with all parties. The permission of the vendor to carry these tests must be sought in advance.

Radiographs of a diagnostic quality need to be taken and interpreted by a veterinarian who is reasonably well versed in radiological interpretation.

The results of all radiographic examinations should be viewed in the light of the clinical and other findings. As part of a clinical investigation radiography is a precise procedure providing detailed information about an area to which attention has already been drawn.

In diagnostic work a lesion is likely to be found and each radiograph is inspected with this in mind. When several areas of a clinically normal horse are radiographed the veterinarian not only has to recognise any changes which are present but also has to assess their present and future significance in the absence of any clinical abnormality.

Reasons for radiography as part of an examination for a purchaser
There are three main reasons for radiography (almost invariably of the limbs):

1. The veterinarian may wish to radiograph a specific area of the horse because of observations made during the clinical examination. In this instance, radiography is performed as in any other clinical investigation and the problems which confront the veterinarian are no more than those of any other case of lameness. If confirmation of the clinical suspicion is obtained radiographically, an opinion can be given depending on the intended use of the horse.

2. The purchaser asks that radiographs should be taken of a clinically normal horse. It is under these circumstances that radiography is often used as a prognostic screening device. Such radiographs will occasionally be of assistance to show (or at least appear to show) that a lesion which

subsequently is diagnosed was not present at the time of examination. On balance, more problems will be caused for the veterinarian by the radiography of clinically normal horses than will be averted.

3. A third possible reason for radiography is at the request of a vendor who wishes, provided that the result is favourable, to be able to demonstrate the benign nature of an abnormality which might otherwise be a cause for concern. This course of action has become prevalent before the auction of expensive yearling thoroughbreds and is even more prevalent in the USA, where facilities to display the radiographs are incorporated. It is the responsibility of the purchaser's own veterinary adviser to view the radiographs and express his opinion accordingly. It has been strongly recommended that it is imprudent to provide both X-rays and an opinion on them on behalf of the vendor.

The examination itself should consist of producing an adequate number of technically adequate radiographs of the appropriate areas and presenting the facts in the form of a report. This report can then be incorporated into the general examination before an opinion on the horse is given. The requirement, as for a clinical examination, is simply that the veterinarian should exercise reasonable care in producing the radiographs and commenting on them.

The date of the examination should be marked on the film, together with a positive means of identification such as the name or brand mark, preferably not in code form.

The same caution must be extended to the use of endoscopy in the apparently normal horse, as the appearance of the larynx of the resting horse may be of little value as to the extent of the airway when the animal is making an extreme respiratory effort. Endoscopy is of considerable use in the evaluation of the cause of suspicious respiratory noises but is of little value in forecasting the athletic potential of the horse.

Particularly where the vendor of the horse is not known to the examining veterinary surgeon, it is prudent to collect a blood sample, which may be examined for the evidence of anti-inflammatory medication. This sample may be either evaluated straight away or may be retained for examination at a later date if there are grounds for suspicion that such medication had been administered.

52

THE LEGAL IMPLICATIONS OF THE PURCHASE OF A HORSE

Introduction

Each time a horse is bought and sold, a contract has been entered into and concluded. It is a common misconception that because nothing has been committed to writing there is no contract. An oral contract is every bit as legal and binding as one which is in writing. Where nothing is in writing – as with most horse sales not at public auction – the ever-present problem is knowing what the terms of the contract are. This is why so many disputes revolve around oral contracts.

By the same token, when a horse is vetted pre-purchase there is a contract between the vet and the person on whose behalf the vetting is undertaken. Where a vet provides a vetting on behalf of a seller, he may incur further liability – to both buyer and seller.

In this chapter we aim to highlight the most common problems, and give some practical advice on the legal implications of buying and selling horses. The majority of problems arise from the lack of committing things to writing, but still most horses are sold – and contracts made – without any written terms. It is important to remember that the law sees a horse in the same way as (say) a car or any other item of goods being bought or sold.

If terms are expressed and confirmed by way of (say) a receipt or warranty, there will be far fewer arguments between buyer and seller. It can be a big help if the buyer simply considers the things which are important to them, writes them down, and asks the seller to consider them on a 'questionnaire' basis. This is no guarantee of satisfaction but will certainly help in the event of a dispute.

In this chapter we will look at the law which applies to sales of horse the important questions to ask; the types of things which commonly go wrong; the remedies available to unhappy buyers; and finally, areas where potential claims against sellers can go awry.

As a buyer, who am I buying from?

This is the most important question to consider, as the answer will govern the rights and remedies the dissatisfied buyer has. Although a private sale from a friend or acquaintance is widely regarded as the most reliable method of purchase, in terms of the comeback the unhappy buyer has his or her protection is limited.

Buying from a private seller

The principal rule in the case of a private sale is *caveat emptor* ('buyer beware'). In the same way as for any private individual buying or selling a car there are (unless expressed in words or writing) no warranties or terms as to quality which apply to a private sale. What this means in practice is asking lots of questions about a prospective purchase.

In other words, if the horse goes lame the day after you bought it and the seller did not make any representations as to its quality, you may have no comeback at all. A representation is something that the buyer (or the buyer's agent) has said about the horse – remember that this may appear in any advertisement for sale.

Examples of representations that the seller might make are:

- Good to box, shoe etc
- Sound in wind and limb
- Novice ride
- Vice free
- (a particular height, age, etc)

The requirements of a misrepresentation claim are: (i) a representation; (ii) reliance on the representation when buyer enters into the contract; and (iii) the representation is false.

If this happens the buyer has the right to reject the horse and claim his or her money back.

So, the animal sold as a 12.2hh first ridden pony, good to box, shoe, etc, suitable for novice rider and vice free' should be just that. If, on the other hand, the seller says nothing about the horse or pony's characteristics and it turns out not as expected, in most cases the buyer will have no comeback because of the important maxim *'caveat emptor'*.

A seller may claim that a buyer would have bought the horse anyway, regardless of any misrepresentation. In that case a claim will not succeed, because it will not be possible to prove that the buyer relied on the (mis) representation in entering into the contract.

It is vital to remember when buying horses that they are not machines. Their behaviour can be very quickly altered by their environment, riders and handlers. The novice ride in the hands of a competent, confident rider can behave quite differently in the hands of an inexperienced rider. When considering a new, unhappy or unsatisfactory partnership this important element should not be disregarded.

Buying from a seller 'selling in the course of a business'
It can be difficult to pinpoint when a seller is 'selling in the course of a business', but it makes a vital difference to the treatment the disappointed seller gets at the hands of the law. This provision applies to horse dealers – many studs who sell some of the progeny of their mares – and some riding schools. It puts the disappointed buyer in a rather better position than in a private sale.

When a seller sells in the course of a business the following terms are implied into the contract:
- The item sold must be fit for the purpose for which it was intended, provided that purpose was made known to the seller;
- The item sold must comply with any description applied to it;
- It must be of 'satisfactory quality';
- The sale must be in accordance with industry custom and practice.

These terms are implied into contracts made by sellers in the course of business, and come from the Sale of Goods legislation, most recently updated in 1994.

The 'satisfactory quality' implied term is subject to two provisos, that there is no breach of the condition in regard to: a defect which is specifically drawn to the buyer's attention prior to purchase; or defects which, if the buyer examines the horse prior to the purchase being made, that examination ought to reveal.

The subtle difference between this part of the law and that which applies to misrepresentation is that no actual representations have to be made for these implied terms to apply.

So if the horse is unsound shortly after purchase, it is likely that the unhappy buyer will have the right to return it on the basis that it was: not of satisfactory quality; and is not fit for the purpose for which it was intended (subject as above).

In respect of a Sale of Goods Act claim, the buyer has a right to reject the horse and claim back the purchase price and associated costs in full. Alternatively he or she may choose not to reject the horse, but claim back the difference in value between the animal that he or she contracted to buy and the animal purchased.

Potential claims regarding horses found to be unsound shortly after sale are (as a rule) more straightforward than horses who are unsuitable because they have behavioural problems. This is where subjective elements intervene – like the animal's stabling arrangements; where it is being asked to go or do and by whom, and the reasonableness of the request given the animal's age and experience.

It is possible to make out a claim on the basis that a horse is (say) not suitable for a novice rider, but the buyer will need expert evidence as to the horse's behavioural problem; and factual evidence as to what the buyer told the seller he or she wanted the horse for. At this stage of a potential claim it can be found that the buyer's expectations were unrealistic.

Sale of Goods Act claims are subject to the same provisos (below) about the timescale for returning the horse.

A final word in this section about Trading Standards, who are entitled to investigate and prosecute anyone falsely advertising good for sale in the course of a business. The dissatisfied buyer may find that they are prepared to help his cause against the seller, although they will not be able to unravel any civil claim.

Buyer at public auction

Where a buyer buys at public auction, the terms on which he buys are the sales company's terms of business which usually appear at the front of the sales catalogue. They usually make specific provisions for the seller of the horse to give warranties (e.g as to soundness, height etc) and also provide for when horses are returnable because of vices like windsucking, box walking and cribbing.

When there is a problem with a horse bought at public auction, the terms and conditions are the first port of call for disappointed buyers. Remember that most of the conditions will contain deadlines about when the sales company must be notified and how long the horse must be allowed to settle in. Deadlines can be particularly stringent so the terms and conditions should be picked up at the earliest possible opportunity. It is also very likely that veterinary evidence will be required, so the unhappy purchaser will need to make sure that the vet sees the horse within the relevant period.

What is a Vice?

A vice has been defined by the Courts as 'either a defect in temperament which makes the horse dangerous or diminishes its usefulness, or a bad habit which is injurious to its health' (Scholefield v Robb, 1839).

In fact, that definition is of only limited value in working out which of many habits horses have (most of which are dangerous and/or injurious to their health) can properly be called a vice.

In the view of the author, crib-biting, windsucking, weaving and box walking can properly be called vices. These are the stable vices which make horses returnable at most reputable horse sales, and the ones which most people regard as properly declarable at the time of sale.

The question of whether biting, kicking, rearing, bucking and napping are vices is moot – still more so those horses with headshaking syndrome or cold backs – none of which, the author believes, can truly be described as vices.

What is Unsoundness?

Soundness has been defined by the Courts as:

'the absence of any disease or seeds of disease in the animal at the time of sale which actually diminishes or, in its progress, would diminish its usefulness.' (Riddell v Burnard, 1847)

In fact this is rather a stringent test which has since been judicially criticised and is, in the author's view, too extreme. What about the horse with degenerative arthritis in its hocks, which only reveals itself two months after purchase? It more than likely fails the 'seeds of disease' test, and yet the seller would have no way of knowing that the problem existed.

Soundness is not an easy concept to grasp, and many clumsy attempts by the Courts at definition have led well advised vets to shy away from the word, with good reason.

In fact the definition of soundness lies within the remit of the vets, and not the lawyers, because every such case will require veterinary evidence to support it.

When can I reject a horse?

The legal answer to this question is: as early as possible. Many futile attempts are made to 'sort out' horses which are found to be badly behaved with their new owner, but these invariably end in disaster with the seller refusing to accept the horse back because it has 'been ruined'.

Of course, horses who occasionally weave or windsuck may settle down after a few days in their new box, but as a general rule if the buyer is unhappy with his or her purchase he should try to return it as early as possible – ideally within a week, but certainly no later than six weeks, depending on the nature of the problem.

So much can go wrong so quickly with horses that it pays to be ultra-cautious. These deadlines are not written into the law (although arguments about 'deemed acceptance' of a horse are common) but have proved a reliable rule of thumb in many claims, and are intended to be of assistance.

Common problems with horse sales

Stable vices are common, as are badly behaved horses or horses who are not suitable for their new owners, and lame or otherwise afflicted animals.

Less common – and more difficult to advise on – are headshakers (whose behaviour is changed according to the season, and who are often sold in winter); mares who turn out to be in foal; or rigs/crypt-orchids. In these cases the advice to be given to the disappointed buyer often depends very much on the facts of the particular case.

Evidence

It will bolster a case enormously to have the right evidence at the right time. Photographs and/or video evidence of the horse doing the thing complained of; or veterinary evidence at the relevant time showing the horse to be lame can be a great help in allowing the potential claimant to set out his or her case to its best advantage. This is something which should be considered at the earliest possible opportunity

Pre-purchase vettings

Every prudent purchaser should have their proposed purchase vetted prior to purchase. This will usually be in the form of the accepted Five Stage Vetting, which is covered in detail in chapter 51. This is a very specific form of Certificate which sets out exactly what examinations the vet has carried out.

It is generally carried out on behalf of the purchaser because (i) only the purchaser knows what they want to use the horse for; and (ii) the examining vet can incur liability to both buyer and seller on the same Certificate if he examines on behalf of the seller rather than only the buyer.

Considering the number of dissatisfied purchasers, vets can count themselves lucky that relatively few of these claims come to their door.

The reasons for this are twofold:
1. The liability of vets on the Five Stage Vetting Certificate is strictly limited. This is a good example of one of the contracting parties setting out his or her part of the bargain clearly and in writing. For example the Certificate will not guarantee freedom from vice.
2. A vet can be wrong and not negligent – and negligent is what he needs to be to found a claim against him.

Veterinary negligence

The legal test for veterinary negligence is the same as for negligence in any other profession. That the professional must do his job using reasonable care and skill to the standard of any competent veterinarian with any particular knowledge and expertise he in fact has. If he falls below that standard he may be negligent.

In effect, the standards are set by the veterinarian's own profession. In order to make out a negligence claim against a vet the prospective claimant will need a report from a fellow vet setting out the ways in which, in his view, the Defendant vet has failed in his duty to his client. This vet may well be expected to give expert evidence at trial.

In the context of the usual pre-purchase examinations the scenarios are usually either:
1. The vet fails to see spot some defect which exists and is apparent at the time of the examination, and any competent veterinarian should have detected. In this case the vet is unlikely to have any defence to the action against him. The Claimant's claim is likely to include the cost of the horse (less any residual or salvage value); wasted veterinary and livery expenses and any extra expenses, such as transport.
2. More interesting is the situation where the buyer complains of a defect which the examining vet claims was not evident at the time of examination, but which may have developed subsequently. Issues like this have to be decided by the Judge as a question of fact based on the evidence available as to where and in what circumstances the problem became

apparent; and on expert evidence as to the way in which, and speed at which, the defect might have developed.

Other golden rules for buyers are:

* Where you are unable to use your own vet, choose your own – do not rely on the seller;
* Make a written note of what, if any, further examinations you have asked to be carried out – and provide it to the vet. This may include endoscopic examination, radiographs, or more routinely, taking blood.
* Always ensure you have the veterinary Certificate duly completed and provided to you before you buy.

Conclusions

The sale and purchase of horses often involves entering contracts whether written or not. The Five Stage Veterinary Examination Certificate is the perfect example of one party to the contract ensuring that his or her side of the bargain is clearly set out. There is no reason why the prospective horse buyer should not employ that principle in the same way.

If there is anything which is particularly important to the potential buyer which the horse should or should not do, or be able to do – like loading or being ridden in traffic – the potential buyer should make careful enquiries of the would-be seller to ensure that his expectations will be fulfilled.

This very process often helps the buyer to address issues which may cause him problems further down the line. It is better if those requirements can be committed to writing in questionnaire form, and (best of all) completed and signed up to by the seller.

53
VETERINARY NURSES IN EQUINE PRACTICE

A person wishing to specialise in working with horses will find a variety of options open to them. Riding schools, local colleges, equine products merchants, veterinary practices and professional training yards all employ people with some experience of handling horses to assist in their day to day running. The work is often hard, tiring, dirty and outdoors; working weekends are common, as horses need looking after seven days a week.

For those interested in the medical aspect of equine care, larger specialist veterinary practices employ and train veterinary nurses. As with any reputable profession, there is a single body for training, assessment and certification of qualified veterinary nurses, which also maintains a membership list. This body is the Royal College of Veterinary Surgeons (RCVS) and the qualification is the Veterinary Nursing Certificate. Only listed veterinary nurses may carry out procedures on animals as declared in Schedule 3 of the Veterinary Surgeons Act 1966.

The RCVS works closely with the British Veterinary Nursing Association (BVNA) in the recruitment of student veterinary nurses and the running of the training scheme. The nurse is trained to a standard that enables them to assist and carry out specialised nursing procedures and assist veterinary surgeons with greater competence and less instruction than untrained staff.

Veterinary Nurse Training
Veterinary nurse training takes place over a minimum of two years. Most students complete their training whilst employed at a veterinary practice that is an RCVS Approved Training and Assessment Centre (ATAC). They must be a minimum of 17 years old.

Veterinary nursing courses are available at a number of colleges of higher education and agricultural colleges. These colleges offer diverse options for the student nurse as they can be run as day-release or full-time residential programmes. They are designed to enhance the practical training that is gained at the veterinary practice.

Entry requirements must be met before an application to the RCVS is made. Passes in five different subject at Grades A, B or C of the General Certificate of Secondary Education (GCSE) shall include a pass in English Language and a pass in either a physical or biological science or in mathematics. Appropriate passes in examinations of a higher or comparable standard may be accepted with approval of the RCVS veterinary nursing committee. Two examinations must be passed prior to qualifying as a Veterinary Nurse (VN). These include written and practical examinations plus submission of work based assessment in the form of a portfolio. Also implemented in 1998 was the first honours degree course in veterinary nursing. It is predicted that other universities and colleges will offer full-time degree courses in the future that incorporate the veterinary nursing certificate.

The Certificate in Equine Veterinary Nursing is a new qualification, which commenced with a pilot study in 1999. This is available initially to qualified veterinary nurses who have at least one year full-time experience in equine practice. The pilot study takes one year to complete for which the student must continue to be employed in equine practice. This course is being run in conjunction with the British Equine Veterinary Association (BEVA).

A two year equine veterinary nurse training course is planned for the future. This will not require veterinary nurse qualification prior to enrolment for those who prefer to work with horses and not small animals. This alternative training course will not be available until after 2002.

Throughout each year many specialist equine practices, universities and BEVA run weekend teaching courses for VNs and auxiliary staff who work in equine practice. They are designed to expose delegates to a wider range of techniques and knowledge than they may experience in their own work. A significant amount of time is devoted to practical training, as this is an area important to the nurse's role in practice. The RCVS encourages qualified VNs to update their skills and knowledge with Continuing Professional Development (CPD).

General Nursing Responsibilities

The equine veterinary nurse is a vital part of the team that provides quality care to patients. This enables the veterinary practice to provide a professional, profitable and efficient service to its clients – crucial for the Practice's reputation.

A regular daily routine should be implemented that provides the nurse with a clear understanding of their role. This is often documented and used as a training aid in the form of 'Standard Operating Procedures'. Nurses are often the first person that a client comes in contact with when a patient is admitted to a hospital. An efficient, understanding and polite manner must be maintained at all times. Especially important is the ability to give sound advice that may have to be delivered over the telephone. A nurse could be expected to give advice on general matters such as feed management, post operative patient and wound care, routine worming and vaccination regime.

When dealing with the equine patient, a nurse must demonstrate confidence and competence in handling, restraint and treatment as the hospitalised horse can be fractious and unpredictable. Economics play a large part in the horse industry and a nurse must be aware that inappropriate advice or poor treatment techniques, such as an improperly applied bandage, could incapacitate a horse and prevent its speedy recovery and return to work.

Patient care
Direct veterinary care of a horse often means working outside normal daylight hours to closely monitor the patient. The occasional sleepless night can be surprisingly rewarding, however, when the patient survives a life-threatening crisis and is on the way to a full recovery. The nurse must be familiar with the normal vital signs of the horse and able to detect subtle changes in its condition. For those who are involved in critical care nursing, disease processes, fluid therapy, haematological/blood biochemistry imbalances and possible complications must be thoroughly understood. Keeping accurate, clear and concise clinical notes is essential in documenting the patient's progress. This combined with a well trained and caring nursing staff is vital in providing the horse and its owner the comfort and assurance they need that the best in care is given.

Diagnostic Techniques
As technological advances impact the veterinary profession, the need for knowledgeable and capable nursing staff to assist in various diagnostic techniques is fundamental. Radiography is essential in aiding the diagnosis of many orthopaedic conditions. As a routine part of most equine practices, the nurse must be particularly aware of the potential risks of ionising radiation. All staff involved are required to wear protective lead gowns, gloves and radiation detection badges. The nurse is usually responsible for ensuring that the standard rules of radiation safety are followed and that doses to those involved are monitored frequently. This is especially true as a horizontal X-ray beam is frequently used, with higher exposure factors than when radiographing small animals, combined with the added unpredictable nature of the horse, increases the risk of exposure to radiation and the need for a professional approach.

The Health and Safety Commission updates the publication 'Working with Ionising Radiation' periodically. This Approved Code of Practice and Guidance (ACOP) should be made available to all staff involved in the radiology of horses. The nurse should be familiar with the relevant regulations and must enforce the rules that are made to safeguard personal safety.

The proficient veterinary nurse will often position the horse and take radiographs for the veterinary surgeon. They must also be competent in developing the films as more errors can occur in the darkroom than whilst taking the radiographs themselves.

The principles of ultrasonography are now widely implemented in equine practice. Both linear and sector scanners are used in orthopaedics, reproduction, medicine, cardiology and surgery. A nurse assisting in this diagnostic technique should be proficient in the patient preparation for an ultrasonographic examination and able to understand how a scanner works. Maintenance of expensive equipment, like an ultrasound scanner, is often left to a nurse and requires care with its delicate components.

The Operating Theatre and Surgical Nursing
When a horse enters an operating theatre a different set of rules must be followed, known as 'sterile technique', to minimise the risk of infection. It is imperative that the theatre nurse is proficient with positioning of the patient, care and maintenance of instrumentation and anaesthetic equipment, sterile technique, and has a good understanding of the surgical procedure. Stock control of all disposable goods and monitoring of sterile packs is just a small part of what is required in managing an operating theatre. It requires a person with a meticulous nature to ensure the smooth running of the daily surgical list. A catastrophe would occur if when the patient was anaesthetised, a vital piece of surgical equipment was found to be non-functional. Most importantly, the theatre nurse is part of a team that must work fast and efficiently to ensure everything is prepared for the next surgical patient as it may require life-threatening emergency surgery.

Anaesthesia
It is important that the veterinary nurse understands the actions of the drugs and volatile agents that are used in an equine general anaesthetic. There are numerous risks to the equine patient (more so than many other species) and the procedure requires careful monitoring from start to finish. All staff involved should be sufficiently trained to assist in resuscitation techniques which, while infrequently used, are vital in treating life threatening respiratory and cardiac arrests.

It is more than likely that the veterinary nurse will be responsible for the upkeep of the anaesthetic machines, monitoring devices and drug stocks. As with surgical instrumentation, all equipment used in association with equine general anaesthesia must be functional and ready for use at short notice.

Medical Nursing
Not all illnesses can be resolved by surgery. Horses with some diseases can require intensive care medical treatment, which may involve a long period of time commitment from the nursing team. As with surgical cases, an understanding of disease processes and their forms of treatments is an important aspect of medical nursing. The care of wounds, changing of dressings,

monitoring intravenous catheters and checking vital signs is just a small part of what is expected from a well trained veterinary nurse. It is important to communicate with the clients to be able to differentiate between a patient's normal behaviour patterns and those of a sick horse. Working closely with a veterinary surgeon enables the nurse to relay information on the subtle changes of their patient which may affect the diagnosis and subsequently the way the horse receives treatment. An enormous amount of responsibility rests with the veterinary nurse when caring for numerous patients at once; common sense and a level head must prevail to maintain the same standards of care for all.

A Personal Note
This overview of the duties and responsibilities carried by the equine veterinary nurses could appear daunting. Veterinary nursing should be considered a profession of which the committed can be proud. In common with most professions, job satisfaction is a key reward element and a prospective nurse should examine their motivation for embarking on a career as a Veterinary Nurse. The training and opportunities exist for the interested person to make a real contribution to the well being of their patients in a profession that is changing and developing.

The following organisations can be contacted for more information or to answer specific questions about the veterinary nursing profession:

British Veterinary Nursing Association
Level 15
Terminus House
Terminus Street
Harlow
Essex CM20 1XA

The Royal College of Veterinary Surgeons
Belgravia House
62-64 Horseferry Road
London SW1P 2AF

Tel: 01279 450567
E-mail: bvna@bvna.co.uk
Website: www.bvna.org.uk

Tel: 020 7222 2001
E-mail: vetnursing@rcvs.org.uk
Website: www.rcvs.org.uk

For more information about health and safety and work practices contact the Health & Safety Executive: The HSE InfoLine Tel: 08701 545500

or write to:

HSE Information Centre
Broad Lane
Sheffield S3 7HQ

Website: www.hse.gov.uk

THE EXAMINATION OF THE HORSE'S MOUTH FOR AGE

The horse's life expectancy

It cannot be stated with any degree of accuracy to what age a horse would live if not subjected to domestication. However, a horse is generally considered to have reached old age at seventeen. Changes in their teeth, such as the wearing away of the molars, appear to prevent many of them from reaching a ripe old age. Instances are on record of horses attaining the age of thirty-five or fifty, and one animal is known to have lived to sixty-three years of age. Bracy Clark (1771-1860), a well-known veterinary surgeon in practice in London, knew a hunter of fifty-two years of age. Youatt (1776-1847), another veterinary surgeon with a high reputation and also in practice in London, knew an owner who had three horses which died at the ages of thirty-five, thirty-seven and thirty-nine; and a colleague of his knew one that received a ball in his neck at the Battle of Preston in 1715, which was extracted at his death in 175 8. Another well-known veterinary surgeon of this period, Percivall, gives an account of a barge horse that died in its sixty-second year. The age at death of some famous racehorses is cited by F. Smith in his *Veterinary Physiology*:

Eclipse	26 years	Ladas	23 years
Touchstone	30 years	Collar	19 years
St Simon	27 years	Pocahontas	33 years
Marcion	23 years	Melton	29 years
Cherry Tree	26 years	Bend Or	26 years
Parrot	36 years	Queen's Birthday	26 years
Hermit	29 years	William III	19 years
King Tom	27 years		

Blaine (1770-1845) in *Outlines of the Veterinary Art* appears to have gone very carefully into the question of old age in horses and he drew the following comparison, which is doubtless very close to the truth:

The first 5 years of a horse may be considered as equivalent to the first 20 years of a man. Thus a horse of 5 years may be comparatively considered as old as a man of 20; a horse of 10 years as a man of 40; a horse of 15 years as a man of 50; a horse of 20 as a man of 60; of 25 as a man of 70; of 30 as a man of 80; and of 35 as a man of 90.

The indications of advanced age in horses are well marked, apart from those connected with the length, shape and colour of the teeth: the edge of the lower jaw becomes sharp, there is a deepening of the hollows over the eyes (supraorbital fossae), and the eyelids become wrinkled. Grey hairs may appear on the face, particularly over the eyes and about the muzzle, and elsewhere, while black horses may turn 'white', although this is unusual. There is a thinness and a hanging down of the lips, a sharpness over the withers, a sinking of the back – a hollowed back is very greatly intensified with age. The joints of the limbs show the effects of work, and the gait loses its elasticity. In Thoroughbred stallions and mares the mean age of death is a little under twenty years. An interesting fact is that horses seldom die quietly.

The teeth

Parts of a tooth A tooth is made up of two parts, one of which is firmly implanted in the socket (alveolus) in the bone which carries it; this part is called the root. The other portion is exposed and its base is surrounded by the gum. The surface of this portion, which is subjected to wear on account of the friction during mastication, is called the table of the crown. The constricted portion of the tooth which separates these two parts is the neck. The extremity of the tooth shows a small perforation opening into a cavity which extends for some distance up the middle of the tooth. This is the pulp cavity.

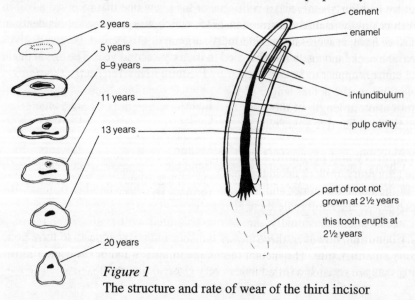

Figure 1
The structure and rate of wear of the third incisor

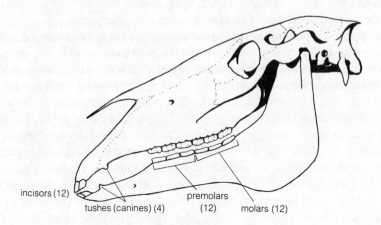

incisors (12)

tushes (canines) (4)

premolars (12)

molars (12)

Figure 2a
A section of the skull showing the location of the teeth in a normal mouth

Three substances enter into the composition of all teeth, namely dentine, enamel and cement. Dentine is the yellowish-white, bone-like material which makes up the greater part of the tooth, and surrounds the pulp cavity. Enamel is the shiny white layer which extends over the exposed portion of tooth, and which is seated upon the underlying dentine. Cement is simply connective tissue converted into bone; it is spread over parts of the exterior of the tooth.

A peculiar feature of the teeth is that as the table of the tooth becomes worn out by friction, the alveolar cavity becomes gradually filled up, so that the tooth is slowly pushed out from its socket. This goes on throughout life, and thus we have, at successive periods of the animal's existence, at first the crown, next the neck, and lastly the root actually in wear. Although in an aged animal the incisors appear to be very long owing to the increase in length of their visible portion, the actual length of the tooth has diminished on account of the diminution in length of the root. The maximum length is attained when the animal is about five years old.

Temporary and permanent teeth Two sets of teeth are developed, namely the temporary, milk or deciduous teeth, and the permanent or persistent teeth.

In the horse the upper and lower jaws carry the same number of teeth. In each jaw of the adult male there are twelve molars, six incisors, two canines or tushes and, occasionally, one or two so-called wolf teeth. In the temporary dentition, however, there are six incisors and only six molars – the first three on either side. The incisor teeth are situated in front; the canine teeth or tushes are situated a little farther back, interrupting the space between the incisors and the premolar or cheek teeth. Canines are usually present only in the male, though small rudimentary ones are quite common in the female, and appear at three-and-a-half to four years; they are fully developed at four-and-a-half to five years. They are absent in a two-year-old. The premolar and molar teeth form the sides of the dental arch and are commonly referred to as the cheek teeth.

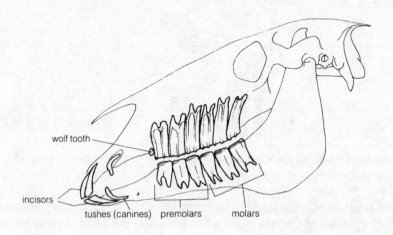

Figure 2b A section of the skull showing the roots of the teeth

Incisors These are in three pairs, termed respectively the centrals, laterals and corners. They are named incisors because they are adapted for cutting. Each is made up of a crown, which is depressed from front to back, and a root, the upper portion of which is somewhat three-sided. A little lower down the root becomes circular, while near the apex it is in the form of an ellipse, the long axis of which lies in an antero-posterior direction. These differences in the shape of the tooth are used as an indication of the age of the animal, because the outline of the free wearing surface will vary according to the part of the tooth which is in use. The table of the crown presents a marked depression called the infundibulum. This was formerly used as an indication of the animal's age, since its gradual disappearance was supposed to occur at a definite rate during the life of the animal. This theory is negated by the fact that considerable variations are met with in the depth of the cavity. The enamel covers the exposed portion of the incisor and also in part the root. It also dips into and lines the infundibulum. Thus when the table has been slightly worn, two rings of enamel are visible on its surface, namely an outer ring by which the whole surface is surrounded and an inner ring surrounding the infundibulum. The cement is deposited in a layer, which presents considerable variations in thickness over the enamel.

Temporary or milk incisors are much smaller and whiter than permanent incisors. They possess a well-defined neck, the anterior part of the crown presents a faint striation and the infundibulum is present at first, but it is very shallow and, as a result, soon disappears as the tooth is worn.

Permanent incisors, on the other hand, are much larger, and on the anterior surface of the crown there is present a well-marked vertical groove.

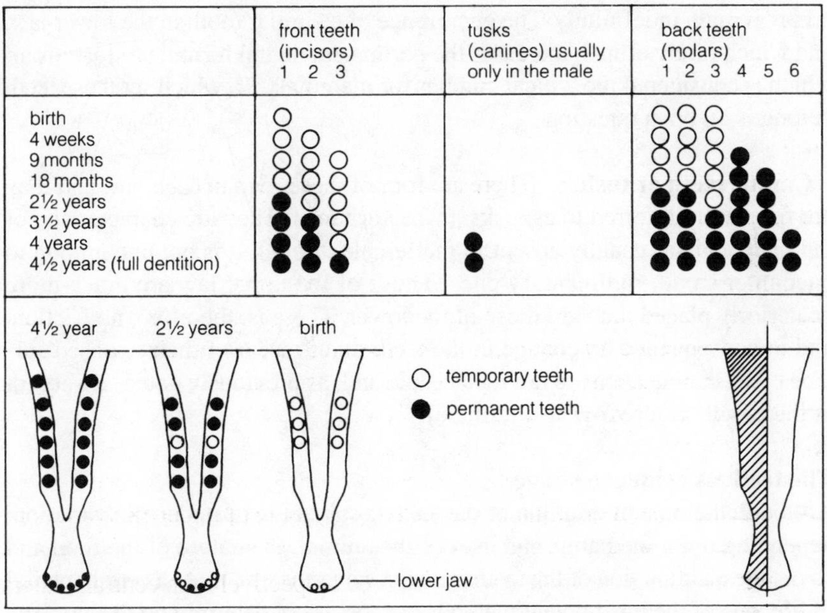
front teeth
(incisors)
1 2 3
tusks
(canines) usually
only in the male
back teeth
(molars)
1 2 3 4 5 6
birth
4 weeks
9 months
18 months
2½ years
3½ years
4 years
4½ years (full dentition)
4½ year
2½ years
birth
temporary teeth
permanent teeth
lower jaw

Figure 3 Teeth eruption on one branch of jaw (lower) i.e. x 4

The tooth tapers gradually from the crown to the root, so that there is no well-defined constriction or neck. The infundibulum is wide and deep, and surrounded by a fairly thick layer of enamel.

Molars In the permanent dentition there are twelve of these in each law, six on either side. The two rows in the upper jaw are more widely separated from one another then are those in the lower. Moreover, the tabular surfaces of the former are directed obliquely downwards and outwards, while those of the latter take an oblique direction which is upwards and inwards. The inner edge of the lower molars is therefore higher than the outer, and the outer edge of the upper molars extends to a much lower level than the inner edge. The roots of some of the molars project into the maxillary sinuses where they are covered by a thin layer of bone. Hence, when diseased and removal is necessary, trephining of the sinus has to be carried out.

Wolf teeth Four teeth are frequently present which are placed one in front of each first molar. These are the wolf teeth. Their exposed portion presents considerable variation in shape: usually they are somewhat tubercular but occasionally one is observed with a crown which resembles a small molar. They are interesting as being the remnants of teeth which were well developed in the eocene ancestors of the horse. A wolf tooth may erupt during the first six months, and is often shed about the same time as the milk tooth behind it, but it may remain indefinitely. The occurrence of a similar tooth in the lower jaw, and which rarely erupts, increases the permanent dental formula to forty-four, which is considered the typical number for mammals. To which set these teeth belong is an open question.

Canine teeth or tushes There are four of these, two in each jaw, and they are frequently referred to as tusks, tushes or fangs. They are characteristic of the male and are usually absent in the female, though it is not uncommon to encounter small, rudimentary ones. Those of the upper law are much more posteriorly placed than are those of the lower. There is, therefore, no friction, and in consequence no change in the teeth due to wear of their exposed surfaces. The canine teeth are not replaceable and, as previously noted, are absent in the mouth of a two-year-old (male).

The teeth as evidence of age
Although the time of eruption of the teeth is subject to considerable variation, depending upon the habits and uses of the animal, the nature of the food and so on, the examination of the teeth remains, nevertheless, up to a certain period of life, one of the most potent methods we possess of determining the age. The times given below are of course only approximate, but they may be reasonably accepted as being the most constant:

At birth Two central incisors. These may not appear until the seventh or tenth day. Three cheek teeth are present.

At 4-6 weeks The lateral incisors.
At 6-9 months The corner incisors.

Figure 4 Teeth at 1 month

Figure 5 Teeth at 6 weeks

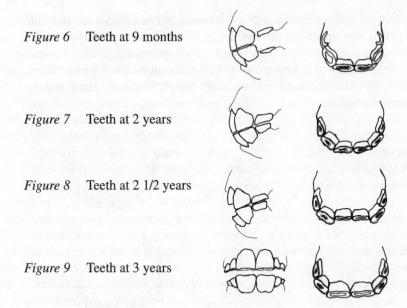

Figure 6   Teeth at 9 months

Figure 7   Teeth at 2 years

Figure 8   Teeth at 2 1/2 years

Figure 9   Teeth at 3 years

At 1 year   All six temporary incisors are present, and four cheek teeth: the three premolars and the first permanent molar. The latter has made its appearance through the gum, but is not so well developed as the other three.

At 2 years   The animal's mouth may present some little difficulty. The incisors are showing signs of wear. The cup-like cavities on their tables have disappeared and the tables themselves are flat and present a faint striation. It is most important to be on one's guard in distinguishing between these and permanent incisors. At this age the molars form the better guide, for an additional permanent molar has made its appearance, so that we now have five present, three of which are temporary and two permanent. In his book *The Examination of Animals for Soundness* R. H. Smythe, MRCVS, states:

> The tail of a 2-year-old is usually shorter than that of a 5-year-old, reaching to just above or level with the hocks. In a 5-year-old it usually reaches to well below the hocks. Even this is a variable feature, and in any case, tails may be pulled or trimmed. Tail length is often a useful guide in moorland ponies running out. Tails are apt to grow faster with good feeding and housing. Tushes or canine teeth in the case of the male will be absent in a 2-year-old but fully developed in a 5-year-old.

At 2 years 6 months   The central temporary incisors are cast and the first pair of permanent incisors burst through the gums.

At 3 years   The two permanent central incisors are up and in wear. The first and second (in position counting from the front, but numbers three and four in age) permanent molars cut through the gums, pushing before them the first and second temporary teeth beneath which they have erupted. These of course are not yet the height of numbers four and five. The supplementary molars, or wolf teeth, are most frequently cast simultaneously with the shedding of these two temporary molars.

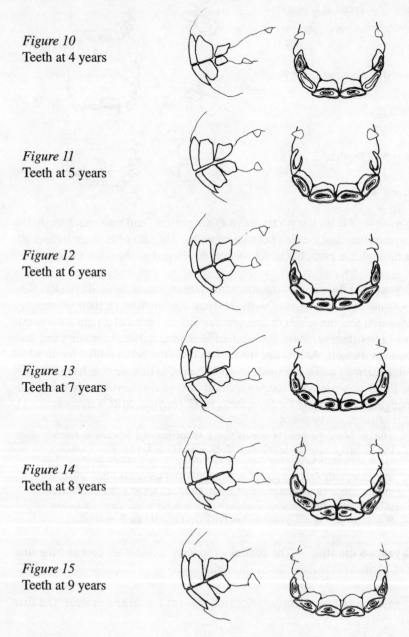

Figure 10
Teeth at 4 years

Figure 11
Teeth at 5 years

Figure 12
Teeth at 6 years

Figure 13
Teeth at 7 years

Figure 14
Teeth at 8 years

Figure 15
Teeth at 9 years

At 3 years 6 months The second pair of permanent incisors (the laterals) appear through the gums and are on a level with those of the first permanent pair when the horse attains the age of four years.

At 4 years 6 months The corner permanent incisors are cut, and when these teeth are well up and the inner and outer edges of their tables are level, the horse is five years old. The last two permanent molars (numbers 3 and 6 in position) in each jaw are cut between the ages of four and five.

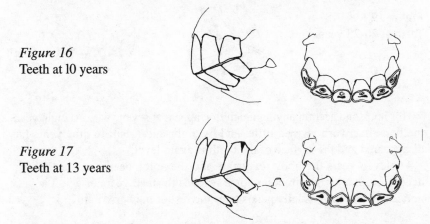

Figure 16
Teeth at 10 years

Figure 17
Teeth at 13 years

At 6 years The corner incisors are exhibiting evidence of wear. The infundibula of the two lateral incisors may have entirely disappeared. This disappearance was formerly regarded as constant at this age, but, for the reasons which have previously been stated, such is not the case and some trace of them is frequently found to remain, although the depressions are much shallower than those in the lateral, or corner, incisors. At this age, in addition, a new feature presents itself on the tabular surface of the central incisors in the form of a blackish or brownish line which runs transversely between the disappearing infundibulum and the anterior edge of the tooth. This is the first appearance of what is known as the dental star, and it indicates the fact that so much of the tooth has been worn away as to bring the upper extremity of the pulp cavity filled with dentine into appearance on the table.

At 7 years The infundibula have disappeared from the central and lateral incisors. The dental star is much better marked in the centrals, and at eight there should be no difficulty in seeing it. At the age of seven a useful guide is furnished by the top corner incisor tooth which does not wear evenly throughout its length, and as a result a projection or hook (sometimes called a dovetail) develops at its posterior edge. As the tooth wears from front to back without reducing the length of the hook, one gets the impression that the tooth carries a projection downwards from its rear edge.

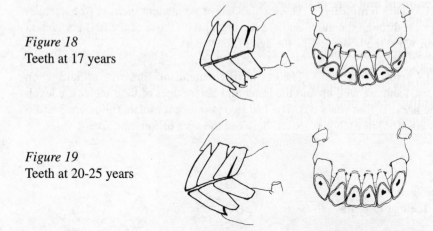

Figure 18
Teeth at 17 years

Figure 19
Teeth at 20-25 years

This hook and accompanying notch first appear at seven years. At eight years the hook has worn away a little, and by eight-and-a-half to nine years has disappeared and the surface of the tooth is again level.

At eleven years the hook reappears and the notch becomes successively deeper, so that by the time the horse reaches thirteen years of age it is very noticeable and then usually persists for the rest of the horse's life.

From 8 years onwards Very little definite evidence can be obtained, but there are a number of changes which assist in arriving at an approximate estimate. At eight the infundibulum has disappeared from all the incisors, and the dental star is clearly appareni in the central incisors. At nine years it appears in the laterals, and at ten to twelve it is present in all the incisors. Attention should also be directed to the shape of the tables, which varies from oval to triangular and then to round as the horse becomes older. In horses up to seven years they are oval, from nine to thirteen triangular, and after thirteen years rounded with a central pulp mark. Once again, the upper corner incisor tooth comes to our assistance by the appearance of a wellmarked longitudinal groove, which first appears as a notch at the outer side of each upper corner tooth just below the gum. As the horse ages, it travels down the tooth as a narrow longitudinal furrow, which is sometimes discoloured (yellow or brown). This is the so-called Galvayne's groove after the well-known horse expert who first drew attention to it, and who is the author of *The Twentieth-Century Book of the Horse*.

This groove makes its appearance at ten years, but quite often its faint commencement can be seen on close inspection at nine years. When it reaches halfway down the tooth the horse is regarded as a fifteen-year-old, and when it has reached the bottom of the tooth, twenty years old. At twenty-five years it has disappeared from the upper half of the tooth, and at thirty years it has disappeared completely.

Treatment and care of the horse's teeth

Regular attention to a horse's mouth ensures healthy teeth and gums, normal mastication, which is essential for good digestion and the assimilation of food, and a responsive mouth. A horse which has difficulty in chewing, drinking or swallowing may be experiencing problems with its teeth. Other signs of dental problems are quidding or the dropping of food, the drooling of saliva, loss of condition, and oral or facial pain, which may be accompanied by facial swelling and frequently a fetid odour.

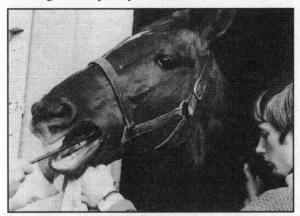

Figure 20   Rasping without a gag

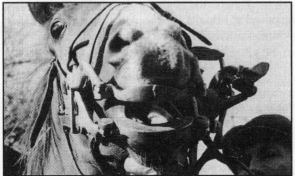

Figure 21   A gag for rasping

As already explained, the horse's incisor and molar teeth continue to grow throughout its life. The rate of growth is normally balanced by an equal rate of wear. However, if the upper and lower tables are not in opposition, there may be loss of grinding action and consequently uneven wear, with unrestricted growth of the unopposed tooth. In cases in which a horse has undergone extraction of a lower permanent molar tooth, it will require regular attention throughout its life to prevent the unopposed molar in the upper arcade becoming overgrown.

The temporary teeth are relatively soft and readily form sharp points along the length of the outer edge of the upper premolars of cheek teeth, particularly the second, and of the inner edge of the lower premolars. With a young horse in the process of mouthing, it is helpful if these sharp edges are smoothed off, thereby reducing the risk of the horse becoming resentful of the bit or hanging on the bit because of oral discomfort. In addition, the action of the snaffle bit forces the cheeks against the leading edge of the upper premolars, and if these have sharp points, the undue pressure will result in bruising and laceration of the inner surface of the cheeks.

It will be seen from Figure 3 that the troublesome period of tooth eruption occurs between two and four years of age. During this period it is a good idea to have the horse's mouth examined two or three times a year and, if necessary, the premolar caps and wolf teeth should be removed and any sharp edges rasped. On conclusion of molar eruption at four years of age and with the development of a level arcade of permanent molar and premolar teeth, regular dental attention may only be necessary once every nine months, unless there are anatomical irregularities such as a narrow mouth, leading to sharp points on the unopposed edges of the molar arcades, or a parrot mouth, leading to excessive growth of the incisors.

Examining the mouth and rasping
Examination of the horse's mouth is performed by grasping the horse's tongue with the left hand through the mandibular space, retracting the tongue, then rotating hand and tongue dorsally. In most instances this causes the horse to open its mouth. The right hand can then be used to draw back the top lip so that the incisor tables can be examined. If a second person holds the horse's head, the operator can inspect all the teeth, using a torch if necessary, and feel for sharp edges. Care should be taken when palpating molar teeth that you do not get your fingers trapped – this is always painful and potentially serious.

If the teeth need rasping, a gag should be used. Sometimes, with difficult subjects, a twitch may also be necessary, but as this tends to interfere with the use of the rasp, it is often better to sedate or tranquillise the patient. The dental rasp is held obliquely against the sharp edges of the molars and parallel to the upper arcade; it is then moved backwards and forwards under pressure to rasp off the excess tooth. When sufficient tooth has been removed the rasping sound will change and the rasp itself will move easily against the teeth.

Overgrown points on upper and lower second premolars and lower third premolars may be removed with a chisel. This procedure should be carried out by a veterinarian.

Major dental operations, such as extractions or the removal of protuberances, require general anaesthesia.

COLOURS AND MARKINGS OF BRITISH HORSES FOR IDENTIFICATION PURPOSES

In 1930 the Royal College of Veterinary Surgeons published a report of a subcommittee set up by the Council in 1928 to prepare a system of description of colours, markings etc of horses for identification purposes. Since that date there have been several revision, the latest issued in 1991 and much of the following is abstracted from that edition. It is not intended to be an exhaustive guide to the colours and markings of British horses but covers the terms and descriptions acceptable to breed societies and others involved in the identification of horses.

The international movement of horses is now commonplace and worldwide travel is considered routine. Certificates of identification are therefore essential and are more likely to be referred to by lay persons and non-professional bodies. As a result, all descriptive terms used in the identification of horses should be readily understandable and accurate.

Body Colours

The principal colours are black, brown, bay, chestnut and grey. If there is any doubt as to the colour the muzzle and eyelids should be carefully examined. This section has been divided into two parts:

a: colours acceptable to Thoroughbred authorities
b: additional colours accepted by non-Thoroughbred authorities

It should be noted that the Thoroughbred authorities now call for all British and Irish bred foals to be microchipped and DNA Parentage Tested, and both are conditions of entry into the General Stud Book.

Microchipping and DNA Partentage Testing

All British and Irish foals born after 1 January 1999 and in training in the United Kingdom should have been microchipped at the foal registration stage. This is evident by the presence of a microchip barcode on the front page and markings page of a passport. However, the presence of a microchip barcode is insufficient by itself as a means of identification and if there is any doubt as to the accuracy of the foal markings your veterinary surgeon should be able to confirm that the barcode present in the passport matches the microchip implanted.

DNA, or deoxyribonucleic acid, is the self-replicating material present in nearly all living organisms and the carrier of genetic information. Since 1 January 2001, Weatherbys, the administrators of racing and the General Stud book have made it a requirement that all foals are DNA Parentage Typed. This follows a two-year programme of gathering DNA samples from registered breeding stock throughout the UK, Ireland and Channel Islands to facilitate the parentage testing of those foals born after January 2001.

In a breed populated by innumerable animals of the same colour, devoid of markings, the introduction of microchipping, DNA typing and subsequent parentage testing represents an extremely accurate means of identification, and the chances of detecting a wrong pedigree has increased from 97% to 99.5%.

SECTION A – COLOURS ACCEPTABLE TO THOROUGHBRED AUTHORITIES

Black – where black pigment is general throughout the coat, limb, mane and tail with no pattern factor present other than white markings.

Brown – where there is a mixture of black and brown pigment in the coat with black limbs, mane and tail.

Bay brown – where the predominating colour is brown with muzzle bay, black limbs, mane and tail.

Bay – bay varies considerably in shade from dull red approaching brown, to a yellowish colour approaching chestnut. It can be distinguished from the chestnut by the fact that the bay has black on the distal parts of the limbs, a black mane and tail, and often black tips to the ears.

Chestnut – this colour consists of yellow-coloured hair in different degrees of intensity, which may be noted. A 'true' chestnut has a chestnut mane and tail which may be darker or lighter than the body colour. Lighter coloured chestnuts may have flaxen manes and tails.

Roan – where the basic body colour has an admixture of many white hairs. Roans are very rare in Thoroughbreds and most which appear to be roan are in the transition to going grey and the intensity of the basic body colour varies according to the seasons. (See Section B). Greys can have chestnut hairs and bays can have white hairs scattered in the coat determining the type of roan.

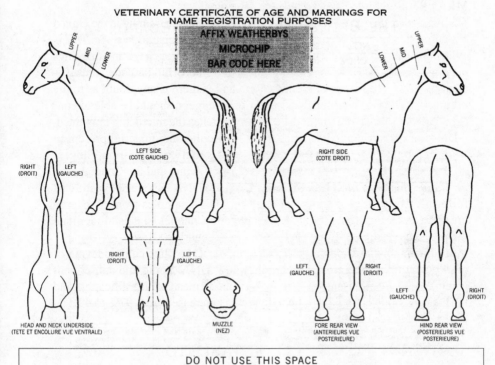

VETERINARY CERTIFICATE OF AGE AND MARKINGS FOR NAME REGISTRATION PURPOSES

AFFIX WEATHERBYS
MICROCHIP
BAR CODE HERE

LEFT SIDE
(COTE GAUCHE)

RIGHT SIDE
(COTE DROIT)

UPPER MID LOWER

UPPER MID LOWER

RIGHT
(DROIT)

LEFT
(GAUCHE)

RIGHT
(DROIT)

LEFT
(GAUCHE)

HEAD AND NECK UNDERSIDE
(TETE ET ENCOLURE VUE VENTRALE)

MUZZLE
(NEZ)

LEFT
(GAUCHE)

RIGHT
(DROIT)

LEFT
(GAUCHE)

RIGHT
(DROIT)

FORE REAR VIEW
(ANTERIEURS VUE
POSTERIEURE)

HIND REAR VIEW
(POSTERIEURS VUE
POSTERIEURE)

DO NOT USE THIS SPACE

*THESE ITEMS ARE BASED ON INFORMATION SUPPLIED BY THE OWNER OR HIS/HER AGENT

*DATE OF BIRTH (ANNEE) / /	COLOUR (ROBE)	SEX (SEXE)	*SIRE (PERE)	*DAM (MERE)
HEAD (TETE)				
NECK (ENCOLURE)				
L.F. (A.G.)				
R.F. (A.D.)				
L.H. (P.G.)				
R.H. (P.D.)				
BODY (CORPS)				
ACQUIRED (MARQUES ACQUISES)				

LIMBS (JAMBES)

FOR OFFICE USE ONLY

FOR BHB OFFICIAL USE ONLY
MARKINGS CHECKED
Stamp Here

SIGNATURE OF VETERINARY SURGEON†
I certify that I *a) inserted a microchip supplied by Weatherbys, which I tested as functioning before and after implantation and I took these markings when I microchipped the horse.
*b) I took markings because on comparing the horse with the markings in the passport/F.I.V.C. I found omission(s)

NAME AND ADDRESS (IN BLOCK CAPITALS)
OF VETERINARY PRACTICE

DATE OF EXAMINATION
/ /

(to be no more then six weeks prior to this form being lodged with Weatherbys)

†Not to be the breeder, owner or trainer of the horse for which the certificate is issued.

*Please delete as appropriate

THE BRITISH HORSERACING BOARD

NC2 - REGISTRATION OF NAME OF HORSE

UNDER THE ORDERS AND RULES OF RACING

	P.P.
	FOR OFFICE USE ONLY

You must enclose the Passport or Foal Identity and Vaccination Certificate for this horse. If you do not have these documents, please contact the Names Section on 01933 440077.

IMPORTANT:- Please tick this box if you are registering this name for Breeding * ☐ **Racing** ☐

* N.B. This form is solely for registration of Name under the Orders and Rules of Racing. If you are registering the name for breeding purposes you may be subject to a further breeding registration fee. Please contact Weatherbys Stud Book Department for full details.

COLOUR	SEX	YEAR OF FOALING	COUNTRY OF FOALING	Name of Sire

Name of Dam	Name of Dam Sire

PROPOSED NAMES (Please give four choices in order of preference, block capitals and leaving spaces where appropriate)

1.
2.
3.
4.

If you feel any of the proposed names are liable to mispronunciation, please indicate the desired pronunciation in the box below. e.g. Caius: pronounced KEYS. Additionally you may be required to provide the desired pronunciation or meaning where it is considered a likelihood of mispronunciation or doubt over the meaning exists.

NUMBER (1,2,3 or 4)	PRONUNCIATION

IF NAME HAS BEEN PREVIOUSLY **RESERVED** PLEASE ENTER RESERVATION NUMBER HERE:

DECLARATION OF NON-PERFORMANCE

I declare that the above horse has not run in a race or races of any type (i.e whether as defined under the Orders and Rules of Racing, any Point to Point Steeplechase, or otherwise).

Signed . . . .(Owner)

OR

DECLARATION OF PERFORMANCE

I confirm that the horse has run in a race or races and attach on a separate sheet details of all such performances together with the name(s) by which the horse was known at the time.

Signed . . . .(Owner)

HORSE NAME REGISTRATION FEES
(Fees valid until 31/12/2000 & inc. VAT)

Under 2 years old £68.68; 2 and 3 years old £98.05; 4 years old and up £89.24
(All name fees include the issue/re-issue of Racing Passport)
Change of name £271.07
Duplicate Racing Passport £68.15

Have you ever had a Weatherbys/British Horseracing Board Account?   Yes/No (delete as appropriate)

☐ I enclose cheque for £ . . . . .made payable to THE BRITISH HORSERACING BOARD LIMITED

☐ Please charge account in the name of . . . .
. . . . .or A/C No. . . . .

DECLARATION A
TO BE COMPLETED IF NEW MARKINGS ARE NOT REQUIRED

I hereby request that the name submitted may be registered in accordance with the Orders and Rules of Racing. I confirm that I have checked the markings contained in the Passport/Foal Identity and Vaccination Certificate or, in the case of an animal for which registration in the General Stud Book or Non-Thoroughbred Register has been applied, the markings which accompanied that application and am satisfied that these **accurately reflect the markings of the horse and that for a foal born in 1999 or thereafter a microchip barcode approved by the Stud Book Authority of Great Britain and Ireland is present within the passport.**

Signed . . . .

Date . . . .

OR

DECLARATION B
TO BE COMPLETED IF NEW MARKINGS HAVE BEEN COMPLETED OVERLEAF

I hereby request that the name submitted may be registered in accordance with the Orders and Rules of Racing, and that up to date veterinary markings have been entered overleaf because (please tick the box or boxes below, as appropriate)
1. The animal is foreign-bred (i.e. not GB/IRE-bred) and/or was foaled since January 1st 1999 and as a result required microchipping ☐
2. The Passport/F.I.V.C. has been lost ☐
3. On comparing the horse with the markings in the Passport/F.I.V.C., I have found an omission(s) in the latter which
(a) whilst not affecting the horse's identity into question, constitutes a difference ☐ OR
(b) gives me cause to doubt its true identity ☐
(Please note there may be a requirement for the horse to be bloodtyped.)

Signed . . . .

Date . . . .

Your name and address details will be verified against or added to the database. It is important that we have your full name and address, including postcode.

Name of Owner (in block capitals) . . . .

Please state title (Mr, Mrs or Miss) . . . . .Daytime Contact Telephone number (in case of query) . . . .

Address of owner . . . .

. . . . .Post Code . . . .

Trainer's Name & Address (if applicable) . . . .

. . . . .Post Code . . . .

To whom should Passport be returned? . . . .

Please return this form to: Names & Passports Section, Racing Administration, Weatherbys, Sanders Road, Wellingborough, Northamptonshire, NN8 4BX.

2/2000

SECTION B – ADDITIONAL COLOURS ACCEPTED BY NON-THOROUGHBRED AUTHORITIES

Blue dun – the body colour is a dilute black evenly distributed. The mane and tail are black. There may or may not be a dorsal band (list) and/or withers stripe. The skin is black.

Yellow dun – there is a diffuse yellow pigment in the hair. There may or may not be a dorsal band (list) and/or withers stripe and bars on the legs. The striping is usually associated with black pigment on the head and limbs. The skin is black.

Cream – the body coat is of a cream colour with unpigmented skin. The iris is deficient in pigment and is often devoid of it, giving the eye a pinkish or bluish appearance.

Piebald – the body coat consists of large irregular patches of black and white. The lines of demarcation between colours is generally well defined.

Skewbald – the body consists of large irregular patches of white and of any definite colour except black. The line of demarcation between the colours is generally well defined.

Odd coloured – the body coat consists of large irregular patches of more than two colours, which may merge into each other at the edges of the patches.

Whole coloured – the term 'whole coloured' is used where there are no hairs of any other colour on the body, head or limbs

Palomino – newly-minted gold coin colour (lighter or darker shades are permissible), with a white mane and tail.

Appaloosian – the body colour is grey, covered with a mosaic of black or brown spots.

Roans – (see previous). Roans are distinguished by the ground colours, all of which are permanent.

Blue-roan – where the body colour is black or black-brown with an admixture of white hair, which gives a blue tinge to the coat. On the limbs from the knees and hocks down the black hairs usually predominate; white markings may be encountered.

Bay or red roan – where the body colour is bay or bay-brown with an admixture of white hairs which give a reddish tinge to the coat. On the limbs from the knees and hocks down black hairs usually predominate; white markings may be encountered.

Strawberry or chestnut roan – where the body colour is chestnut with an admixture of white hairs. On the limbs from the knees and hocks down chestnut hairs usually predominate; white markings may be encountered.

Markings

The variations in markings of horses are infinite and cannot be described accurately by a limited number of terms without certain arbitrary groupings. In some cases a combination of the terms given below must be employed. All certificates of identification should, in conformity with later remarks, consist of a narrative accompanied by a sketch on which the markings are indicated accurately.

Whorls

Whorls are formed by changes in direction of flow of the hair. Their recording is one of the oldest methods of identifying horses from birth, since their site and character vary to some degree in every animal. They may take various forms, depending on the interface at which two or more flows of hair meet, eg, simple, tufted, linear, crested, feathered and sinuous.

A guide to the recognition of the various types of whorl is:

Simple – a focal point into which the hairs seem to converge from different directions; this requires only the term 'whorl' in the narrative.
Tufted – as for a simple whorl, but the hair converges and piles up into a tuft.
Linear – two opposing sweeps of hair meet from diametrically opposite directions along a line.
Crested – as for linear, but the hair from each of the two directions rises up to form a crest.
Feathered – two sweeps of hair meet along a line but the direction of flow of each sweep is at an angle to the other so that together they form a feathered pattern.
Sinuous – two opposing sweeps of hair meet along an irregular curving line.

In all cases, whether there are white marks or not, the whorls on the head and crest should be described in the narrative and indicated in the sketch. If there are few or no white markings, at least five head, neck or body whorls must be noted.

The position of head whorls should be clearly specified with reference to the midline and eye level, to white markings and to each other if two or more occur in close proximity. The description invariably begins at the forehead.

White marks

If the boundary of a white mark is not clearly defined, of the following descriptions should be used.

Mixed – to be used to describe a white marking which contains varying amounts of hairs of the general body colour.

Bordered – to be used where any marking is circumscribed by a mixed border, e.g. 'bordered star', 'bordered stripe'.

Flesh marks – patches where the pigment of the skin is absent should be described as 'flesh marks'

Head

Star – any white mark on the forehead: size, shape, intensity, position and coloured markings (if any) on the white to be specified. Should the marking in the region of the center of the forehead consist of a few white hairs only it should be so described and not referred to as a star.

Stripe – the narrow white marking down the face, not wider that the flat anterior surface of the nasal bones. In the majority of cases the star and stripe are continuous and should be described as a star and stripe conjoined. Where there is a gap in the length of the stripe it should be described as an interrupted stripe. Where a stripe is separated from the star it should simply be noted that a stripe is present and where no star is present the point of origin of the stripe should be indicated. The termination of all stripes and any variation in breadth, direction and any markings on the white should be so stated, e.g., broad stripe, narrow stripe, inclined to left, terminating at upper right nostril, etc.

Blaze – a white marking covering almost the whole of the forehead between the eyes and extending beyond the width of the nasal bones and usually to the muzzle. Any variations in direction, termination and any markings on the white should be stated.

White face – where the white covers the forehead and front of the face, extending laterally towards the mouth. The extension may be unilateral or bilateral, in which case it should be described accordingly.

Snip – an isolated white marking, independent of those already named and situated between or in the region of the nostrils. Its size, position and intensity should be specified (see Flesh marks).

Lip markings – should be accurately described whether embracing the whole or a portion of either lip (see Flesh marks).

White muzzle – where the white embraces both lips and extends to the region of the nostrils.

Other Characteristics

Acquired marks – there are many adventitious marks (i.e. not congenital marks) which are permanent, eg saddle marks, girth marks and other harness marks, permanent bandage marks, firing and branding marks, surgical scars, tattoo marks etc. Wherever these occur they should be described in the narrative and their location indicated in the sketch by an arrow. The presence of white hairs should be mentioned. If a horse is docked or has nicked ears this fact should be mentioned.

Congenital abnormalities – any congenital marks or other abnormalities should be clearly described in the certificate and indicated on the sketch where possible.

Wall-eye – this term should be used exclusively where there is such a lack of pigment, either partial or complete, in the iris as usually to give a pinkish-white or bluish-white appearance to the eye. Any other important variations should be noted.

Showing the white of the eye – where some part of the white sclera of the eye shows between the eyelids.

The Prophet's Thumb Mark – this is a muscular depression seen usually in the neck, but sometimes in the shoulders and, occasionally, in the hindquarters. More often found in Arabs and Thoroughbreds. It should be indicated on the sketch by a triangular mark and mentioned in the narrative.

Body

Grey-ticked – where white hairs are sparsely distributed through the coat or any part of the body.

Flecked – where small collections of white hairs occur distributed irregularly in any part of the body. The degrees of flecking may be described by the terms 'heavily flecked', 'lightly flecked'.

Black marks – this term should be used to describe small areas of black hairs among white or any other colour.

Spots – where small, more or less circular, collections of hairs differing from the general body colour occur, distributed in various parts of the body. The position and colour of the spots must be stated.

Patch – this term should be used to describe any larger well-defined irregular area (not covered by previous definitions) of hair differing from the general body colour. The colour, shape, position and extent should be described.

Zebra marks – where there is striping on the limbs, neck, withers or quarters.

Mane and tail – the presence of differently coloured hairs in mane and tail should be specified.

List – a dorsal band of black hairs which extends from the withers backwards.

Limbs

Hooves – any variation in the colour of the hooves should be noted. If a horse has few other identifying characteristics the hoof colour should be specified, even if black. In the case of grey the colour of each hoof should be stated.

White markings on limbs – white markings on limbs should be accurately defined and the extent precisely state, eg, 'white to half pastern', white to below the fetlock' etc. The use of such terms as 'sock' and 'stocking' is not acceptable.

APPENDIX 1:
PROPRIETARY MEDICINES

Listed below is a selection of drugs listed in the text together with their trade names where applicable

Abbreviations used:-

(NLH)   Not Licensed for Horses
(H)   Licensed for humans only
(country)   Country where product is licensed if no licensed product available in the UK

Products with any of the above abbreviations against them, may only be used in accordance with the 'Cascade' system as defined in *the British Veterinary Association*: Code of Practice on Medicines.

Where products are licensed in other countries, for horses, a 'Special Treatment Authorisation' may be applied for, to the VMD.

A

acepromazine (acetylpromazine): ACP Injection, Tablets, Sedazine Paste and Sedalin Gel

adrenaline (epinephrine): Adrenaline (1 in 1000)(H)

altrenogest: Regumate

amikacin: Amikin (H)

amoxycillin: Amoxypen (NLH)

ampicillin: Amfipen

ascorbic acid (vitamin C): Ascorbic Acid Injection or Tablets, Combivit

aspirin (acetylsalicylic acid): Aspirin Tablets (H), Rheumatine (NLH)

atropine (sulphate): Atrocare Injection

autogenous vaccines: Vaccine generated from the animals own tissue and injected back into the same animal

B

benzoic acid/salicylic acid preparation: Dermisol Cream and Solution

benzyl benzoate: Killitch, Sweet Itch Plus

benzyl penicillin: Crystapen

betamethasone: Betsolan Injection and Soluble

biotin containing hoof care preparations: Biometh-Z, Bio-Trition,

boric acid: Calciject

butorphanol: Torbugesic

C

calcium alginate: Algisite, Kaltogel, Sorbsan

camphor: Camphor, Green Oils
  Healing Gel
carbamazepine: Carbamazepine (H),
  Tegretol (H)
carprofen: Zenecarp/Rimadyl Granules
  and Injection
catechu: Catechu
cetrimide: Cetavlex cream (H), Cetream,
  Hibicet
charcoal: Activated Charcoal,
  Carbomix (H)
chlorhexidine: Hibiscrub, Nolvasan,
  Savlon
chloramphenicol: Chloromycetin V
  Redidrops (NLH), Chloramphenicol
  (H), Kemicetine (H)
chlortetracycline hydrochloride:
  Aureomycin Soluble Powder (NLH),
  Aureomycin Ointment (H)
chondroitin sulphate: Component in
  several preparations including
  Cosequin and Cortaflex
cimetidine: Cimetidine Tablets (H),
  Tagamet Tablets, Syrup and
  Injection (H)
clenbuterol: Ventipulmin Granules, Syrup
  and Injection
clostridium botulinum antitoxin:
  Botulism Antitoxin (H)
cloxacillin: Orbenin (NLH)
codeine: Codeine Phosphate Tablets,
  Syrup and Linctus (H)
copper sulphate: Copper Suphate
  (powder), to be used as a solution
coumaphos: Asuntol (Austral & NZ),
  Negasunt (discontinued, no UK
  licensed alternative available)
cypermethrin: Barricade, Deosan Deosect
cyproheptadine: Periactin (H)

D
danthron: Bilex (Austral)
detomidine hydrochloride: Domosedan
dexamethasone: Colvasone, Dexadreson,
  Opticorten
dimethyl sulphoxide: DMSO (Topical)
diminazine diaceturate: Berenil
dipyrone (Metamizole Sodium):
  Dipyrone 50% Injection, Buscopan
  Compositum
doxapram hydrochloride: Dopram V

E
enilconazole: Imaverol
equine chorionic gonadotrophin, eCG
  (Serum Gonadotrophin): Folligon
  (NLH), Fostim 6000 (NLH), PMSG-
  Intervet (NLH)

erythromycin: Erythromycin (H),
  Erythromycin Ethyl Succinate
  (Suspension)(H)
etamiphylline camsilate: Millophyline-V
eucalyptus oil: Eucalyptus Oil (H), Green
  Oils Healing Gel (ingredient within)

F
febantel: Bayverm Pellet 1.9%
fenbendazole: Panacur, Equine Guard,
  Paste, Suspension and Granules
flunixin meglumine: Finadyne Paste,
  Granules and Solution, Binixin,
  Cronyxin, Meflosyl
follicle-stimulating hormone (FSH):
  Super-OV (NLH)
framycetin sulphate: Framomycin (NLH)
frusemide (Furosemide): Frusemide
  Tablets BP(Vet), Lasix 5% Solution,
  Lasix Tablets (NLH)

G
gelatin: Gelofusine Veterinary, Haemaccel
gentamicin: Pangram 5% (NLH),
  Gentoject (Eire)
glucosamine: contained in Cosequin,
  Cortaflex
gonadotrophin releasing hormone
  (GnRH): Buserelin– Receptal,
  Deslorelin– Ovuplant (Austral)
griseofulvin: Fulvin (H), Norofulvin,
  Dufulvin Paste and Granules

H
haloxon: Organophosphorus compound
  used as an anthelmintic, (see
  Metriphonate)
heparin: Heparin Injection (H)
human chorionic gonadotrophin (hCG):
  Chorulon
hyaluronic acid (Sodium hyaluronate):
  Hyonate, Hylartil, Hyalovet
hydrochlorothiazide: HydroSaluric
  (MSD)(H)

hydrocortisone: Efcortesol (H),
Hydrocortone (H), Solu-Cortef (H)
hyoscine: Hyoscine (H), Buscopan
composition

I

imidicarb dipropionate: Imizol
(Austral, Eire)
influenza vaccines: Duvaxyn Plus,
Equip F, Prevac Pro
insulin: Insuvet (NLH), Caninsulin (NLH)
iodine (strong iodine, weak iodine):
Aqueous Solution of Iodine
iridium wires: Radio Isotopes (special
licence required to use)
isoxsuprine hydrochloride: Navilox,
Oralject Circulon
ivermectin: Eqvalan, Furexel, Panomec,
Eraquell

K

kaolin: Kaogel

L

levamisole: Levacide, Levadin
luteinizing hormone (LH): Chorulon

M

magnesium oxide: Milk of magnesia
(Magnesium hydroxide mixture)
(NLH)
magnesium sulphate: Epsom Salts
mebendazole: Telmin Paste and Granules
meclofenamic acid: Arquel V Granules
methionine (+ Biotin):Biometh-Z,
Biotrition, Farrier's Formula
methylthioninium chloride: Methylene
blue
metriphonate trichlorphon: Neguvon
(Austral)
mineral oil: Liquid Paraffin
morphine: Morphine Suphate (H)
moxidectin: Equest, Cydectin (NLH)

N

naproxen: Naprosyn (H), Nycopren (H),
Synflex (H)
neomycin
sulphate/ Prednisolone/ Nitrofurazone:
Dermobion Green
neomycin Sulphate: Neobiotic Pump,

Nivemycin (H)
niclosamide: Yomesan (H), Mansonil-M
(NZ)

O

oestradiol: Oestradiol benzoate
(UK-NLH), Oestradiol
Benzoate(Austral, Eire, NZ)
oestrogen: Diethylstilbestrol (H),
Ethinyloestradiol (H) (see oestradiol)
oxfendazole: Autoworm(NLH), Parafend
(NLH), Systamex (NLH)
oxibendazole: Lincoln Horse and Pony
Wormer
oxidized cellulose: Oxycel (H), Surgicel
(H)
oxyclozanide: Zanil Fluke Drench (Eire)
oxytocin: Oxytocin, Oxytocin-S

P

penicillin; Penicillin G (see
Benzylpenicillin); Procaine Penicillin:
Duphapen, Depocillin
permethrin: Coopers Fly Repellent Plus
for Horses, Louse Powder, Switch
pethidine hydrochloride: Pethidine
Injection 50mg/ml
phenylbutazone: Equipalazone Powder,
Paste and Injection, Pro-Dynam
phosphate enema: Fletchers' Phosphate
Enema (H)
piperazine: Piperazine Citrate BP (Vet),
Piperazine Worm Powder (Austral)
polysulphated glycosaminoglycans:
Adequan
potassium chloride: Crystals, Potassium
Chloride Solution Strong (H)
potassium iodide: Potassium Iodide
BP (H)
povidone iodine: Pevidine, Vetasept,
Betadine (H)
praziquantel: Droncit (NLH), Adtape
(NZ)
prednisolone: Prednicare (NLH), Pred-X
(Austral); methylprednisolone: Depo-
Medrone V
progesterone: Progesterone Injectable
(NLH), Progesterone (Austral),
Proluton Depot(H)
promethazine hydrochloride:
Phenergan (H)

prostaglandin; Cloprostenol: Estrumate; Dinoprost: Lutalyse; Luprostiol: Proslvin

pyrantel (pyrantel embonate): Pyratape P, Strongid P

pyrethrin: Dermoline Shampoo, Sweet Itch Lotion, Radiol Insecticidal Shampoo

pyrimethamine: Daraprim (H)

Q

quinidine: Quinidine Sulphate (H), Kinidin Durules(H)

R

rafoxanide: Flukex (Eire (NLH)), Ridafluke (Eire (NLH)

rhinopneumonitis vaccine: Duvaxyn EHV

rifampicin: Rifampicin (H), Rifadin (H)

romifidine: Sedivet

S

sarcoid cream: ref Phillip Leverehulme, Large Animal Hospital, Liverpool University

selenium: Aquatrace Selenium (NLH), Deposel Injection(NLH)

silver nitrate: Avoca (H), Veterinary Caustic Pencil 95% BP

silver sulphadiazine: Flamazine (H)

sodium acetate: Sodium Acetate

sodium acid phosphate: Hexamine and Sodium Acid Phosphate Tablets (NLH)

sodium bicarbonate: Sodium Bicarbonate (H)

sodium calcium versenate (sodium calcium edetate): Sodium Calciumedetate (Strong) (NLH), Ledclair (H)

sodium chloride: Salt Crystals, Various IV fluids

sodium cromoglycate: Cromovet (Eire)

sodium hyaluronate: Hylartil, Hyalovet, Hyonate

sodium iodide: Sodide (Austral)(NLH), Sodium Iodide (USA)(NLH)

sodium phosphate: Phosphate-Sandoz (H), Foston (NLH)

strangles vaccines: not available in the UK, USA licensed vaccine.

streptomycin: Devomycin

sulphadiazine (with trimethoprim); Duphatrim, Equitrim, Norodine,

Trimediazine

sulphamethoxazole (with trimethoprim): Co-trimoxazole (H)

sulphanilamide powder: Negasunt (no longer available)

sulphonamides: Sulphadimidine – Vesadin (NLH) Potentiated sulphonamides – see Sulphadiazine

sulphur: Preparations Golden Mane, Kerect (NLH), Tarlite (NLH)

suramin: Germanin (Ger)

T

tannic acid: Tannin

testosterone: Methyltestosterone; Orandrone (NLH): Testosterone Esters; Durateston (NLH), Supertest (Austral)

tetanus antitoxin: Tetanus Antitoxin Behring

tetanus toxoid: Duvaxyn T, Equip T, Tetanus Toxoid Concentrate

triamcinolone: Kenalog (H), Triamolone Forte (Austral), Vetalog (USA)

triclabendazole: Fasinex (NLH)

trimethoprim: see sulphadiazine with trimethoprim

tuberculosis vaccine: BCG (Bacillus Calmette –Guerin) vaccine (H)

V

vasopressin: Pitressin(H)

veterinary poultice/Wound dressing (Tragacanth, Boric Acid): Animalintex

vitamin K1 (Phytomenadione): Konakoin (H)

vitamins A and D: Duphafral, Multivitamin 9, Multivitamin

W

white soft paraffin: Vaseline (H)

warfarin sodium: Warfarin (H)

X

xylazine: Chanazine, Rompun, Virbaxyl

Z

zinc carbonate: Calomine Lotion (H)

zinc oxide: Calomine Lotion (H)

APPENDIX 2:
FEI PROHIBITED SUBSTANCES

Horses taking part in a competition must be healthy and compete on their inherent merits. The use of a Prohibited Substance might influence a horse's performance or mask an underlying health problem and could falsely affect the outcome of a competition. The list of Prohibited Substances has been compiled to include all categories of pharmacological action.

1. Prohibited Substances are substances originating externally, whether they are endogenous to the horse or not.

Substances acting on the nervous system.
Substances acting on the cardiovascular system.
Substances acting on the respiratory system.
Substances acting on the digestive system **other than certain specified substances used exclusively for the oral treatment of gastric ulceration – see Note 1.**
Substances acting on the urinary system.
Substances acting on the reproductive system.
Substances acting on the musculoskeletal system.
Substances acting on the skin (e.g. hypersensitising agents).
Substances acting on the blood system.
Substances acting on the immune system, other than those in licensed vaccines.
Substances acting on the endocrine system, endocrine secretions and their synthetic counterparts.
Antipyretics, analgesics and anti-inflammatory substances.
Cytotoxic substances.

2. List of substances for which maximum threshold levels or ratios have been established (Note 1).

Salicylic acid	750 micrograms per millilitre in urine or 6.5 micrograms per millilitre in plasma
Total Arsenic	0.3 microgram per millilitre in urine
Available Carbon Dioxide	37 millimoles per litre in plasma
Dimethyl sulfoxide	15 micrograms per millilitre in urine or 1 microgram per millilitre in plasma
Hydrocortisone	1 microgram per millilitre in urine
Nandrolone	free and conjugated 5α-oestrane-3 ,17α-diol to 5(10)-oestrene-3ß,

	17α-diol in urine at a ratio of 1 or less.
Testosterone	free and conjugated testosterone
(geldings)	0.02 microgram per millilitre
	in urine
Testosterone	free and conjugated testosterone to
(fillies and mares)	epitestosterone
	12:1 or less in urine
Theobromine	2 micrograms per millilitre in urine

Note 1: Oral treatment by the histamine H2-receptor antagonist Ranitidine is permitted and will not necessitate the use of a medication form. The decision to permit this option will be reviewed annually by the FEI.

After *Annexe IV of the Veterinary Regulation published by the FEI* (September 2000). The 2001 Assembly also approved the inclusion of omeprazole as a permitted treatment for gastric ulceration (Bulletin FEI 5-2001).

APPENDIX 3:
NOTIFIABLE DISEASES

The following diseases in horses are notifiable under The Infectious Diseases of Horses Order, 1987. Article 4 of this Order requires any owner, veterinary surgeon or laboratory that suspects the presence of any of these diseases to notify the Divisional Veterinary Manager (DVM) with all practicable speed.

African horse sickness
contagious equine metritis
dourine
epizootic lymphangitis
equine infectious anaemia
equine viral encephalomyelitis
glanders (including farcy)

Further to the above The Equine Viral Enteritis Order, 1995, requires any suspicion of Equine Viral Enteritis to be notified to the DVM.

The zoonotic diseases, anthrax and rabies, are also notifiable.

GLOSSARY

The following is not intended to be a comprehensive list, but a useful guide to the terminology commonly used throughout the book. More detailed definitions can be obtained by reference to a veterinary dictionary.

Acute Sudden in onset
Aerobe A micro-organism which requires oxygen to exist
Aetiology The causes of disease
Anaemia Reduction of red cells and/ or haemoglobin within the blood
Anaerobe A micro-organism which is able to exist without oxygen
Analgesic An agent which alleviates pain without causing loss of consciousness
Anaphylaxis Immediate hypersensitivity to a foreign protein or a drug
Anterior Towards the front
Arrhythmia Variation from the normal rhythm of the heart beat
Ataxia Incoordination of muscular activity
Atelectasis Incomplete expansion of the lungs
Atrophy Wasting; reduction in size
Azoturia Excess nitrogen in urine, associated with destruction of skeletal muscle

Biopsy The removal of a portion of tissue for diagnostic purposes
Bradycardia Decreased heart rate

Carcinoma A malignant tumour, consisting of epithelial cells
Cardiovascular Relating to the heart and blood vessels
Congenital Existing at, or before, birth
Chronic Of long duration

Diuretic A substance that promotes the excretion of urine
Dysrhythmia Disturbance of rhythm
Dystocia Difficulties associated with birth

Ectoparasites Parasites which live on the exterior of their hosts
Empyema The presence of pus in a body cavity, e.g. guttural pouch
Endocrine Relating to the glands of internal secretion
Endoscope An instrument for visualising the inside of cavities
Enterotomy An incision into the intestine
Epiphysis Portion of bone separated from the main bone by cartilage
Epistaxis Bleeding from the nose
Excoriation Abrasion of a portion of the skin
Exostosis A cartilage capped protuberance from the surface of bone

Fibrosis An increase in fibrous connective tissue

Globulins A group of proteins which are insoluble in water

Haematology The nature, functions and diseases of blood
Haematoma A collection of blood which forms a mass
Hemiplegia Paralysis affecting one side only

Immunoglobulin A protein with antibody activity

Laparotomy An incision through the abdominal wall
Lateral Towards the side
Lesion Any alteration caused by disease or injury
Leucocyte One of the white cells of the blood
Lymphangitis Inflammation of vessels

Medulla The innermost portion of an organ or structure
Micturition Urination

Necrosis The death of cells
Nephritis Inflammation of the kidney
Neuritis Inflammation of nerves
Neuroendocrine Involving the relationship of the nervous and endocrine systems
Neuroma A tumour of the nervous system

Oedema Swelling, caused by an accumulation of fluid
Ophthalmia Inflammation of the eye
Ophthalmoscope Instrument for examining the interior of the eye
Osteochondritis Inflammation of bone and cartilage
Osteocytes Bone cells

Paresis Partial paralysis
Pathogenesis The development of disease
Pathogenic Capable of producing disease
Pathology The study of the nature of disease
Periosteum Connective tissue covering bone surfaces
Periostitis Inflammation of the periosteum
Peristalsis Muscular movement consisting of successive wave-like contractions
Physiology The study of functions of the living organism
Plasma Portion of blood which is straw-coloured prior to clotting
Posterior Towards the back
Prognosis Prediction of the course and outcome of a condition
Prophylaxis Measures to prevent the development or spread of disease
Pyrexia Abnormal elevation of body temperature

Resection Removal of a portion of organ or tissue

Serum Amber-coloured liquid which separates from clot when blood coagulates
Sloughing Casting off necrotic tissue
Synovia Clear fluid found in joints, bursas and sheaths of tendons
Systemic Involving the whole body

Tachycardia Increased heart rate

INDEX

Note: numbers in italics refer to illustrations

erythrocytes 107
Escherichia coli 396, 439-43, 465, 471, 481, 653
eucalyptus oil 577
Eustachian tubes 60, 183, *184*
event horses 267
examination
of eye 177-8
of heart 90-5
for lameness
at exercise 195-7
at rest 194-5
of mouth, for age 826-36
for respiratory problem 74-5
of skin 134
Examination of Animals for Soundness, The 831
excitement 72
excretion 51, 114, 151
exercise 61, 68-9, 72-3, 86, 95-8, 103, 104, 193, 246-7, 257, 269, 300, 336
examination at 195-7
intolerance 57, 61, 69, 70, 74, 76
newborn foal and 435-6
exercise-induced pulmonary haemorrhage (EIPH) 86, 451, 778-80, 795-6
exercise physiology 773-89
blood 779, 781
cardiovascular system 781-2, 796
dietary requirements 783-4
locomotion 789
muscular system 782-3
respiratory system 777-81, 794-6
exercise psychology 100
exercise videoendoscopy 799
exertional rhabdomyolysis 783, 794
exfoliative dermatitis 150
exhalation 71
exocrine gland 56
exostosis 204, 210
expectorant drugs 78
expiration 74
extension 345
extensor carpi obliquus muscle 13
extensor carpi radialis muscle 12, 13
distension of tendon sheaths of 238
extensor process 13, *265*

fracture of 303
extensor tendon 14
of carpi obliquus muscle 13
external abdominal oblique 12
external intercostals 12
extracellular fluid 111
extrauterine v. intrauterine life (table) 427
exuberant granulation tissue 654
eye(s) 1, 63, 67, 131, 169, 172-82
birth defects 181
chambers and segments of 175
conditions of 178-81
congenital abnormalities 739-40
defects rendering horse unfit for purchase 802
discharges 177, 178, 179, 180
examination of 177-8
lotions 577
sore 178
tumours 178
ulcers 178, 180
eyeball 173, 176, 180-1
eyelashes 174, 179
eyelid(s) 149, 158, 174, 177, 178, 180
injuries to 178, 179, 180
retraction of 476

face flies 146-7
facial catheter 64
facial crest 12, 173, *174*
facial nerve 158, 186
facial paralysis 158, 186
facial swelling 44, 63, 64
faecal egg counts 514-20, 524-9
Fallopian tubes 375, *376*, 378-9
infundibulum of *377*
false bursa
see acquired/false bursae
false rig 362
faradism 193, 199
farm poisons 602
farrier-made shoes 349-59
fascile 264, *265*
fascicular membrane *265*
Fasciola hepatica 547
fat 49, 52, 56, 173
fatigue fractures 210
fatty liver syndrome 287
feathered whorl 842
feed 692-4

see also food; nutrition and feeding
feeding horses 79, 120
excessive 102, 149
hunters 757-60
and NMS 497
feeding programmes 694-7
broodmares 695-6
mature horses at maintenance 694
orphan foals 696
weanlings 696-7
working horses 694-5
feeling 154
loss of 157, 159
feet 283-308, *284, 288*
conditions of 285-308
examination of 616-17
functional anatomy of 282-3
infection in 293-4
lameness of 189, 191, 192, 195
of newborn foals 436
pain in 194
poor trimming of 191
preparing for shoeing 347-8
sore 285-7
soundness and conformation 720-1
weightbearing surfaces of 350-1
female genital organs 373-80
feminization, testicular 735
femoropatellar joint 255
femur 12, *253*
fractures of 220
fenbendazole 82, 524
ferric/ferrous compounds 577
fertility 367-8, 484
fescue toxicosis 604-5fetlock
conditions of 201, 231-5
distension of *see* articular windgall
notching of contour 263
sinking of 272
fetlock joint 11, 12, 145, 212, 262, 345
angular deformity 332-3, *332*
arthritis of 232-3
chip fractures in 234
condylar fractures 235
flexural deformity of 330-1
sprain of 232
fetlock varus 332-3, *333*